Stylianos Papadakos

T

HR

-DP/DT

HR

T

HR.

*Cardiac Catheterization
and Angiography*

# Cardiac Catheterization and Angiography

*Edited by* WILLIAM GROSSMAN, M.D.

Dana Professor of Medicine, Harvard Medical School;
Chief, Cardiovascular Division,
Beth Israel Hospital, Boston, Massachusetts

THIRD EDITION

LEA & FEBIGER   PHILADELPHIA

LEA & FEBIGER
*600 Washington Sq.*
*Philadelphia, Pa.   19106–4198*
*U.S.A.*

Library of Congress Cataloging in Publication Data

Main entry under title:
Cardiac catheterization and angiography.

Includes bibliographies and index.
1. Cardiac catheterization.     2. Angiography.
I. Grossman, William, 1940–          [DNLM:
1. Angiocardiography.     2. Heart Catheterization.
WG141.5.C2 C267]
RC683.5.C25C37  1985          616.1'207575          85-4545
ISBN 0-8121-0994-5

*First Edition, 1974*
*Second Edition, 1980*
*Reprinted, 1985*

PRINTED IN THE UNITED STATES OF AMERICA

Print number   3

TO MY WIFE, MELANIE, AND MY CHILDREN
JENNIFER, EDWARD, AND JESSICA

# Preface

THIS textbook in both its conception and design is aimed at the instruction of physicians training to become cardiologists. The intent was to compile a book that would be practical and that would bring together clear and concise descriptions of the major techniques currently employed in cardiac catheterization and angiography. No effort was made to be exhaustive or to construct a compendium of every technique that has been reported; instead, we have concentrated on the detailed description of a few methods that are moderately successful, that are practical, and whose strengths and weaknesses are well known.

The book begins with a section on general principles of cardiac catheterization and angiography. This has been substantially revised from the second edition, and contains information on proper utilization of radiologic and cineangiographic equipment and the incidence, causes, and prevention of complications of cardiac catheterization.

The second section deals with techniques of catheter placement, including discussions of arteriotomy, percutaneous catheterization, transseptal catheterization, balloon-tipped flow-directed catheters, and special considerations in the catheterization of infants and children. Subsequent sections on hemodynamic principles and angiographic techniques attempt to cover basic knowledge in these areas, with an emphasis on practical application and on avoidance of commonly encountered mistakes and pitfalls.

Discussion of the interpretation of hemodynamic and angiographic findings has been largely separated from the description of techniques. Interpretation is discussed and illustrated at the end of the book in the chapters on profiles of characteristic hemodynamic and angiographic abnormalities in specific disorders (Part VI). This separation is purposeful, and serves to emphasize the importance of considering hemodynamic and angiographic data together when analyzing the physiologic and anatomic abnormalities presented by a given disorder.

A unique section on "Evaluation of Cardiac Function" offers pragmatic discussions of recent advances and the current state of the art in evaluation of systolic and diastolic ventricular function, atrial pacing, ventricular volume analysis, myocardial blood flow, dynamic and isometric exercise, and electrophysiologic techniques.

In the third edition, the section on "Special Catheter Techniques" (Part VII) has been greatly expanded and now contains chapters on coronary angioplasty, percutaneous placement of intraaortic balloon pump, endomyocardial biopsy, placement of temporary and permanent pacemakers, and application of lasers and coronary angioscopy in the cardiac catheterization laboratory. These chapters reflect many of the exciting developments in cardiology in recent years, and give practical instruction aimed at assisting the cardiologist and cardiology trainee in the application of these advances to clinical practice.

This book could not have been written without the help of many individuals whose names do not appear in the list of contributors. In particular, I am grateful to Dr. Eugene Braunwald; my many colleagues in the Departments of Medicine at Harvard Medical School and the Beth Israel and Brigham and Women's Hospitals, who gave me encouragement and advice; to our Cardiology Fellows whose thoughtful questions and comments stimulated me to undertake this task in the first instance; and to the technicians and staff of our laboratory whose hard work and dedication allow the precepts of this book to be transformed into action each day.

I hope that this book will be of value not only to those involved in the daily practice of cardiac catheterization and angiography but to all who are involved in the care of patients with serious heart disease. Most of all, I sincerely hope that the lessons of this book will benefit the patients themselves; without this final result, it will have been a sterile venture.

WILLIAM GROSSMAN, M.D.
*Boston, Massachusetts*

# Contributors

JULIAN M. AROESTY, M.D.
Associate Clinical Professor of Medicine,
Harvard Medical School;
Cardiovascular Division,
Beth Israel Hospital,
Boston, MA

DONALD S. BAIM, M.D.
Assistant Professor of Medicine,
Harvard Medical School;
Director, Invasive Cardiology,
Beth Israel Hospital,
Boston, MA

JOSEPH R. BENOTTI, M.D.
Associate Professor of Medicine,
University of Massachusetts Medical Center;
Associate Director,
Cardiac Catheterization Laboratory,
University of Massachusetts Medical Center,
Worcester, MA

ARLENE BRADLEY, M.D.
Assistant Professor of Medicine
Division of Cardiology,
University of Texas Health Science Center at
San Antonio,
San Antonio, TX

BLASE A. CARABELLO, M.D.
Professor of Medicine,
Medical University of South Carolina,
Charleston, SC

STAFFORD I. COHEN, M.D.
Associate Clinical Professor of Medicine,
Harvard Medical School;
Cardiovascular Division,
Beth Israel Hospital,
Boston, MA

JOHN P. DiMARCO, M.D., Ph.D.
Associate Professor of Medicine,
Director, Clinical Electrophysiology
Laboratory,
Cardiology Division,
University of Virginia School of Medicine,
Charlottesville, VA

DAVID P. FAXON, M.D.
Associate Professor of Medicine,
Boston University School of Medicine;
Director, Cardiac Catheterization Laboratory,
University Hospital,
Boston, MA

MICHAEL A. FIFER, M.D.
Instructor in Medicine,
Harvard Medical School;
Cardiovascular Unit,
Massachusetts General Hospital,
Boston, MA

ROBERT E. FOWLES, M.D.
Adjunct Associate Professor of Medicine,
University of Utah College of Medicine;
Director, Noninvasive Laboratory,
University of Utah Medical Center,
Salt Lake City, UT

MICHAEL D. FREED, M.D.
Associate Professor of Pediatrics,
Harvard Medical School; Senior
Associate in Cardiology, The
Children's Hospital Medical Center,
Boston, MA

PETER GANZ, M.D.
Assistant Professor of Medicine,
Harvard Medical School;
Associate Director, Cardiac
Catheterization Laboratory,
Brigham and Women's Hospital
Boston, MA

WILLIAM GANZ, M.D., C.Sc.
Professor of Medicine, University of
California at Los Angeles School of
Medicine; Senior Research Scientist,
Department of Cardiology, Cedars-
Sinai Medical Center, Los Angeles, CA

WILLIAM GROSSMAN, M.D.

Dana Professor of Medicine,
Harvard Medical School;
Chief, Cardiovascular
Division, Beth Israel
Hospital, Boston, MA

L. DAVID HILLIS, M.D.

Associate Professor of Internal Medicine,
University of Texas Southwestern Medical
School;
Director, Cardiac Catheterization Laboratory,
Parkland Memorial Hospital,
Dallas, TX

JOHN F. KEANE, M.D.

Associate Professor of Pediatrics,
Harvard Medical School; Senior
Associate in Cardiology;
Co-Director, Cardiac Catheterization
Laboratory, The Children's Hospital
Medical Center, Boston, MA

BEVERLY H. LORELL, M.D.

Assistant Professor of Medicine,
Harvard Medical School;
Co-Director, Hemodynamic
Research Laboratory,
Beth Israel Hospital,
Boston, MA

ROBERT MARCO, R.T.

Technical Coordinator,
Department of Radiology,
Beth Israel Hospital,
Boston, MA

RAYMOND G. McKAY, M.D.

Assistant Professor of Medicine,
Harvard Medical School;
Associate Director,
Coronary Care Unit,
Beth Israel Hospital,
Boston, MA

RICHARD C. PASTERNAK, M.D.

Assistant Professor of Medicine,
Harvard Medical School;
Director, Coronary Care Unit,
Beth Israel Hospital,
Boston, MA

SVEN PAULIN, M.D.

Stoneman Professor of Medicine,
Harvard Medical School;
Chairman, Department of Radiology,
Beth Israel Hospital,
Boston, MA

J. RICHARD SPEARS, M.D.

Assistant Professor of Medicine,
Harvard Medical School;
Director, Cardiac Laser Laboratory,
Beth Israel Hospital,
Boston, MA

H.J.C. SWAN, M.D. PH.D., F.R.C.P.

Professor of Medicine, University of
California at Los Angeles School of
Medicine; Director, Department of
Cardiology, Cedars-Sinai Medical
Center, Los Angeles, CA

# Contents

—

## PART IV: Angiographic Techniques

## PART V: Evaluation of Cardiac Function

# PART VI: Profiles of Hemodynamic and Angiographic Abnormalities in Specific Disorders

# PART VII: Special Catheter Techniques

# PART I
## *General Principles of Cardiac Catheterization and Angiography*

## chapter one

# Cardiac Catheterization: Historical Perspective and Present Practice

WILLIAM GROSSMAN

I T IS difficult to imagine what our concepts of heart disease might be like today if we had to construct them without the enormous reservoir of physiologic and anatomic knowledge derived during the past 30 years in the cardiac catheterization laboratory. As Andre Cournand remarked in his Nobel Lecture of December 11, 1956: "the cardiac catheter was . . . the key in the lock."[1] By turning this key, Cournand and his colleagues led us into a new era in the understanding of normal and disordered cardiac function in man.

## HISTORICAL REVIEW

According to Cournand,[2] cardiac catheterization was first performed (and so named) by Claude Bernard in 1844. The subject was a horse, and both the right and left ventricles were entered by a retrograde approach from the jugular vein and carotid artery. An era of investigation of cardiovascular physiology in animals then followed, resulting in the development of many important techniques and principles (pressure manometry, the Fick cardiac output method), which awaited direct application to the patient with heart disease.

Although others had previously passed catheters into the great veins, Werner

Forssmann is generally credited with being the first person to pass a catheter into the heart of a living person—himself.[3] At age 25, while receiving clinical instruction in surgery at Eberswalde, near Berlin, he passed a catheter 65 cm through one of his left antecubital veins, guiding it by fluoroscopy (he looked through a mirror held by his nurse in front of the fluoroscope screen) until it entered his right atrium. He then walked to the Radiology Department (which was on a different level, requiring that he climb stairs), where the catheter position was documented by a chest roentgenogram (Fig. 1-1). During the next two years, Forssmann continued to perform catheterization studies, including six additional attempts to catheterize himself. Bitter criticism, based on an unsubstantiated belief in the danger of his experiments, caused Forssmann to turn his attention to other concerns, and he eventually pursued a career as a urologist.

It is of interest that Forssmann's primary goal in his catheterization studies was to develop a therapeutic technique for the direct delivery of drugs into the heart. He wrote: "If cardiac action ceases suddenly, as is seen in acute shock or in heart disease, or during anesthesia or poisoning, one is forced to deliver drugs locally. In such cases the intracardiac injection of drugs may be life saving. However, this may be a dangerous pro-

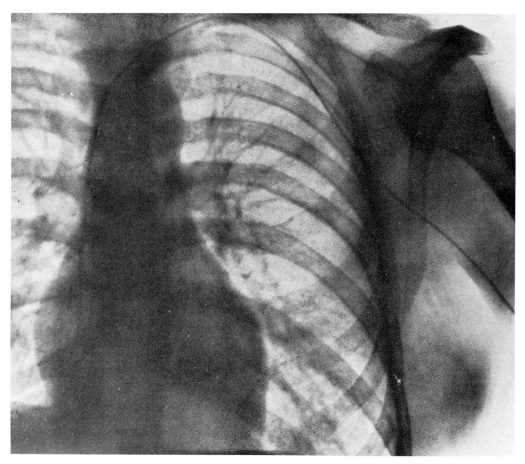

**Fig. 1-1**  The first documented cardiac catheterization. At age 25, while receiving clinical instruction in surgery at Eberswalde, Werner Forssmann passed a catheter 65 mm through one of his left antecubital veins until its tip entered the right atrium. He then walked to the Radiology Department, where this roentgenogram was taken.[2] (Klin Wochenschr 8:2085, 1929. © Springer-Verlag Berlin, Heidelberg, New York)

cedure because of many incidents of laceration of coronary arteries and their branches leading to cardiac tamponade, and death. . . . Because of such incidents, one often waits until the very last moment and valuable time is wasted. Therefore I started to look for a new way to approach the heart, and I catheterized the right side of the heart through the venous system."[3]

The potentials of Forssmann's technique as a diagnostic tool were appreciated by others. In 1930, Klein reported 11 right heart catheterizations, including passage to the right ventricle and measurement of cardiac output using Fick's principle.[4] The cardiac outputs were 4.5 and 5.6 L/min in two patients without heart disease. In 1932 Padillo and co-workers reported right heart catheterization and measurement of cardiac output in two subjects.[2] Except for these few studies, application of cardiac catheterization to study of the circulation in normal and disease states was fragmentary until the work of Andre Cournand and Dickinson Richards, who separately and in collaboration produced a remarkable series of investigations of right heart physiology in man.[5-7] In 1947 Dexter reported his studies on congenital heart disease.[8] He went further than his predecessors by passing the catheter to the pulmonary artery, and in addition he mentioned some observations on "the oxygen saturation and source of pulmonary capillary blood" obtained from the pulmonary artery "wedge" position.[9] Subsequent studies from Dexter's laboratory[10] and by Werko[11] elaborated on this pulmonary artery "wedge" position, and pressure measured at this position was reported to be a good estimate of pulmonary venous and left atrial pressure. During this exciting early period, catheterization was used to investigate problems in cardiovascular physiology by McMichael in England,[12] Lènegre in Paris,[13] and Warren, Stead, Bing, Dexter, Cournand, and others in this country.[14-23]

Further developments came rapidly. To touch briefly on some of the highlights: Retrograde left heart catheterization was first reported by Zimmerman[24] and Limon Lason[25] in 1950. The percutaneous technique developed by Seldinger in 1953[26] was soon applied to cardiac catheterization of both the left and right heart chambers.[26] Transseptal catheterization was first developed in 1959 by Ross[27] and Cope[28] and quickly became accepted as a standard technique. Selective coronary arteriography was developed by Sones in 1959 and perfected to a remarkable excellence over the ensuing years.[29,30] This technique was modified for a percutaneous approach by Ricketts and Abrams[31] in 1962 and Judkins[32] in 1967. In 1970 a practical balloon-tipped flow-guided catheter technique was introduced by Swan and Ganz, making possible the applicability of catheterization outside the catheterization laboratory.[33]

In the more recent past, investigators have focused once again on the therapeutic potential of the cardiac catheter. In 1977, Grüntzig introduced the technique of coronary angioplasty.[34,35] In the ensuing years, the method was widely applied and with rapidly evolving technology appears to be developing a firm position rivaling coronary bypass surgery as a therapeutic modality for coronary artery disease. Intracoronary administration of thrombolytic agents in patients with acute myocardial infarction was introduced in the late 1970s, and rapidly gained acceptance as a treatment for acute myocardial infarction due to coronary thrombosis.[36-38]

There are many other landmarks that could be mentioned, and many individuals whose contributions should be recognized. The interested reader is referred elsewhere for details.[39-40]

## INDICATIONS FOR CARDIAC CATHETERIZATION

As performed today, cardiac catheterization may be defined as a combined hemody-namic and angiographic procedure undertaken for diagnostic or therapeutic purposes.

As with any invasive procedure, the decision to perform cardiac catheterization must be based upon a careful balance of the risk of the procedure against the anticipated benefit to the patient. Cardiac catheterization is generally recommended when there is a need to confirm the presence of a clinically suspected condition, define its anatomic and physiologic severity, and determine the presence or absence of associated conditions. This need most commonly arises when the clinical assessment suggests that the patient is approaching the stage of rapid deterioration, incapacitation, and death when viewed in the context of the natural history of his or her specific disorder. Cardiac catheterization may yield information that will be crucial in defining the need for cardiac surgery, coronary angioplasty, or other therapeutic interventions as well as timing, risks, and anticipated benefit in a given patient.

***Is Cardiac Catheterization Necessary in All Patients Being Considered for Cardiac Surgery?*** Although few would disagree that consideration of heart surgery is an adequate reason for the performance of catheterization, there are differences of opinion about whether *all* patients being considered for heart surgery should undergo preoperative cardiac catheterization. In this regard, at least one recent study[41] concluded that routine cardiac catheterization is unnecessary before valve replacement but can be reserved for specific indications in some patients. There has been sharp disagreement with this conclusion by at least two authorities,[42-43] who pointed out that information concerning concomitant coronary artery obstruction, pulmonary hypertension, and other associated conditions cannot be precisely obtained without cardiac catheterization. In a study of 108 consecutive patients referred for cardiac catheterization, noninvasive evaluation led to diagnostic predictions that were completely correct in 86% of patients.[44] A "management strategy" (choice of (1) no catheterization, no operation; (2) no catheterization, operation; (3) cardiac catheterization required before decision regarding operation) was decided upon, based on the clinical and noninvasive evaluation, and this management strategy was subsequently evaluated by comparison with the findings of the actual cardiac catheterization, which followed noninvasive evaluation in every pa-

**TABLE 1-1** *Correctness of Suggested Management Strategies Based on Clinical and Full Noninvasive Studies in 108 Patients*

| Suggested Strategy | Number of Patients | Errors |
|---|---|---|
| No catheterization; no operation | 19/108 (18%) | 3/19 (16%) |
| No catheterization; operation | 30/108 (28%) | 0/30 (0%) |
| Catheterization | 59/108 (54%) | 0/59 (0%) |

tient.[44] The results are summarized in Table 1-1.

Thus, although clinical and noninvasive evaluation are usually adequate for clinical decision making, there was a 16% error rate in devising an appropriate management strategy in one category of strategy. In this regard I would emphasize that the risks of catheterization are small compared to those of cardiac surgery in a patient with an incorrect clinical diagnosis or in a patient in whom the presence of an unsuspected additional condition greatly prolongs and complicates the planned surgical approach. *The operating room is not a good place for surprises:* cardiac catheterization can provide the surgical team with a precise and complete roadmap of the course ahead and thereby permit a carefully reasoned and maximally efficient operative procedure. Furthermore, information obtained by cardiac catheterization may be invaluable in the assessment of crucial determinants of prognosis, such as left ventricular function and the patency of the coronary arteries. For these reasons, I recommend cardiac catheterization in virtually all patients in whom heart surgery is contemplated.

There are other major therapeutic considerations besides heart surgery that may depend upon the type of information afforded by cardiac catheterization. For example, pharmacologic intervention with heparin in suspected acute pulmonary embolism, or with high doses of propranolol and/or calcium antagonists in suspected hypertrophic subaortic stenosis might well be considered decisions of sufficient magnitude to warrant confirmation of the diagnoses by angiographic and hemodynamic investigation.

A second broad indication for performing cardiac catheterization is to diagnose obscure or confusing problems in heart disease, even when a major therapeutic decision is not imminent. Currently, the most common instance of this indication in our laboratory is presented by the patient with chest pain of uncertain etiology, about whom there is confusion regarding the presence of obstructive coronary artery disease. Both management and prognosis of this difficult problem are greatly simplified when it is known, for example, that the coronary arteries are widely patent. Another example within this category might be the symptomatic patient with a suspected diagnosis of cardiomyopathy. Although some may feel satisfied with a clinical diagnosis of this condition, the implications of such a diagnosis in terms of prognosis and therapy (such as long-term bed rest or chronic anticoagulant therapy) are so important that I feel it worthwhile to be aggressive in ruling out potentially correctable conditions with certainty (e.g., pericardial effusive-constrictive disease), even though the likelihood of their presence may appear remote on clinical grounds.

***Research.*** On occasion, cardiac catheterization is performed primarily as a research procedure. Although research is conducted to some degree in nearly all routine diagnostic studies performed in our laboratory, this is quite different from catheterization for the sole purpose of a research investigation. Such studies should be carried out only under the direct supervision of an experienced investigator who is expert in cardiac catheterization, using a protocol that has been carefully scrutinized and approved by the Human Studies Committee at the investigator's institution, and after a thorough explanation has been made to the patient detailing the risks of the procedure and the fact that the purpose of the investigation is to gather research information.

## CONTRAINDICATIONS

If it is important to carefully consider the indications for cardiac catheterization in each patient, it is equally important to determine whether there are any contraindications. Over the past several years, our concepts of contraindications have been modified because patients with acute myocardial infarction, cardiogenic shock, intractable ventricular tachycardia, and other extreme conditions have tolerated catheterization and coronary arteriography surprisingly well. At present the only absolute contraindication to cardiac catheterization in our laboratory is the refusal of a mentally competent patient to consent to the procedure.

A long list of *relative* contraindications must be kept in mind, however, and these include all intercurrent conditions that can be corrected and whose correction would improve the safety of the procedure. These relative contraindications are listed in Table 1-2. For example, ventricular irritability can increase the risk and difficulty of left heart catheterization and can greatly interfere with interpretation of ventriculography (see Chapter 14); it should be suppressed medically prior to catheterization. Hypertension increases predisposition to ischemia and/or pulmonary edema, and should be controlled prior to and during catheterization. Other conditions that should be controlled prior to elective catheterization include intercurrent febrile illness, decompensated left heart failure, correctable anemia, digitalis toxicity, and hypokalemia. *Allergy to radiographic contrast agent* is a relative contraindication to cardiac angiography, but with proper pre-medication the risks of a major adverse reaction can be substantially reduced, as discussed in Chapter 3.

*Anticoagulant therapy* is more controversial as a contraindication. Some authors have cautioned against the use of anticoagulants, particularly when percutaneous techniques are utilized;[45–48] others suggest that their use may be safe or even desirable.[49–50] As pointed out in Chapters 5 and 13, heparin may lower the incidence of thromboembolic complications during coronary angiography. It is important to distinguish anticoagulation with oral anticoagulants (e.g., coumadin) from that with heparin. Heparin anticoagulation can be reversed rapidly during catheterization if necessary (e.g., perforation of the heart or great vessels, uncontrolled bleeding from femoral or brachial sites). Reversal of the prolonged prothrombin time of oral anticoagulation represents a more complex problem. *I strongly oppose acute reversal of oral anticoagulation with parenteral vitamin K* because of the occasional induction of a hypercoagulable state. This in turn may result in thrombosis of prosthetic valves or thrombus formation within cardiac chambers, arteries, or veins. If reversal of oral anticoagulation is required, I recommend administration of fresh frozen plasma. For patients chronically anticoagulated with an oral agent, I routinely recommend discontinuation of the oral anticoagulant 48 hours prior to cardiac catheterization, with heparin given during these 48 hours for the patients who have a strong indication for continuous

---

**TABLE 1-2** *Relative Contraindications to Cardiac Catheterization and Angiography*

1. Uncontrolled ventricular irritability: the risk of ventricular tachycardia/fibrillation during catheterization is increased if ventricular irritability is uncontrolled.

2. Uncorrected hypokalemia or digitalis toxicity.

3. Uncorrected hypertension: predisposes to myocardial ischemia and/or heart failure during angiography.

4. Intercurrent febrile illness.

5. Decompensated heart failure: especially acute pulmonary edema, unless catheterization can be done with patient sitting up.

6. Anticoagulated state: prothrombin time >18 seconds.

7. Severe allergy to radiographic contrast agent.

8. Severe renal insufficiency and/or anuria: unless dialysis is planned to remove fluid and radiographic contrast load.

anticoagulation (e.g., mechanical cardiac valve prosthesis). I prefer to have the prothrombin time less than 18 seconds and no heparin administration for 4 hours prior to the catheterization. If anticoagulant therapy cannot be interrupted at all, I prefer heparin for the reasons just mentioned.

## FACTORS INFLUENCING CHOICE OF APPROACH

Of the various approaches to cardiac catheterization, certain ones have only historical interest (transbronchial approach, posterior transthoracic left atrial puncture, suprasternal puncture of the left atrium). In this book we will discuss in detail only (a) catheterization by direct exposure of artery and vein, and (b) catheterization by percutaneous approach (including transseptal catheterization). Left ventricular puncture will be mentioned briefly, although this has not been required in our laboratory in several years.

By either the direct or percutaneous approach (or a combination of both), the great vessels and all cardiac chambers can be entered in nearly all cases. Each method has its advantages and disadvantages, its adherents and detractors. In reality, the methods are not mutually exclusive but rather complementary, and the physician performing cardiac catheterization should be well versed in both methods.

***Advantages of the Brachial Approach.*** The direct exposure approach usually utilizes cutdown on the brachial artery and basilic vein at the elbow, whereas the percutaneous approach of Seldinger traditionally involves entry of the femoral artery and vein at the groin.[26] In recent years, percutaneous right heart catheterization from the internal jugular vein has been widely applied. The direct brachial approach may have advantages in a patient with peripheral vascular disease involving the abdominal aorta, iliac, or femoral arteries, suspected femoral vein or inferior vena caval thrombosis, or coarctation of the aorta. The direct brachial approach may also have advantages in the very obese patient, in whom the percutaneous femoral technique may be technically difficult and bleeding hard to control after catheter removal. Some prefer the brachial approach in patients who have significant hypertension, aortic regurgitation, or wide pulse pressure from other causes, or who are receiving anticoagulants. In these three circumstances, an increased hazard of bleeding has been reported with the percutaneous femoral technique. Other advantages frequently cited for the direct brachial approach include greater catheter control, greater potential selection of catheters (end-hole, side-hole), use of a single left heart catheter/Sones catheter) for left ventriculography and coronary angiography, and greater ease of catheter exchange in case of a clotted catheter.

***Advantages of the Femoral Approach.*** In contrast, the percutaneous femoral approach has its own broad set of advantages and indications. Arteriotomy and arterial repair are not required; it can be performed repeatedly in the same patient at intervals, whereas the brachial approach can rarely be repeated more than two or three times with safety; infection and thrombophlebitis at the catheterization site are rare; and there is no need for surgical (suture) closure of the skin. It is clearly the method of choice in a patient with absent or diminished radial and brachial pulsations, or when direct brachial approach has been unsuccessful. This last indication is important, for example, in the patient with tight aortic stenosis in whom retrograde catheterization may prove impossible; in this circumstance, percutaneous transseptal catheterization of the left atrium and ventricle is helpful (see Chapter 5). In the rare instance when retrograde arterial and transseptal catheterization have not been successful in gaining entry into the left ventricle, direct transthoracic puncture of the left ventricle may be considered.

## DESIGN OF THE CATHETERIZATION PROTOCOL

Every cardiac catheterization should have a protocol, that is, a carefully reasoned sequential plan designed specifically for the individual patient being studied. Although this protocol may exist only in the mind of the operator, it is our practice to prepare a written protocol and post it in the catheterization suite so that all personnel in the laboratory may be aware of exactly what is planned and thus may be reasonably expected to anticipate the needs of the operator.

Certain *general principles* should be considered in the design of a protocol. *First,* we prefer to have an arterial monitor line present in virtually all cases; when complications develop (and they do, no matter how skilled the operator), it is helpful to be able to monitor arterial pressure continuously. In our laboratory, an arterial monitor line (usually a percutaneously introduced radial artery cannula) is placed at the start of each brachial cardiac catheterization. For catheterizations done by the percutaneous femoral approach, we use introducer arterial sheaths (see Chapter 5), and the sidearm of the sheath serves to monitor arterial pressure. *Second,* hemodynamic measurements should precede angiographic studies, whenever possible, so that the physiologic values may be as basal as possible at the time of crucial pressure and flow measurements. *Third,* pressures and oxygen saturations should be measured and recorded in each chamber immediately after entry and before passing on to the next chamber. If problems should develop during the later stages of a catheterization procedure (atrial fibrillation or other arrhythmia, pyrogen reaction, hypotension, or reaction to contrast material), the investigator will wish that he had measured pressures and saturations "on the way in," rather than waiting until the time of catheter pullback. A *fourth principle* is that pressure and cardiac output measurements should be made as simultaneously as possible. A simple routine for recording pressure during the cardiac output measurement can be learned by the laboratory personnel and performed efficiently in every case.

Beyond these general guidelines, the protocol will reflect individual differences from patient to patient. With regard to angiography, it is important to keep Sutton's Law* in mind, and order the contrast injections in relation to what are the most important diagnostic considerations in a given patient.

---

*When once asked why he robbed banks, Willie Sutton is reported to have replied: "because that's where the money is."

# PREPARATION AND PREMEDICATION OF THE PATIENT

It goes without saying that the emotional as well as the "medical" preparation of the patient for cardiac catheterization is the responsibility of the operator. We believe it is our firm obligation to fully explain the proposed procedure in such terms that the patient will be in a position to give truly informed consent. We *always* tell the patient and his family that there is some risk involved, although we generally reassure them we do not anticipate any special problems in their case. Out consent form lists these specific risks and informs the patient that "there is a less than 1% risk of serious complications (stroke, heart attack, or death)." If the patient and his family want to know more about these risks, they will ask for details. We do not understate the discomfort or duration of the procedure and believe that to do so runs the risk of losing one's credibility. We have been quite satisfied with this overall approach and can heartily recommend it.

Once the question of indications and contraindications has been dealt with and the patient's consent obtained, attention can be directed toward the matter of medications. As mentioned earlier, we prefer to have the prothrombin time less than 18 sec and no heparin administered for 4 hours. For patients on chronic anticoagulation, we discontinue oral anticoagulants the day prior to hospitalization (or 48 hours prior to study for outpatient catheterizations) and on admission we begin intravenous heparin, which is stopped after midnight on the night preceding the catheterization. Heparin and oral anticoagulants are reinstituted following the catheterization, and heparin is stopped once adequate prothrombin time prolongation has been achieved. This may be unnecessary, since reports previously mentioned have suggested that it is safe to perform cardiac catheterization on a patient receiving anticoagulants. Further studies are needed to clarify this issue.

The question of administering antibiotics prophylactically is frequently raised, and some laboratories routinely administer them prior to catheterization.[30] We do not administer antibiotics prophylactically before cardiac catheterization, and we know of no controlled studies to support their use.

A wide variety of sedatives has been employed for premedication. We routinely use diazepam (Valium), 5 to 10 mg p.o., and diphenhydramine (Benadryl), 25 to 50 mg p.o., one-half hour prior to starting the procedure. For coronary angiography, atropine, 0.4 mg subcutaneously, is recommended by some.[51] In a patient in whom unusual anxiety or discomfort is anticipated, meperidine (Demerol) may be added in doses from 25 to 100 mg IM, depending on body size.

It is probably worthwhile to have both antecubital fossae scrubbed with pHisoHex the night prior to catheterization if the brachial approach is to be used and to have one or both groins shaved if a femoral approach is planned. It is our practice to have the patient fasting (except for his oral medications) after midnight, but many laboratories allow a light tea and toast breakfast without ill effects. It is important to have complete vital signs recorded by the nurse before the patient leaves the ward, so that the procedure may be aborted if a change has occurred in the patient's condition during the night. The patient should be sent to the catheterization laboratory with his or her eyeglasses and dentures (if any) when Fick cardiac output and Douglas bag collection of expired air are planned.

In a typical patient, our precatheterization orders might be:

1. To Cardiac Catheterization Laboratory at 7:00 AM tomorrow by stretcher; patient to be in hospital gown, and with eyeglasses and dentures, if any.
2. Fasting after midnight except for regularly scheduled oral medications.
3. Scrub both antecubital fossae with pHisoHex, and prepare the right groin.
4. Have patient void before leaving for catheterization laboratory.
5. Record complete vital signs before patient leaves for catheterization laboratory.
6. Premedication: Valium 10 mg p.o. and Benadryl 50 mg p.o. as the patient leaves the floor.

This list must be regarded as a general procedure guide and obviously will have to be modified as the details of specific situations require.

## THE CARDIAC CATHETERIZATION FACILITY

A modern cardiac catheterization laboratory requires an area of 500 to 700 sq. feet, within which will be housed a conglomeration of highly sophisticated electronic and radiographic equipment. Reports of the Inter-Society Commission for Heart Disease Resources on optimal resources for cardiac catheterization facilities have appeared in 1971, 1976, and 1983. In the 1983 report,[52] a variety of issues are dealt with, some of which are listed:

1. Location of a catheterization laboratory: within a hospital vs. freestanding
2. Outpatient catheterization
3. Administration, staff organization, and criteria for professional privileges
4. Optimal annual caseload for physicians and for the laboratory
5. Radiation safety and radiologic techniques
6. Physiologic measurements, patient safety

The reader is referred to this report[52] for detailed discussion of these issues. Certain points, however, are worth repeating here.

*Outpatient cardiac catheterization* has been demonstrated by a variety of groups to be safe, practical, and highly cost-efficient. In properly selected cases, outpatient catheterization should be encouraged as part of an overall effort to use hospital facilities more efficiently and to contain the costs of medical care. Most laboratories that have had extensive experience with outpatient catheterization[53] have utilized the brachial approach, which allows the patient to be ambulatory within minutes of the completion of the catheterization study.

A second issue addressed in the Inter-Society report concerns the question of proximity and availability of *cardiac surgical facilities*. The report states that "Optimally, cardiovascular catheterization laboratories should be located only in institutions with well organized and closely related programs of cardiovascular surgery. Exceptions will exist, but should be rare."[52] Immediately available cardiac surgical back-up is particularly critical for laboratories performing coronary angioplasty, endomyocardial biopsy, transseptal catheterization, or studies on patients suspected to have left main coronary

**TABLE 1-3**  *Inter-Society Recommendations for Catheterization Laboratory and Physician Caseloads*[52]

| | |
|---|---|
| 1. Adult Catheterization Laboratories | $\geq$300 cases/year |
| 2. Pediatric Catheterization Laboratories | $\geq$150 cases/year |
| 3. Physician Caseload: | |
|     Adult catheterizations | $\geq$150 but $\leq$600 |
|     Pediatric catheterizations | $\geq$50 |

Note: The report indicates that physicians with extensive experience (e.g., more than 1000 independently performed catheterizations) can perform fewer catheterizations to maintain their skill levels.

artery disease, severe aortic stenosis, or other conditions that increase the risk of the catheterization procedure.

*Utilization levels* as well as optimal *physician caseload* represent a third issue of general interest addressed in the Inter-Society report.[52] The report recommends certain levels of utilization for cost-effectiveness and maintenance of skills (Table 1-3). It is important to note that there is an upper limit as well as a lower limit to the optimal caseload. This is important, since a cardiologist should not have such an excessive caseload that it interferes with proper precatheterization evaluation of the patient and adequate postcatheterization interpretation of the

data, report preparation, patient follow-up, and continuing medical education.

Having carefully considered indications and contraindications, chosen a method of approach, designed the catheterization protocol and prepared the patient, the next step is to perform the cardiac catheterization itself and thereby gain the anatomic and physiologic information needed in the individual case. Chapters 4 to 6 offer detailed descriptions of how this may be done. These descriptions are not proposed as the *only* correct approaches, but rather as methods that have proven moderately successful, that are practical, and whose strengths and weaknesses are known.

# REFERENCES

1. Cournand AF: Nobel Lecture, December 11, 1956. *In* Nobel Lectures, Physiology and Medicine 1942–1962. Amsterdam, Elsevier Publishing Co., 1964. p 529.
2. Cournand A: Cardiac catheterization. Development of the technique, its contributions to experimental medicine, and its initial application in man. Acta Med Scand Suppl 579:1–32, 1975.
3. Forssmann W: Die Sondierung des rechten Herzens. Klin Wochenschr 8:2085, 1929.
4. Klein O: Zur Bestimmung des zerkulatorischen minutens Volumen nach dem Fickschen Prinzip. Munch Med Wochenschr 77:1311, 1930.
5. Cournand AF, Ranges HS: Catheterization of the right auricle in man. Proc Soc Exp Biol Med 46:462, 1941.
6. Richards, DW: Cardiac output by the catheterization technique in various clinical conditions. Fed Proc 4:215, 1945.
7. Cournand AF, et al: Measurement of cardiac output in man using the technique of catheterization of the right auricle or ventricle. J Clin Invest 24:106, 1945.
8. Dexter L, et al: Studies of congenital heart disease. II. The pressure and oxygen content of blood in the right auricle, right ventricle, and pulmonary artery in control patients, with observations on the oxygen saturation and source of pulmonary "capillary" blood. J Clin Invest 26:554, 1947.
9. Dexter L, Burwell CS, Haynes FW, Seibel RE: Oxygen content of pulmonary "capillary" blood in unanesthetized human beings. J Clin Invest 25:913, 1946.
10. Hellems HK, Haynes FW, Dexter L: Pulmonary "capillary" pressure in man. J Appl Physiol 2:24, 1949.
11. Lagerlöf H and Werkö L: Studies on circulation of blood in man. Scand J Clin Lab Invest 7:147, 1949.
12. McMichael J, Sharpey-Schafer EP: The action of intravenous digoxin in man. Q J Med 13:1123, 1944.
13. Lenègre J, Maurice P: Premiers recherches sur la pression ventriculaire droits. Bull Mem Soc Med d'Hôp Paris 80:239, 1944.
14. Stead EA Jr, Warren JV: Cardiac output in man:

analysis of mechanisms varying cardiac output based on recent clinical studies. Arch Intern Med 80:237, 1947.

15. Stead EA Jr, Warren JV, Brannon ES: Cardiac output in congestive heart failure: analysis of reasons for lack of close correlation between symptoms of heart failure and resting cardiac output. Am Heart J 35:529, 1948.

16. Bing RJ, et al: Catheterization of coronary sinus and middle cardiac vein in man. Proc Soc Exp Biol Med 66:239, 1947.

17. Bing RJ, et al: Measurement of coronary blood flow, oxygen consumption, and efficiency of the left ventricle in man. Am Heart J 38:1, 1949.

18. Vandam LD, Bing RJ, Gray FD Jr: Physiologic studies in congenital heart disease. IV. Measurements of circulation in 5 selected cases. Bull Johns Hopkins Hosp 81:192, 1947.

19. Bing RJ, Vandam LD, Gray FD Jr: Physiological studies in congenital heart disease. I. Procedures. Bull Johns Hopkins Hosp 80:107, 1947.

20. Burchell HB: Cardiac catheterization in diagnosis of various cardiac malformations and diseases. Proc Mayo Clin 23:481, 1948.

21. Wood EH, et al: General and special techniques in cardiac catheterization. Proc Mayo Clin 23:494, 1948.

22. Burwell CS, Dexter L: Beri-beri heart disease. Trans Assoc Am Physicians 60:59, 1947.

23. Harvey RM, et al: Some effects of digoxin upon heart and circulation in man: digoxin in left ventricular failure. Am J Med 7:439, 1949.

24. Zimmerman HA, Scott RW, Becker ND: Catheterization of the left side of the heart in man. Circulation 1:357, 1950.

25. Limon-Lason R, Bouchard A: El Cateterismo Intracardico; Cateterizacion de las Cavidades Izquierdas en el Hombre. Registro Simultaneo de presion y Electrocadiograma Intracavetarios. Arch Inst Cardiol Mexico 21:271, 1950.

26. Seldinger SI: Catheter replacement of the needle in percutaneous arteriography: a new technique. Acta Radiol 39:368, 1953.

27. Ross J Jr: Transseptal left heart catheterization: a new method of left atrial puncture. Ann Surg 149:395, 1959.

28. Cope C: Technique for transseptal catheterization of the left atrium: preliminary report. J Thoracic Surg 37:482, 1959.

29. Sones FM Jr, Shirey EK, Prondfit WL, Westcott RN: Cine-coronary arteriography. Circulation 20:773, 1959 (abstract).

30. Sones FM Jr: Cine Coronary Arteriography. *In* Hurst JW, Logue RB (eds): The Heart. 2nd edition. New York, McGraw Hill Book Co., 1970. p 377.

31. Ricketts JH, Abrams HL: Percutaneous selective coronary cine arteriography. JAMA 181:620, 1962.

32. Judkins MP: Selective coronary arteriography: a percutaneous transfemoral technique. Radiology 89:815, 1967.

33. Swan HJC, et al: Catheterization of the heart in man with use of a flow directed balloon-tipped catheter. N Engl J Med 283:447, 1970.

34. Grüntzig A, et al: Coronary transluminal angioplasty. Circulation 56:II-319, 1977 (abst).

35. Grüntzig A, Senning A, Siegenthaler WE: Nonoperative dilatation of coronary artery stenoses. Percutaneous transluminal coronary angioplasty. N Engl J Med 301:61, 1979.

36. Rentrop P, et al: Selective intracoronary thrombolysis in acute myocardial infarction and unstable angina pectoris. Circulation 63:307, 1981.

37. Ganz W, et al: Intracoronary thrombolysis in evolving myocardial infarction. Am Heart J 101:4, 1981.

38. Markis JE, et al: Myocardial salvage after intracoronary thrombolysis with streptokinase in acute myocardial infarction. N Engl J Med 305:777, 1981.

39. Zimmerman HA (ed): Intravascular Catheterization. 2nd ed. Springfield, Ill., Charles C Thomas, 1966.

40. Warren JV: Fifty years of Invasive Cardiology. Werner Forssmann (1904–1979). Am J Med 69:10, 1980.

41. St. John Sutton MG, et al: Valve replacement without preoperative cardiac catheterization. N Engl J Med 305:1233, 1981.

42. Robert WC: Reasons for cardiac catheterization before cardiac valve replacement. N Engl J Med 306:1291, 1982.

43. Rahimtoola SH: The need for cardiac catheterization and angiography in valvular heart disease is not disproven. Ann Intern Med 97:433, 1982.

44. Alpert JS, Sloss LJ, Cohn PF, Grossman W: The diagnostic accuracy of combined clinical and non-invasive evaluation: comparison with findings at cardiac catheterization. Cathet Cardiovasc Diagn 6:359, 1980.

45. O'Brien KP, Glancy DL, Brandt PWT: Cardiac catheterization: indications, current techniques, and complications. Aust Radiol 14:378, 1970.

46. Mendel D: A Practice of Cardiac Catheterization. Oxford, Blackwell Scientific Publications, 1968. p 119.

47. Braunwald E, Swan HJC (ed): Cooperative study on cardiac catheterization. Circulation 37(Suppl. III):98, 1968.

48. Mortensen, JD: Clinical sequelae from arterial needle puncture, cannulation, and incision. Circulation 35:1118, 1967.

49. Kloster FE, Bristow JD, Seaman AJ: Cardiac catheterization during anticoagulant therapy. Am J Cardiol 28:675, 1971.

50. Walker WJ, Mundall SL, Broderick HG, Prasad B, Kin J, Ravi JM: Systemic heparinization for femo-

ral percutaneous angiography. N Engl J Med 288:826, 1973.

51. Green GS, McKinnon CM, Rosch J, Judkins MP: Complications of selective percutaneous transfemoral coronary arteriography and their prevention. Circulation 45:552, 1972.

52. Friesinger GC, et al: Intersociety Commission for Heart Disease Resources: Report on Optimal Resources for Examination of the Heart and Lungs: Cardiac catheterization and radiographic facilities. Circulation 68:893A–930A, 1983.

53. Fierens E: Outpatient coronary arteriography. A report on 12,719 studies. Cathet Cardiovasc Diagn 10:27, 1984.

## chapter two

# Radiographic Principles and Practice

ROBERT MARCO *and* SVEN PAULIN

T HE CARDIOLOGIST who performs catheterizations has, by virtue of previous training, profound knowledge and experience in human circulatory physiology, readily recognizes the clinical expressions of pathophysiologic conditions, and is well prepared to handle emergency situations. The cardiologist is also well educated in the technical aspects of how to measure hemodynamic and metabolic parameters. On the other hand, he or she frequently has not received training in diagnostic radiology and lacks experience in both radiographic techniques and radiation protection. If technical problems occur, such as total equipment failure or inadequate image quality, the cardiologist is not well prepared to troubleshoot or to make appropriate observations to the technical experts. The same holds true for situations when one may have suggestions for procedural improvements, design of alternative methodology, or patient convenience and safety. The purpose of this chapter is to familiarize the reader with some essential radiographic principles, the equipment components currently available for cardiac angiography, and the generally accepted programs for radiographic quality assurance and radiation protection.

## THE ANGIOGRAPHIC ROOM

Incorporation of radiographic equipment adds space demands to a room that might be used exclusively for catheterization purposes and other cardiologic invasive procedures such as pacemaker placement, EKG mapping, or myocardial biopsies. The room should be at least 500 sq feet (47 sq meters) with a ceiling height of at least 10 feet (3 meters). Depending on the complexity of the examinations that are expected to be performed, such as emergency examinations requiring balloon pump assist, thrombolytic interventions during the early stages of an acute myocardial infarction, or emergency angioplasty in unstable angina, the space requirements should be appropriately increased in relation to the additional equipment components selected. A room ≥600 sq feet is preferable to allow for future needs of additional equipment (e.g., digital computers, nuclear camera).

Installation of radiographic equipment mandates that the walls of the room be shielded with lead to a minimum height of 7 feet. It is advisable to locate radiologic controls as well as physiologic recording and monitoring equipment to ensure that personnel are shielded from direct and scatter radiation. Protection can be accomplished with a cockpit configuration with large, lead-containing glass windows that permit direct visual contact. If this equipment is housed inside the room, proper protection with additional shields is mandatory. Heavy radiographic equipment components such as the x-ray transformer, power module, and cine pulse unit are not affected by radiation exposure and thus can be incorporated into the room in a location that interferes minimally with ongoing activities. It is vital that the radiographic equipment be positioned to ensure that high voltage cables be short, not more than 60 feet (20 meters); constant potential equipment should have cables less than 40 feet (13 meters) in length.

The need for radiographic equipment varies with the nature of the examinations that the laboratory is expected to perform. Multipurpose rooms that frequently include large radiographic film changers, spot film cameras, and biplane equipment have greater space needs. In the following pages, an outline is given for the technical installation of radiographic cine equipment in single plane, the most common installation in most cardiac catheterization laboratories.

## X-RAY CINEMATOGRAPHY

Historically, the first cinematographic recordings of x-ray images were performed using long (lasting several seconds), high current exposures that illuminated a fluorescent screen, the image of which was photographed with a conventional movie camera. Introduction of image intensifiers reduced the x-ray exposure considerably. Nevertheless, the x-ray exposure occurred continuously while the camera shutter opened up intermittently; more than 50% of the x rays were generated wastefully. The incorporation of cine pulsing systems has overcome this problem, since they permit control of the length of exposure and regulate x-ray photon flow from the radiographic tube to the image intensifier input surface in synchronization with the action of the cine camera. This regulation can be accomplished by using either of two different systems. One uses a grid incorporated into the x-ray tube that controls directly the electron flux from the cathode to the anode target by applying appropriate voltage. The other system consists of a high vacuum switching tube located in the x-ray generator. Both systems provide a wide range of control of exposure times and deliver optimal energy waveforms that are capable of producing maximum film blackening per unit of time.

## RADIOGRAPHIC EXPOSURES

The duration of each single exposure is of great importance in cardiac radiology be-cause of movement blurring. In selective coronary arteriography, for example, short exposure times are particularly crucial; the small arterial branches are submitted to phasically occurring rapid heart motion with peak values for spatial displacement of 200 mm/sec or more. Exposure times of 3 to 6 msec eliminate the motion blurring that might arise as a result of this movement. Since the shortest exposure time of single-phase equipment systems is 6 msec, and three-phase systems can deliver bursts as short as 1 msec, the superiority of the latter for cardiac examinations is evident.

In addition to the exposure time, two other factors determine the quality of x-ray exposure for each individual pulse and greatly influence the characteristics of the image. The first is the *electrical current expressed in milliamperes (mA), which determines the number of x-ray photons generated per unit time.* The higher the current, the greater the photon flux. If the photon flux is marginal for a given object, the image deteriorates because of increased quantum mottle. Quantum mottle is a randomly occurring graininess in a projected movie film that is perceived as a continuously changing pattern, similar to the events that one may expect to see in a recently disturbed ant hill. Higher photon flux obtained by using increased current would solve this problem, but is hindered because the capacity of the x-ray tubes and tetrode switches is limited. Excessive radiation exposure to the patient must also be considered.

The second factor is *the level of kilovolt (kV), which determines the energy spectrum of the x-ray photons produced.* The higher the kV, the shorter the wave length of radiation, which increases the penetrating power of the photons. Considering that angiographic contrast agents contain iodine, the ideal energy level of the radiation beam would be approximately 70 kV, preferentially in a narrow, monochromatic spectrum. This would ensure maximal x-ray attenuation by the iodine-containing agent with which the vessels are filled, resulting in optimal contrast against other structures in the object, such as parenchymal organs and soft tissues with a density similar to that of water or of bone, which contains calcium. The technology presently available does not permit this resolution, since technically unattainable high currents are required that impose unacceptable skin radiation levels to the patient.

Higher kV peak levels ranging from 90 to 110 kV (up to 125 kV in very heavy patients) are currently used. At this level the photons penetrate more effectively and result in more film blackening at a given current, but produce lower contrast. Increased scatter also results, which causes a higher gray background level on the film, generated by non-image-producing photons.

## AUTOMATIC EXPOSURE CONTROL

Modular generator controls facilitate the selection of components necessary for appropriate exposure. Generator controls for cineradiography can be simplified to contain a limited number of preset programs. It is essential for cardiac angiography to incorporate an *automatic brightness stabilization system* that will compensate rapidly for changes in x-ray attenuation. Since the relatively small size of the image intensifier field is not capable of encompassing the entire human heart, panning is unavoidable and results in changing film exposures, particularly when the field includes segments of the easily penetrated surrounding lung fields.

The use of manual control by even an experienced radiologic technologist is unreliable. Automatic exposure control is preferable and can be accomplished by a variety of approaches. The simplest and still most widely used method is to vary by direct feedback system the number of emitted photons at preset kV levels, either by changing the current or the exposure time of each pulse. Since doubling of either time or milliamperage increases film blackening only to what is achieved by an increase of 6 to 8 kV, the range of variation within this system is limited, relatively slow, and frequently reaches the upper limit of capacity. A kV control system has a rapid response, since minor changes in tube potential greatly affect film blackening and have relatively little effect on contrast. Combination systems are presently considered to be optimal; in these systems, the optimal mA setting for a given piece of radiographic equipment is preselected and kV varies automatically to regulate film blackening.

## GENERATOR

The x-ray generator is basically a step-up transformer that provides the high voltage necessary to accelerate electrons in the x-ray tube. Incoming power for a generator to be used in cineangiographic laboratories should be 400 to 480 volts in the form of a three-phase alternating current. The basic construction of a generator consists of transformer wires that are placed in a large tank and submerged in oil for cooling and insulation. Incorporated into the system are rectifiers, which convert the alternating current needed for step-up transformation into direct current that feeds the x-ray tube. The most powerful x-ray generators on the market are those that satisfy the needs for rapid large film serial radiography with an output of more than 100 kV at 100 kV, which is provided by either a 3-phase 12-pulse or a constant-potential generator. When combined with pulsing systems, these generators permit powerful currents of 600 mA or more, with precise timing down to 1 msec bursts, which guarantees reliable constant power delivery with optimal photon flux delivery throughout the exposure time. In cinematography, which uses electron acceleration in an image intensifier, generators of such power are not necessary. Since the requirement for electric current output for these systems is generally considered to be 1½ to 2 times the cine pulse output, a level at which voltage fluctuations during pulsing are minimal, less powerful generators may suffice. Silicone-controlled, rectifier-contacting 12-pulse generators of comparably low kW rating (60 kW) can provide sufficient cine current and voltage output in the range needed for cardiac cinematography and thus represent a more economic alternative. It should be noted that limitations regarding a higher current and the subsequent increased x-ray photon flux during the short exposure pulse are found primarily in the x-ray tubes, which are not capable of coping with either higher energy intensity at the small anode target or the problems of heat dissipation.

## X-RAY TUBES

The primary design consideration in the construction of an x-ray tube is its heat-loading capability (Fig. 2-1). Electrons emitted from a heated tungsten filament are accelerated across the x-ray tube until they hit the anode, where they are rapidly decelerated through interaction with the atoms of the target material. This conversion process is

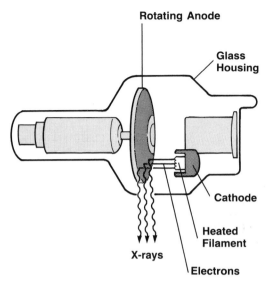

**Fig. 2-1.** Schematic illustration of an x-ray tube. Electrons liberated from the heated filament of the cathode are accelerated toward the slanted surface of the rapidly rotating anode. On impact with the target material, the electron flow generates x-ray photons leaving the x-ray tube in the direction of the tube window.

inefficient in the extreme—less than 0.6% of the electric energy provided to the tube with a tungsten target at 80 kV is converted to x rays; the rest generates heat. Therefore, in the design of an x-ray tube, great consideration is given to increasing its heat-loading capability. The amount of heat generated per unit time is primarily a function of tube current. Although it is possible to obtain equal film blackening at lower milliampere current, and thus lessen heat load by increasing kV, deterioration in image quality due to lower contrast may result. Given the optimal values for tube tension (70 to 80 kV) and exposure time (3 to 6 msec) for cardiac angiography, x-ray tubes capable of high current (600 to 1000 mA) are desirable.

The greatest heat problem arises at the anode target, which is the small area at which the electron beam is concentrated. The target material therefore has to have a high melting point (tungsten or tungsten alloys) and is often backed up with lighter material of good thermal conductivity such as graphite. Furthermore, heat tolerance is increased significantly by using rotating anodes with large diameters (100 to 120 mm) capable of up to 20,000 rpm, so that the elec-

trons use a band-shaped, circular target. In addition, all materials included in the tube are selected and designed to maximize the conduction, convection, and radiation of heat away from the anode. Under very high heat load applications, water cooling devices may supplement the heat dissipation provided by the insulating oil in which the tube is immersed.

X-ray tubes frequently have two or three focal spots of varying size that increase their flexibility. For this purpose, the face of the anode is beveled at different angles with respect to the electron flow. Given equal focal spot sizes, a decreased target angle will increase the heat-loading capability, but will reduce the angle at which the emitted x-ray photons diverge out toward the imaging plane, thus producing a smaller radiographic field (Fig. 2-2). In addition, the anode heel effect, which is a reduction in radiation intensity on the anode side of the radiographic field due to absorption of photons by the anode itself, will be more noticeable. In cineradiography, the anode heel effect rarely causes a problem except when very large field image intensifiers are used or tube malalignment has occurred. A 6- to 9-degree target angle on a 100 mm diameter anode provides adequate field coverage for cardiac examinations at the usual imaging distances (70 to 100 cm) with small image intensifiers (5 to 7 inch), and provides two or more times the output capacity of a conventional 15- to 17-degree target angle x-ray tube. It should

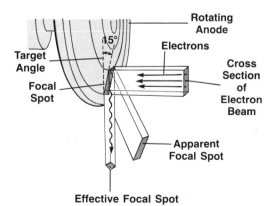

**Fig. 2-2.** Illustration of relationship between anode target angle, electron beam dimension, and effective focal spot, which by definition is specified in the direction perpendicular to the electron beam. The apparent size of a focal spot depends upon the direction from which it is viewed.

be noted that the benefit of increased geometric sharpness deriving from a small focal target can be easily offset by inappropriate increases of the distance between the object and the intensifier input service. Likewise, intentional efforts to accomplish angiographic magnification by placing the object closer to the x-ray tube and farther away from the image plane must use ultra-small focal spots. However, since tubes with lower capacity will require longer exposure times, the degree of motion unsharpness associated with cardiac studies may greatly degrade image quality.

It has been suggested that optimal anode angle and focal spot size combinations should be specifically designed for different types of examinations as well as some disease processes. However, the number of tubes required for such a strategy would be a luxury that few institutions could afford. In general, a bifocus tube with a 0.6/1.0 mm focal spot size combination, rated at 30/80 kW and used with a small to moderate field size image intensifier is considered to be satisfactory for cardiac angiography.

## IMAGE INTENSIFIERS

The introduction of image intensifiers into medical radiology in the early 1950s revolutionized radiologic diagnosis. They quickly replaced direct fluoroscopy, which had to be performed in a darkened room. Although radiation exposure to the patient per time of observation has not been significantly altered, the patient can now be examined conveniently in a lightened room, and observations can be made more accurately on bright television screens. These observations can be seen by several observers simultaneously. In addition, videotape recording for instant replay or storage has become an option.

Because the image intensifier reduces the radiation level at which a rapid sequence of images can be obtained, it is perhaps the most important component of radiographic systems that aim to produce motion pictures of biologic events. Therefore, the importance of the image intensifier for imaging the heart and its function is self-evident.

An image intensifier consists basically of a highly evacuated glass tube with a large input surface and a small output surface

(Fig. 2-3). For the purpose of x-ray conversion, the input surface contains a layer of phosphor, made either of zinc cadmium sulfide crystals or cesium iodide, separated from the photocathode by a thin transparent membrane. Visible light generated by the phosphor passes through the thin membrane and is absorbed by the photocathode, thereby generating low energy electrons. These low energy electrons travel with increasing speed toward the anode, which has a high positive charge. During this passage, several electrostatic focusing lenses, arranged in circular fashion in the intensifier, control their proper radial path through a common point on the central axis of the tube and produce an inverted image on the output screen. Intensification of the image is achieved both by minification and electronic gain, which result from the kinetic energy that the electrons have received from the high voltage applied to the anode. The overall gain in brightness of image intensifiers may vary between 2400 and 6000 times.

Image intensifiers are available in different sizes. The smaller ones have an input diameter of 12 to 17 cm (5 to 7 in) and are preferred for selective coronary angiography because of their better resolution power. Their small field size is a disadvantage, and this is further reduced by so-called overframing within the optical system; a center rectangular area of the round field is used for cine imaging only. Appropriate panning of the patient during the examination overcomes this problem. Larger field size is necessary for studies not well suited to panning,

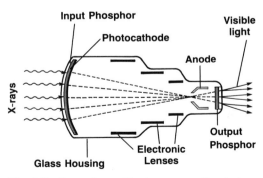

**Fig. 2-3.** Image intensifier in cross-sectional view. The path of x rays, electrons released by the photocathode and accelerated toward the anode to hit the small output phosphor, is illustrated.

such as selective left ventriculography. Larger image intensifiers with an input diameter of 22 to 25 cm (9 to 10 in) can be used for these studies; however, lesser resolution of detail is accomplished. Dual mode intensifiers that allow instant switching from small to large field size are available and are convenient. For a given intensifier system, there is a trade-off between resolution and gain. In angiography, resolution is more important and the intensifier tube should be selected accordingly. Image intensifiers of the smaller variety should provide a resolution in combination with an optical system of not less than four line pairs per millimeter (LP/mm). The larger ones, as mentioned above, have less resolution power, which, however, should still be at a level of 3 LP/mm.

The small output image is matched with an optical system. The system usually consists of a collimator lens and a camera lens, both of which should be matched for tandem operation. Since the best films for cardiac cinematography have a relatively slow speed, it is essential that the optical system provide good light input. The F-stop openings should be at least two stops smaller than maximum. Still smaller openings do not improve image quality significantly and should not be used, as they would require either increased radiation or faster film. For coronary angiography, a small image intensifier with a radiation input of 30 to 40 microroentgens per frame is recommended.

Since the images on the movie film are rectangular (18 × 24 mm), total documentation of the circular intensifier input field would result in a small image with an area of wasted film. Varying degrees of overframing are commonly used, resulting in cutoff of some of the circle's fringes, and a larger presentation of the essential central area (Fig. 2-4). Total overframing implies that the rectangular film frame is projected totally within the circular field of the intensifier. It reduces the effective field and is therefore recommended for special magnification purposes only.

For clinical examinations, particularly in adults, 35-mm cameras are used primarily. Sixteen mm cameras, which have been advocated for high speed motion studies in the past, have poorer image quality. Although 35-mm cameras can be run up to a speed of 80 frames per second, they are usually operated at 24 to 50 frames per second.

| Framing Mode | | Film Area Used |
|---|---|---|
| Exact Framing | 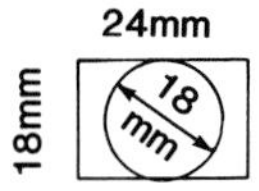 24mm / 18mm / 18 mm | 58% |
| Mean Diameter Overframing | 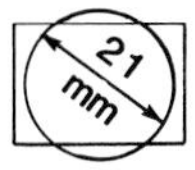 21 mm | 73% |
| Maximum Horizontal Overframing | 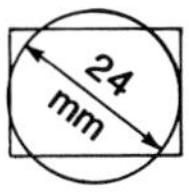 24 mm | 88% |
| Total Overframing | 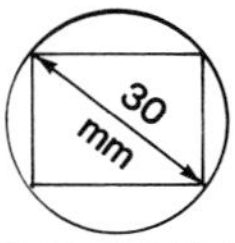 30 mm | 100% |

**Fig. 2-4.** Relationship of framing method to field size reduction in cinefluoroscopy. (Modified from Friesinger GC, et al: Report of Inter-Society Commission for Heart Disease Resources. Circulation 68(4):893A, 1983.)

An effective television system is essential for fluoroscopic surveillance during catheterization, which frequently includes test injections. Television display of the angiographic events being recorded on the film also contributes greatly to patient safety. For this purpose, semitransparent mirrors are interposed to divert a small portion of the image information to the television camera.

Videotape recording is used widely for instant replay and for review prior to film development. A well-designed 525-line 10 to 15 MHz bandwidth television camera system takes advantage of the high resolution of modern cesium iodide intensifiers. High resolution television viewing systems with line scan rates of 800 or more might be preferable if the television information is used for long-term image recording and storage.

## EXAMINATION TABLE AND EQUIPMENT SUPPORT

The patient is placed in a recumbent position on an examination table, the top of which should be as radiolucent as possible. Carbon-fiber tops combine adequate strength with little radiation absorption. For panning purposes, the top must be floating, so that the tabletop can be moved easily in both longitudinal and lateral directions by manual control.

Historically, cinematographic equipment consisted of a fixed tube under the table with the x-ray beam directed toward a ceiling-mounted intensifier above the patient's chest. The patient had to be rolled on his or her side to obtain oblique views. This shortcoming was corrected by the introduction of patient support cradles that are placed on the tabletop and facilitate patient rotation by means of electrical motor drive (Fig. 2-5). In addition, compared to the hard flat tabletop, the cradle reduced patient discomfort by providing more even distribution of body weight.

For many years the support cradle was the only available device for the practice of coronary cinematography. Disadvantages of this system included changes of reference points for simultaneously performed hemodynamic

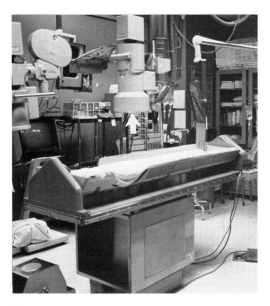

**Fig. 2-5.** Patient support cradle mounted on x-ray table. This device permits rotation of patient within a fixed vertically directed x-ray tube-intensifier cine system. The x-ray tube is positioned under the table and encapsulated in steel housing. White arrow identifies input surface of ceiling mounted intensifier in overhead position.

examinations, such as pressure recordings, and the inability to angulate the x-ray equipment in relation to the patient's long axis. The latter shortcoming was particularly noticeable in the angiographic delineation of certain anatomic areas, such as the proximal left anterior descending and circumflex branches close to the left main coronary artery bifurcation, where either one was markedly foreshortened in the conventional oblique projections. Angiographers tried to solve this dilemma by practicing a so-called sit-up view, a very inconvenient process that required the patient to be propped up on large pillows or wedges. Another arrangement, available to owners of biplane equipment, was to offset the horizontal unit of the cine equipment and to rotate the patient correspondingly. Although successful in individual cases, these technical improvisations were inconvenient and disruptive.

The first equipment that permitted more convenient performance of cranially angulated views was the Philips Cardio-Diagnost (designed for the Cleveland Clinic), which has a rotating C-arm support of the x-ray equipment and a flat tabletop. Modified patient support carts on wheels permitted changes of the patient's longitudinal axis within the system.

In our own search for an angiographic unit with the greatest possible freedom of projections, we developed, in collaboration with XRE Corporation, a larger version of a so-called parallelogram stand that had proved successful in the performance of neuroradiologic examinations. This principle of suspension permits the x-ray tube and the intensifier to be pivoted in circular motion around the patient, but it can also be angulated in craniocaudal direction up to 45 degrees (Fig. 2-6). This cardiac unit, now known as the Poly-Diagnost C (Philips Corporation), permits excellent freedom of motion and rapid positioning by means of motor drives. Since the isocentric point of the equipment and the relatively small image field cannot be compensated for totally by panning, it is essential that the patient supporting table be adjustable in height. In contrast to C-Arm, U-Arm, and the L-U devices, the parallelogram principle has another advantage in that it does not angle the images on film or on television. Because the patient remains constantly in flat recumbent position, reproducibility of different angulations can be accom-

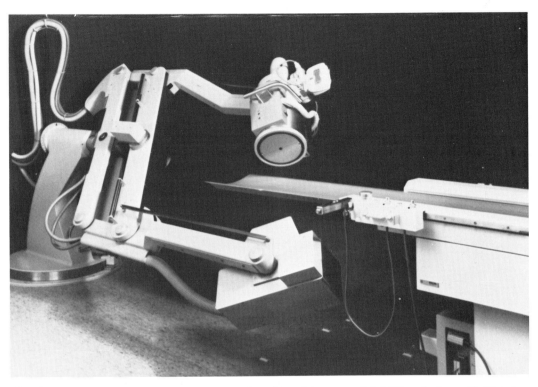

**Fig. 2-6.** Modern x-ray equipment support stand positioned to accomplish LAO projection with 35-degree cranial tilt when patient is supine. This parallelogram system is an innovative extension of the U-arm concept, performing both isocentric left and right rotation around the horizontal axis and isocentric angulation about the transverse axis.

plished easily. For that purpose, graded degree scales are displayed on the unit in both directions of motion.

It should be remembered that major degrees of angulation in relation to the patient's long axis unavoidably increase the object thickness. This further taxes the capability of the radiographic equipment.

To avoid confusion and to enhance communication between different laboratories, it is advisable to adhere to a terminology that is widely recommended and accepted (Fig. 2-7).

## CINE FILM AND PROCESSING

Unlike direct large film radiography, patient exposure in cineradiography is affected by film speed only to a minor degree, as film blackening is controlled mostly by the F-stop of the camera lens and interchangeable aperture diaphragms of varying diameters. Each of the major film manufacturers produces films with different speed, contrast, and latitude characteristics. Proper film selection and manipulation of processing parameters will result in images tailored to the personal preference of the laboratory director (Fig. 2-8).

Recently, there have been general trends toward slower speed films because their better resolution and wider latitude yield increased diagnostic information. However, changes in any one component of the imaging chain must be made with great care because of the marked interdependence of all system components. For example, the inherent contrast of a cine film one finds desirable may greatly depend on the image contrast yielded by the image intensifier. The basic steps of film processing—development, fixation, washing, and drying—are similar to those used for large film processing, but a high quality cine film requires far more stringent processing controls.

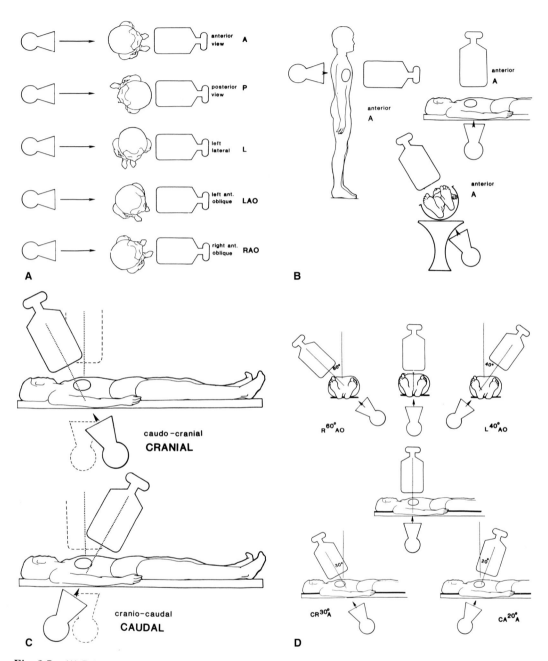

**Fig. 2-7.** (A) Principle of radiographic nomenclature for different projections around the patient's long axis. The object's (patient's) surface facing the observer determines the identification for a specific view. (B) The terminology for radiographic projections relates to the patient's body and not to the orientation in space. Thus, all three illustrated situations—standing, recumbent, recumbent in turned cradle—represent posteroanterior projections. (C) Angulations in relation to the patient's long axis. In accordance with nomenclature principles based on direction of x rays, the upper illustration represents a cranial and the lower a caudal projection or view. (D) Angulations in cranial or caudal direction can occur in combination with any of the conventional projections. The center row illustrations represent the true posteroanterior view with 0 degree angulation. Degree of angulation can be expressed numerically in elevated position following the corresponding symbols as exemplified in illustrations to left and right.

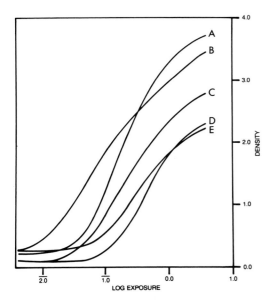

**Fig. 2-8.** Density curve characteristics of several different cine films (A to E), each processed as recommended by manufacturers. Curves farther to left are obtained by using more sensitive or "faster" films. The steeper the slope of the curves, the greater the inherent "content" of the film, but the narrower the exposure latitude for obtaining satisfactory information.

The human eye has a persistence vision of about 0.2 seconds; given the high frame rate at which cine films are viewed, the eye is integrating five or more images per second. Minute physical defects or small changes in tonal value of the film can seriously degrade apparent image quality. Immersion time, temperature, agitation/replenishment, recirculation, and cleanliness are therefore far more critical factors than they are with large film processing. Cinefluorographic processing, therefore, is a task that requires meticulous operation, should be conducted by a qualified professional, and must be submitted to a quality assurance program that guarantees the highest image quality and consistency. The following description includes points that are essential in the effective operation of one of the commercially available dedicated automatic cine film processing units.

A precondition for any successful processing quality control program is a thoroughly cleaned processor loaded with fresh, properly mixed chemicals, in which all of the electromechanical components have been checked for proper function and any excessively worn parts have been replaced. Temperature gauges and the replenishment and recirculation pumps should be checked and calibrated, and the transport system speed should be checked for accuracy and consistency. The functions of the processor for any particular film should be set according to the film manufacturer's recommendations. It is important to assure that lighting conditions in the film processing room are safe and that they match conditions that are recommended—some cine films require complete darkness.

Special precautions are necessary for the proper establishment and maintenance of photographic film processing. The responsible technician will, therefore, periodically measure the volume rate of solution replenishment with a graduated cylinder, check film transport speed and different immersion times with a stopwatch, determine the appropriate temperature of solutions with the aid of a high-precision thermometer, and check on the accurate responses of the different thermostats.

The most important control instruments for film processing are a high quality *sensitometer* and a *densitometer*. The *sensitometer* consists of an accurately calibrated light source that delivers constant exposures. A built-in step pattern with increasing light attenuation (21 steps preferred) results in a scale of decreasing blackening transferred on the film test strip, which is then processed in the unit. The *densitometer* permits accurate measurement of the optical densities at different steps on the processed film strip, the results of which can be plotted against optical density units. For practical purposes, control film strips should be obtained in sufficient number and selected from the laboratory's film supply so that they will appropriately represent a certain film batch or shipment. Test strips should be run daily at approximately the same time as the processor unit warm-up. Additional tests must be done when processor performance is in question. For the daily film density check, three determinations are recommended: speed index, contrast index, and base + fog density. The latter is measured with the densitometer on an unexposed area of the processed control strip. This value is usually low, in the magnitude of 0.1 to 0.2 optical density units. It is further recommended that out of the exposed scale pattern on the film test the density step with a value of 0.85 optical density above the base + fog level should be chosen as the speed index. The third densitometric measurement is performed on the step representing approximately twice the light exposure of the speed index step. Subtraction of the optical density value of the speed index step from this higher value represents the contrast index, and any deviation from its value would indicate differences in film contrast or latitude.

Daily monitoring of these factors is performed rather quickly and permits highly accurate maintenance of the initially established optimal processing conditions. Speed and contrast indices should not vary by more than ±0.1, and the base + fog by not more than 0.02. Even slight variations beyond this range should alert the responsible unit operator to a possible problem.

Parallel comparison of two film strips is recommended when changing to a new film supply or a different brand, as this will readily detect film inconsistencies or changes in characteristics. Periodically (once a month) a full determination of the film characteristics curve that includes all 21 steps should be performed, which will allow comparison with previous tests to assure overall consistency.

## IMAGING EQUIPMENT QUALITY ASSURANCE

Effective monitoring and control of proper and consistent film processing is a prerequisite for appropriate surveillance of long- and short-term performance of the entire chain of imaging equipment. The gross performance of the system should be checked at the start of each day. The responsible radiologic technician is assigned to perform these basic tests on each image intensifier unit in the laboratory. The two factors to be determined are cine on-frame optical density and resolution. The performance of these tests must be standardized as much as possible to minimize extraneous variations. Thus, source to image distance (SID), degree of collimator opening, exposure values, and x-ray tube focal spots should be chosen in a manner that assures easy replication.

The *cine on-frame density* is determined densitometrically on a test film that has been exposed under conditions that simulate the examination of the average patient, using a phantom (copper plate) as a patient equivalent. A standard phantom, provided by the Society for Cardiac Angiography to its membership laboratories, attenuates the x-rays uniformly and permits interdepartmental comparison of equipment performance. The phantom is imaged on a cine run that lasts several seconds, and the procedure is repeated for each mode of a multimode intensifier. The optical density is measured on the frame center of the processed film. Results reported from the central laboratory of the Society for Cardiac Angiography,* which monitors the performance of laboratories at 70 institutions, showed that the average optical density value was 0.90 optical density units, with 84% falling within the range of 0.65 to 1.15. Although the optimum value will be established according to a particular institution's preference, the optical density determinations for each unit should not vary by ±0.15, nor should it vary between units by more than ±0.1 density units. Again, the film processor must operate precisely within narrow tolerance limits to assure that these measurements are reliable.

The determination of *the cine on-frame resolution* measures the spatial resolution power of the x-ray tube/image intensifier/ camera/film system. Again, under standardized exposure conditions, a cine resolution test pattern is radiographed, and the on-frame appearing image is analyzed. A suitable resolution test pattern is provided by the Society for Cardiac Angiography, which consists of eight 45 degree sections of copper mesh ranging from 30 to 100 mesh holes per inch. Alternatively, patterns may be constructed from commercially available materials. These test patterns, which are to be placed close to the intensifier input surface, frequently require removal of the grid. The evaluation is performed subjectively by an observer who examines several frames of the cine film in front of a brightly illuminated viewbox with a 7X magnifying glass. According to definition, the value for resolution will be determined by the finest mesh that can be identified clearly along the length of the corresponding mesh segment from the center to

*Society for Cardiac Angiography, 9500 Euclid Avenue, Cleveland, OH 44106.

the edge of the image field (Fig. 2-9). The determination is made by examining several frames from the middle of the run. The value will be expressed in the dimensions of the test pattern (line pairs per mm, mesh holes per inch, etc.). Deviations in the results of cine on-frame density and resolution in this routine fashion indicate significant malfunction in one or more of the system's components.

In addition to the daily controls, periodic in-depth testing of the system's various components should be performed by a qualified radiation physicist (Table 2-1). Acceptance testing of new equipment is highly recommended before purchase to assure a level of performance in accordance with specifica-

tions. These results will provide the standards for comparison with subsequent tests of current operating conditions. If no such institutional standards exist, test results can be compared to those obtained by the Society for Cardiac Angiography.

## RADIATION SAFETY

It is an institutional responsibility to assign a knowledgeable and experienced person to function as radiation safety officer. The responsibilities of this position include the tasks of enforcing existing laws and regulations, informing and educating the personnel involved, and making continuous ef-

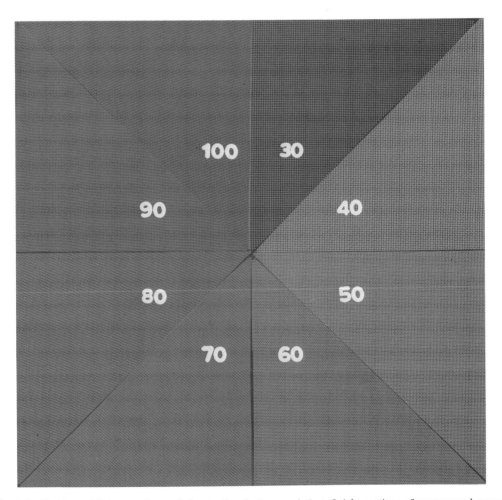

**Fig. 2-9.** Radiographic image of a resolution testing device consisting of eight sections of copper mesh screening, each with differing numbers of line pairs per inch, as indicated by the numbers 30-100.

**TABLE 2-1.** *Parameters to Be Checked on Cineradiographic Equipment*

| Item | Personnel Category | Testing Required: | | | | |
|---|---|---|---|---|---|---|
| | | On Installation | After Repair | As Necessary | A | S |
| Beam restriction | P | X | X | X | | X |
| System alignment | P | X | X | X | | X |
| System resolution | P | X | X | X | | X |
| Exposure rate | P | X | X | X | | X |
| Automatic exposure control | P | X | X | X | | X |
| Camera/film | P/R | X | X | X | | Every film change |
| Optical cleaning | P/R | X | X | X | X | |
| Camera shutter | P/R | X | X | X | X | |

P = physicist or engineer; R = radiographer or technician.
A = annually; S = semiannually.

forts to eliminate all sources of unnecessary radiation exposure.

**Radiation Units.** The units of x-ray exposure appearing in the relevant literature are *roentgen (R)*, *rad*, or *rem*. The *roentgen* unit is defined in terms of the amount of ionization created per unit volume of air. The *rad* (radiation absorbed dose) is a unit of absorbed dose and is defined as the amount of energy deposited per unit mass of irradiated material. Under experimental conditions, the heat generated by the absorbed x-ray quanta converted into energy of motion of ions and electrons is measured and defined as the energy deposited for each gram of irradiated material. The relationship between the exposure expressed in R to the absorbed dose in rads varies with the type of tissue exposed. An exposure of 1 R that irradiates soft tissue by either direct beam or scatter x-rays will result in an absorbed dose of about 0.99 rad. Bone, which absorbs more, would receive a dose of 4 rads. Rem (radiation equivalent man) is the unit of dose used in the state and federal radiation control regulations to specify the maximum allowable doses. The rem is intended to account for different types of radiation that produce varying damage for the same absorbed dose. For radiation due to alpha particles or neutrons, the number of rems would be different than the number of rads; however, for x-rays and gamma rays used in diagnostic imaging, rem and rad are practically identical.

**Population Exposure to Radiation.** In an effort to improve understanding of radiation exposure risks in the catheterization-angiography laboratory, we quote here data that present estimates of ionizing radiation to which the entire population is exposed. This exposure derives mainly from two sources: natural and man-made. Among the man-made sources, medical exposures play the greatest role (Table 2-2). For example, the estimates made by the Public Health Service in 1964 indicate that the genetically significant dose of medically administered radiation was 55 mrem per year (millirem = $\frac{1}{1000}$ of a rem per year) as compared to the naturally occurring average whole body dose of approximately 100 mrem/year. It is obvious that man-made exposure levels have increased during recent times and may well increase further. The

**TABLE 2-2.** *Radiation to Population*

| Source | Dose mrem/Year |
|---|---|
| *Natural* | |
| Cosmic | 38–70 |
| Terrestrial | 40–60 |
| Internal | 18–25 |
| *Man-made* | |
| Medical | 55–70 |
| Occupational | 2 |
| Residual fallout | 2 |
| *Total* | 170–200 |

Figures are approximations compiled from estimates by the National Academy of Science and Bureau of Radiological Health of the Food and Drug Administration.

importance of vigilant control and protection as well as research that will elucidate the effects on biologic organisms is self-evident.

The biologic effects of radiation can be divided into two categories: genetic and somatic. Genetic effects are produced by mutations in the reproductive cells and affect later generations. Immediate somatic effects on patients are unlikely to occur at the dose levels of diagnostic and interventional radiologic procedures. The somatic effects depend not only on the amount of radiation but also on the time when they were received. Since growing organisms are more sensitive, children (and particularly the unborn fetus) are in general more susceptible to radiation injury.

***Recommended Radiation Limits.*** It is not known as yet whether there exists a minimum or threshold dose of radiation below which there is no risk. For regulatory purposes, the concept of maximum permissible dose has been developed. The recommended limits for nonoccupational personnel are 0.5 rem per year; for radiologic personnel, 5 rem per year. Although these limits cannot guarantee complete elimination of any hazard, they represent doses below which the risks are very small. No maximum permissible dose limit has been established for the patient; it is therefore the responsibility of the physician to determine the balance between the potential damage deriving from the radiation exposure and the expected benefit that the examination or procedure entails. Although radiation risk at levels used in medical diagnosis are minor, the trained radiologist must always observe the general concept of "as low as practicable" whether he acts as supervisor, performer, or consultant for radiographic examinations.

***Film Badges and Monitoring of Radiation Exposure.*** Monitoring of radiation to occupationally exposed personnel is mandatory. Any dose exceeding the level of 5 rem per year constitutes an overexposure and requires investigation by the regulatory agency. No dose beyond 3 rem should be allowed during any three-month period. An occupationally exposed person who is pregnant cannot receive more than 0.5 rem to the fetus during the entire gestation period. A review of exposure history to date should be undertaken as soon as a pregnancy is confirmed to see if special steps must be taken to achieve 0.5 rem or less. For all personnel potentially exposed, a radiation safety officer keeps a record of the values deriving from the monthly measured film badges and may investigate the reasons for any exposure above such levels. Standard practice is to monitor the level of total body exposure represented by *film badges,* carried at the trunk and under the apron. In addition to the whole body maximal exposure limitations, limits have also been established for various organs, such as thyroid, eyes, or hands. In order to measure these exposure levels, additional badges may be used in accordance with special protocols.

***Protection against Radiation.*** Within the shielded procedure room, cinefluoroscopy and angiography produce radiation that is present throughout that room. In fact, scatter radiation levels from cardiac catheterization procedures are the highest of any commonly performed diagnostic x-ray study. Enforcement of the three traditional methods used to reduce radiation exposure is mandatory. They consist of the following: minimize the time that x-ray exposure occurs; maximize the distance between personnel and the patient; use optimal shielding devices.

Since the total fluoroscopic exposure is directly proportional to the total fluoroscopic time, it has to be used most effectively. The term "heavy foot" appropriately describes the novice operator who has not as yet learned to release the fluoroscopic pedal as soon as possible. Although exposure values in fluoroscopy are much less than they are during cine runs, the exposure by scatter radiation cannot be neglected. During cardiac catheterization procedures, fluoroscopic scatter rays have been measured[6] at levels of 25 mR, 10 mR, 2 mR per hour (mR = milliroentgen, $\frac{1}{1000}$ R) for the angiographer, the nearby assistant, and the second assistant at the foot of the table, respectively. Since the dose level during angiography is higher (depending on technique, 10- to 20-fold), it is advisable for the catheter operator to temporarily increase the distance as much as possible or to step behind a shielding device. Data derived from the same source exemplify the importance of distance on the level of scatter radiation during x-ray cinematography decreasing from 140 mR/h at 2 feet to 13 mR at a 6-foot distance from the x-ray beam center.[6]

Shielding can be accomplished by many different devices. In the catheterization laboratory, the most common device is the protective apron, which consists of a layer of lead covered with vinyl or cloth. Heavy aprons with a lead equivalent of 0.5 mm thickness are recommended for operators who are positioned close to the patient. These aprons protect about 80% of the active bone marrow and the gonads, assuming that the person always faces the patient. For those who need to turn their backs to the patient during the procedure, wraparound aprons are recommended. As these aprons are quite heavy and consist of two pieces, dividing the burden between shoulders and hips is recommended. Less than 0.5 mm lead layer aprons should not be used. Careful handling, storage, and periodical inspection of aprons for mechanical damages are mandatory.

Additional shielding devices that may be worn by personnel are a lead neck wrap for the thyroid and leaded eyeglasses for lens protection. These are very effective, particularly when encapsulating the body part from all directions; however, they are relatively heavy and inconvenient and may hamper the ease with which operators can work effectively. Therefore, devices of the so-called barrier type are often preferred; these are mounted to the x-ray equipment or interposed between table, equipment, patient, and operators. Examples of effective devices are steel overhangs or "lips," which are attached to the bottom of the image intensifier housing, or ceiling-mounted steel frames containing lead glass. The latter device can be encapsulated in a sterile transparent plastic bag so it will not contaminate the field of operation. Movable floor-based leaded barriers with glass windows of different sizes can also be used effectively to give additional protection to laboratory personnel or observers present in the room during the examination.

A special word of caution is appropriate for the cardiac catheterization laboratory, where the radiographic equipment installations have undergone significant changes in

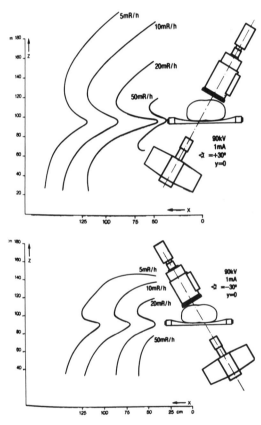

**Fig. 2-10.** Isoexposure curves representing radiation exposure to the operator during cardiac catheterization using U-arm or C-arm systems. The upper panel represents a 30-degree LAO view; the lower panel shows a 30-degree RAO view. The operator is standing to the patient's right, and the patient's feet are toward the reader. Radiation is highest at the level of the table and patient due to radiation scatter. (Reprinted from Balter S, Sones FM Jr, Brancato R: Radiation exposure to the operator performing cardiac angiography with U-arm systems. Circulation 58:925, 1978, with permission.)

design. This refers primarily to the different equipment mounts that permit angulation and projections in almost all conceivable directions. With a conventional system, the x-ray tube is enclosed and located under the patient table and the image intensifier is placed above the patient. Patient rotation within the beam results in little if any changes in the radiation scatter environment. With the new C-Arm, U-arm, or parallelogram supports, the patient remains in unchanged supine position on the table while the x-ray tube-image intensifier system is rotated and angulated in the desired direction. This maneuver implies a change in the direction of the x-ray center beam with con-comitant change in back scatter of radiation bouncing off the patient. The latter is most marked when the tube is positioned close to the operator firing in a direction away from him with rebounds of scatter being twice as high as with conventional technique. Therefore, dose level lines within the room should be determined by a radiation physicist whenever a new installation takes place and, if necessary, the appropriate shielding devices should be added. A diagram illustrating the effect of angular views on radiation exposure to the operator is shown in Figure 2-10, based on the work of Balter and co-workers.[10]

# REFERENCES

1. Friesinger GC, et al: Report of Inter-Society Commission for Heart Disease Resources. Optimal resources for examination of the heart and lungs: Cardiac catheterization and radiographic facilities. Circulation 68(4), 893, 1983.
2. Judkins MP: Angiographic equipment: The cardiac catheterization laboratory. *In* Abrams HL (editor): Coronary Arteriography: A Practical Approach. Boston, Little, Brown and Company, 1983.
3. Kodak: Films for cinefluorography. Eastman Kodak, 1983 brochure.
4. Levin D, Dunham L: Angiography: Principles underlying proper utilization of radiologic and cineangiographic equipment. *In* Grossman W (editor): Cardiac Catheterization and Angiography, second edition. Philadelphia, Lea & Febiger, 1980.
5. Moore RJ: The Physics of Cardiac Angiography. Myrle C. Enterprises, Inc., 1983.
6. Moore RJ: Society for Cardiac Angiography cine testing results: 1982. Myrle Co. Radiological Physics, Inc., 1982.
7. Schulz RJ: Diagnostic X-ray Physics. GAF Corporation Publication No. 9636-125, 1977.
8. Quality assurance in diagnostic radiology. A guide prepared following a workshop held in Nuremberg, Federal Republic of Germany, 20–24 October 1980. World Health Organization, Geneva, Switzerland, 1982.
9. Paulin S: Terminology for radiographic projections in cardiac angiography. Letter to the Editor. CCD 7:341, 1981.
10. Balter S, Sones FM Jr. Brancato R: Radiation exposure to the operator performing cardiac angiography with U-arm systems. Circulation 58:925, 1978.

## chapter three

# Complications of Cardiac Catheterization: Incidence, Causes, and Prevention

WILLIAM GROSSMAN

I N SUPPORT of the principle that if anything can go wrong it will, there is an extensive literature describing a wide array of complications that have been associated with cardiac catheterization.* Although many reports detail the complications of coronary angiography or other specific subtypes of cardiac catheterization, relatively few reports deal with complications of all types of cardiac catheterization procedures. Two multicenter studies are of particular interest in this regard: (1) the Cooperative Study on Cardiac Catheterization,[1] which represented a prospective study of all catheterization procedures (n = 12,367) in 16 laboratories over a 24-month period, and; (2) the Registry report from the Society for Cardiac Angiography,[2] which represented the experience of 66 laboratories that studied 53,581 patients over a period of 14 months. The Cooperative Study involved a small group of major medical centers at a time when the caseload involved primarily valvular heart disease; coronary angiography was a part of the catheterization procedure in only 27% of the patients in that report. In contrast, the Registry report from the Society for Cardiac Angiography,[2] based on self-reporting from a mixture of academic and private laboratories, covered a time period when suspected or known coronary artery disease was the commonest indication for catheterization: 41,204 of the 53,581 patients (77%) were studied by coronary angiography and did not have valvular, congenital, or other types of coronary disease.

Major complications (including death, myocardial infarction, stroke, serious arrhythmias, vascular injury) occurred in 1.82% of cases in the Registry report,[2] less than the 3.4% serious complication rate in the Cooperative Study.[1] While this difference may represent improvement in the safety of cardiac catheterization in the 14 years separating the two studies, it is worth noting that in the Registry report at least 28% of the patients studied had either minimal or no cardiac disease. Thus, laboratories where the percentage of normal or nearly normal studies is lower may expect to have a higher rate of death and other major complications than 1.8%.

## DEATH

Death occurred in 75 of 53,581 cases (0.14%) in the Registry report,[2] and was much more common in infants under 1 year of age (1.7%). In the Registry report and in

---

*The term *cardiac catheterization* will be taken to include catheterization and related angiography (e.g., left ventriculography, coronary angiography).

other reported series death in adult patients undergoing cardiac catheterization is more likely to occur in the elderly, especially in women over 70 years of age. Features that increase the risk of death are listed in Table 3-1.

The mortality rate associated with coronary angiography has improved considerably in the last 15 years. Previously, this rate was in excess of 1% in many laboratories,[3-6] but with improvement in technique and widespread use of heparinization the death rate with coronary angiography has fallen to its current low level of 0.1 to 0.3%, depending on case mix.

Similarly, the older literature often showed a difference in mortality between brachial and femoral approaches to coronary angiography,[3,6,7] with the femoral approach having a greater risk. However, recent studies[2] show comparable risk for both brachial and femoral techniques, probably reflecting in part the value of systemic heparinization with the percutaneous femoral approach.[8-11]

In cardiac catheterization laboratories today, deaths are most common in the subset of patients with *left main coronary artery disease* undergoing left heart catheterization and coronary arteriography. Bourassa has emphasized this, and in his institution the mortality rate in such patients was 6% in a series reported in 1976.[12] Others have re-ported mortality rates of 10%,[13] and 15%[14] in patients with significant lesions of the left main coronary artery. In the Registry report of the Society for Cardiac Angiography, 22 of the 2452 patients with ≥50% obstruction of the left main coronary artery died in association with cardiac catheterization. This considerably lower death rate (0.86%) was nevertheless more than 20 times higher than the death rate for patients with 1 vessel coronary disease (0.03%) in that series.

*Prevention of a fatal outcome* in patients with one or more of the "risk factors" listed in Table 3-1 requires that catheterization and cardiac surgical schedules should be coordinated so that patients at highest risk can be moved from the catheterization laboratory directly to the operating room. During the procedure itself, keeping the volume of radiographic contrast to a minimum, especially in patients known to have depressed left ventricular contractile function (ejection fraction of echocardiogram or radionuclide scan ≤30%) and increased pulmonary capillary pressure (≥30 mm Hg), is important. If physiologic measurements (e.g., pressures and output) routinely precede angiography, such high risk patients will be identified more easily and can be "pretreated" with intravenous furosemide, oxygen, and a vasodilator (e.g., nitroglycerin, sodium nitroprusside) prior to performing angiographic

**TABLE 3-1** *Patient Characteristics Associated with Increased Mortality From Cardiac Catheterization*

1. *Age:* Infants (<1 year old) and the elderly (>65 years old) are at increased risk of death during cardiac catheterization. Elderly women appear to be at higher risk than elderly men.

2. *Functional Class:* Mortality in Class IV patients is more than 10 times greater than in Class I–II patients.

3. *Severity of Coronary Obstruction:* Mortality for patients with left main disease is more than 10 times greater than for patients with 1 or 2 vessel disease.

4. *Valvular Heart Disease:* Especially when combined with coronary disease is associated with a higher risk of death at cardiac catheterization than coronary artery disease alone.

5. *Left Ventricular Dysfunction:* Mortality for patients with LV ejection <30% is more than 10 times greater than if ejection fraction is ≥50%.

6. *Severe Non-Cardiac Disease:* Patients with renal insufficiency, insulin-requiring diabetes, advanced cerebrovascular and/or peripheral vascular disease, and severe pulmonary insufficiency appear to have an increased incidence of death and other major complications from cardiac catheterization.

studies. We have found that a *tilting* cardiac catheterization table, which allows rapid transition to Trendelenberg position (for hypotension) or reverse-Trendelenberg (for pulmonary congestion/edema), is valuable in helping to get very sick patients through cardiac catheterization and angiography.

*Careful entry* of the coronary catheter into the left coronary ostium is important in all patients, but it is mandatory in those suspected of having left main coronary artery disease in whom preformed catheters are being used. Meticulous attention to *all the details* of technique is important in preventing deaths in the cardiac catheterization laboratory, since even a minor complication (e.g., vasovagal reaction, arrhythmia) may be fatal in a patient with limited cardiac reserve. Despite all such measures, it seems likely that a certain irreducible mortality rate will be associated with cardiac catheterization in patients with the characteristics enumerated in Table 3-1.

## MYOCARDIAL INFARCTION

Myocardial infarction as a complication of cardiac catheterization was not examined specifically by the Cooperative Study.[1] That study, which covers the years 1966 to 1968, may not be relevant with regard to this specific complication, since only 14.5% of the patients in that study had arteriosclerotic coronary heart disease. Myocardial infarction as a complication of the procedure has been reported in 0.09%,[12] 0.45%,[7] 0.61%,[15] 0.07%,[2] 1.2%,[3] and 2.6%[5] of patients undergoing cardiac catheterization and angiography.

Factors predisposing to myocardial infarction are *unstable angina* (including crescendo pattern and angina at rest), *recent subendocardial infarction*, and *insulin-requiring diabetes mellitus*. Documentation of myocardial infarction when it is less than transmural in extent may be difficult following cardiac catheterization, since intramuscular injections (e.g., lidocaine) and the soft tissue trauma of the catheterization may lead to increases in serum enzyme levels (LDH, GOT, total CPK) often used to assess the presence or absence of myocardial infarction.[16,17] Such elevations of enzyme levels may be seen with either brachial or femoral approaches. In a study of CPK isoenzymes following uncomplicated cardiac catheterization, although total CPK was increased in nearly all patients, none had elevation of CPK-MB activity.[18] Thus, an increase in serum CPK-MB activity is necessary for the diagnosis of myocardial infarction following cardiac catheterization.

*Prevention of myocardial infarction* involves the same principles discussed under prevention of deaths, particularly (1) the use of heparin during coronary angiography; (2) immediate recognition and treatment of vagal reactions, arrhythmia, angina, or hypotension; (3) full medical therapy prior to and during catheterization in patients with unstable angina (adequate use of beta-adrenergic blocking agents, oxygen, nitrates, and control of blood pressure); and (4) intraaortic balloon counterpulsation in patients who remain unstable despite full medical therapy.

## CEREBROVASCULAR COMPLICATIONS

Cerebrovascular complications occurred in 0.2% of patients reported in the Cooperative Study,[1] 0.23% of studies in the survey of Adams et al.[7] and 0.07% of studies in the Registry report.[2]

*Prevention of cerebrovascular complications* can be accomplished largely by systemic anticoagulation (especially if polyurethane catheters are used), paying meticulous attention to proper technique of catheter flushing, wiping guidewires free of blood before insertion, and restricting the time for use of guidewires to two minutes at a stretch (after which the wire is removed and wiped, and the catheter aspirated and flushed before re-entry of the wire) even in the patient who has received systemic heparinization. In addition, it is probably wise to avoid advancing the left heart catheter out to the left ventricular apex in patients with suspected left ventricular aneurysm or recent myocardial infarction and possible mural thrombus. Patients with known cerebrovascular disease, diminished or absent carotid pulsations, bruits over the carotids, subclavian, or vertebrobasilar arteries are probably at increased risk for cerebrovascular complications of catheterization. Careful avoidance of unnecessary catheter or guidewire entry into the carotid and vertebrobasilar arteries should reduce the risk of stroke in these patients.

# LOCAL BRACHIAL AND FEMORAL COMPLICATIONS

Local arterial complications of cardiac catheterization are a frequently discussed problem.[1,2,8,15,19–30] Campion reported a 9.6% brachial artery re-exploration rate at the Mayo Clinic.[20] Machleder, Sweeney, and Barker reported a 5.4% brachial re-exploration rate.[22] Brener and Couch[25] reported a 6% incidence of local femoral arterial problems and a 28% incidence of brachial arterial problems. In a report from Judkins' laboratory,[15] local femoral complications occurred in 16 out of 445 consecutive cases (3.6%). There were no serious sequelae in 15 of these patients, but one died during an operative attempt to correct the problem. Sones has reported 2% to 3% segmental occlusion at the site of arteriotomy.[31] Judkins has emphasized that serious femoral complications are related to the presence of preexisting iliofemoral disease, and that in such patients it is best to avoid a percutaneous femoral approach.[15] Nearly all laboratories have noted that women have a significantly higher incidence of both femoral and brachial arterial thrombosis following cardiac catheterization.[12,24]

A much lower rate of vascular complications (0.56%) was noted in the Registry report,[2] perhaps reflecting technical improvements in recent years.

***Brachial Approach.*** The types of local complication differ with the brachial and femoral approaches. With the brachial approach, arterial thrombosis accounts for the great majority of local complications. This is often related to formation of a thrombus in the proximal arterial segment during the catheterization procedure and failure to effectively remove it prior to arterial repair. Prevention of this complication can be accomplished by routinely using a Fogarty catheter prior to arterial repair, followed by instillation of a heparin solution into the proximal and distal arterial segments to prevent thrombus formation during closure of the arteriotomy. Brachial arterial thrombosis may also develop secondary to an intimal flap that is not properly "tacked down" or removed at the time of arterial repair and creates a small pocket of stasis where a thrombus can form. Occasionally, arterial spasm developing in the hours immediately following catheterization and successful arterial repair will result in secondary arterial thrombosis and convert an initially bounding radial pulse into one that is weak or absent six hours postcatheterization.

*Prevention of brachial artery thrombosis* can best be accomplished by meticulous attention to the details of arterial repair, which are discussed in Chapter 4. In my practice adequate heparinization includes systemic administration of heparin (5000 units intravenously) shortly after initial arterial entry and local administration of heparin (1000 to 1500 units into both proximal and distal arterial segments) at the time of arterial repair. Inspection of the arteriotomy site, trimming of any free intimal flaps, and avoidance of arterial narrowing (as frequently occurs with a purse-string closure) will minimize arterial thrombosis. I do not reverse anticoagulation with protamine at the end of a brachial catheterization; if the arterial repair has been done properly, there should not be any local bleeding.

Other potential local complications of brachial arterial catheterization include injury to the median nerve during cutdown and isolation of the artery, delayed dehiscence of arterial sutures with late arterial bleeding, bacterial arteritis, and local cellulitis-phlebitis associated with the cutdown itself. Injury to the median nerve is rare and should not occur if the dissection is careful. Rarely, postcatheterization bleeding within the brachial wound may lead to hematoma formation and compression of the nerve. This responds to prompt evacuation of the hematoma. Mild injury to the median nerve results in numbness and weakness of the thenar aspect of the hand, which almost always returns to normal within three to four weeks. Local cellulitis-phlebitis is most likely to occur if (1) there is extensive soft tissue dissection during the brachial cutdown; (2) large veins are used and tied off; (3) the catheterization procedure is long; (4) seroma or hematoma forms in the incision; (5) nonviable tissue (e.g., fat deprived of its blood supply) is left in the incision; and (6) there is poor surgical technique or violation of sterile procedure. The routine used of a potent germicidal agent (e.g., 1% povidone-iodine solution) for wound irrigation prior to skin closure substantially reduces the incidence of infection. Prophylactic antibiotics are not necessary in the routine case, but I recommend their use in any situation in which a high probability of wound infection exists (e.g., a long procedure in which a known breach of sterile technique occurred). In such instances, oxacillin 500 mg p.o. every six hours for five days beginning at the time of wound closure (initial loading dose given intravenously) is generally adequate.

***Femoral Approach.*** With regard to the femoral approach, potential local complications include arterial or venous thrombosis, distal embolization, false aneurysm, hematoma with vascular and neural compression, and delayed hemorrhage.[1,8–11,15,23–25,27–29,32]

In general, femoral arterial thrombosis requires urgent surgical intervention. Failure to accomplish this may result in propagation of thrombus into smaller distal branches of the femoral arterial tree, making ultimate restoration of normal perfusion to the limb impossible and necessitating amputation. Distal embolization represents a difficult problem, which is fortunately rare with the routine use of anticoagulants.

False aneurysm, which represents pulsating encapsulated hematoma in communication with a ruptured artery, generally develops when there has been improper groin compression following removal of the arterial catheter. These aneurysms are painful and almost invariably rupture, although rupture may not occur until several days (or even weeks) following catheterization. Surgical intervention is necessary to correct the problem in all cases. An example of a false aneurysm of the femoral artery is shown in Figure 3-1.

Delayed hemorrhage may result from false aneurysm, but more commonly it results from either poor clot formation or premature ambulation. Patients with defective platelet function (e.g., those with uremia) or who are receiving systemic anticoagulants may exhibit delayed bleeding or hemorrhage.[23] Premature activity, particularly if it is associated with a substantial rise in blood pressure, may dislodge the platelet-fibrin plug from the arterial puncture site and cause arterial bleeding. Most laboratories require at least 6 hours

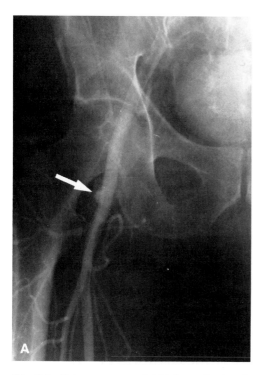 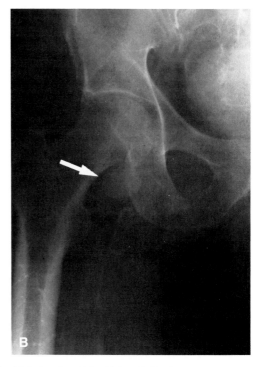

**Fig. 3-1.** False aneurysm of right femoral artery (arrows) which developed 4 to 5 days following percutaneous retrograde femoral arterial catheterization complicated by a significant postcompression local hematoma after groin compression. A. Arterial injection. B. Residual contrast seen in the aneurysm during the washout phase.

of bed rest following femoral arterial catheterization, and many require 12 to 18 hours of bed rest.

Femoral venous thrombosis is a potential complication of right heart catheterization from the femoral venous approach, and I have seen an instance of pulmonary embolism in one such case. Iliac vein thrombosis may be more common in pediatric practice, especially where repeated venous catheterization procedures may be done in cyanotic, polycythemic patients. Thrombosis of the lower portion of the inferior vena cava, iliac, or femoral veins was reported in 22 children out of a total of 1043 (2.1%) who had undergone serial cardiac catheterizations.[33]

Local infection is rare with the percutaneous femoral approach.

Local arterial complications can be minimized by paying meticulous attention to the details of arterial entry and repair. It is generally acknowledged that the incidence of thrombosis is related to the duration of the procedure (especially the "arterial time"), the number of catheters used, and the presence of underlying atherosclerotic disease. Claudication of the arm or leg following cardiac catheterization is not unheard of, and if distal arterial pulses are feeble or absent following catheterization, surgical exploration should be performed.

## PERFORATION OF THE HEART OR GREAT VESSELS

Perforation of the heart or intrathoracic great vessels has been reported with cardiac catheterization. In the Cooperative Study,[1] 100 patients (0.8%) had perforation of the heart or great vessels. Seventy-six of these were cardiac perforations (0.6%), and the most common sites were right atrium (33 cases), right ventricle (21 cases), left atrium (10 cases), and left ventricle (12 cases). Thirty of the 33 right atrial perforations were related to transseptal catheterization; thus, the right ventricle is the commonest site of cardiac perforation in patients undergoing catheterization by techniques other than transseptal. In our experience, the risk of cardiac perforation is greatest in elderly women (≥65 years) undergoing right heart catheterization. Stiff catheters (such as NIH or Gorlin pacing catheters) should be avoided in these patients, and inexperienced individuals (e.g., trainees with less than four months' experience in right heart catheterization) should defer to senior personnel in such cases. Perforation of the subclavian artery, iliac artery, abdominal aorta, or great veins has been reported and is generally associated with excessive catheter manipulation. In many such instances, catheter manipulation was continued despite resistance to passage or complaints by the patient of pain related to the catheter passage.

Eshagy and co-workers[34] reported mediastinal and retropharyngeal hemorrhage as a complication of retrograde brachial left heart catheterization in two patients. Both patients were receiving anticoagulants prior to catheterization (prothrombin times were 42 and 23 seconds), and in both cases there was difficulty in catheter manipulation from the subclavian artery to the ascending aorta. Treatment with maintenance of an adequate airway, correction of hypoprothrombinemia, and blood replacement was successful in both cases.

Perforation of the heart is the main hazard of transseptal catheterization, since the procedure actually entails controlled perforation of the interatrial septum. Unintentional perforation of the aorta, atrial wall, coronary sinus, or right atrial appendage may occur, leading to cardiac tamponade. Perforation of the heart is the major complication of endomyocardial biopsy and will be discussed in Chapter 32.

## VASOVAGAL REACTIONS

Vasovagal or so-called vagal reactions are common and may be serious. They are frequently (but not always) incited by *pain* in a tense, anxious patient and consist of nausea, hypotension, and bradycardia. In older patients the entire picture of a vagal reaction may be present *without the bradycardia*. The mechanism of the reaction is presumed to be sudden peripheral vasodilatation involving arterioles and venules, unaccompanied by a compensatory increase in cardiac output.[34a] Vagal reactions respond dramatically to intravenous atropine, 0.5 to 1.0 mg (*and* to cessation of catheter manipulation) if they are recognized promptly. Elevation of the legs is a helpful adjunct to the treatment of vagal hypotension in the supine patient and will generally result in partial correction of hypotension within 10 to 15 seconds; by this time the atropine is usually taking effect. If the hypotension and bradycardia of a vagal reaction are permitted to persist for any period of time, serious arrhythmias or irreversible shock may develop, particularly in patients with ischemic heart disease or aortic stenosis.

## ARRHYTHMIA AND CONDUCTION DISTURBANCE

Major arrhythmias occurred in 1.2% of cardiac catheterizations in the Cooperative Study,[1] and included ventricular fibrillation (59 cases, 0.4%), ventricular tachycardia (12 cases, 0.10%), asystole or marked bradycardia (37 cases, 0.30%), complete heart block (7 cases, 0.06%), and supraventricular arrhythmia (35 cases, 0.28%), among other arrhythmias. In studies reflecting the current predominance of patients with coronary artery disease in catheterization laboratories, ventricular fibrillation was reported in 1.28% (600 instances in a total of 46,904 cases) of patients undergoing coronary angiography in the survey of Adams and co-workers.[7] Ventricular fibrillation, tachycardia, or asystole occurred in 0.77% of 5,250 patients undergoing left heart catheterization and coronary arteriography at the Montreal Heart Institute between 1970 and 1974.[12] In the Registry report from the Society of Cardiac Angiography,[2] arrhythmias requiring treatment occurred in 0.56% of patients (58% ventricular fibrillation, 26% ventricular tachycardia, 16% bradycardia).

Arrhythmias may occur with either right or left heart catheterization. Balloon-flotation right heart catheterization is by no means free of risk of serious arrhythmias. In a prospective study of 150 bedside pulmonary artery catheterizations using balloon-flotation catheters,[35] ventricular salvos (3 to 5 consecutive ventricular depolarizations) occurred in 30% of insertions, nonsustained ventricular tachycardia (5 to 30 ventricular premature beats in a row) occurred in 22% of insertions, "sustained" ventricular tachycardia (>30 beats in sequence) occurred in 3%, and 2/150 insertions were complicated by ventricular fibrillation. A new right bundle branch block was noted in 5% of insertions and lasted an average of 9.5 hours.

In general, serious ventricular arrhythmias occur in two situations: (1) with excessive catheter manipulation within the left or right ventricular chambers, especially in a patient with resting ventricular irritability, or (2) suddenly, following coronary artery contrast injection, especially of the right coronary artery. Those that occur in the second situation give the impression of being idiosyncratic reactions, since the patients may have normal coronary anatomy. Their incidence may be reduced by injecting the smallest amount of radiographic contrast agent sufficient to opacify the arterial tree.

Complete heart block has been reported from several laboratories as a complication of cardiac catheterization.[36,37] It is most commonly seen during right heart catheterization in a patient with preexisting left bundle branch block (LBBB), when the sudden development of transient right bundle branch block (RBBB) during passage of a catheter from the right ventricle to the pulmonary artery leaves the patient with no mechanism for conduction of atrial impulses to the ventricles. Unless an adequate ventricular escape focus takes over, profound hypotension and asystole may occur. The availability of a standby pacemaker is mandatory in such cases, and we commonly use a pacing catheter (e.g., the 7 French Gorlin) for right heart catheterizations in patients with preexisting LBBB. Alternatively, the use of a Swan-Ganz balloon-tipped catheter for right heart catheterization in such patients may reduce the risk of heart block, but as just mentioned some risk of transient right bundle branch block is present even with the balloon-flotation catheter.[35]

Atrial arrhythmias that occur during cardiac catheterization are generally atrial fibrillation or flutter. Again, a common precipitating cause is excessive catheter manipulation in the right atrium, where multiple atrial extrasystoles commonly precede the development of atrial fibrillation or flutter. Both arrhythmias usually revert spontaneously to sinus rhythm, but external cardioversion may be necessary in some cases. In patients requiring a right heart or coronary sinus catheterization who are felt to have a higher risk for developing atrial fibrillation (e.g., a history of paroxysmal atrial fibrillation, frequent atrial extrasystoles at rest, increased left or right atrial pressures), a single dose of quinidine or procainamide 1 to 2 hours prior to the scheduled catheterization procedure may help prevent atrial fibrillation.

## PHLEBITIS, INFECTIONS, FEVER

Phlebitis, fever, or local infection occurs in fewer than 1% of cardiac catheterizations, and some of the causes and predisposing factors have been discussed previously. The phlebitis, usually minor, almost always responds to hot soaks and elevation of the affected limb. Fever is rare and usually transient; it may represent pyrogen reaction, allergy to contrast agent, or systemic reaction to local phlebitis or infection. Bacterial endocarditis as a complication of cardiac catheterization is rare. As mentioned previously, although some laboratories routinely use antibiotic prophylaxis, most do not, and I do not favor routine use of antibiotics before catheterization. Paying careful attention to sterile technique and cleansing the brachial wound with copious quantities of sterile saline followed by 1% aqueous iodine-povidone solution will minimize the incidence of these complications.

## PYROGEN REACTIONS

Pyrogen reactions are not commented upon in most reported series of cardiac catheterization. The Cooperative Study mentions two cases.[1] Pyrogen reactions result from the introduction of foreign protein, endotoxin, or other antigenically active substances into the blood. A series of cases occurring within a single laboratory should raise suspicion of contamination in the catheter or instrument sterilization procedures. In one such epidemic,[38] an increase in the incidence of fever and chills in association with cardiac catheterization was traced to contamination of the hospital distilled water reservoir with acinetobacteria calcoaceticus and a pseudomonas species. Sterilization killed the bacteria but left endotoxin coated on the internal lumen of the catheters, and when this was flushed into the circulation during catheterization and angiography, a pyrogen reaction resulted. Endotoxin may be detected with either the limulus lysate assay or a rabbit pyrogen test.[38]

A typical pyrogen reaction consists of rigors with subsequent development of fever and may follow intravascular injections or angiograms by intervals ranging from 1 to 60 minutes. The rigors can be severe, and temperatures in excess of 102°F may be seen. In my experience the clinical manifestations of these reactions have often responded dramatically to small intravenous doses of morphine (e.g., 2 to 4 mg IV), repeated as necessary. Catheterization should be discontinued with the development of such reactions, since the source of the pyrogenic material is rarely immediately obvious. The incidence of pyrogen reactions may be reduced substantially by using disposable catheters, stopcocks, and other equipment. However, careful cleaning and preparation of catheters and instruments is generally all that is required to minimize the occurrence of these reactions.

## HYPOTENSION

Hypotension during cardiac catheterization is generally a consequence of one of the complications already discussed (such as vagal reaction or myocardial infarction). However, hypotension may develop following left ventriculography due to the vasodepressor properties of the contrast agent (dilation of systemic arterioles and venules) as well as its myocardial depressant properties. Such hypotension is usually transient and passes within 30 seconds. On occasion it may persist longer and usually responds to elevation of the legs and expansion of intravascular volume with half-normal saline solution.

Postcatheterization hypotension may develop in the patient who has received large amounts of radiographic contrast agent at catheterization, in whom postcatheterization diuresis (the hyperosmolar contrast material acts as an osmotic diuretic) combines with continued vasodepressor effect to cause relative hypovolemia. The hypotension of such patients is associated almost invariably with *normal* or *increased warmth of the skin*, suggesting that paresis of vasomotor regulation persists as long as contrast agent remains in the circulation. Such postcatheterization hypotension virtually always has a major orthostatic component and usually responds promptly to fluid administration and the supine or Trendelenberg position. In my experience, women of aesthenic build with a history of chronic "low blood pressure" are particularly susceptible to this complication and may exhibit blood pressures of 70 to 80 mm Hg during the first six hours following catheterization and angiography. The administration of colloid-containing solutions (Plasmanate, dextran) may be helpful in cases that fail to respond to increased rate of crystalloid administered intravenously. The hypotension usually resolves after the radiographic contrast agent is "washed out" of the circulation by way of the kidneys.

Other causes to be considered in the patient with postcatheterization hypotension include delayed cardiac tamponade due to gradual leak from unrecognized cardiac perforation produced at the time of catheterization and blood loss due to hemorrhage from the arterial puncture site or from an internal vascular perforation.

## ELECTRICAL HAZARDS

Electrical hazards have been reported in association with cardiac catheterization, including fatal ventricular fibrillation.[39–42] With the present standard use of isolation transformers and equipotential environment, such events are rare.

## OTHER COMPLICATIONS

*Pulmonary edema* developing during cardiac catheterization is rare and is usually related to (1) a new untoward cardiac event (e.g., acute myocardial infarction): (2) the stress of angiographic contrast material; (3) the recumbent position; or (4) other factors in a patient with already compromised left ventricular function. The Cooperative Study[1] described four patients who experienced this complication. Bourassa reports this complication in four patients (0.1%) following coronary angiography at the Montreal Heart Institute.[12] This complication usually responds promptly to (1) helping the patient to sit up, (2) administering an intravenous diuretic (e.g., 20 to 40 mg furosemide), and (3) oxygen by mask. If there is not prompt evidence of major improvement (within three minutes), consideration of more ag-

gressive therapy (e.g., sodium nitroprusside if the arterial systolic pressure is 120 mm Hg or more, and intraaortic balloon counterpulsation if there is associated hypotension) is in order.

*Pulmonary artery perforation and pulmonary hemorrhage* associated with use of the flow-directed balloon-tipped catheter have been reported from several laboratories.[43–48] Several of these cases were fatal. Overinflation of the balloon and excessive time in "wedge" (balloon inflated) position appear to have been factors. This complication seems to be more likely to occur in women, elderly persons, and those with pulmonary hypertension. Giving careful attention to the instructions of Drs. Ganz and Swan in Chapter 7 of this textbook for use of their catheter will prevent this complication. Other complications reported in association with the flow-directed balloon-tipped catheter include arrhythmias (discussed above), ruptured chordae of the tricuspid valve,[49] pulmonary thromboembolism,[50] and intracardiac knotting of the catheter.[51] Again, careful adherence to proper technique (Chapter 7) should prevent (or at least minimize) the occurrence of such complications with this catheter.

*Coronary artery dissection* is a rare complication of cardiac catheterization.[52–55] This seems to be more common with the right coronary artery and may result from vigorous injection of a jet of contrast agent against an atherosclerotic plaque, or from excessive force of catheter tip entry into the coronary ostium.

Morise and co-workers have reported 3 cases of coronary artery dissection secondary to coronary angiography and have reviewed 39 additional cases reported in the literature.[55] Their 3 patients were young women (37, 40, and 42 years old), without significant atherosclerotic coronary narrowing. From their cases and review of the literature they concluded that catheter-induced coronary dissection can occur with either brachial or femoral approach and is more likely to occur in the right coronary artery and in women under age 45 with minimal atheromatous disease. Most left coronary dissections result in infarction.

*Cholesterol embolization* leading to renal failure has occurred from retrograde femoral arterial catheterization of the aorta.[56] Characteristically the renal insufficiency develops slowly (weeks to months) and progressively following the catheterization, and renal biopsy specimens show intravascular cholesterol crystals. Evidence of peripheral embolization, such as livido reticularis or ischemia of the toes, may be present: again, these commonly develop only after a considerable time interval (weeks) following catheterization. Eosinophilia is often present and episodic hypertension is also a frequent finding. The prognosis is not good, and renal insufficiency commonly progresses to complete and permanent renal failure.

*Systemic or pulmonary embolization of vegetations* is a potential hazard of cardiac catheterization in patients with endocarditis of the left- or right-sided cardiac valves. Although often discussed, there is little if any evidence that catheter-induced dislodgement of vegetations occurs. Welton and co-workers reviewed their experience with 35 patients who underwent catheterization for severe heart failure (30 patients) and persistent sepsis or recurrent embolization (5 patients) during active endocarditis. Catheterization-induced embolization did not occur in any of these 35 patients.[57] They concluded that catheterization can be performed safely and yields important information in patients with active endocarditis who are being considered for surgical intervention.

*Pulmonary embolism* can occur after cardiac catheterization, and a study comparing the incidence of new focal pulmonary embolism after brachial and femoral catheterization has been reported.[57a] Using ventilation-perfusion scans before and one day after catheterization, an 8.3% incidence of new perfusion defects was seen after retrograde femoral catheterization (combined left and right heart), but no new defects occurred with brachial catheterization.

*Severe protamine reactions* that simulate anaphylaxis have been reported in association with cardiac catheterization.[57b] These reactions tend to occur immediately after administration of protamine intravenously, which is used for reversing systemic heparinization after percutaneous femoral catheterization. The reactions consist of profound hypotension with dyspnea, wheezing, and circulatory collapse. Death may ensue, although most patients respond to epinephrine and supportive measures. Protamine reactions are much more likely to occur in diabetics who have been receiving NPH insulin,

and may occur in 27% of these patients.[57b] Patients who have been receiving NPH insulin, as well as those with a history of allergy to fish, should not receive protamine if at all possible.

## GENERAL CONSIDERATIONS

*Caseload.* At least one report has found an inverse correlation between the *caseload* of a cardiac catheterization laboratory and its incidence of major complications.[7] With regard to coronary angiographic procedures, the mortality rate in institutions performing fewer than 100 procedures per year was eight times higher than in institutions performing more than 400 procedures per year.[7] These data were interpreted to mean that greater caseload per physician leads to greater skill and technical proficiency and fewer complications. This important conclusion, which has influenced the ICHD report on optional resources for cardiac catheterization and angiography,[58] has been challenged by a study of eight cardiac catheterization laboratories in the State of Washington.[59] That study found an extremely low rate of major complications in association with coronary angiography, even though the caseload/laboratory (average 50 to 250 cases/year) and caseload/angiographer (average 65 cases/year) was low. These authors suggest that skill can be maintained even without a large caseload and that the low complication rates of some laboratories with high volume may primarily reflect liberal indications for the procedure and relatively small numbers of patients with high-risk conditions (e.g., left main coronary disease, unstable angina, overt left ventricular failure). This complex and important issue cannot be resolved on the basis of current data.

*Speed.* The *speed* with which a catheterization procedure is accomplished is also widely regarded to be a determinant of the risk of complications. Unfortunately, there are few data on this subject. The Cooperative Study[1] analyzed the duration of catheterization procedures in 16 participating laboratories and found that there was a bell-shaped curve with the most common duration being 2.0 to 3.0 hours (5022 cases, 41% of total procedures, median = 2.5 hours), with 4207 procedures (34%) lasting 1.0 to 2.0 hours, and

2054 procedures (17%) lasting between 3.0 and 4.0 hours. Procedures accomplished under one hour and those that took longer than five hours accounted for 1.9% and 2.8% of total cases, respectively. Although no comparable data have been published in recent years, it is my impression that improvements in technique have shortened the duration of cardiac catheterization as currently practiced. No attempt was made in the Cooperative Study[1] to relate duration of procedure to major complications. Duration of a cardiac catheterization procedure may be prolonged by factors that tend to be associated with a high risk of complication. For example, the elderly patient with extensive atherosclerosis and arterial tortuosity may have a long procedure because of technical difficulties associated with catheter passage in such patients. There may also be an increased risk of complications in such patients because they frequently have more extensive disease and diminished reserve. In this instance the high risk is not necessarily due to the increased duration of the procedure: the two are "true, true; unrelated." Similarly, a young patient with normal vessels and minimal cardiac disease may have a rapid catheterization procedure, but speed of the procedure in this instance cannot fairly be credited with the low risk. In my view,

duration of the procedure is an important "independent" risk factor only when it can clearly be related to lack of skill or inexperience of the operator or when severe cardiac decompensation requires that the patient spend minimal time in the supine position.

***Pseudocomplications.***   Finally, a word relevant to "pseudocomplications" of cardiac catheterization is in order.[60,61] Patients suffering from serious cardiac disease experience major cardiac events (myocardial infarction, ventricular arrhythmia, systemic embolus) as part of the natural history of their disease. If one of these events happens to occur during or within 24 hours of a scheduled cardiac catheterization, is it fair to always regard it as a complication of the procedure? Hildner and co-workers[60,61] examined events that occurred from 24 hours before to 72 hours after scheduled catheterizations. The incidence of "pseudocomplications" or events occurring in the 24 hours prior to catheterization was 0.81%, including 0.24% deaths. During the same period there was a 0.81% incidence of catheterization procedure-related complications with no deaths. Thus it is clear that the incidence of complications after cardiac catheterization is influenced by rate of occurrence of unexpected major cardiac events and the natural history of the patient's basic cardiac disease.

## REFERENCES

1. Braunwald E, Swan HJC (eds): Cooperative study on cardiac catheterization. Circulation 37 (Suppl. III):1, 1968.
2. Kennedy JW, et al: Complications associated with cardiac catheterization and angiography. Cathet Cardiovasc Diagn 8:5, 1982.
3. Chahine RA, Herman MV, Gorlin R: Complications of coronary arteriography: comparison of the brachial to the femoral approach. Ann Intern Med 76:862, 1972.
4. Takaro T, Pifarre R, Wuerflin RD: Acute coronary occlusion following coronary arteriography: mechanisms and surgical relief. Surgery 72:1018, 1972.
5. Walson WJ, Lee GB, Amplatz K: Biplane selective coronary arteriography via percutaneous transfemoral approach. Am J Roentgen 100:332, 1967.
6. Takaro T, Hultgren HN, Littman D, Wright EC: An analysis of deaths occurring in association with coronary arteriography. Am Heart J 86:587, 1973.
7. Adams DF, Fraser DB, Abrams HL: The complications of coronary arteriography. Circulation 48:609, 1973.

8. Freed MD, Keane JF, Rosenthal A: The use of heparinization to prevent arterial thrombosis after percutaneous cardiac catheterization in children. Circulation 50:565, 1974.
9. Judkins MP, Gander MP: Prevention of complications of coronary arteriography. Circulation 49:599, 1974.
10. Eyer KM: Complications of transfemoral coronary arteriography and their prevention using heparin. Am Heart J 86:428, 1973.
11. Walker WJ et al: Systemic heparinization for femoral percutaneous coronary arteriography. N Engl J Med 288:826, 1973.
12. Bourassa MG, Noble J: Complication rate of coronary arteriography. A review of 5250 cases studied by percutaneous femoral technique. Circulation 53:106, 1976.
13. Lavine P, Kimbiris D, Segal BL, Linhart JW: Left main coronary artery disease: clinical, arteriographic and hemodynamic appraisal. Am J Cardiol 30:791, 1972.
14. Cohen MV, Cohn PF, Hermann MV, Gorlin R: Diagnosis and prognosis of left main coronary ar-

tery obstruction. Circulation 46(Suppl. 1): 57, 1972.

15. Green GS, McKinnon CM, Rosch J, Judkins MP: Complications of selective percutaneous transfemoral coronary arteriography and their prevention. Circulation 45:552, 1972.

16. Burckhardt D, Vera CA, LaDue JS, Steinberg I: Enzyme activity following angiography. Am J Roentgen 102:406, 1968.

17. Michie DD, Conley MA, Carretta RF, Booth RW: Serum enzyme changes following cardiac catheterization with and without selective coronary arteriography. Am J Med Sci 260:11, 1970.

18. Roberts R, Ludbrook PA, Weiss ES, Sobel BE: Serum CPK isoenzymes after cardiac catheterization. Br Heart J 37:144, 1975.

19. Mortensen JD: Clinical sequelae from arterial needle puncture, cannulation, and incision. Circulation 35:1118, 1967.

20. Campion BC, et al: Arterial complications of retrograde brachial arterial catheterization. Mayo Clin Proc 46:589, 1971.

21. Jeresaty RM, Liss JP: Effects of brachial artery catheterization on arterial pulse and blood pressure in 203 patients. Ann Heart J 76:481, 1968.

22. Machelder HI, Sweeney JP, Barker JF: Pulseless arm after brachial artery catheterization. Lancet 1:407, 1972.

23. Bristow JD, et al: Late, heparin-induced bleeding after retrograde arterial catheterization. Circulation 37:393, 1968.

24. Kloster FE, Bristow JD, Griswold HE: Femoral artery occlusion following percutaneous catheterization. Am Heart J 79:175, 1970.

25. Brener BJ, Couch NP: Peripheral arterial complications of left heart catheterization and their management. Am J Surg 125:521, 1973.

26. Nicholas GG, DeMuth WE: Long term results of brachial thrombectomy following cardiac catheterization. Ann Surg 183:436, 1976.

27. Takahashi O: The effects of transfemoral cardiac catheterization on limb blood flow in children. Chest 71:159, 1977.

28. Rosengart R, Nelson RJ, Emmanoulides GC. Anterior tibial compartment syndrome in a child: an unusual complication of cardiac catheterization. Pediatrics 58:456, 1976.

29. Lang EK: A survey of the complications of percutaneous retrograde arteriography. Seldinger technique. Radiology 81:257, 1963.

30. Baker LD, Lesin SJ, Mathur VS, Messer JV: Routine Fogarty thrombectomy in arterial catheterization. N Engl J Med 279:1203, 1968.

31. Sones FM Jr: Cine coronary arteriography. *In* Hurst JW, Logue RB, (eds): The Heart. 2nd ed. New York, McGraw-Hill Book Company, 1970, p 377.

32. Stanger P: Complications of cardiac catheterization of neonates, infants and children. Circulation 50:595, 1974.

33. Mathews RA, et al: Iliac venous thrombosis in infants and children after cardiac catheterization. Cathet Cardiovasc Diagn 5:67, 1979.

34. Eshagy B, et al: Medastinal and retropharyngeal hemorrhage: a complication of cardiac catheterization. JAMA 226:427, 1973.

34a. Weissler, AM Warren JV: Vasodepressor syncope. Am Heart J 57:786, 1959.

35. Sprung CL, et al: Advanced ventricular arrhythmias during bedside pulmonary artery catheterizations. Am J Med 72:203, 1982.

36. Gupta PK, Haft JI: Complete heart block complicating cardiac catheterization. Chest 61:185, 1972.

37. Stein PD, Mathur VS, Herman MV, Levine HD: Complete heart block during cardiac catheterization of patients with pre-existent bundle branch block. Circulation 34:783, 1966.

38. Reyes MP, et al: Pyrogenic reactions after inadvertent infusion of endotoxin during cardiac catheterizations. Ann Intern Med 93:32, 1980.

39. Bousvaros GA, Conway D, Hopps JA: An electrical hazard of selective angiocardiography. Can Med Assoc J 87:286, 1962.

40. Starmer CF, Whalen RE, McIntosh HD: Hazards of electric shock in cardiology. Am J Cardiol 14:537, 1964.

41. Mody SM, Richings M: Ventricular fibrillation resulting from electrocution during cardiac catheterization. Lancet 2:698, 1962.

42. Starmer CF, McIntosh HD, Whalen RE: Electrical hazards and cardiovascular function. N Engl J Med 284:181, 1971.

43. Golden MS, Pinder T Jr, Anderson WT, Cheitlin MD: Fatal pulmonary hemorrhage complicating use of a flow-directed balloon-tipped catheter in a patient receiving anticoagulant therapy. Am J Cardiol 32:865, 1973.

44. Lapin ES, Murray JA: Hemoptysis with flow directed cardiac catheterization. JAMA 220:1246, 1972.

45. Chun CHM, Ellestad MH: Perforation of the pulmonary artery by a Swan-Ganz catheter. N Engl J Med 284:1041, 1971.

46. Pope LA, et al: Fatal pulmonary hemorrhage after use of the flow-directed balloon-tipped catheter. Ann Intern Med 90:344, 1979.

47. Foote GA, Schabel SI, Hodges M: Pulmonary complications of the flow-directed balloon-tipped catheter. N Engl J Med 290:927, 1974.

48. McDaniel DD, et al: Catheter-induced pulmonary artery hemorrhage. J Thorac Cardiovasc Surg 82:1, 1981.

49. Smith WR, Glauser FL, Jemison P: Ruptured chordae of the tricuspid valve: The consequence of flow directed Swan Ganz catheterization. Chest 70:790, 1976.

50. Goodman DJ, Rider AK, Billingham ME, Schroeder JS: Thromboembolic complications with the indwelling balloon tipped pulmonary arterial catheter. N Engl J Med 291:777, 1974.

51. Lipp H, O'Donoghue K, Resnekov L: Intracardiac knotting of a flow-directed balloon-tipped catheter. N Engl J Med 284:220, 1972.

52. Meller J, Friedman S, Dack S, Herman MV: Coronary artery dissection—a complication of cardiac catheterization without sequelae: case report and review of the literature. Cath Cardiovasc Diagn 2:301, 1976.

53. Haas JM, Peterson CR, Jones RC: Subintimal dissection of the coronary arteries: a complication of selective coronary arteriography and the transfemoral percutaneous approach. Circulation 38:678, 1968.

54. Guss SB, et al: Coronary occlusion during coronary angiography. Circulation 52:1063, 1975.

55. Morise AP, Hardin NJ, Bovill EG, Grundel WD: Coronary artery dissection secondary to coronary arteriography. Cathet Cardiovasc Diagn 7:283, 1981.

56. Smith MC, Ghase MK, Henry AR: The clinical spectrum of renal cholesterol embolization. Am J Med 71:174, 1981.

57. Welton DE, et al: Value and safety of cardiac catheterization during active infective endocarditis. Am J Cardiol 44:1306, 1979.

57a. Gowda S, Bollis AM, Haikal AM, Salem BI. Incidence of new focal pulmonary emboli after routine cardiac catheterization comparing the brachial to the femoral approach. Cathet Cardiovasc Diagn 10:157, 1984.

57b. Stewart WJ, McSweeney SM, Kellet MA, Faxon DB, Ryan TJ. Increased risk of severe protamine reactions in NPH insulin dependent diabetics undergoing cardiac catheterization. Circulation 70:788, 1984.

58. Friesinger GC, et al: Optimal resources for examination of the heart and lungs. Cardiac catheterization and radiographic facilities. Circulation 68:893A, 1983.

59. Hansing CE, et al: Cardiac catheterization experience in hospitals without cardiovascular surgery programs. Cathet Cardiovasc Diagn 3:207, 1977.

60. Hildner FJ, Javier RP, Ramaswamy K: Psuedocomplications of cardiac catheterization. Chest 63:15, 1973.

61. Hildner FJ, Javier RP, Tolentino A, Samet P: Pseudo-complications of cardiac catheterization: update. Cathet Cardiovasc Diagn 8:43, 1982.

# PART II
*Techniques of Cardiac
Catheterization*

*chapter four*

# Cardiac Catheterization by Direct Exposure of Artery and Vein

WILLIAM GROSSMAN

A FTER the question of indications and contraindications has been settled and the properly premedicated patient arrives at the laboratory, the catheterization protocol is transformed into action. This chapter and Chapters 5 and 7 will deal with techniques predominantly used in the catheterization of adults and older children. Special considerations in infants and smaller children will be discussed in Chapter 6.

In our laboratory the patient is usually transferred from the stretcher to a flat carbon-fiber table top that is comfortably padded. Electrocardiogram (ECG) leads are placed, and the patient is then draped. The pertinent areas (antecubital fossae, groins) are scrubbed with 1% povidone-iodine solution or another suitable antiseptic solution.

Before proceeding to the actual catheterization, it is our policy to obtain a full 12-lead ECG at this point and to place an intravenous line in the arm opposite that through which the catheterization is planned. These tasks can be accomplished by the catheterization laboratory nurse or a properly trained technician. The intravenous line can be used for administering drugs (such as heparin or atropine) during catheterization and fluids following catheterization. The ECG should be examined by the physician who will perform the catheterization, and the procedure is aborted if any significant changes (e.g.,

evidence of new myocardial infarction, arrhythmia) have developed since the last previous ECG.

## INCISION, ISOLATION OF VESSELS, AND CATHETER INSERTION

With the direct brachial approach I favor a single cutdown in the right antecubital fossa through which both right and left heart catheterizations are performed. The brachial artery is identified by palpation (Fig. 4-1), and local anesthesia is induced (I use 2% lidocaine), first through a short 25- or 27-gauge needle to raise an intradermal bleb, and then through a long (1½-inch) 22-gauge needle to infiltrate the subcutaneous, deep fascial, and periosteal tissues.

When inducing local anesthesia, it is important to remember that *slow injection* is less painful and produces better tissue infiltration. We use liberal amounts of lidocaine, 5 to 15 ml initially, repeating frequently so that 15 to 20 ml are commonly administered in the course of a catheterization. If anesthetization is done properly, the catheter insertion site ought to be virtually painless throughout the procedure.

Next, a transverse incision is made with a number 15 surgical blade just proximal to

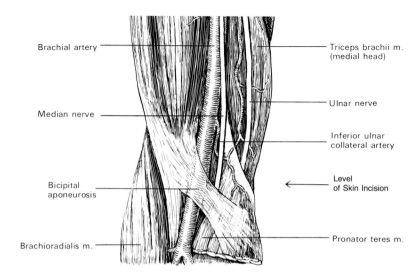

Brachial artery

Triceps brachii m. (medial head)

Median nerve

Ulnar nerve

Inferior ulnar collateral artery

Bicipital aponeurosis

← Level of Skin Incision

Brachioradialis m.

Pronator teres m.

**Fig. 4-1.** Anatomy of antecubital fossa illustrating course of the brachial artery. The artery is best sought at or slightly above the antecubital skin crease, medial to the bicipital aponeurosis. Care must be taken not to disturb the median nerve, which usually lies medial to the brachial artery. (From Clemente, C.: Gray's Anatomy of the Human Body, 30th American ed. Philadelphia, Lea & Febiger, 1985.)

the flexor crease. If right and left heart catheterizations are contemplated, the incision is wide and made over the palpable brachial artery; if right heart study alone is planned, the incision is narrow and made directly over a previously identified *medial* vein. Those who ignore this latter dictum soon learn that the large plump veins of the lateral antecubital fossae usually drain into the cephalic system, through which it may be difficult to navigate the catheter into the right atrium. The medial veins drain either into the basilic or brachial venous systems, both of which join the axillary vein by direct continuation and are thus easy routes to the superior vena cava and right atrium (Fig. 4-2).

The operator should stand between the patient's arm and chest during the cutdown, so that his line of vision within the incision is angled from medial to lateral. This is important, since the brachial artery usually lies below the bicipital aponeurosis and will be visualized only as the aponeurosis is lifted and retracted laterally. Standing at the outside (lateral) aspect of the arm makes it more likely that the first structure seen and isolated by the operator will be the median nerve, and this must be avoided.

The tissues are separated by blunt dissection with a curved hemostat, and an appropriate vein is brought to the surface, separated from adjacent nerves and fascia, and tagged proximally and distally with 3-0 or 4-0 silk. The brachial artery is similarly brought to the surface with a curved hemostat, isolated from adjacent nerves, veins, and fascia, and tagged proximally and distally with moistened umbilical tape or silicone elastomer surgical tape * (Fig. 4-3). In isolating the brachial artery, I like to use a small, self-retaining retractor and a short right-angle vascular clamp (e.g., 6¼-inch Kantrowitz clamp, Fig. 4-4).

Before proceeding with the right heart catheterization, we routinely place an arterial monitor line in the left radial or right femoral artery, using percutaneous technique (see Chapter 5 for details of technique of percutaneous entry). A 4F or 5F catheter-introducer, advanced over an appropriate J guide wire, is adequate to monitor arterial pressure during the catheterization procedure. The usefulness of such an arterial monitor line cannot be overstated. It need not be kept sterile, can be used during the catheterization to obtain arterial blood samples during the Fick cardiac output determinations, to withdraw arterial blood during indicator-

*Retract-o-tape. Med-Pro Ltd., Sun Prarie, WI.

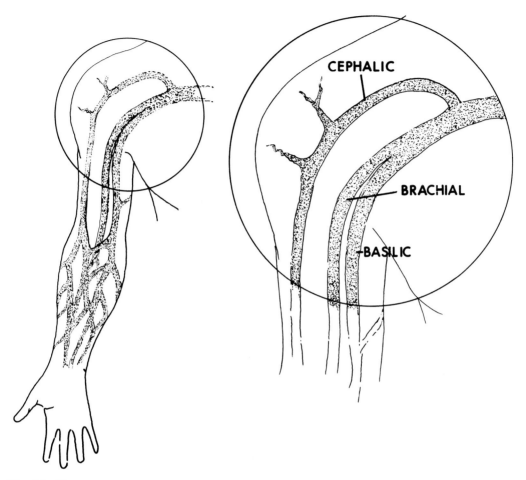

**Fig. 4-2.** Venous anatomy of the arm. Brachial and basilic veins are medial to the cephalic vein within the antecubital fossa. Note that the brachial and basilic veins continue directly into the axillary and subclavian system, whereas the cephalic system frequently joins the subclavian vein at a right angle. Passage of a catheter from the cephalic system to the right atrium may thus be quite difficult; the medial veins provide the straightest pathway.

dilution studies, and to monitor arterial pressure nearly continuously. Although catheterization can be done without such a line, the presence of an arterial monitor line can be of great value, especially if trouble develops (e.g., hypotension, arrhythmias, perforation).

After placing the arterial monitor line and isolating the brachial artery and basilic or brachial vein, it is time to proceed with the right heart catheterization. An appropriate catheter is selected (see next section) such as a Goodale-Lubin or Cournand, and flushed vigorously with heparinized solution (concentration, 3000 IU heparin per liter of 5% dextrose in water or normal saline solution). A transverse incision is made in the vein with small scissors, and the catheter is introduced with the aid of either curved tissue forceps without teeth or a small plastic catheter introducer.* I occasionally place the vein over a "bridge" formed by straight forceps to enable better control and to diminish oozing during passage of the catheter (Fig. 4-3).

Once the catheter has been introduced and passed a short distance, blood is aspirated, and the catheter is again flushed with heparinized solution. The catheter may then be connected by means of flexible plastic

*Catheter Introducer, Becton Dickinson and Company, Rutherford, NJ.

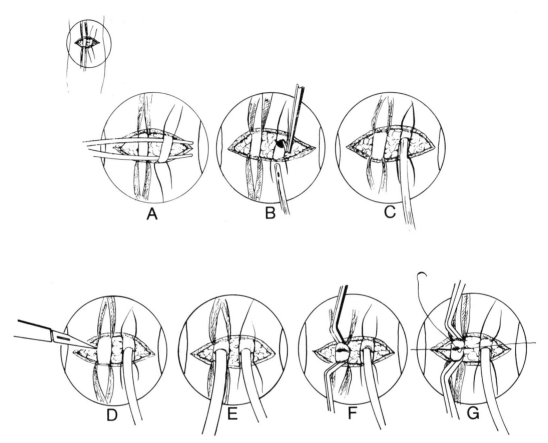

**Fig. 4-3.** Catheterization by direct exposure of brachial artery and vein. (A) Artery and vein have been isolated. Both are tagged proximally and distally; the artery with moist umbilical or silicone-elastomer tape, the vein with 3-0 silk. The vein has been placed over a "bridge" formed by a straight forceps to enable better control. (B) The vein has been incised with a small scissors, and the catheter is about to be inserted with the aid of a plastic catheter introducer (see text). (C) Passage of the right heart catheter. (D) Incision of the brachial artery with a number 11 surgical blade. The cutting edge of the blade is facing upwards, and the point approaches the artery from the side and at an angle of ~10 to 20 degrees to the horizontal to avoid perforating the posterior wall. (E) Passage of the left heart catheter. (F) In preparation for arterial repair, concentrated heparinized saline solution is "locked" in the vessel by placing bulldog clamps as far above and below the arteriotomy as possible (see text). (G) Closure of the arteriotomy by continuous or running stitch. Stay sutures are placed at each end of the arteriotomy (see text).

tubing to either the side port of a Paley manifold* (at whose end port is a pressure transducer), or more directly via a manifold to a sterile pressure transducer (see Chapter 9). We have chosen the latter system because of its better frequency-response characteristics and the resultant superior quality pressure tracings. The interposed manifold allows entry of heparinized flush solution, and by turning the stopcock the operator can have

*United States Catheter and Instrument Corporation, Billerica, MA.

intermittent pressure monitoring and catheter flush.

After passage of the right heart catheter, which will shortly be discussed in detail, the brachial artery is cleaned and incised transversely with a number 11 surgical blade (Fig. 4-3). An appropriately selected left heart catheter (see the following section), which has been flushed as described, is then inserted and passed retrograde a short distance before it is aspirated, flushed with heparinized solution, and connected to a pressure measurement, intermittent flush

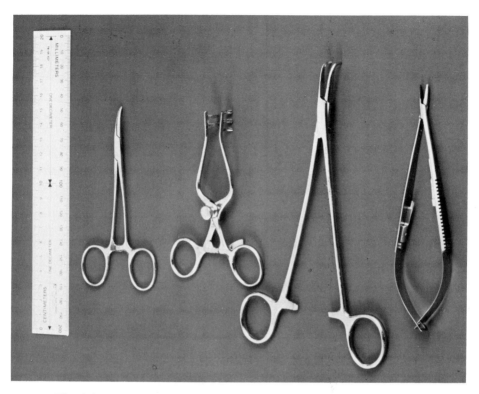

**Fig. 4-4.** Instruments useful in brachial arterial catheterization, including (from top to bottom) a Castro-Viejo type needle holder, right-angle vascular clamp, Weitlaner self-retaining retractor, and small curved "mosquito" hemostat. The right-angle vascular clamp is helpful in isolating the artery from surrounding structures and bringing it up to the surface, where it can be cleaned and tagged. The special needle holder has a delicate hold and release mechanism and is widely used in ophthalmologic and vascular surgery as an aid in the fine control of suture placement.

system similar to that described for the right heart catheter. When the catheter is flushed manually, the barrel of the flush syringe should *always* be vertical, with the hub facing downward. The catheter should be aspirated first until there is a free return of blood, and only 2 to 3 ml of flush solution need be injected, although the syringe should contain more than this. These precautions will greatly reduce the hazard of air embolism. Many laboratories routinely administer heparin solution (e.g., 3000–5000 IU heparin) into the distal brachial artery; this may reduce the incidence of arterial thrombosis. In my own practice, I do not give heparin locally into the artery; instead, I administer 5000 IU of heparin intravenously after the arterial catheter has been passed to the central aorta.

## CATHETER SELECTION

Catheter selection depends on the demands of the protocol. Right heart catheters usually are utilized for measurement of right atrial, right ventricular, pulmonary artery, and pulmonary capillary wedge pressures. For the latter purpose, only an end-hole catheter is adequate, although the catheter may in addition have side holes in close proximity to the tip. I use either a Goodale-Lubin or Cournand catheter* as the initial right heart catheter, although many will prefer a flow-directed balloon-flotation catheter for routine right heart catheterization (see Chapter 7). If atrial pacing is planned, a Gorlin elec-

*United States Catheter and Instrument Corporation, Billerica, MA.

trode catheter* (modification of the Goodale-Lubin for pacing) is effective; it is especially useful for coronary sinus sampling and pacing.

Passage of the right heart catheter occasionally is accompanied by transient right bundle branch block. Should this occur in a patient with pre-existing left bundle branch block, bilateral or complete heart block will develop and may require emergency ventricular pacing. A Swan-Ganz balloon-tipped catheter may be used in patients with left bundle branch block, as it is less likely to cause trauma to the right bundle. Alternatively, a pacing catheter may be used so that immediate ventricular pacing can be instituted should complete heart block develop.

For right-sided angiography, a closed-end catheter that has multiple side holes and is easy to pass to the pulmonary artery should be chosen, and for this purpose I frequently use the Eppendorf catheter.* Other frequently employed right heart catheters include the standard Lehman catheter* (not to be confused with the Lehman ventriculography catheter*), which is similar to the Cournand catheter but has a larger lumen, and many types of tapered end-hole catheters used when a percutaneous approach is employed (see Chapter 5).

Left heart catheters utilized when the direct brachial approach is employed include both open-end and closed-end multiple side-hole catheters, which are used for both pressure measurement and angiography. The *Sones* catheter is commonly used as a left heart catheter, and it can be most helpful at times in crossing a tight aortic valve when other catheters have failed. It has a tendency to recoil during ventriculography, and it may produce myocardial staining when used by an inexperienced operator.

The polyurethane Sones catheter, marketed by Cordis Corporation† (see Chapter 13), is particularly easy to manipulate into the ascending aorta, coronary arteries, and left ventricle, and it is a commonly used left heart catheter in our laboratory. This catheter has a variety of curves (I generally use

---

*United States Catheter and Instrument Corporation, Billerica, MA.

†80 cm Cordis brachial coronary A, Sones technique, type II. Cordis Corporation, Miami, FL.

‡Millar Instruments, Houston, TX.

the type II), and in 7 and 8 French sizes tapers to a 5 French external diameter near its tip. It has an end-hole and four side-holes within 7 mm of the tip. The catheter will accept an 0.035-inch guide wire, which is often helpful in navigating through a tortuous subclavian artery into the ascending aorta. It is an excellent catheter for crossing a tight aortic valve, with or without the added help of a straight guide wire.

Because the Sones catheter frequently causes ventricular extrasystoles during left ventriculography, I occasionally use a closed-end, multiple side-hole catheter for left ventriculography and initial hemodynamic measurements. In this regard, the polyurethane 7F or 8F NIH catheter made by Cordis Corporation is easy to use and to advance into the left ventricle. The Eppendorf catheter (USCI) is similar to the NIH catheter and may be used for ventriculography. Some operators prefer to use a pigtail catheter from the brachial approach; the tip of this catheter must be straightened out by a guide wire prior to entry at the arteriotomy site. The catheters I use most frequently for right and left heart catheterization are shown in Figure 4-5.

When high-fidelity artifact-free tracings are needed, a micromanometer-tipped catheter may be chosen, such as the Mikro-tip‡ (see Chapter 9). The Mikro-tip catheter is available in a modification (PC481, 471) with multiple side holes through which angiography can be performed. It is also available with a "pigtail" end for percutaneous placement.

Other left heart catheters include the Gensini* (usually employed with percutaneous technique; see Chapter 5), the Lehman ventriculography catheter,* the Rodriguez-Alvarez* catheter, and the Shirey catheter* (which may be used for a retrograde approach to the left atrium).

## ADVANCING THE RIGHT HEART CATHETER

Both right and left heart catheters should be advanced as soon as possible after introduction into the vascular system, since letting them sit in the bloodstream at body temperature results in loss of catheter stiffness

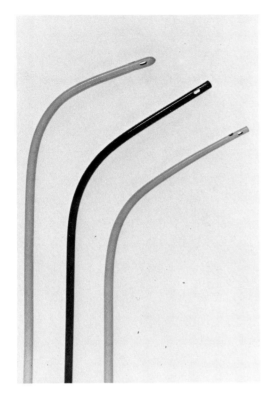

**Fig. 4-5.** Catheters that I use routinely when doing right and left heart catheterization. The Goodale-Lubin catheter (middle) has an end-hole and 2 side-holes and is ideal for right heart catheterization, including measurement of pulmonary capillary wedge pressure. The polyurethane NIH catheter (left) is a closed-end catheter with multiple side-holes, ideal for left ventriculography (see Chapter 14) and aortography. The polyurethane Sones catheter (right) tapers to a 5F tip with an end-hole and 4 side-holes; it is useful for coronary angiography and also for left ventriculography (at low flow rates).

and diminishes catheter control. The right heart catheter is advanced under fluoroscopic control to the right atrium. If there is difficulty entering the superior vena cava, it is sometimes helpful to try the following maneuvers: have the patient take a deep breath; raise the right arm and shoulder toward the head (ask the patient to shrug his right shoulder); turn the patient's head to the extreme left; remove the patient's pillow. If the catheter tip consistently points in a cephalad direction, try to *gently* form a loop proximal to the tip, which then may buckle and prolapse into the superior vena cava. In the last suggestion, the word *gently* must be

emphasized; a catheter should *never* be forcibly advanced against a resistance. On occasion, a guide wire may be helpful in passing from the subclavian vein into the superior vena cava. If these maneuvers do not meet with prompt success, try a different catheter. Each catheter has a slightly different bend, and generally one will be just right for a given patient.

A word is offered here concerning *venous spasm*, which may develop in any patient but is especially common in women. If spasm develops, do not try to advance the catheter, but instead withdraw it for a distance of 10 to 20 cm and then briskly move it to and fro in short (approximately 5-cm) strokes. This will commonly "break" the spasm, and the catheter may then be freely advanced to the right heart. *If spasm persists, a smaller catheter must be used.* Right heart catheterization in adults can be accomplished with 5 French or 6 French catheters, and a percutaneous femoral venous approach can be used if this is not successful. Persisting in the presence of spasm produces pain, vagal reactions, and hypotension, and a minor problem can thus be converted into a catastrophe. The same approach, by the way, applies equally to *arterial spasm*.

When the catheter tip has been advanced to the superior vena cava (SVC), I generally draw a blood sample for oximetry. If the SVC blood oxygen saturation is substantially lower than the pulmonary artery oxygen saturation, a full oximetry run should be done (Chapter 12). Such an oxygen "step-up" may be the only clue to unsuspected atrial septal defect. To accomplish all these tasks successfully requires 1 to 2 minutes. The catheter tip is next advanced to the right atrium, where pressure is recorded prior to advancing the catheter to the pulmonary artery.

In navigating from the right atrium to right ventricle and pulmonary artery, the J-loop technique should be tried first. The catheter is advanced so that its tip catches on the lateral right atrial wall and the catheter looks like the letter J on fluoroscopy (Fig. 4-6). The catheter is next rotated counterclockwise so that the tip of the J sweeps the anterior right atrial wall (thus avoiding the coronary sinus, whose ostium lies posterior to the tricuspid valve) and jumps across the tricuspid valve into the right ventricle. At this point, the technician monitoring the patient's ECG will frequently note extrasystoles and call these

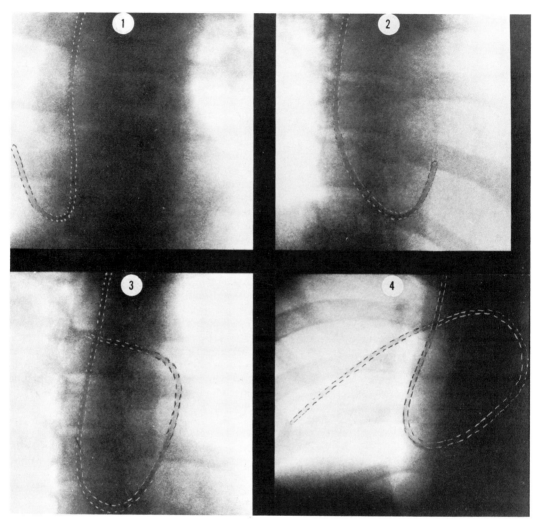

**Fig. 4-6** Advancing the right heart catheter. In navigating from right atrium to pulmonary artery, the J-loop technique should be tried first. (1) The catheter is advanced so that its tip catches on the lateral right atrial wall and forms the letter J. (2) It is then rotated counterclockwise so that the catheter tip sweeps the anterior right atrial wall (thus avoiding the coronary sinus) and jumps across the tricuspid valve into the right ventricle. (3) The catheter tip, pointing towards the right ventricular outflow tract, can be easily advanced into the pulmonary artery. (4) The patient takes a deep breath, and the catheter is advanced to the "wedge" position (see text).

off to the operator; this is a sign that the catheter has entered the right ventricle. Since the catheter usually still retains its J curve (woven Dacron catheters have a "memory" and will retain an imposed shape for a short time after the imposing force has been removed), its tip will now be pointing toward the right ventricular outflow tract and can easily be advanced into the pulmonary artery. Right ventricular pressure may

be recorded during the transit, or it may be recorded subsequently during the catheter pull-back.

If the catheter tip meets any resistance during its transit through the right ventricular outflow tract, *do not advance it.* Pull back until the tip is free, and again gently try to advance to the pulmonary artery. It is easy to perforate the right ventricular outflow tract and end up in the pericardial space. In this regard, it should be pointed out that older women (e.g., >65 years of age) seem particularly susceptible to this complication, and we therefore use 7 French (or smaller) catheters routinely in these patients.

With the catheter now in the pulmonary artery, pressure is again measured and blood is sampled for oximetry. Next, the catheter is advanced to the "wedge" position. This can be done simply by having the patient take a deep breath and hold it while the catheter is advanced until its tip will go no farther (Fig. 4-6) and does not pulsate with the heart. Having the patient cough at this time will frequently advance the catheter tip into a true "wedge" position. The catheter loop may need to be pulled back slightly at this point to avoid coiling up in the right ventricle and atrium.

Pressure is measured and the pressure waveform is examined. If there is any doubt that a true wedge position has been achieved, blood is sampled from the catheter. The pressure is accepted as a true wedge pressure only if completely (≥95%) saturated blood can be aspirated from the catheter.[1] When mitral stenosis is not expected to be present, the wedge pressure may be "confirmed" simply by its typical waveform and by its match against simultaneous left ventricular diastolic pressure. If an unexpected diastolic gradient is detected between left ventricular and pulmonary wedge pressures, the wedge position should be confirmed by blood sampling. Blood oxygen saturation from a true wedge position should be ≥95%, unless the catheter is wedged in a lung segment with poor aeration (e.g., atelectatic lobe, pneumonia, pulmonary edema). If a Swan-Ganz catheter is used to obtain pulmonary capillary wedge pressure, it often will be necessary to aspirate and discard the 5 to 15 ml of pulmonary artery blood that lies between the balloon and the pulmonary capillary bed before bright red pulmonary capillary blood can be sampled. When using a Cournand, Goodale-Lubin or Lehman (end-hole) catheter to obtain a wedge pressure, it is our practice to leave the catheter in the wedge position, flushing *intermittently* at three-minute intervals (continuous flushing in the wedge position frequently causes the patient to develop violent coughing), and proceed with the left heart catheterization. We perform cardiac output determinations with right heart pull-back to the pulmonary artery only after simultaneous pulmonary capillary wedge and left ventricular pressures have been recorded. A different practice must be followed when the Swan-Ganz or other balloon catheter is used as a right heart catheter. These catheters must *never* be left in the wedge (balloon-up) position for any significant period of time. Failure to observe this rule may cause pulmonary infarction and/or rupture of the pulmonary artery, as is discussed in Chapter 7.

The Cournand catheter is somewhat stiffer than the Goodale-Lubin, and it may be easier to control in the right heart and to advance to wedge position. Stiffer right heart catheters (such as the Cournand and Gorlin catheters) may also be more dangerous, particularly in elderly women, in whom perforation of the heart can easily occur (see Chapter 3). One way of temporarily stiffening a Goodale-Lubin or other catheter, is to advance a 0.038- or 0.045-inch guide wire (soft end first) to within 2 to 3 inches of the catheter's tip. This maneuver commonly gives the added stiffness necessary to get to wedge position. The guide wire should not remain in the catheter for more than 2 to 3 minutes, after which it is removed and the catheter is carefully aspirated and flushed.

## ADVANCING THE LEFT HEART CATHETER

After the right heart catheter has been advanced to the pulmonary artery or wedge position, an appropriately selected left heart catheter is inserted into the brachial artery as described previously. This catheter is then advanced into the ascending aorta just above the aortic valve. If there is difficulty navigating from the subclavian or innominate arteries into the ascending aorta, the operator may try all the maneuvers suggested for guiding the right heart catheter into the superior vena cava. These include having the patient take a deep breath, shrug his right shoulder, turn his head to the extreme left, removing his pillow, and extending the right arm by manual traction on the wrist. If the tip consistently points in a cephalad direction, the operator may try to *gently* prolapse the part of the catheter just proximal to its tip into the ascending aorta. If the patient experiences any pain during this latter maneuver, the operator should desist immediately, lest a dissection or perforation result. It has been my impression that passage of a left heart catheter from the subclavian artery to the central aorta is easier when the patient is lying on a flat-topped table, as opposed to the cradle-type table. The cradle often forces the shoulders forward and distorts the arterial anatomy, such that more bends and curves need to be negotiated in navigating from brachial artery to central aorta.

As with right heart catheterization, *if the catheter does not pass after a relatively brief attempt at manipulation, resist the temptation to become more vigorous.* When using an end-hole catheter (e.g., the Sones catheter, pigtail catheter, or Gensini catheter) a soft J-tipped spring guide wire may be advanced through the catheter tip to lead the way. The 0.035-inch-diameter guide wire can be used with the Cordis Sones catheter, and larger sizes with the pigtail or Gensini catheters. On rare occasions, the ascending aorta cannot be entered via the right brachial artery, necessitating a percutaneous femoral approach or left brachial artery cutdown.

Once in the ascending aorta, central aortic pressure is measured and recorded simultaneously with arterial monitor pressure. The catheter is then advanced across the aortic valve into the left ventricle. This usually can be accomplished by producing to-and-fro excursions of the catheter while gradually rotating it through 360 degrees, so that the catheter tip moves up and down on the aortic valve over its entire plane.

As mentioned previously, the Cordis polyurethane NIH catheter is often used as a left heart catheter in our laboratory when the brachial approach is employed. This soft tipped catheter may be advanced directly (tip first) into the left ventricle, or it may be prolapsed across the aortic valve, loop first, as illustrated in Figure 4-7. Once in the ventricle it is usually quite stable when curved directly in front of the mitral valve (Fig. 4-7). This is also an excellent angiographic position for the NIH or Eppendorf catheters and rarely results in artifactual mitral regurgitation.

On occasion, it may be difficult to enter the left ventricle, particularly when dealing with severe aortic stenosis. In this circumstance, one should try several catheters of different types (we have had good results with the Sones catheter which occasionally

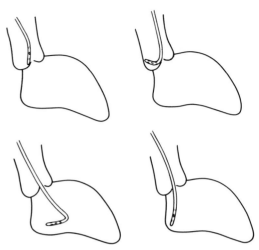

**Fig. 4-7.** Diagrammatic representation of retrograde left ventricular catheterization with the NIH or Eppendorf catheters. These soft-tipped catheters may be advanced directly (tip first) into the left ventricle or may be prolapsed across the aortic valve, loop first (as shown in the sequence upper left, upper right, and lower left). Once in the ventricle either catheter is usually quite stable when curved directly in front of the mitral valve (lower right). This is also an excellent angiographic position for the NIH or Eppendorf catheters, and rarely results in artifactual mitral regurgitation.

will pass a tight aortic valve easily), or utilize a straight-tipped guide wire approach before abandoning the attempt. When crossing a stenotic aortic valve retrograde, it is often helpful to view the aortic root and valve in left anterior oblique projection. This view shows the calcified leaflets well and may demonstrate the location of the orifice that will provide a target for repeated to-and-fro excursions of the catheter tip or straight-tipped guide wire. If a guide wire is used, the catheter is advanced over the guide wire into the ventricular chamber, and following removal of the guide wire, the catheter is then aspirated vigorously and flushed. With a guide wire–facilitated entrance into the left ventricle, there is a danger that the guide wire tip may pass under endocardial trabeculations, so that the catheter subsequently advanced over the guide wire is not free in the ventricular chamber. This can lead to serious myocardial staining during power injection of contrast, but should be detectable from appearance of the catheter tip and from the washout of contrast after a test injection. Success in crossing a tight aortic valve depends on experience, luck, and sheer determination.

A special purpose left heart catheter was developed by Dr. Earl Shirey for retrograde catheterization of the left atrium. The Shirey catheter* is a tapered, multiple side-hole woven Dacron catheter that resembles the Sones catheter. It can be prolapsed loop-first into the left ventricle, so that its tip faces the aortic and mitral valves (Fig. 4-8) rather than the left ventricular apex. Withdrawal of the redundant loop frequently guides the catheter tip into the left atrium.

Once the left ventricle has been entered and a stable position is found, it is advisable to immediately obtain simultaneous recordings of critical pressures, such as left ventricular, peripheral arterial (through the arterial monitor line), and pulmonary capillary wedge pressures. Although these pressures will be recorded again during the cardiac output determinations, arrhythmias or other unanticipated problems may develop, greatly altering the basal physiologic state and possibly requiring catheter withdrawal. In such circumstances, the operator will sorely regret not having measured the pressures earlier.

## REPAIR OF VESSELS AND AFTERCARE

After the completion of diagnostic studies, the left heart catheter is removed and the brachial arteriotomy is repaired. Repair may be done in many ways (purse-string, interrupted, continuous), but I will describe only my own approach.

The proximal and distal portions of the artery are checked for vigorous and free bleeding, and a Fogarty embolectomy catheter† is employed.[2] The use of a Fogarty catheter routinely in all brachial catheterizations has resulted in an extremely low incidence of diminished radial pulse and arterial insufficiency.

When good proximal flow has been established, 10 to 15 ml of a concentrated solution

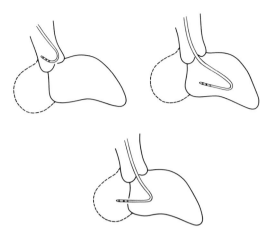

**Fig. 4-8** Diagrammatic illustration of retrograde catheterization of the left atrium using the Shirey catheter. It can be prolapsed loop-first into the left ventricle (upper left), so that its tip faces the aortic and mitral valves (upper right) rather than the left ventricular apex. Withdrawal of the redundant loop frequently guides the catheter tip into the left atrium (lower panel).

of heparinized saline (3000 IU of heparin in 30 ml normal saline) are infused into the proximal artery through the Sones or NIH catheter; this solution is "locked" in the vessel by immediately placing a vascular bulldog type clamp‡ as far above the arteriotomy as possible (Fig. 4-3). The same procedure is then repeated for the distal segment (i.e., use of Fogarty catheter, administration of heparin, placement of bulldog clamp). At this point, a stay suture is placed at each end of the arteriotomy, which is then closed using a continuous or running stitch (Fig. 4-3) with fine nonwettable suture material such as 6-0 Tevdek.§ The stay suture at one end of the incision is the start of the running stitch, and the stitch is completed by tying to the other stay suture. The advantage of a continuous suture is that it tightens as the artery expands after the clamps are removed.[3]

I prefer to use a special needle holder (Castro-Viejo type), with a delicate hold and release mechanism when doing the arterial repair. Needle holders of this type (Fig. 4-4) are commonly used in ophthalmologic and

---

*USCI, Billerica, MA.

†Arterial embolectomy catheter; 3 French, 40 cm. Shiley Laboratories, Irvine, CA.

‡DeBakey peripheral vascular bulldog clamps with 45-degree to 60-degree angled jaws, V. Mueller, Chicago, IL.

§Tevdek, Deknatel Company, Queens Village, NY.

vascular surgery and are an aid in the fine control of suture placement.

After suturing the artery, the distal bulldog clamp is removed first, and the forearm is massaged from the wrist toward the elbow, to milk out any air within the lumen of the artery before releasing the proximal bulldog clamp. The proximal clamp is then removed, and any minor leaks are controlled by direct finger pressure, which must be sufficiently gentle so that the radial pulse can be palpated. If leaking does not stop within a few minutes of such finger pressure, an additional suture or two may be required. It is important that the radial pulse be palpable and essentially of the same amplitude as prior to the arteriotomy. If it is absent or greatly diminished, the artery should be reopened and a Fogarty catheter passed *proximally and distally*. When this is unsuccessful, prompt consultation should be obtained from an experienced vascular surgeon (if possible while the wound is still open), who usually will be able to identify and correct the problem. The operator should carefully watch the vascular surgeon and learn from him exactly what the problem was, how it was corrected, and how it might have been prevented.

After successfully repairing the arteriotomy, the vein utilized in the right heart catheterization may be tied off or repaired like the arteriotomy, depending on the needs of the individual case. The wound is then flushed out with copious quantities of fresh sterile saline solution followed by 10% povidone-iodine solution.* Currently, we close the wound using a subcuticular stitch of an absorbable suture (4-0 Dexon "S" on a cutting needle) thereby avoiding the need for suture removal. Alternatively, the skin may be closed with interrupted mattress sutures of 4-0 nylon. These sutures must then be removed seven to ten days later. Antibiotic ointment is placed on the suture line and covered with a firm dressing (although not so firmly that it diminishes the radial pulse).

The patient is usually instructed to drink 1 to 2 quarts of water or juice by 6:00 PM, to compensate for the diuretic action of the angiographic contrast material, as well as to help wash this myocardial and vascular de-

---

*Pharmadine, Sherwood Pharmaceutical, Mahwah, NJ.

pressant out of his vascular system. If there is any question about the patient's ability to drink the required fluid, an equivalent amount should be administered intravenously. We have rarely seen pulmonary congestion from this regimen, but have frequently seen hypotension when this instruction was not followed or was countermanded by a well-meaning but uninformed house officer. In patients with poor left ventricular function and/or pulmonary capillary wedge pressures ≥25 mmHg, or in whom little or no radiographic contrast was used, the fluid orders should be correspondingly reduced.

In a typical case, our postcatheterization orders might read:

1. Resume all previous medications.
2. Blood pressure (specify arm), pulse, and inspection of dressings every 15 minutes ×4, then every 1 hour ×4, then every 4 hours.
3. Call intern *and* catheterization laboratory (specify phone number) for any problems (such as bleeding, loss of pulse, or hypotension).
4. Encourage p.o. fluids: 1–2 L over 6–8 hours.
5. Pain medication (e.g., codeine, meperidine, Demerol).

There is no need for the patient to be kept flat or motionless in bed following the procedure. The patient may sit up, eat, and (if no groin procedure has been done) get out of bed (with assistance) to go to the bathroom. The operator should see the patient later in the afternoon in order to check the dressing, peripheral pulses, and general condition of the patient. This may also be a suitable time to discuss with the patient and his family the results of the investigation and recommendations for further treatment (e.g., surgical procedures) if any. In a patient in whom the catheterization was done as an outpatient procedure, the patient may be discharged to home following check of the radial pulse and antecubital fossa incision.

In less than 1% of cases, a radial pulse has been absent by the time we have seen the patient on late afternoon rounds. In such cases, I usually administer 1 aspirin and watch the patient overnight, with a plan to bring the patient to the catheterization laboratory the next morning for re-exploration by me and the Cardiology Fellow who had done the catheterization with me. In about one third of the cases there is a strong pulse the next morning, and the absence of a pulse on evening rounds is attributed to spasm or a transient thrombus. In two thirds of the cases, the radial pulse is still weak or absent, and these patients come to the laboratory where under local (2% xylocaine) anesthesia, I reopen the incision, take down the arterial repair, pass a Fogarty catheter in both directions (usually getting a sizeable thrombus) and remove any intimal fronds or flaps that are visible. Heparin is administered systemically (5000 IU) and locally into the proximal and distal segments of the artery, and the artery is repaired using 6-0 Tevdek in a continuous suture, as before. Using this approach, I have not had a single patient in whom corrective intervention by a vascular surgeon has been required in 5 years.

It is important to emphasize that the complications of a catheterization should be managed *by the physicians who have done the catheterization.* Not only are these individuals the ones most likely to understand the genesis of a specific problem, but this is clearly the best method of continuing education to ensure the prevention of future complications.

## DIRECT LEFT VENTRICULAR PUNCTURE

As mentioned earlier, the great vessels and chambers of the heart can usually be entered by techniques described in this chapter or in Chapter 5. On rare occasions, it will be impossible to enter the left ventricle by either retrograde or transseptal approaches, and direct left ventricular puncture will have to be considered. This consideration may arise in the patient with severe aortic stenosis or in the patient with prosthetic valves (e.g., Bjork-Shiley) in both mitral and aortic positions. In the 12,367 procedures reviewed by the Cooperative Study on Cardiac Catheterization, direct left ventricular puncture was employed in only 260.[4]

An excellent historical review and detailed description of technique is given by Zimmerman.[5] He recommends that the puncture be performed by a thoracic surgeon and describes both the subxiphoid and apical techniques. Without stating an absolute prefer-

ence, he points out that cardiac tamponade is four times more frequent with the subxiphoid approach. Pain and vasovagal reactions are common,[5,6] and therefore premedication with atropine and Demerol is desirable. After local anesthesia, a 9-inch number 18 gauge blunt-end needle with removable stylet, over which a Teflon catheter is fitted, is inserted through a small stab wound made in the skin overlying the apex beat. The needle is directed toward the second right costochondral junction and slightly posteriorly, so that when advanced it will enter the left ventricle parallel to its long axis. After entering the left ventricle, the Teflon catheter is advanced over the needle and the latter is removed. Once pressure is recorded and blood is withdrawn for oxygen analysis, left ventriculography may be performed either through the Teflon catheter[5] or through a Gensini catheter that has been exchanged for the Teflon one using a guide wire technique.[6] Complications reported with this procedure include cardiac tamponade, ventricular fibrillation, pneumothorax, hemothorax, intramyocardial injection of contrast medium, reflex hypotension, and chest pain.

One group has reported left ventricular puncture and angiography in 22 patients, 19 of whom had aortic and mitral valve prostheses (Starr-Edwards).[7] There were no deaths; 2 fully anticoagulated patients had hemothorax, 2 had transient neurologic events, and 1 had a myocardial stain.

In another report a technique is described for using echocardiography to guide transthoracic left ventricular puncture.[8] Seven patients with either Bjork-Shiley or Starr-Edwards aortic prostheses were studied successfully using this approach. The interested reader is referred to the original description for details.[8] The use of ultrasound has proven useful in guiding pericardiocentesis and should be of considerable value in the patient requiring transthoracic left ventricular puncture.

## REFERENCES

1. Rapaport E, Dexter L: Pulmonary "capillary" pressure. *In* Methods in Medical Research. Year Book Publishers 7:85, 1958.
2. Baker LD, Leshin SJ, Mathur VS, Messer JV: Rou-

tine Fogarty thrombectomy in arterial catheterization. N Engl J Med 279:1203, 1968.

3. Mendel D: A Practice of Cardiac Catheterization. Oxford, Blackwell Scientific Publications, 1968. pp 124–125.

4. Braunwald E, Gorlin R: Total population studied, procedures employed, and incidence of complications. *In* Cooperative Study on Cardiac Catheterization. Circulation 37(Suppl. III): 36, 1968.

5. Zimmerman HA: Intravascular Catheterization. 2nd edition. Springfield, Ill., Charles C Thomas, 1966. pp 38–62.

6. Semple T, McGuinness JB, Gardner H: Left heart catheterization by direct ventricular puncture. Br Heart J 30:402, 1968.

7. Morton MJ, McAnulty JH, Rahimtoola SH, Ahuja N: Risks and benefits of postoperative cardiac catheterization in patients with Ball valve prostheses. Am J Cardiol 40:870, 1977.

8. Vignola PA, Swaye PS, Gosselin AJ: Safe transthoracic left ventricular puncture performed with echocardiographic guidance. Cathet Cardiovasc Diagn 6:317, 1980.

*chapter five*

# Percutaneous Approach and Transseptal Catheterization

DONALD S. BAIM *and* WILLIAM GROSSMAN

I N CONTRAST with the direct brachial technique, the percutaneous approach to left and right heart catheterization involves achieving vascular access via needle puncture,[1] obviating surgical isolation of the vessel during either the introduction or subsequent withdrawal of the cardiac catheter.[1] Once the needle has been positioned within the vessel lumen, a flexible guide wire can be advanced through the needle and well into the central vasculature.[2] When this needle is withdrawn, the guide wire remains in its intravascular position and provides a means of introducing the desired catheter. Although most catheters may be inserted directly over the guide wire, it is now more common to place an introducing sheath over the guide wire,[3,4] and then advance the catheter through this sheath. With appropriate skill and knowledge of regional anatomy, the percutaneous technique can be adapted to catheter insertion from a variety of entry sites. Venous catheterization can be performed via the femoral, internal jugular, subclavian, or median antecubital vein, whereas arterial catheterization can be performed via the femoral,[3,4] brachial,[5] or axillary[6] artery. At the termination of the procedure, the catheters and introducing sheaths are withdrawn, and bleeding from the puncture sites is controlled by the application of direct pressure.

## CATHETERIZATION VIA FEMORAL ARTERY AND VEIN

### Selection of Puncture Site

The adjacent femoral artery and vein (Fig. 5-1) are the most commonly used vessels for percutaneous diagnostic cardiac catheterization. Vessel puncture should be achieved between 1 and 3 cm below the inguinal ligament, which can be easily palpated as it courses from the anterior superior iliac spine to the pubic tubercle. While some operators rely on the location of the inguinal skin crease rather than the inguinal ligament for the selection of the puncture site, skin crease position can be misleading in obese patients, but the iliac spine and ligament continue to be reliable anatomic landmarks. The femoral artery typically lies at the midpoint of the inguinal ligament and can be palpated over a several centimeter span distal to the ligament. The femoral vein lies approximately one fingerbreadth *medial* to the artery, along a parallel course.

Most difficulties in entering the femoral artery and vein—and most vascular complications—arise as the result of inadequate identification of these landmarks prior to attempted vessel puncture. Punctures of the artery at or above the inguinal ligament

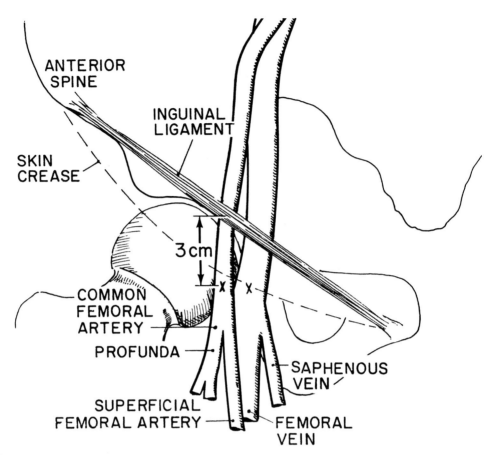

**Fig. 5-1.** Regional anatomy relevant to percutaneous femoral arterial and venous catheterization: The right femoral artery and vein are shown coursing underneath the inguinal ligament, which runs from the anterior superior iliac spine to the pubic tubercle. The arterial skin nick (indicated by X) should be placed approximately 3 cm below the ligament and directly over the femoral arterial pulsation, and the venous skin nick should be placed at the same level but approximately one fingerbreadth more medial. Although this level corresponds roughly to the skin crease in most patients, anatomic localization relative to the inguinal ligament provides a more constant landmark (see text for details).

make catheter advancement difficult and predispose to inadequate compression, hematoma formation, and/or intraperitoneal bleeding following catheter removal. Punctures of the artery more than 3 cm below the inguinal ligament increase the chance that the femoral artery will have divided into its profunda and superficial femoral branches. Puncture in the crotch between these two branches fails to enter the arterial lumen, and puncture of either one of the branches increases the risk of a thrombotic occlusion due to smaller vessel caliber. Because the superficial femoral artery frequently overlies the femoral vein, low venous punctures may pass inadvertently through the superficial

femoral artery, leading to excessive bleeding and the possible formation of an arteriovenous fistula.

## Local Anesthesia

Adequate local anesthesia is absolutely necessary for a successful catheterization. It cannot be overemphasized that poor anesthetization leads to poor patient cooperation and makes a long morning in the catheterization laboratory for both patient and operator. Once the inguinal ligament and femoral artery have been identified, the femoral artery is palpated along its course using the three middle fingers of the left hand, with the uppermost finger positioned just below the inguinal ligament. Without moving the left hand, a linear intradermal wheal of 1 or 2% lidocaine is raised slowly following tangential insertion of a 25- or 27-gauge needle along a course overlying both the femoral artery and vein at the desired level of entry.

With the left hand remaining in place, transverse skin punctures are made over the femoral artery and vein, using the tip of a #11 scalpel blade. The smaller needle is replaced by a 22-gauge 1 ½-inch needle, which is used to infiltrate the deeper tissues along the intended trajectory for arterial and venous entry. As this needle is advanced, small additional volumes of lidocaine are infiltrated by *slow* injection. Each incremental infiltration should be preceded by aspiration so that intravascular boluses can be avoided. If the anesthetic track passes through the artery or vein, infiltration should be suspended until the tip of the needle has passed out of the back wall of the vessel and then continued to the full length of the needle or to the point where the needle tip contacts the periosteum. Approximately 10 to 15 ml 1% xylocaine administered in this fashion usually provides adequate local anesthesia. The patient should be warned that he may experience some burning as the anesthetic is injected but that the medication will abolish any subsequent sharp sensations.

Once local anesthesia has been achieved, the small skin nicks can be enlarged and deepened, using the tips of a curved "mosquito" forceps. This procedure decreases the resistance that is encountered during subsequent advancement of the Seldinger needle and catheter and assures that any vascular bleeding will become manifest as oozing through the puncture rather than hidden in the formation of a deep hematoma.

## Femoral Vein Puncture

Femoral venous puncture is usually performed prior to arterial puncture. This provides secure venous access for the administration of fluids or drugs and shortens the arterial catheter time by allowing completion of the right heart catheterization before introduction of the arterial catheter. With the left hand palpating the femoral artery along its course below the inguinal ligament, the Seldinger needle (Fig. 5-2) is introduced through the more medial skin nick. This 18-gauge thin-walled needle consists of a blunt, tapered external cannula through which a sharp solid obturator projects. The needle should be grasped so that the index and middle fingers lie below the lateral flanges of the needle, with the thumb resting on the top of the solid obturator, and should be advanced along the sagittal plane angled approximately 45 degrees cephalad (Fig. 5-3). While this needle can occasionally be advanced up to its hub, the tip of the needle will usually stop more superficially as it encounters the periosteum of the pubic tubercle. The periosteum is well innervated and may be quite tender if the initial lidocaine infiltration failed to reach this level. Accordingly, forceful contact with the periosteum is neither necessary nor desirable. If the patient experiences significant discomfort, some operators will remove the obturator from the Seldinger needle and infiltrate additional lidocaine into the deep tissues through the outer cannula.

At this point, it is hoped that the Seldinger needle has transfixed the femoral vein. The obturator is removed, and a 10-ml syringe is attached to the hub of the cannula. The syringe and cannula are depressed so that the syringe lies closer to the anterior surface of the thigh (Fig. 5-3) and the needle is more parallel (rather than perpendicular) to the vein. Gentle suction is applied to the syringe, and the whole assembly is slowly withdrawn toward the skin surface. In doing so, it is helpful to control the needle with both the left hand (which also rests on the patient's leg for support) and the right hand (which also controls the aspirating syringe). As the tip of the cannula is withdrawn into the venous lumen, free flow of blood into the syringe will be evident. With the left hand stabilizing the needle, the right hand is used to remove the syringe and to advance a 0.035- or 0.038-inch J guide wire into the hub of the needle. In doing so, the wire tip may be straightened by hyperextension of the wire shaft in the right hand or by leaving the tip of the wire within the plastic introducer supplied by the manufacturer. The wire should slide through the needle and 10 to 15 cm into the vessel with no perceptible resistance. Fluoroscopy should then show the tip of the

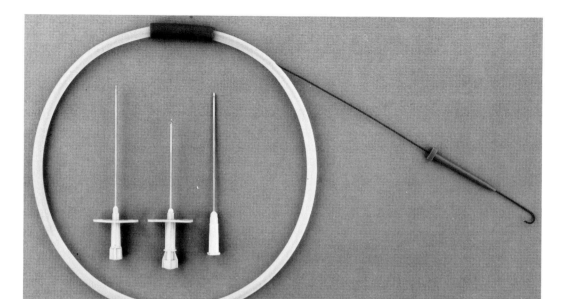

**Fig. 5-2.** Percutaneous needles and guide wire. Left, a Seldinger needle with its sharp solid obturator in place. Center, a Potts-Cournand needle, which differs in the fact that its obturator is hollow and therefore allows the operator to see blood flashback as the artery is punctured. Right, 18-gauge thin-wall needle used for internal jugular vein puncture. The percutaneous needles are surrounded by an 0.038 inch, 145 cm J guide wire.

guide wire just to the left (patient's right) of the spine.

*If difficulty is encountered in advancing the guide wire, it should never be overcome by the application of force.* Fluoroscopy may simply reveal that the tip of the wire has entered a small lumbar branch and that it can be drawn back slightly and redirected or gently prolapsed up the iliac vein. When resistance to advancement is encountered at or just beyond the tip of the needle, however, even greater care is required to avoid vascular injury. This resistance may simply be due to apposition of the tip of the needle to the back wall of the vein, which can be corrected by further depression of the needle hub, with or without slight withdrawal of the needle shaft. If this maneuver fails to allow free advancement of the wire, however, the wire should be removed and the syringe should be reattached to the needle hub to ensure that free flow of venous blood is present before additional wire manipulation is attempted—the wire should not be reintroduced unless free flow is obtained. If the wire still cannot be advanced, the needle cannula should be withdrawn, and the punc-

ture site should be compressed for one to three minutes. The anatomic landmarks should be reconfirmed, and puncture reattempted. In some cases, venous puncture during a Valsalva maneuver may help by distending the femoral vein and making clean puncture more likely.

At this point, the needle is removed, leaving the wire within the vein and secured at the skin entry site by the left hand. The protruding wire is wiped with a moistened gauze pad, and its free end is threaded into the lumen of a sheath and dilator combination adequate to accept the intended right heart catheter. While conventional sheaths and dilators (USCI "888" or equivalent) are frequently used to introduce the venous catheter, our laboratory now uses a sheath equipped with a backbleed valve and sidearm connector (Fig. 5-4, USCI "Hemaquet" or Cordis sheath) to control bleeding around the catheter shaft and to provide a means of administering extra fluid during the right heart catheterization. Whichever device is used, it is important to ensure that one has control of the proximal end of the guide wire, which is held in a fixed position, as the

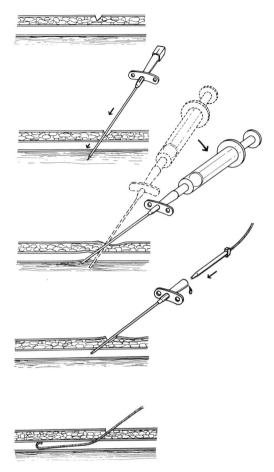

**Fig. 5-3.** Seldinger technique for venous puncture. A skin nick has been created overlying the desired vein, which is punctured through and through by a Seldinger needle with its solid obturator in place. In the center panel, the obturator is removed and the needle cannula is attached to a syringe. Depression of the syringe toward the surface of the skin tents the vessel slightly and facilitates axial alignment of the cannula at the moment that slow withdrawal brings the tip of the cannula back into the vessel lumen. This is recognized by the sudden ability to withdraw venous blood freely into the syringe, which is then removed from the needle cannula to permit advancement of the J guide wire (shown here with a plastic straightener in place). Once the guide wire has been advanced safely into the vessel, the needle cannula can be removed.

dilator is introduced through the skin. The sheath and dilator are rotated as they are advanced progressively through the soft tissues. If excessive resistance is encountered, it may be necessary to remove the dilator from the sheath and to introduce the dilator

alone before attempting to introduce the combination. If inspection shows that initial attempts have created significant burring at the end of the sheath, a new sheath should be obtained.

## Catheterizing Right Heart from Femoral Vein

Once the sheath is in place, the wire and dilator are removed, and the sheath is flushed by withdrawal of blood and administration of heparinized saline solution. In our laboratory we usually connect the sidearm of the venous sheath to a one liter bag of normal saline solution, using a sterile length of intravenous extension tubing. The desired venous catheter is then flushed, attached to the venous manifold, introduced through the sheath, and advanced up the vena cava. We commonly use a 7 Fr Swan-Ganz catheter because of its ease of passage, low risk of injury to the right heart chambers, and its ability to perform thermodilution measurements of cardiac output. Often, however, we use a conventional woven Dacron (Goodale-Lubin or Cournand) catheter when thermodilution outputs are not desired or when greater catheter control is needed.

Deviation of the catheter tip from its paraspinous position during advancement suggests entry into a renal or hepatic vein, which can be corrected by slight withdrawal and rotation of the catheter. Once the catheter is above the diaphragm and within the right atrium, it is rotated counterclockwise to face the lateral wall of the right atrium (Fig. 5-5). Additional counterclockwise rotation and gentle advancement allow passage of the catheter tip into the superior vena cava, which is contiguous with the posterolateral wall of the right atrium. In contrast, anterior orientation of the catheter tip at this point may result in its entrapment in the right atrial appendage and inability to reach the superior vena cava. Once in position, a baseline superior vena caval blood sample is obtained for measurement of oxygen saturation and comparison with the subsequently measured pulmonary arterial blood $O_2$ saturation, to screen for unsuspected left-to-right shunts. The catheter is then flushed with heparinized saline solution and withdrawn to the right atrium for pressure measurement.

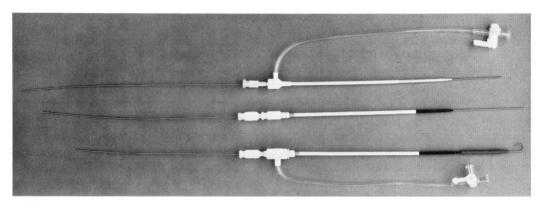

**Fig. 5-4.** Vascular sheaths. Center, conventional sheath and dilator assembly (USCI "888"). Two arterial-venous introducers equipped with backbleed valves and sidearm attachment; top, a Cordis sheath; bottom, a USCI Hemaquet. Each device is inserted over a conventional guide wire as a unit, following which the inner Teflon dilator is removed to permit catheter introduction. The two side-arm sheaths also permit fluid infusion and an additional site for pressure monitoring with the catheter in place.

The principles of advancing a catheter from the femoral vein to the pulmonary artery apply to either the Swan-Ganz or stiffer woven Dacron catheters. With the tip of the catheter positioned at the lower portion of the lateral right atrial border, clockwise rotation will cause the catheter tip to sweep the anterior and anteromedial wall of the right atrium, along which the tricuspid valve is located (Fig. 5-5). As the catheter tip passes over the tricuspid orifice, slight advancement will cause it to enter the right ventricle where pressure is again recorded. If the right atrium is enlarged, greater curvature of the catheter may be necessary: a large J loop may be formed by engaging the tip of the catheter against the lateral right atrial wall or in the ostium of the hepatic vein just below the diaphragm. This larger loop can then be rotated clockwise in the atrium as described above, and usually it will enter the right ventricle.

Simple advancement of the catheter in the right ventricle will cause the tip to move toward the apex of that chamber and will not usually result in catheterization of the pulmonary artery. To achieve this latter end, the catheter must be withdrawn slightly so that its tip lies horizontally and just to the right (patient's left) of the spine. In this position, clockwise rotation will cause the tip of the catheter to point upwards (and slightly posteriorly) in the direction of the right ventricular outflow tract (Fig. 5-5). The catheter should be advanced only when it is in this orientation to minimize the risk of ventricular arrhythmias or injury to the right ventricle. Advancement may be facilitated if performed as the patient takes a deep breath. If these maneuvers fail to achieve access to the pulmonary artery due to enlargement of the right atrial and ventricular chambers, the catheter may be withdrawn to the right atrium and formed into a large "reverse loop," which allows the tip of the catheter to cross the tricuspid valve in an upward orientation more likely to enter the outflow tract (Fig. 5-5, bottom right). When manipulated appropriately, the catheter tip should cross the pulmonic valve and advance to a wedge position without difficulty. Having the patient take a deep breath and cough during advancement will often be of assistance in achieving a wedge position. While catheters advanced from the leg are more likely to seek the left pulmonary artery than catheters advanced from above, either pulmonary artery can be catheterized by appropriate manipulation or careful introduction of a curved J guide wire. Following measurement of the wedge pressure, the catheter is withdrawn to the proximal left or right pulmonary artery, and a second blood saturation is obtained.

Attempts to perform right heart catheterization occasionally result in entry into other structures. If a woven Dacron catheter is advanced in the right atrium with a posteromedial orientation, it may cross a patent foramen ovale and enter the left atrium. This

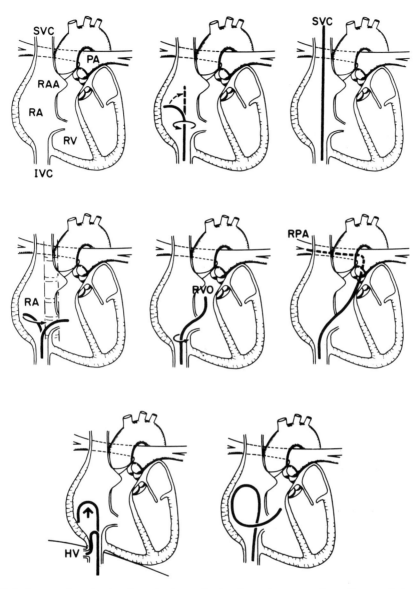

**Fig. 5-5.** Right heart catheterization from the femoral vein, shown in cartoon form. Top panel, the right heart catheter is initially placed in the right atrium (RA) aimed at the lateral atrial wall. Counterclockwise rotation aims the catheter posteriorly and allows advancement into the superior vena cava (SVC). Although not evident in the figure, clockwise catheter rotation into an anterior orientation would lead to advancement into the right atrial appendage (RAA), precluding SVC catheterization. Center row, the catheter is then withdrawn back into the right atrium and aimed laterally. Clockwise rotation causes the catheter tip to sweep anteromedially and cross the tricuspid valve. With the catheter tip in a horizontal orientation just beyond the spine, it is positioned below the right ventricular outflow tract (RVO). Additional clockwise rotation causes the catheter to point straight up, allowing for advancement into the main pulmonary artery and from there into the right pulmonary artery (RPA). Bottom row, two manuevers useful in catheterization of a dilated right heart. A larger loop with a downward directed tip may be required to reach the tricuspid valve and can be formed by catching the catheter tip in the hepatic vein (HV) and advancing the catheter quickly into the right atrium. The reverse loop technique (bottom, right) gives the catheter tip an upward direction, aimed toward the outflow tract.

can be recognized by a change in the atrial waveform, position of the catheter tip across the spine, and the ability to withdraw fully oxygenated blood from the catheter tip. Although more unusual, it is also possible for a woven Dacron catheter to enter the ostium of the coronary sinus, inferiorly and posteriorly to the tricuspid orifice. Again there will be continued presence of an atrial waveform, but saturation sampling will disclose a far lower value (20 to 30%) than was present in the superior vena cava. The most important points about these sidetrips off the beaten path to the right ventricle are that the operator should recognize that the tip of the catheter is *not* in the right ventricle (i.e., one should not attempt to get to the pulmonary artery) and should decide where the catheter is (by pressure monitoring, saturation analysis, or injection of a small amount of contrast agent) before withdrawing the catheter to the right atrium and proceeding with the right heart catheterization.

*Unsuspected anatomic abnormalities* can frequently be detected by an unusual catheter position or course. In Figure 5-6, the appearance of the right heart catheter course in three such congenital abnormalities (persistent left superior vena cava, patent ductus arteriosus and anomalous pulmonary venous return) is depicted. The commonest abnormality, atrial septal defect, is sometimes hard to detect by catheter position alone, since the catheter appearance in the left atrium or ventricle may be indistinguishable (in the anteroposterior view) from its course during usual right heart catheterization. Measurement of pressure and blood oxygen saturation, together with hand injection of radiographic contrast and use of oblique and lateral views, should allow the operator to sort out the anatomy.

In patients with elevated right heart pressures, those undergoing specialized procedures (endomyocardial biopsy, coronary sinus catheterization), or those in whom prolonged post-procedure monitoring with a balloon-flotation catheter is desired, the right internal jugular vein offers an excellent alternative to the femoral vein. The technique for jugular puncture is described in Chapter 32, and the method of advancing the right heart catheter to the pulmonary artery is identical to that described in Chapter 4. On occasion, percutaneous right heart catheterization is performed from the subclavian or median basilic vein, using a similar technique.

## Femoral Artery Puncture

The femoral artery is punctured by inserting the Seldinger needle through the more lateral skin nick. Again, the needle is inserted at approximately 45 degrees, along the axis of the femoral artery as palpated by the three middle fingers of the left hand. The experienced operator may feel the transmitted pulsations as the tip of the needle contacts the wall of the femoral artery, but it is customary to advance the needle completely through the artery until the periosteum is encountered. If a single wall puncture is desired, the operator may prefer a Potts-Cournand needle (Fig. 5-2), in which the obturator has a small lumen that transmits a flashback of arterial blood as the vessel is entered. Once the obturator is removed, the hub of the needle may be depressed slightly toward the anterior surface of the thigh. Because arterial pressure makes it unnecessary to attach a syringe to the cannula, both hands can be used to stabilize the needle as it is slowly withdrawn. As the needle comes back into the lumen of the femoral artery, vigorous pulsatile flow of arterial blood should be evident. A 145 cm 0.035- or 0.038-inch J guide wire should then be advanced carefully into the needle and should move freely up the aorta, which is located to the right (patient's left side) of the spine on fluoroscopy, to the level of the diaphragm.

If wire motion ceases to be free after several centimeters, or if the patient complains of any discomfort during wire advancement, subintimal position of the wire is a distinct possibility. The wire should be withdrawn slightly under fluoroscopic control, and the needle should be removed as the left hand is used to stabilize the wire and control arterial bleeding. After the wire is wiped with a moist gauze pad, a small (5 Fr) dilator can be cautiously introduced up to the point where the wire had advanced without difficulty. The wire is then withdrawn from the dilator, which is aspirated to ensure free flow of blood and flushed carefully. A small bolus of

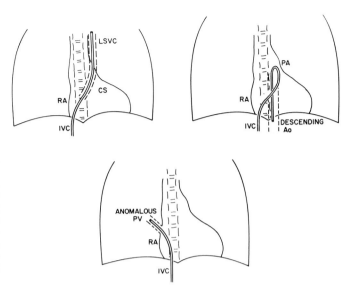

**Fig. 5-6.** Unsuspected anatomic abnormalities frequently can be detected by an unusual catheter course or position. Upper left panel, the course of a catheter passed from the femoral vein to inferior vena cava (IVC), right atrium (RA), coronary sinus (CS), and up into an anomalous left superior vena cava (LSVC). Upper right panel, the catheter crossing from pulmonary artery (PA) to descending aorta (Ao) by way of a patent ductus arteriosus. Bottom panel, the catheter entering an anomalous pulmonary vein draining into the right atrium.

contrast medium is then injected gently under fluoroscopic monitoring. This injection will usually disclose the anatomic reason for difficult wire advancement—either iliac tortuosity, stenosis, or dissection. If dissection is present, retrograde left heart catheterization should be relocated to the other femoral artery or to the brachial artery, and the patient should be observed for signs of progressive dissection or arterial compromise, both of which are fortunately rare with retrograde guide wire dissections. If tortuosity or stenosis is the problem, more specialized guide wires (a large 15 mm J, floppy or movable core J) may be carefully reintroduced through the dilator in an attempt to reach the descending aorta.

If difficulty in advancing the guide wire is encountered at or just beyond the tip of the needle and if this difficulty is not corrected by slight depression or slight withdrawal of the needle, the guide wire should be withdrawn to ensure that vigorous arterial flow is present before any further wire manipulation. If flow is not brisk or if the wire can still not be advanced, the needle should be removed and the groin should be compressed for 5 minutes. The operator should verify the correctness of the anatomic landmarks and attempt repuncture of the femoral artery. If the second attempt is unsuccessful in allowing wire advancement, a third attempt on the same vessel is unwise.

## Catheterizing Left Heart from Femoral Artery

Once the guide wire has been advanced to the level of the diaphragm, the needle cannula is removed. The left hand is used to stabilize the wire and control arterial bleeding while the wire is wiped with a moistened gauze pad to remove any adherent blood. If the catheter is to be introduced directly into the artery, it is customary to dilate the soft tissues by brief introduction of a Teflon arterial dilator one Fr size smaller than the intended catheter, before introducing the left heart catheter itself. In our laboratory, however, essentially all left heart catheterizations from the femoral approach are performed using a 7 Fr or 8 Fr sheath equipped with a backbleed valve and sidearm tubing, as described above. This is introduced over the guide wire (the proximal end of which is held in a straightened, fixed position) with a rotational motion, following which the guide wire and dilator are removed, and the sheath is aspirated, flushed, and connected by its sidearm to a manifold for monitoring arterial pressure. This sheath should be reflushed immediately after each catheter is introduced or withdrawn and every 5 minutes during the catheterization to avoid encroachment of blood and potential thrombus formation within the sheath. The desired left heart catheter is then flushed and loaded with a 145 cm J guide wire. The tip of the catheter is straightened manually to facilitate introduction into the backbleed valve. The soft end of the guide wire is then advanced carefully through the catheter, out the end of the sheath, and to the level of the diaphragm before the catheter itself is advanced. If the back end of the wire is extended straight down the patient's leg and held fixed to the leg, this will ensure that the wire remains in constant position within the aorta during catheter advancement. The guide wire is then removed, the catheter is connected to the arterial manifold and double flushed (withdrawal and discarding of 10 ml of blood, followed by vigorous injection of heparinized saline solution). Full intravenous heparinization (5000 U) is established immediately after the left heart catheter is inserted.

If any difficulties were encountered during the initial advancement of the guide wire, a slightly different technique is advisable. The operator may choose to leave the tip of the guide wire at the diaphragm while the dilator is removed from the sheath and the left heart catheter is introduced, thereby avoiding the need to renegotiate complex iliofemoral anatomy with the guide wire. Similarly, all subsequent left heart catheters may be introduced with the aid of a short exchange-length (180 cm) guide wire, the tip of which can be left in place at the diaphragm as one catheter is removed and the second is reintroduced, rather than withdrawing one catheter and inserting the second catheter and wire through the sheath de novo. Of course, if the left heart catheterization is being performed without the aid of a sheath, it is mandatory to leave the tip of the wire in the abdominal aorta during the removal of the first catheter and the introduction of a second catheter in order to retain access to the vessel.

The initial left heart catheter in most cases is a pigtail catheter with multiple side holes. This catheter can be advanced to the ascending aorta without difficulty, at which point the ascending aortic and femoral arterial (sheath side arm) pressures are recorded simultaneously (Fig. 5-7).[3,4] The systolic peak in the femoral waveform may be slightly delayed and accentuated compared to the ascending aortic pressure trace, but the diastolic and mean pressures should be

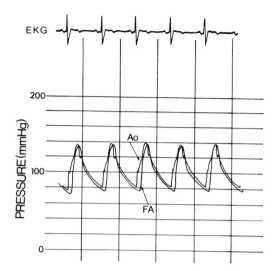

**Fig. 5-7.** Central aortic pressure (Ao) measured through a 7.3 French pigtail catheter (Cook) and femoral artery (FA) pressure measured from the sidearm of an 8 French arterial sheath (Cordis). Only minimal damping of the femoral artery pressure is seen, blunting its systolic overshoot, which frequently exceeds central aortic systolic pressure (see Chapter 9). With larger (7.5 French and 8 French) catheters, more damping may occur in the sidearm pressure. Catheter and sidearm are connected to small volume-displacement transducers without intervening tubing.

virtually identical. The pigtail catheter is then advanced across the aortic valve and into the left ventricle. If the aortic valve is normal and the pigtail is oriented correctly, it will usually cross the valve directly. In many cases, however, it may be necessary to advance the pigtail down into one of the sinuses of Valsalva so as to form a secondary loop (Fig. 5-8). As the catheter is withdrawn slowly, this loop will span the diameter of the aorta and often fall across the valve (Fig. 5-8).

If significant aortic stenosis is present, the pigtail must be advanced across the valve with the aid of a straight 0.038-inch guide wire. Approximately 6 cm of the guide wire is advanced beyond the end of the pigtail catheter, and the catheter is withdrawn slightly until the tip of the guide wire is leading (Fig. 5-8). The position of the tip of the guide wire within the aortic root can then be controlled by rotation of the pigtail catheter and adjustment of the amount of wire that protrudes; less wire protruding directs the wire tip toward the left coronary ostium,

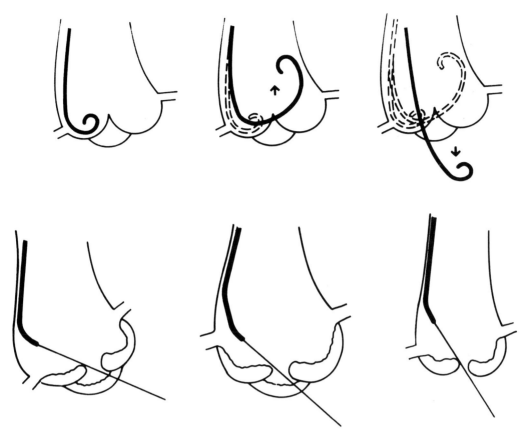

**Fig. 5-8.** Crossing the aortic valve with a pigtail catheter. Although a correctly oriented pigtail catheter will frequently cross a normal aortic valve directly, it may also come to rest in the right or noncoronary sinus of Valsalva (top row, left). Further advancement of the catheter enlarges the loop to span the aortic root (top row, center) and positions the catheter so that slow withdrawal causes it to sweep across the aortic orifice, and fall into the left ventricle (top row, right). To cross a stenotic aortic valve, the pigtail catheter must be led by a segment of straight guide wire (bottom row, left). Increasing the length of protruding guide wire straightens the catheter curve and causes the wire to point more towards the right coronary ostium; reducing the length of protruding wire restores the catheter curve and causes the wire to point more toward the left coronary. Once the correct length of wire and the correct rotational orientation of the pigtail catheter have been found, repeated advancement and withdrawal of both the catheter and guide wire as a unit will allow the wire to cross the valve. In a dilated aortic root, an angled pigtail provides more favorable wire positions (bottom row, center). In a small aortic root (bottom row, right), a Judkins right coronary catheter may be preferable.

whereas more wire protruding directs the wire toward the right coronary ostium. With the wire tip positioned so that it is directed towards the aortic orifice, the tip of the wire will usually quiver in the systolic jet. Wire and catheter are then advanced as a unit until the wire crosses into the left ventricle. If the wire buckles in the sinus of Valsalva instead of crossing the valve, the system is withdrawn slightly and readvanced with or without subtle change in the length of protruding wire or the orientation of the pigtail catheter. Alternatively, some operators pre-fer to leave the pigtail catheter fixed and move the guide wire independently in attempts to cross stenotic aortic valves. During attempts to cross the aortic valve, the wire should be withdrawn and cleaned and the catheter should be double-flushed vigorously every three minutes despite systemic heparinization. If promising wire positions are not obtained, the process should be repeated using a different catheter: an angled pigtail (USCI, Cordis) if the aortic root is dilated or a Judkins right coronary catheter if the aortic root is unusually narrow. Once the tip of the guide wire is across the aortic valve, additional wire should be inserted before the catheter itself is advanced; otherwise the catheter may be diverted into the sinus of Valsalva and flip the wire out of the left ventricle. Once the catheter is in the left ventricle, the wire is immediately withdrawn and the catheter is aspirated vigorously, flushed and hooked up for pressure monitoring, so that a gradient can be measured even if the catheter is rapidly ejected from the left ventricle or must be withdrawn because of arrhythmias.

At the termination of the left heart catheterization, heparin is usually reversed by the administration of protamine (1 ml = 10 mg of protamine for every 1000 U of heparin). The operator should be watchful for potential adverse reactions to protamine, characterized by hypotension and vascular collapse, as discussed in Chapter 3. Protamine reactions are especially common in insulin-dependent diabetics. After administration of protamine, the arterial catheter and sheath are removed, and firm manual pressure is applied using three fingers of the left hand positioned sequentially up the femoral artery beginning at the skin puncture. With the fingers in this position, there should be no ongoing bleeding into the soft tissues or through the skin puncture, and it should be possible first to obliterate the pedal pulses and then release just enough pressure to allow them to barely return. This pressure is gradually reduced over the next 10 to 15 minutes, at the end of which time pressure is removed completely. The venous sheath is usually removed 5 minutes after compression of the arterial puncture has begun, with gentle pressure applied over the venous puncture using the right hand. In some laboratories, the groin is compressed by a mechanical device (Compressar, Instromedix, Beaverton, OR), but continuous presence of a trained person is required to ensure that the device is providing adequate control and is not compromising distal perfusion. The puncture site and surrounding area are then inspected for hematoma formation and active oozing, and the quality of the distal pulse is assessed before application of a bandage.

It is our policy to keep the patient at bed rest with the leg straight overnight following percutaneous femoral catheterization, with a sandbag in place over the puncture site for the first 6 hours after catheter removal. In patients at higher risk for rebleeding (those with hypertension, obesity, or aortic regurgitation) application of a pressure bandage in addition to the sandbag may be of value. Although the patient should be instructed not to move the leg for at least 6 hours following the catheterization procedure, this does not mean that the patient must lie flat during this time. Elevation of the head and chest to 30 to 45 degrees by the electrical or manual bed control, without muscular effort by the patient, will greatly increase the patient's comfort and will not increase the risk of local bleeding. The only reason to insist that the patient lie completely flat is if there is significant orthostatic hypotension. Prior to ambulation, the puncture site should again be inspected for recurrent bleeding, hematoma formation, development of a bruit suggestive of pseudoaneurysm or A-V fistula formation, or loss of distal pulses.

## Relative Contraindications to Femoral Artery Catheterization

Although hemostasis is usually obtained easily after removal of a percutaneous arterial catheter, it should be emphasized that patients with a wide pulse pressure (e.g., severe aortic incompetence or systemic hypertension) have more problems with bleeding than do patients with normal blood pressures. In addition, gross obesity and poor femoral artery pulsations may make percutaneous femoral artery catheterization extremely difficult.

Complications of percutaneous retrograde arterial catheterization are fortunately infrequent and usually not life-threatening. These complications, as well as their causes and prevention, are discussed in Chapter 3.

## BRACHIAL OR AXILLARY ARTERY CATHETERIZATION

The techniques described above for percutaneous insertion of a femoral catheter also can be used successfully from the brachial or axillary artery, with or without an introducing sheath. The smaller caliber of these vessels, potential difficulties in controlling the catheterization site at the end of the procedure, and the tendency for hematomas at these locations to be poorly tolerated make them less desirable than femoral catheterization unless the latter is unsuccessful or contraindicated (by severe distal aortic or peripheral vascular disease or prior aortofemoral grafts) and an operator experienced in the conventional direct brachial approach (described in Chapter 4) is not available.

## TRANSSEPTAL LEFT HEART CATHETERIZATION

With the development of retrograde left heart catheterization, the use of transseptal puncture for access to the left atrium and left ventricle[7,8] has become an infrequent procedure in most adult cardiac catheterization laboratories. In these laboratories, transseptal puncture is reserved for situations in which direct left atrial pressure recording is desired (pulmonary venous disease), in which it is important to distinguish true idiopathic hypertrophic subaortic stenosis (IHSS) from catheter entrapment, in which retrograde left heart catheterization has failed (e.g., due to severe peripheral arterial disease or aortic stenosis), or is dangerous due to the presence of a certain type of mechanical prosthetic valve (e.g., Bjork-Shiley or St. Jude valves). The infrequency with which the procedure is needed has made it difficult for most laboratories to maintain operator expertise and to train cardiovascular fellows in transseptal puncture and has given the procedure an aura of danger and intrigue. Although insufficient attention to technique during transseptal catheterization *may* lead to serious and potentially lethal complications, the mortality in experienced centers is less than 0.1%. Complications can be minimized by avoiding patients with distorted anatomy due to congenital heart disease, right atrial enlargement, significant chest or spine deformity, or inability to lie flat, as well as patients with ongoing anticoagulant therapy, left atrial thrombus, or suspected left atrial myxoma. While there is no substitute for extensive hands-on experience, we offer this review of the basic approach to transseptal catheterization as a guide for the inexperienced or infrequent operator.

The goal of transseptal catheterization is to cross from the right atrium to the left atrium through the fossa ovalis. In approximately 10% of patients, this maneuver is performed inadvertently during right heart catheterization with a woven Dacron catheter, due to the presence of a probe-patent foramen ovale, but in the remainder mechanical puncture of this area with a needle and catheter combination is required to enter the left atrium. While puncture of the fossa ovale itself is quite safe, the danger of the transseptal approach lies in the possibility that the needle and catheter will puncture an adjacent structure. To minimize this risk, the operator must have a detailed familiarity with the regional anatomy of the atrial septum (Fig. 5-9). As viewed from the feet with the patient lying supine, the plane of the atrial septum runs from 1 o'clock to 7 o'clock. The area of the fossa ovalis is bounded anteriorly and superiorly by the aortic root and posteriorly by the posterior free wall of the right atrium. The fossa ovalis is located superiorly and posteriorly to the ostium of the coronary sinus and well posterior of the tricuspid annulus and right atrial appendage. The fossa ovalis is approximately 2 cm in diameter and is bounded superiorly by a ridge—the limbus.

Transseptal catheterization is performed *only* from the right femoral vein. We utilize a 70 cm curved Brockenbrough needle, (USCI, Billerica, MA) which tapers from 18 gauge to 21 gauge at the tip (Fig. 5-10). It is usually inserted into the matching catheter with an obturator (Bing stylet) protruding slightly beyond the tip of the needle to avoid abrasion or puncture of the catheter wall during needle advancement. The hub of this needle is equipped with a metal flange, which indicates the orientation of the needle curve and serves as a reference point for monitoring the position of the needle tip relative to the tip of the catheter. Prior to insertion, a sterile ruler is used to measure the distance between the needle flange and the catheter hub under two conditions: first, with the tip of the Bing stylet at the tip of the catheter, and second, with the tip of the Brockenbrough needle itself at the tip of the catheter (Fig. 5-11). Measurements should be recorded for later reference as the needle is being introduced.

Venous entry is performed as described above, except that no sheath is used. An 0.038 inch 145 cm J guide wire is advanced

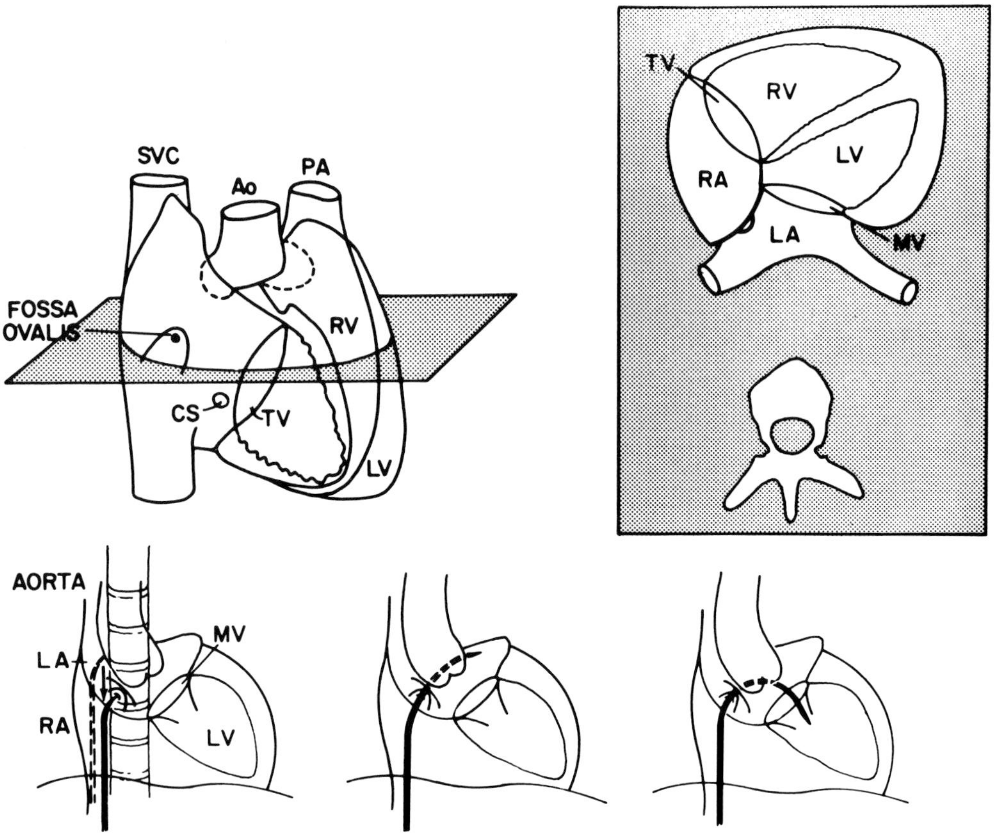

**Fig. 5-9.** Regional anatomy for transseptal puncture. Upper left, the position of the fossa ovalis is shown relative to the superior vena cava (SVC), aortic root (Ao), coronary sinus (CS), and tricuspid valve (TV). Upper right, a cross section through the fossa (looking up from below) demonstrating the posteromedial direction of the interatrial septum (bold line) and the proximity of the lateral free wall of the right atrium. Bottom row, the appearance of the transseptal catheter as it is withdrawn from the SVC in a posteromedial orientation. As the catheter tip slides over the aortic root (bottom left, dotted position) it appears to move rightward on to the spine. Slight further withdrawal leads to more rightward movement into the fossa (solid position). Puncture of the fossa with advancement of the catheter into the left atrium (bottom row, center), and advancement into the left ventricle with the aid of a curved tip occluder (right). (Redrawn from Ross J Jr: Considerations regarding the technique for transseptal left heart catheterization. Circulation 34:391, 1966.)

well up into the vena cava, the introducing needle is then removed, and the protruding guide wire is wiped with a moistened gauze pad. The previously calibrated transseptal catheter (usually a 70 cm, 8 Fr Teflon Brockenbrough catheter (USCI, Billerica, MA) with six side holes and an end hole, and a 2.5 or 3.0 cm distal curve) is then inserted into the superior vena cava over the guide wire. A 2.5 cm catheter curve is adequate for normal sized left atria, with larger curves needed when there is left atrial enlargement. Once the catheter is in position, the guide wire is

removed, and the catheter is vigorously double flushed.

The next step is the advancement of the Brockenbrough needle and Bing stylet up to, but not beyond, the tip of the catheter. As the needle and its stylet are advanced into the catheter with stylet in place, the patient may experience a slight sensation of pressure. The progress of the needle tip should be monitored fluoroscopically, looking for any sign of perforation of the catheter by the needle. It is essential to allow the needle to rotate freely during advancement so that it

**Fig. 5-10.** The Brockenbrough system. Left to right, catheter, needle, and Bing stylet. (Redrawn from Ross J Jr: Considerations regarding the technique for transseptal left heart catheterization. Circulation 34:391, 1966.)

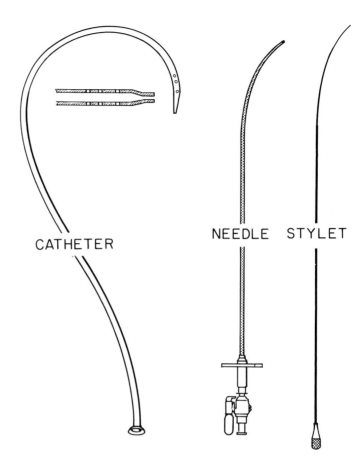

CATHETER     NEEDLE    STYLET

may follow the curves of the catheter; the hub of the needle should never be grasped and rotated at this point. As the tip of the Bing stylet approaches the tip of the catheter (indicated by measurement of the distance between the needle flange and the catheter hub), the stylet should be removed and the needle itself should be advanced to the tip of the catheter, again monitored by fluoroscopy and ruler measurement. The needle is connected to a pressure manifold, using a three-way stopcock and a short length of pressure tubing, and double flushed. The superior vena caval pressure should then be recorded through the needle, and the needle should be rotated so that the direction indicator points anteriorly with the patient lying absolutely flat.

Under continuous fluoroscopic and pressure monitoring, the needle and catheter are held in constant relationship and are withdrawn slowly using both hands and firmly controlling the direction indicator with the right hand. During this withdrawal from the

superior vena cava, the direction indicator is rotated clockwise so that the arrow is oriented posteromedially (4 o'clock when looking from below) as the tip of the catheter enters the right atrium. The needle and catheter are maintained in their posteromedial orientation and continue to be withdrawn slowly; this withdrawal will cause the catheter tip to slip over the bulge of the ascending aorta and move rightward (toward the patient's left) so as to overlie the vertebrae in the anterior projection (Fig. 5-9). Slight further withdrawal is associated with a second rightward movement as the catheter tip "snaps" into the fossa ovalis. If the foramen is patent, the catheter may cross into the left atrium spontaneously at this point, as indicated by a change in atrial pressure waveform and the ability to withdraw oxygenated blood from the needle. Otherwise, the catheter is advanced slightly so as to engage the limbus at the superior portion of the foramen ovale. If the operator is satisfied with the position of the catheter, the Brockenbrough

**Fig. 5-11.** The Brockenbrough system with the needle and stylet inserted into the catheter. Ruler measurement of the distance from the catheter hub to the needle flange is shown with the tip of the stylet at the tip of the catheter (position 1) and with the stylet withdrawn and the needle tip extended to the tip of the catheter (position 2). (Redrawn from Ross J Jr: Considerations regarding the technique for transseptal left heart catheterization. Circulation 34:391, 1966.)

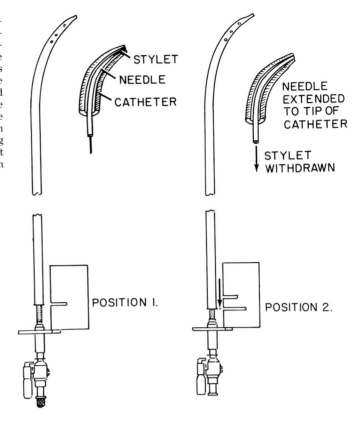

needle is then advanced abruptly so that its point emerges from the tip of the catheter and perforates the atrial septum. Successful entry into the left atrium is confirmed by both the recording of a left atrial pressure waveform *and* the withdrawal of oxygenated blood. Once the operator is confident that the needle tip is across the interatrial septum, the needle and catheter are then advanced as a unit a *short* distance into the left atrium, taking care to control their motion so that the protruding needle does not injure left atrial structures. Once the catheter is across the atrial septum, the needle is withdrawn and the catheter is double-flushed vigorously and connected to a manifold for pressure recording.

The main risk during transseptal catheterization is inadvertent puncture of the aortic root, coronary sinus, or posterior free wall of the right atrium, rather than the fossa ovalis. As long as the patient is not anticoagulated and perforation is limited to the 21-gauge tip of the Brockenbrough needle (i.e., perforation is recognized and the catheter itself is

not advanced), this is usually benign. However, if the 8F catheter is advanced into the pericardium or aortic root, potentially fatal complications may occur, underscoring the need for the operator to monitor closely the location of the transseptal apparatus by fluoroscopic, pressure, and oxygen saturation at each stage of the procedure. If the initial attempt at transseptal puncture is unsuccessful, the operator may wish to repeat the catheter positioning procedure by removing the transseptal needle from the catheter, withdrawing the catheter slightly, and reinserting the 0.038 inch guide wire into the superior vena cava. *One should never attempt to reposition the catheter-needle combination in the superior vena cava in any other way, since perforation of the right atrium or atrial appendage is a distinct possibility during such maneuvers.*

Once the catheter is safely in the left atrium, additional manipulation may be required to enter the left ventricle. If the tip of the catheter has entered an inferior pulmonary vein (as evident by its projection outside the posterior heart border in the right anterior oblique projection), the left ventricle can be approached by torquing the catheter 180 degrees in a counterclockwise direction so that its tip moves anteriorly as it is withdrawn slightly. As the catheter tip moves anteriorly and downward, further advancement will usually allow it to cross the mitral valve and enter the left ventricle. If not, it may be necessary to insert a curved tip occluder into the catheter through an o-ring sidearm adaptor, so as to tighten the tip curve and facilitate advancement into the ventricle. By converting the Brockenbrough catheter from an end- and side-hole to a side-hole only device, the tip occluder also minimizes the chance for left ventricular staining and perforation during contrast ventriculography. However, contrast angiography at 8 to 10 ml/sec for 40 to 50 ml total injection (as with the Sones catheter) can usually be accomplished safely without a tip occluder, if desired. Following the completion of hemodynamic and angiographic evaluation, the Brockenbrough catheter is withdrawn in the usual manner during continuous pressure recording. If the procedure has not been complicated by perforation of the right or left atrium or puncture of the aorta, heparin can be administered. Alternatively, the transseptal puncture can be delayed until the end of a procedure, when heparin given prior to angiography has been reversed by the administration of protamine.

While the above procedure is the most widely applied approach to transseptal catheterization, we should point out that other systems are used for transseptal catheterization with considerable success. These include the Paulin catheter, whose out-of-plane tip curvature facilitates entry of the left ventricle, and the Mullins transseptal sheath,[9] an elongated version of the conventional femoral sheath and dilator which can be advanced into the left atrium over a Brockenbrough needle and thereby permit the insertion of any conventional catheter (electrode catheter, micromanometer catheter, or pigtail catheter) into the left atrium.

# REFERENCES

1. Seldinger SI: Catheter replacement of the needle in percutaneous arteriography, a new technique. Acta Radiol 39:368, 1953.
2. Judkins MP, Kidd HJ, Frische LH, Dotter CT: Lumen-following safety J-guide for catheterization of tortuous vessels. Radiology 88:1127, 1967.
3. Barry WH et al: Left heart catheterization and angiography via the percutaneous femoral approach using an arterial sheath. Cathet Cardiovasc Diagn 5:401, 1979.
4. Hillis LD: Percutaneous left heart catheterization and coronary arteriography using a femoral artery sheath. Cathet Cardiovasc Diagn 5:393, 1979.
5. Pepine CJ, et al: Percutaneous brachial catheterization using a modified sheath and new catheter system. Cathet Cardiovasc Diagn 10:637, 1984.
6. Velix B, et al: Selective coronary arteriography by percutaneous transaxillary approach. Cathet Cardiovasc Diagn 10:403, 1984.
7. Ross J Jr.: Considerations regarding the technique for transseptal left heart catheterization. Circulation 34:391, 1966.
8. Brockenbrough EC, Braunwald E: A new technique for left ventricular angiocardiography and transseptal left heart catheterization. Am J Cardiol 6:1062, 1960.
9. Laskey WK, et al: Transseptal left heart catheterization: use of a sheath technique. Cathet Cardiovasc Diagn 8:535, 1982.

## chapter six

# Cardiac Catheterization in Infants and Children

JOHN F. KEANE *and* MICHAEL D. FREED

C ARDIAC catheterization in infants and children allows a unique opportunity to study physiologic effects of simple and complex lesions in a population with almost invariably normal coronary arteries. While morbidity from catheterization is low and mortality is almost negligible in older infants and children, the risks are higher among infants under the age of 4 months, many of whom are seriously ill at the time of the study.[1,2] With continued emphasis on complete repair rather than palliation, even in early infancy, our surgical colleagues justifiably expect meticulous, detailed anatomic and physiologic diagnoses even in the youngest patients. In addition, in recent years there has been an increase in therapeutic procedures undertaken in the catheterization laboratory such as dilatation of stenotic valves and vessels. There has also been an increase in the use of such diagnostic techniques as electrophysiologic studies and endomyocardial biopsies. Catheterization and these newer techniques, particularly in the young infant, should be undertaken only by physicians and technicians experienced in this field, using the best equipment available.

## GENERAL CATHETERIZATION PROTOCOL

In the past five years 3137 cardiac catheterizations have been performed at The Children's Hospital in Boston. The following approach, also taking into account a major commitment to the training of pediatric cardiologists, represents our current views based largely on this experience.

***Physiologic Measurement.*** The initial phase of the catheterization study is generally a physiologic one. A right heart catheterization is performed first, with measurement of superior vena caval oxygen saturation, followed by recordings of pressures and saturations in the midlateral right atrium, the inflow and outflow portions of the right ventricle, the main, right, and left pulmonary arteries, and finally in the pulmonary capillary wedge position. The catheter is withdrawn to the right atrium, the atrial septum is explored, and if traversed, pressure and saturation are recorded in the left atrium and ventricle and at least one pulmonary vein. The catheter is then withdrawn while recording pressure to the right atrium and is repositioned in a distal pulmonary artery. An arterial catheter is then placed, and pressure, saturation, and blood gases are recorded in the ascending aorta. The patient is then heparinized at a dose of 100 IU/kg, to a maximum dose of 5000 IU. If the left ventricle has not already been entered through the mitral valve, the retrograde catheter is passed across the aortic valve; pressure and oxygen saturation are recorded, together with a simultaneous pulmonary capillary wedge pressure. The catheter is then withdrawn to the descending aorta while pressure is being recorded. Oxygen consumption is then measured, during which a right-sided withdrawal series of pressures and saturations are obtained for computation of pulmonary and systemic flow and resistance determinations.

***Angiographic Measurement.*** The next phase of the study consists of angiography, with particular emphasis on appropriate patient positioning for optimum visualization of defects and for ventricular volume determinations. Finally, special procedures, such as valve or vessel dilatations, endomyocardial biopsies, or coil occlusions of appropriate vessels, are undertaken. In some children, however (e.g., those with WPW and SVT), extensive electrophysiologic data collections are the prime objectives of the study, and these are undertaken initially, followed by physiologic and angiographic studies where necessary at the conclusion. The renal shadows are then filmed, the catheters are removed, and because most of the procedures are performed percutaneously by way of the femoral vessels, bleeding is controlled within approximately 15 minutes by applying gentle local pressure, without the use of protamine sulfate.

Since babies under four months of age, particularly newborn infants, are frequently very ill at the time of the study, the catheterization procedure differs somewhat from that for older children, and both approaches are now presented in greater detail.

# Infants

Babies with heart disease often have either cyanosis or congestive heart failure, and many are acidotic. Prior to arrival in the catheterization laboratory, in addition to obtaining a routine electrocardiogram and chest roentgenogram, we have found that echocardiography has been of increasing value in arriving at a more accurate tentative diagnosis, thus enabling a more rational approach to the study. Chloral hydrate (50 mg/kg p.o.) may be given approximately one-half hour before the catheterization in infants over one month of age.

On arrival in the laboratory, the baby is positioned on a heating blanket; an electronic rectal thermometer is inserted for continual temperature monitoring. Whenever possible in those less than one week of age, an umbilical artery catheter is placed (at least size 5 French for later angiographic

purposes) for monitoring of systemic blood gases throughout the study, enabling acidosis to be recognized and treated. Blood has been obtained prior to the study for grouping and cross matching (for later transfusion purposes during the study). The umbilical catheter is connected to a pressure transducer for continuous pressure monitoring. If the infant is less than 72 hours old, the umbilical stump is prepared and draped in addition to both inguinal areas, and a brief attempt initially is made to catheterize the umbilical vein. A small hand injection of dilute contrast material is valuable to determine patency and location of the ductus venosus. Although the advent of balloon catheters has improved access to the various chambers by way of the umbilical vein, maneuverability within the heart is generally easier from a femoral venous approach. Most of the catheterizations in our laboratory are performed from the inguinal area and are accomplished percutaneously. Because they are probably safer, we tend to use balloon catheters in neonates.

Our general approach is to record rapidly right heart oxygen saturations and pressures from the superior vena cava to the pulmonary capillary wedge position. It is important to mention that if tetralogy of Fallot or critical pulmonary stenosis is suspected, especially if there is evidence of ventricular right-to-left shunting, *no attempt whatever is made to enter the pulmonary artery*, as this may precipitate a severe cyanotic-acidotic episode. In addition, it is usually possible to cross the atrial septum, to record saturations and pressures in the left atrium and ventricle and pulmonary vein. If an umbilical arterial line is not already in place, the femoral artery is cannulated, percutaneously in the majority of cases, usually with a short Teflon cannula, and the patient is given heparin.[3] Oxygen consumption is then measured by the continuous flow-through method,[4] during which a right-sided pull-back series of oxygen saturations and pressures is recorded, together with systemic arterial saturation, pressure, and blood gas determinations.

Angiography is then performed. For transvenous angiography we generally use a Berman balloon catheter (Critikon, Inc., Tampa, FL), which is advantageous both because of its maneuverability and avoidance of myocardial staining. However, if lesions associated with a large degree of left-to-right shunting are encountered, the practically obtainable injection flow rates with this catheter are often insufficient to allow precise visualization of the defects. In these situations (for example, a large ventricular septal defect or truncus arteriosus), we have found a specially designed 3.2 or 4 French pigtail catheter (UMI, Ballston Spa, NY) introduced in retrograde fashion to be particularly useful.[5,6]

Nearly all cineangiography is performed using biplane equipment, with particular attention being given to proper positioning of the baby for optimal visualization of the suspected defect.[7,8] The contrast material used generally is Renovist (ER Squibb and Sons, Princeton, NJ), but if end-diastolic pressures are particularly elevated, then a contrast material with very little sodium, such as Cardiograffin, is substituted. Although the toxic dose of contrast in these infants is uncertain, every effort is made not to exceed a total dose of contrast medium of 4 ml/kg for the whole study. We replace precisely all blood losses, generally at the conclusion of the procedure, carefully observing the right atrial pressure during the transfusion.

## Children

All patients over the age of one year receive Demerol Compound as premedication one hour prior to the study, the dosage being based on weight and degree of cyanosis. Demerol compound contains chlorpromazine (Thorazine 6.25 mgm/ml), promethazine (Phenergan 6.25 mgm/ml) and meperidine (Demerol 25 mgm/ml) and is widely used for premedication in pediatric cardiac catheterization. The dose is based on degree of cyanosis, weight, and age, although we do not use this medication in infants under one year of age. In a noncyanotic patient, we give 1 ml/20 lb (1 ml/9 kg) to a maximum of 2 ml. We use 1 ml/30 lb (1 ml/13.6 kg) if mild or moderate cyanosis is present, and 1 ml/40 lb (1 ml/18 kg) if cyanosis is severe. Those under one year receive chloral hydrate by mouth, (50 mg/kg). The main exceptions to the foregoing schedule are cyanotic patients suspected of having tetralogy of Fallot; these children are premedicated with morphine sulfate, 0.1 mg/kg, especially if cyanotic spells have occurred in the past.

In our laboratory, virtually all catheterizations in children are performed percutaneously from the inguinal area. One advantage of this method is that the same vessel can be used for later studies. In general, an end-hole Lehman catheter (USCI, Billerica, MA), size 5 to 8 French, depending on the size of the child, is used for the right heart study. Oxygen saturation and pressure are recorded in sequential fashion from superior vena cava to the pulmonary wedge position. Most patients also undergo a retrograde arterial study, generally utilizing thin-walled Teflon pigtail catheters (UMI, Ballston Spa, NY), and all receive heparin, as this has been shown to be effective in preventing arterial thrombosis in children.[3] An advantage of the thin-walled Teflon pigtail catheters is that they permit high flow rates of angiographic contrast material, which is particularly important when one is dealing with large shunts or single large mixing chambers. For example, a 6-French 80-cm thin-walled Teflon pigtail catheter can easily deliver contrast at 35 ml/sec, whereas the same catheter in size 8 French can deliver contrast agent at 45 to 50 ml/sec. Oxygen consumption is measured in all, using either expired air collected in a Douglas bag or a continuous flow-through method. Alternatively, cardiac output may be measured by thermodilution.[9] Again, during cardiac output determination, standard left and right heart pull-back series of oxygen saturations and pressures are recorded.

## ANGIOGRAPHY

Biplane cineangiography is then carried out, utilizing appropriate angulation both for the optimal visualization of defects and for ventricular volume calculations. Again, a total volume of contrast material of 4 ml/kg should not be exceeded.

***Equipment.*** Biplane equipment is important for the safe study of infants and enables the operator to keep the volume of contrast medium to be used as low as possible while obtaining the maximum amount of information. While either cineangiography or full size cutfilm may be used satisfactorily in the majority of patients, we have found that in our laboratory where we have both capabilities available we now use cineangiography exclusively.

***Patient Position.*** For many years angiographic diagnoses had been made using primarily frontal and lateral projections. In recent years, however, compound projections using cranial and oblique angulations have been found to be more effective in the precise definition of underlying defects.[7,8] We find the combination of 70 degrees left anterior oblique and 25 degrees cranial angulation to be particularly useful in membranous and muscular ventricular septal defects, subvalvular aortic stenosis, and subpulmonary stenosis in d-transposition and that 40 degrees cranial angulation alone clearly outline the pulmonary arteries in tetralogy of Fallot (Figs. 6-1, 6-2). The four-chambered or heptoclavicular view using 45 degrees left anterior oblique and some 40 degrees cranial angulation is particularly useful in those with a complete atrioventricular canal, tricuspid atresia, or truncus arteriosus.

## Balloon Occlusion Angiography

In the past few years, balloon occlusion angiography has been introduced for improving anatomic details. This technique is especially useful in lesions involving the aortic arch, such as coarctation (Fig. 6-3) or interruption, and also in babies with tetralogy of Fallot and pulmonary atresia. In the group with arch anomalies, the catheter (5 French Berman balloon angiographic catheter) is passed antegrade through a patent ductus arteriosus, and the balloon is inflated in the midthoracic aorta for about 5 sec during which the angiogram is recorded. In those with tetralogy of Fallot and pulmonary atresia, this same catheter is passed antegrade across the aortic valve, again to the midthoracic aorta just below the origin of the collaterals, and the angiogram is recorded using the same technique.

## Coronary Arteriography

In the past, angiography in the ascending aorta was the technique used to delineate the proximal coronary arteries in the infant and child. With the recent availability of smaller catheters, such as 4.5F right and left modified Judkins catheters (Cook Inc., Bloomington, IN), selective coronary arteriograms are being performed increasingly, particularly in infants and children with Kawasaki's disease. The techniques used are the same as for adults except the amounts of contrast medium injected are of course much smaller. The catheters are usually introduced via a sheath in the femoral artery.

## SPECIAL PROCEDURES

A variety of special procedures are utilized in pediatric cardiac catheterization, some of which are presented briefly.

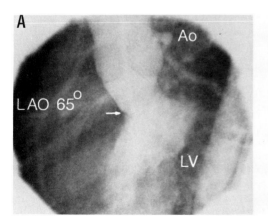 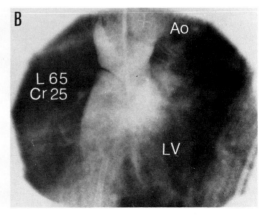

**Fig. 6-1.** Membranous subvalvular aortic stenosis. (A) barely visible (arrow) using standard left oblique (LAO) projection, but (B) clearly identified using compound left oblique and cranial (Cr) view. (From Fellows KE, Keane JF, Freed MD: Angled views in cineangiocardiography of congenital heart disease. Circulation 56:485, 1977.)

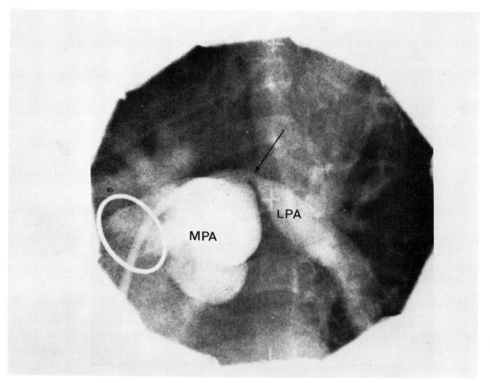

**Fig. 6-2.** Tetralogy of Fallot. Severe stenosis (arrow) at origin of left (LPA) from main pulmonary artery (MPA). Lesion not visualized on previous standard A-P and lateral projections, but now clearly identified using compound left oblique and cranial view.

## Balloon Atrial Septostomy

Since the introduction of balloon atrial septostomy by Rashkind,[11] it has remained an integral part of the catheterization of babies less than one month of age with transposition of the great arteries, particularly in those with an intact ventricular septum. This procedure, by virtue of the atrial septal tear it creates, produces increased mixing between the systemic and pulmonary circuits, which in transposition are arranged in parallel rather than in series. In the majority of cases, the result is an immediate and dramatic increase in systemic oxygen saturation, with alleviation of acidosis. The septostomy catheter may be introduced into the umbilical vein or femoral vein percutaneously (often requiring a 7 French sheath because of the balloon size), or by way of a cutdown approach using either the proximal bulb of the saphenous vein or the superficial femoral vein. The balloon septostomy catheters that we use are either the 5 French Miller balloon atrial septostomy catheter (American Edwards Laboratories, Santa Ana, CA) or the 6 French Rashkind catheter (USCI, Billerica, MA) with the recessed balloon.

The balloon is placed in the left atrium, biplane fluoroscopy being essential to document the leftward high and posterior position, particularly when a single lumen catheter is used. The Miller balloon is inflated quickly with up to 4 ml of dilute Renovist (the Rashkind with 1.5 to 2 ml), then withdrawn sharply to the right atrial/inferior vena cava junction, then quickly advanced to the mid-right atrium, and deflated as rapidly as possible. This maneuver usually is repeated at least twice. Oxygen saturation and pressure measurements are then made, and a satisfactory response is manifested by a rise in arterial oxygen saturation, increased bidirectional shunting at the atrial level, and elimination of any pressure gradient between the atria.

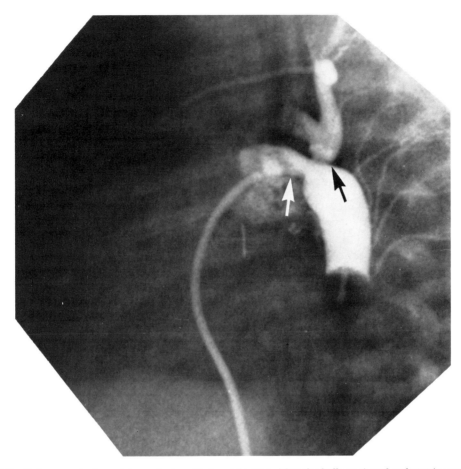

**Fig. 6-3.** Balloon occlusion aortography in a 20-day-old infant. After the balloon-tipped catheter is passed via right heart chambers through a patent ductus arteriosus into the aorta, the balloon is inflated with $CO_2$, occluding the descending aorta and preventing antegrade flow, with retrograde outlining of coarction (dark arrow) and patent ductus arteriosus (light arrow).

## Blade Atrial Septostomy

An alternative method of septostomy, for use in the catheterization laboratory in infants beyond one month of age, has been introduced by Park et al. in recent years.[12] This procedure, not entirely without risk, utilizes a 5 French catheter that has an extrudable blade at its tip and is introduced via a #7 French sheath from the femoral vein. The blade is opened carefully in the left atrium using biplane fluoroscopy and then withdrawn slowly across the septum into the right atrium. Following this, a standard balloon septostomy is done to further enlarge the hole.

## Balloon Dilatation

There has been increasing interest in recent years in the use of balloon dilatation of a number of obstructive lesions seen in pediatric cardiology. To date, discrete valvular pulmonary stenosis in these patients, 1 year of age or more, appears to be the lesion most successfully relieved by this therapeutic modality[13,14] (Fig. 6-4). Other lesions in children that have been so treated with some success include postoperative aortic coarctation and pulmonary artery stenosis, congenital (Fig. 6-5) or acquired.[15-17]

With regard to methodology, in valvular pulmonary stenosis, for example, the diame-

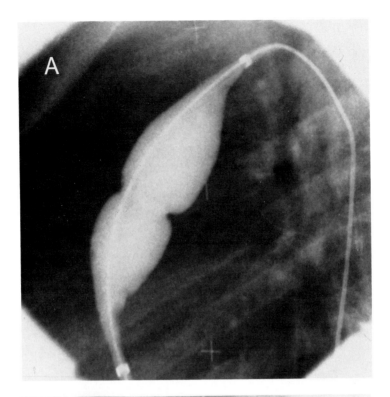

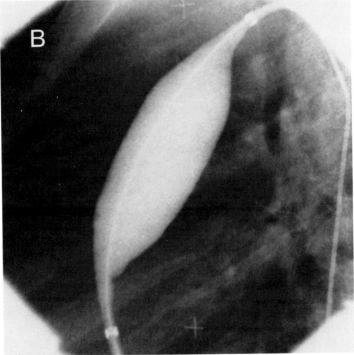

**Fig. 6-4.** Dilatation of stenotic pulmonary valve using balloon dilatation catheter filled with dilute contrast material. (A) Waist produced by stenotic valve as balloon is inflated. (B) Obliteration of waist when balloon is fully inflated.

PRE

POST

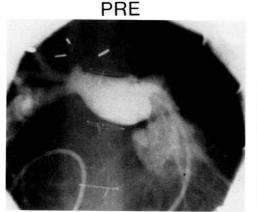
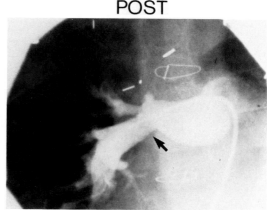

**Fig. 6-5.** Dilatation of stenotic right pulmonary artery. (PRE) Stenosis at origin of lower lobe pulmonary artery. (POST) Enlargement of vessel diameter following dilatation (arrow).

ter of the valve annulus is first measured from the lateral cineangiogram. A balloon dilatation catheter (Meditech, Watertown, MA) is then chosen which is 20 to 30% greater than the diameter measured. In a 4-year-old child this would often be a 20-mm balloon which is wrapped around the end of a 9F catheter. This catheter is introduced percutaneously into the femoral vein over a long 0.038 inch J-guide wire, the end of which has already been positioned distally in the left lower lobe. The balloon is then placed so that it straddles the valve annulus and then is rapidly inflated with dilute contrast material until the "waist" produced by the stenotic valve disappears (Fig. 6-4). Approximately 5 seconds of inflation time are all that are required. That this technique is effective is supported by our own observation of the reduction of a 76 mmHg gradient at age 5 years to 6 mmHg a year later. In our oldest patient, age 42 years, a valve gradient of 102 mmHg was reduced to 30 mmHg at the conclusion of the study using a 20-mm balloon.

While pulmonary valve dilatations appear to be safe to date, it should be noted that occasional deaths have been reported with other lesions.

## Coil Occlusion

Patients with tetralogy of Fallot and pulmonary atresia often have collateral vessels arising from the thoracic aorta which con-

tribute to pulmonary blood flow. At the time of intracardiac repair, these are often inaccessible to the surgeon, since the operation is performed via an anterior approach. Many of these, especially those that are long, relatively straight, and with distal stenoses, may be occluded by the introduction of one or more coils.[18]

In terms of methodology, a selective cineangiogram is first recorded in a collateral vessel. An end-hole catheter is then introduced from the femoral artery into the proximal segment of this collateral vessel. An occluding spring embolus (Cook Inc., Bloomington, IN) whose diameter when extruded is slightly larger than that of the vessel is then advanced using a soft 0.038 inch guide wire through the catheter and out into the vessel. After a 10-minute waiting period for clot formation around the coil, a selective cineangiogram is repeated. If occlusion is incomplete, additional coils may be placed (Fig. 6-6).

## Prostaglandin E

Prostaglandin E relaxes newborn ductal muscle and is currently being used extensively in newborns.[19,20] We and others have found it most useful as a temporary preoperative measure in maintaining patency of the ductus arteriosus, particularly in newborn infants with pulmonary atresia who depend on an open ductus arteriosus for maintenance of pulmonary blood flow. Infusion of

## PRE

## POST

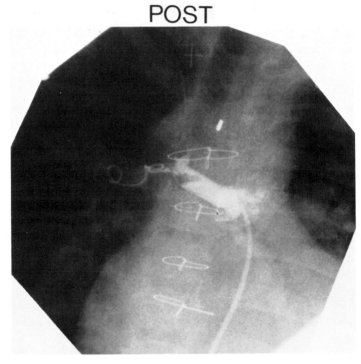

**Fig. 6-6.** Coil occlusion in pulmonary atresia with tetralogy of Fallot. The catheter is advanced up the descending aorta to the left of the spine, and its tip is placed in a large collateral vessel that gives off sizeable arteries to the right upper, middle, and lower pulmonary lobes. The native pulmonary arteries are not seen. The anatomy is shown before (PRE) and after (POST) occlusion of the collateral vessel by a wire coil.

prostaglandin $E_1$ (0.1 $\mu$g/kg/min) in the arterial or venous system generally results in a dramatic rise in systemic arterial oxygen saturation, with alleviation of acidosis resulting in a much more stable cardiac status preoperatively. In critically ill newborn infants with severe coarctation or interruption of the aortic arch, infusion results in dilatation of the constricted ductus and restores systemic cardiac output, again resulting in a much more stable preoperative cardiac status.[20]

## Pulmonary Vein Wedge Injections

Pulmonary vein wedge injection has usually been used in patients with pulmonary atresia to outline pulmonary arteries not otherwise visualized by thoracic aortography or by selective injections in collateral vessels. With an end-hole catheter in a pulmonary vein, either with the balloon inflated or wedged, contrast material (0.3 ml/kg), followed by an equal amount of flush solution, is injected by hand. One must be careful to avoid extravasation into the lung parenchyma by too forceful an injection. The parenchymal pulmonary artery is usually well outlined by this method (Fig. 6-7). More importantly, especially if blood flow is very diminished, it is sometimes possible to backfill the mediastinal ipsilateral pulmonary artery and on occasion the main and contralateral pulmonary arteries if they are in continuity.

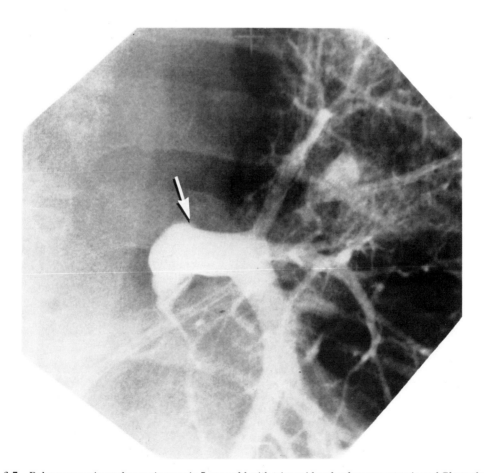

**Fig. 6-7.** Pulmonary vein wedge angiogram in 5-year-old with tricuspid and pulmonary atresia and Glenn shunt. Retrograde filling of large proximal left pulmonary artery (arrow) and hypoplastic main pulmonary artery following injection in left upper lobe pulmonary vein.

## Transatrial Septal Puncture (Transseptal Left Heart Catheterization)

The availability of biplane fluoroscopy has significantly reduced the complications associated with this procedure and the introduction of the Mullins transseptal sheath (USCI, Billerica, MA) has been helpful.[21] This sheath allows the introduction of a variety of catheters into the left atrium, including the Park blade, septostomy, and a variety of angiographic catheters. In addition, we have found that initially outlining the left atrial margins on the fluoroscopy screen (following a pulmonary artery biplane cineangiogram) has been helpful. We also prefer to attach the needle lumen to a syringe containing contrast material rather than to pressure as the latter frequently becomes damped when the precise needle tip position is uncertain. We use the Brockenbrough technique and have used this procedure for all ages of children, including infancy, for a variety of lesions, mainly aortic stenosis. The use of a deflector wire (Cook Inc., Bloomington, IN) has been useful when difficulty has been encountered in crossing the mitral valve.

## Electrophysiologic Studies

The number of electrophysiologic studies both pre- and postoperatively is increasing. The methodology is similar to that described in Chapter 22, the only major difference being the use of smaller electrode catheters (5F) in infants and children.

## Endomyocardial Biopsies

Endomyocardial biopsies of left and right ventricles are also increasing. Methodology is described in Chapter 31, the only differences being all our studies are performed from the femoral approach, preformed 6F right and left heart long sheaths are used, and the bioptome utilized is 5F in size (Cordis Corp. Miami, FL).

## REFERENCES

1. Braunwald E, Swan HJC: Cooperative study on Cardiac Catheterization. American Heart Association Monograph No. 20. Circulation 37 (Suppl. 3):1, 1968.
2. Stanger P, et al: Complications of cardiac catheterization of neonates, infants and children. Circulation 50:595, 1974.
3. Freed MD, Keane JF, Rosenthal A: The use of heparinization to prevent arterial thrombosis after percutaneous cardiac catheterization in children. Circulation 50:569, 1974.
4. Lees MH, Bristow JD, Way C, Brown M: Cardiac output by Fick Principle in infants and young children. Am J Dis Child 114:144, 1967.
5. Keane JF, Freed MD, Fellows KE, Fyler DC: Pediatric cardiac angiography using a 4 French catheter. Cathet Cardiovasc Diagn 3:313, 1977.
6. Keane JF, Fellows KE, Lang P, Fyler DC: Pediatric arterial catheterization using a 3.2 French Catheter. Cathet Cardiovasc Diagn 8:201, 1982.
7. Elliott LP, et al: Axial cineangiography in congenital heart disease: Section II. Specific lesions. Circulation 56:1084, 1977.
8. Fellows KE, Keane JF, Freed MD: Angled views in cineangiocardiography of congenital heart disease. Circulation 56:485, 1977.
9. Freed MD, Keane JF: Cardiac output by thermodilution in infants and children. J Pediatr 92:39, 1978.
10. Denham B, Ward OC, McCann P, Blake N: Aortography in infantile coarctation: A simple and effective technique. Arch Dis Child 54:717, 1979.
11. Rashkind WJ, Miller WW: Creation of an atrial septal defect without thoracotomy. A palliative approach to complete transposition of the great arteries. JAMA 196:991, 1966.
12. Park SC, et al: Blade atrial septostomy: Collaborative study. Circulation 66:258, 1982.
13. Labibidi Z, Wu J-R: Percutaneous balloon pulmonary valvuloplasty. Am J Cardiol 52:560, 1983.
14. Kan JS, et al: Percutaneous transluminal balloon valvuloplasty for pulmonary valve stenosis. Circulation 69:554, 1984.
15. Kan JS, et al: Treatment of restenosis of coarctation by percutaneous transluminal angioplasty. Circulation 68:1087, 1983.
16. Lock JE, et al: Balloon dilatation angioplasty of aortic coarctations in infants and children. Circulation 68:109, 1983.
17. Lock JE, Castaneda-Zuniga WR, Fuhrman BP,

Bass JL: Balloon dilatation angioplasty of hypoplastic and stenotic pulmonary arteries. Circulation 67:962, 1983.

18. Fuhrman BP, et al: Coil embolization of congenital thoracic vascular anomalies in infants and children. Circulation 70:285, 1984.

19. Lang P, et al: The use of protaglandin E, in an infant with interruption of the aortic arch. J Pediatr 91:807, 1977.

20. Freed MD, et al: Prostaglandin E1 in infants with ductus arteriosus-dependent congenital heart disease. Circulation 64:899, 1981.

21. Mullins CE: Transseptal left heart catheterization: Experience with a new technique in pediatric and adult patients. Pediatr Cardiol 4:239, 1983.

*chapter seven*

# Balloon-Tipped Flow-Directed Catheters

PETER GANZ, H.J.C. SWAN, *and* WILLIAM GANZ

DIAGNOSTIC catheterization of the right side of the heart with semirigid cardiac catheters requires fluoroscopic guidance and substantial skill. Abnormal positions of the heart chambers and of the great vessels associated with cardiac dilatation or with congenital malformation present difficulties even to experienced laboratory cardiologists. These problems have been largely overcome by the introduction of balloon-tipped flow-directed catheters,[1-3] which allow for rapid and relatively safe catheterization of the pulmonary artery without fluoroscopy. It was through the application of these catheters in the intensive care unit that the many pitfalls in the clinical assessment of hemodynamic disturbances became apparent. It was learned in patients with acute myocardial infarction that the value of central venous pressure (or jugular venous pressure) is limited by the fact that it reflects the functional state of the right ventricle, which frequently does not parallel that of the left ventricle.[4] Although S3 gallop sounds may be useful in the clinical recognition of chronic ventricular failure, their presence or absence has limited predictive value in estimating left ventricular filling pressure in myocardial infarction.[5,6] Similarly, serious discrepancies have been noted between radiologic evidence of heart failure and the level

of pulmonary wedge pressure when rapid hemodynamic changes take place.[7,8] These observations have been extended to critically ill medical[9] and surgical[10] patients without acute myocardial infarction. Balloon-tipped catheters have made an important contribution in extending the applicability of hemodynamic monitoring to the bedside. Information derived from right heart catheterization is often pivotal in the evaluation of hemodynamic disorders, in directing treatment, and in monitoring the results of therapy in critically ill patients.

## BASIC FEATURES AND CONSTRUCTION

An inflated balloon at the tip of the catheter is carried by the circulation and guides the catheter from the right atrium into the pulmonary artery or to other sections of the vascular bed in patients with congenital cardiac malformations. The inflated balloon protrudes beyond the tip of the catheter and protects the tip from impinging on the myocardium, thereby preventing it from damaging the endocardium and producing arrhythmias or heart block.

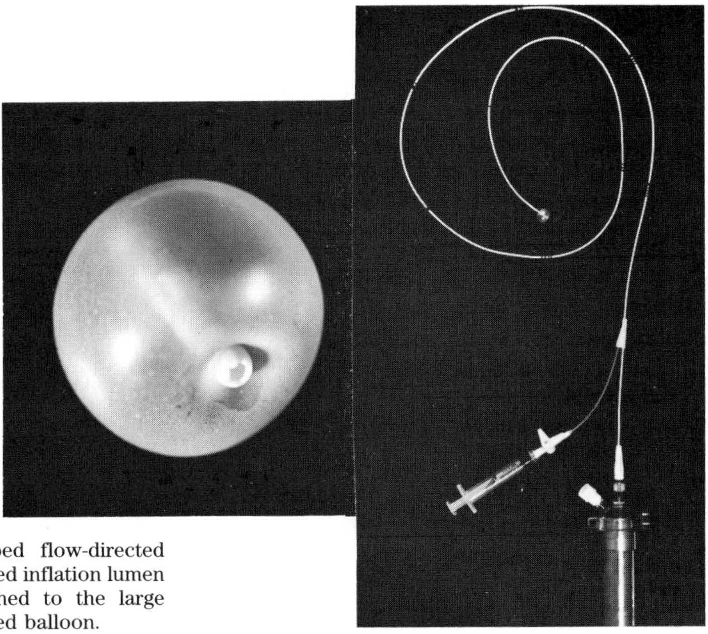

**Fig. 7-1.** Standard balloon-tipped flow-directed catheter with inflated balloon, closed inflation lumen and a pressure transducer attached to the large lumen. Close-up view of the inflated balloon.

The most widely used catheter* is constructed from polyvinylchloride and has a soft pliable shaft which softens further at body temperature (Fig. 7-1). A balloon is fastened 1 to 2 mm from the tip. The standard catheter is 110 cm long and is color-coded according to size from 5, 6, to 7 French in external diameter. As the deflated balloon extends slightly outside the shaft, the venous sheath used to introduce the catheter may have to be 0.5 French larger than the stated catheter size.

Most catheters have a preformed J curvature at the distal end to facilitate passage from the superior vena cava through the right ventricle. A catheter with an "S" tip has also been designed for femoral vein insertion. Catheters intended for long-term use are available with heparin coating to reduce thromboembolic complications. Triple-lumen catheters are available with distal and proximal ports (the third lumen being for balloon inflation), which allow simultaneous measurement of right atrial and pulmonary artery or pulmonary capillary wedge pressures. The proximal port terminates either 20

or 30 cm proximal to the catheter tip, facilitating location in the right atrium under varying conditions of cardiac size and anatomy. Additional lumens may carry thermistor wires for thermodilution studies, pacing electrodes, or venous infusion ports. The catheters are all radiopaque and can be visualized easily by fluoroscopy or plain-film chest roentgenography.

## TECHNIQUE OF FLOW-DIRECTED CATHETERIZATION

Before insertion, the integrity of the balloon must be tested by inflating under sterile liquid (e.g., saline solution) to the volume specified by the manufacturer, while observing for gas leakage. The antecubital, femoral, internal jugular, and subclavian veins may be used as insertion sites, the latter two being utilized particularly outside the catheterization laboratory. After entry into the selected vein, the catheter is advanced until the tip is in or near the right atrium. This usually occurs after advancement of 15 cm from the jugular or subclavian vein, 40 cm from the right and 50 cm from the left antecubital area, and about 30 cm when a femoral vein is

*Swan-Ganz™ Flow-Directed Catheter, Edwards Laboratories, Santa Ana, CA.

used. An increase in respiratory fluctuation of the intravascular pressure monitored from the catheter confirms intrathoracic location of the catheter tip. At this time the balloon is inflated to its specified volume (this volume is printed on the catheter by most manufacturers).

Air may be used for balloon inflation, but carbon dioxide should be used when there is any possibility that the catheter may enter the arterial circulation. Injection of carbon dioxide into the arterial circulation in the event of balloon rupture is free of the hazard of serious consequences, since the solubility of $CO_2$ in blood is about 20 times that of air at normal body temperature. The balloon may have to be refilled every few minutes, because carbon dioxide slowly diffuses through the wall of the latex balloon.

The catheter-tip pressure and surface electrocardiogram are monitored as the catheter proceeds through the right ventricle and pulmonary artery into a "wedge" position (Fig. 7-2). That the catheter is truly in the wedge position can be recognized by several methods: (1) ascertaining fluoroscopically that the catheter is located peripherally and that it stops "bobbing" with each cardiac cycle, (2) demonstrating clearcut A and V waves in the wedge tracing (in sinus rhythm), (3) doc-

umenting a fall in pressure from mean pulmonary artery to mean wedge, and (4) demonstrating a wedge oxygen saturation equal to or greater than that in a systemic artery (e.g., ≥95%). If the wedge pressure is obtained from a large pulmonary artery, it may be necessary to discard 5 to 15 ml of "pulmonary artery" blood before fully oxygenated capillary blood is sampled. This "dead space" blood is sitting in the pulmonary artery between the catheter tip and the capillary network and must be withdrawn before oxygenated blood from the pulmonary capillary can reach the catheter.

As the catheter softens with time, the contractions of the right ventricle may diminish the transcardiac catheter loop and advance the catheter tip into a smaller branch of the pulmonary artery. In such cases inflation of the balloon to full capacity will cause overdistension with potential damage to the pulmonary arterial wall and/or high pulmonary wedge pressure reading (due to compression of the catheter lumen). To avoid potential damage to the vessel wall and recording of inaccurate pressures, it is *imperative* that inflation of the balloon for obtaining wedge pressure be performed *gradually* under continuous monitoring of the pulmonary artery pressure and that the inflation of the balloon

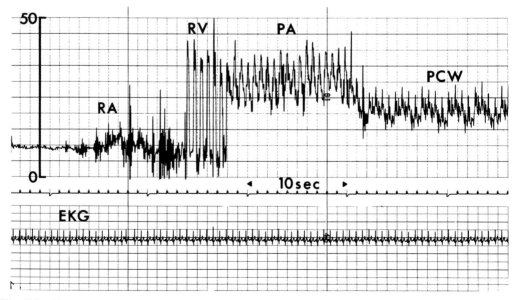

**Fig. 7-2.**  Pressures recorded during insertion of a balloon-tipped flow-directed catheter. *RA* = right atrial pressure, *RV* = right ventricular pressure, *PA* = pulmonary arterial pressure, *PCW* = pulmonary capillary wedge pressure. The scale at the left calibrates pressure from 0 to 50 mm Hg.

be stopped when the change from pulmonary artery to pulmonary wedge pressure configuration is noted.

Passage of the balloon flotation catheter is more difficult in patients with right-sided chamber enlargement, especially in face of low forward cardiac output. Deep inspiration, use of the Valsalva maneuver, and stiffening of the catheter by slow perfusion with 5 to 10 ml of sterile cold saline solution may facilitate passage into the pulmonary artery.

Because femoral vein insertion of the standard J-curved balloon catheter points the tip of the catheter at the right ventricular apex, gentle rotation under fluoroscopy to orient the tip into the right ventricular outflow tract is often required. If difficulty in positioning the catheter persists, a suitable guide wire may be inserted to stiffen the catheter. It is preferable not to advance the guide wire beyond the catheter tip to avoid damaging intracardiac structures. On occasion it is useful to form a 270 degree loop against the lateral wall of the right atrium, directing the tip of the catheter at the outflow tract, but take care not to form a knot.

## MEASUREMENT OF PULMONARY ARTERY AND WEDGE PRESSURES

In a series of comparisons in the catheterization laboratory and in the animal laboratory, there was no noteworthy difference between the pressures recorded from the tip of the flow-guided catheter after occlusion of a pulmonary artery branch by the inflated balloon and those obtained by conventional end-hole catheters advanced more peripherally to the true wedge position.*

The pulmonary capillary wedge pressure provides information about two important determinants of cardiopulmonary function. First, the level of this pressure is a factor in the genesis of pulmonary congestion by regulating the transfer of fluid from the pulmonary capillaries into the interstitial space and the alveoli. Second, the pulmonary wedge pressure accurately reflects the mean left atrial pressure and therefore in the absence of mitral valvular disease closely approximates left ventricular mean diastolic pressure, an index of left ventricular preload. In the absence of pulmonary vascular disease, generally the pulmonary arterial end diastolic pressure is only 1 to 3 mm Hg higher than the mean pulmonary wedge pressure; it can therefore be used as an indicator of the mean wedge pressure in patients without preexisting pulmonary hypertension and avoid the need for frequent balloon inflations. Differences between the pulmonary arterial end diastolic and pulmonary wedge pressure in excess of 5 mmHg suggest a primary pulmonary vascular disorder. In patients with severe mitral regurgitation and large V waves in the left atrial and pulmonary capillary pressures, the mean wedge pressure may exceed pulmonary artery end diastolic pressure as the V wave is averaged into the mean wedge but not into the pulmonary artery diastolic pressure.

As soon as the wedge pressure reading has been taken, the balloon should be deflated. Leaving the balloon inflated, particularly if the catheter tip is in a distal pulmonary artery, may lead to erosion of the pulmonary artery wall with consequent pulmonary artery perforation and massive hemoptysis.

## MEASUREMENT OF CARDIAC OUTPUT BY THERMODILUTION

Flow-directed thermodilution catheters allow for rapid determinations of cardiac output by injection of a known amount of cold sterile solution into the right atrium and measurement of the resultant change in blood temperature in the pulmonary artery by the catheter thermistor.[11,12] (See Chap. 8.)

## TEMPORARY VENTRICULAR PACING AND RECORDING OF INTRACAVITARY ELECTROGRAMS

Rapid insertion of bipolar balloon flow-directed catheters into the right ventricle usually can be accomplished without fluoroscopy, by electrocardiographic monitoring. A unipolar electrocardiogram can be recorded

---

*True wedge pressure is usually confirmed by visual inspection of the pressure waveform and its diastolic tracking of a simultaneously measured LV pressure. If there is any doubt about the waveform, or if an unexpected diastolic gradient is present, the wedge position may be confirmed by blood sampling as described on p. 53. If this is not possible, attempt to wedge the catheter with the balloon deflated, or use another right-heart catheter.

from the distal tip electrode by connection to the V lead of the electrocardiogram (ECG). Entry of the catheter into the right atrium is indicated by a large atrial complex. At this point the balloon is inflated and again immediately deflated once the catheter has entered the right ventricle to avoid flotation into the right ventricular outflow tract. Entry of the catheter into the right ventricle is indicated by a marked decrease in the amplitude of the atrial complex and an increase in the ventricular complex. The catheter is advanced several centimeters into the right ventricle until elevation of the ST segment is observed, indicating endocardial contact. The catheter is available in two modifications: The first is designed for insertion from the femoral vein and is J curved distally for stable placement in the apex. The second type, designed for insertion via the superior vena cava, is straight.

Flow-directed catheters are now available which, in addition to recording pulmonary artery, pulmonary capillary wedge and right atrial pressures, and thermodilution cardiac outputs, allow for atrial and ventricular pacing and intracavitary ECG monitoring.* The unique feature of these catheters entails a bend at the site of the ventricular electrodes which forces the electrodes against the endocardium for firm contact. When used in patients during cardiac surgery, atrial pacing could be achieved in 85% of patients, ventricular pacing in 94%, and sequential pacing in 82%.[13] The stated percentages would be expected to decrease with time in awake mobile patients. These catheters have been used for A-V sequential pacing for hemodynamic reasons and for diagnosis or overdrive of arrhythmias. The intracardiac electrograms are relatively insensitive to muscle tremor and to electrical interference and can be used for initiation of intraaortic balloon pumping even in face of electrocautery.[14] The availability of stable atrial and ventricular complexes should facilitate computer analysis of cardiac rhythm disturbances.

## APPLICATIONS IN ADULTS

***Cardiac Catheterization Laboratories.*** Catheterization of the right ventricle and pulmonary artery with the balloon-

*Swan-Ganz Pacing TD Catheter, Edwards Laboratories, Santa Ana, CA.

tipped flow-guided catheter can frequently be accomplished in the same or less time than that required for semirigid nonfloating catheters and at a lower risk of serious arrhythmias. For these reasons catheterization with flow-directed balloon-tipped catheters has become routine in most cardiac catheterization laboratories.[1,15]

Recent special applications of the balloon flow-directed catheter have included its use in transseptal left-heart catheterization.[16] Unlike with conventional methods, it is easier to advance the catheter into the left ventricle and also into the aorta. Balloon-tipped catheters have also been utilized to occlude temporarily a patent ductus arteriosus or an atrial septal defect, thus defining the size and hemodynamic importance of the shunt.[17] The use of the catheter for balloon-wedge angiography is discussed below.

***Coronary Care Units.*** The hemodynamic status of patients with acute myocardial infarction cannot always be defined correctly by the clinical evaluation.[18] Catheterization of the pulmonary artery permits rapid and accurate assessment of cardiac performance. With the data derived from measurements of cardiac output and pulmonary capillary wedge pressure, one can define hemodynamic subsets that determine both the prognosis and the appropriate therapeutic intervention.[18]

Recording pressures from the right atrium, right ventricle, pulmonary artery, and pulmonary wedge position and sampling blood from the right heart chambers for oxygen saturation also may allow the physician to recognize specific complications of acute myocardial infarction such as acute mitral regurgitation, ventricular septal rupture,[19] right ventricular infarction,[20,21] or cardiac tamponade.[22]

***Intensive Care Units.*** Right-heart catheterization is used widely to monitor patients without acute myocardial infarction who are critically ill from a variety of other causes.[9,10] In a group of medical patients who were not responding to initial therapy, the information provided by right heart catheterization prompted a change in therapy in almost 50% of the cases.[9] Hemodynamic monitoring is essential to detect left ventricular failure in patients with adult respiratory distress syndrome.[23]

Interpretation of hemodynamic data may pose difficulty in patients on mechanical ventilators. Intrathoracic pressure becomes positive during the forced inspiration driven by the ventilator and falsely elevates intravascular pressure. These effects are usually obvious on examination of the phasic wedge tracing, which shows obliteration of the normal A and V wave pattern when the capillary bed is compressed by increased intraalveolar pressure. It has been recommended that pressures be recorded at end-expiration for patients on ventilators.[24,25] The additional effects of positive end-expiratory pressure (PEEP) on the measured intraluminal pressures will depend in part upon pulmonary compliance; patients with decreased compliance may not have intrapleural (and thus intrapericardial) pressures elevated significantly by PEEP. In such cases, an elevated measured-LV filling pressure would likely be accurate. When large disparity is found in intravascular filling pressures on vs off PEEP, it is better to rely more on the thermodilution cardiac output determinations and their response to volume-loading or volume-reduction (e.g., diuresis) as a means of assessing adequacy of left heart filling pressure. On occasion when the accurate determination of filling pressure is deemed important, esophageal balloons or intrapleural catheters have been employed for measurement of intrapleural (and thus intrapericardial) pressure,[26] which is then subtracted from the measured pulmonary wedge pressure.

### *Surgery and Anesthesiology.*

The clinical outcome of patients undergoing major operations, such as abdominal aortic surgery, is greatly influenced by the risk of cardiac decompensation. Major stresses on the cardiovascular system involve sudden shifts in intravascular volume, third space accumulation of fluid, and alterations in systemic vascular resistance due to anesthesia. A safer perioperative course with the ability to modulate hemodynamic variables has been reported with the use of pulmonary artery catheterization.[27]

## APPLICATIONS IN CHILDREN AND INFANTS

Smaller (4 French size) and more flexible catheters, including catheters for measurement of cardiac output by thermodilution, are available for pediatric use. The following indications for the use of the flow-directed balloon-tipped catheters have been reported.

1. Catheterization of children in whom the exact anatomy and position of the cardiac chambers prior to catheterization are not known.
2. Manipulation of the catheter into chambers and vessels not readily accessible by conventional means; for instance, entry into the pulmonary artery from the left or common ventricle and entry into the aorta from the right or common ventricle in transposition of the great vessels.[28-31]
3. Passage of the catheter through an interatrial communication into the left atrium, left ventricle, and aorta in order to avoid retrograde arterial catheterization and an arteriotomy.
4. Obtaining pulmonary arterial wedge pressure in patients in whom wedge pressure might otherwise be difficult to obtain. Obtaining pulmonary arterial wedge arteriograms and visualization of the relevant pulmonary vein by rapid washout of contrast medium following sudden deflation of the balloon, particularly in partial or total anomalous venous connection.
5. In patients liable to have arrhythmias initiated by catheter manipulation, as in patients with Wolff-Parkinson-White syndrome or Ebstein's anomaly.

Caution must be exercised when the catheter is in the aorta or any large artery because the arterial flow may carry the inflated balloon distally until it occludes a major vessel, such as the carotid artery or descending aorta. This complication can be avoided by continuous pressure monitoring and partial deflation of the balloon in order to maintain its position.

## SIGNIFICANCE OF LARGE PULMONARY V WAVES

The phasic contour of the pulmonary wedge tracing may yield important diagnostic information. The V wave in the left atrial and pulmonary wedge tracing normally represents filling of the left atrium during systole against a closed mitral valve. An abnormally large V wave is sometimes defined as being 10 mmHg greater than mean pulmonary wedge pressure.[32,33] The most common cause of large V waves is mitral regurgitation. It has been pointed out recently that large V waves are not specific for mitral regurgitation and that its other important causes include left ventricular failure, mitral stenosis, and ventricular septal defects.[32,33] To understand the mechanisms of large V waves, the major determinants of their height have to be considered:

1. The size of the V wave is in part determined by the amount of blood entering the left atrium during systole. Increased blood enters the left atrium retrograde in mitral regurgitation, or antegrade from shunts that increase pulmonary venous return as in ventricular septal defects.

2. The pressure-volume relationship of the left atrium is curvilinear (Fig. 7-3), whereby changes in volume produce little change in pressure when the left atrial pressure is low but a similar change in volume is associated with a large change in pressure at the high pressure end of the curve. Thus, atrial inflow during systole results in large V waves when the left atrial pressure is elevated as in left ventricular failure or mitral stenosis. Conversely, large V waves may be absent in patients with severe mitral regurgitation who are hypovolemic. Patients with acute mitral regurgitation may have particularly steep pressure-volume curves signifying noncompliance of the small left atrium and such patients often exhibit giant V waves (i.e., peak V wave more than twice the mean wedge pressure). The value of the V wave in diagnosing mitral regurgitation is discussed in Chapter 23.

## PULMONARY WEDGE ANGIOGRAPHY

Injection of contrast medium into the pulmonary vascular bed through a catheter in the wedge position yields a standstill, high resolution angiogram.[34,35] By injecting distal to the inflated balloon, it is possible to evaluate an entire segment of lung.[34] Finding of an elevated pulmonary vascular resistance by hemodynamic criteria in patients considered for cardiac surgery may not distinguish increased vascular reactivity from structural morphologic damage. Pulmonary wedge angiography has been used to evaluate the extent of structural pulmonary vascular disease, especially in patients with congenital heart disease. Wedge angiograms have shown progressively more abrupt tapering of the pulmonary arteries in patients who have both increasingly abnormal pulmonary hemodynamics and increasingly severe structural changes in lung biopsy tissue. Methods for quantifying such pulmonary artery taper have been described.[34] The degree of filling of small peripheral arteries that become obliterated in this disease process also can be estimated.

Pulmonary wedge angiography has also been used to diagnose pulmonary emboli,[36,37] and this is discussed in detail in Chapter 15. When performed at the bedside with portable x-ray equipment, some studies have suggested a high incidence of false negatives and false positives. This is not surprising in view of the small portion of the lung vasculature visualized through the use of relatively low resolution x-ray equipment. The predictive power of this method is likely to be improved when there has been the prior suggestion of multiple embolic events by radionuclide methods or when a high resolution wedge angiogram is performed on a specific segment of the lung to further clarify the findings from routine pulmonary angiography.

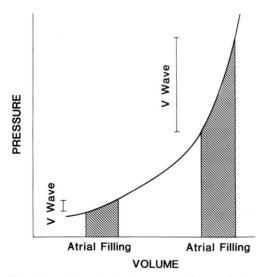

**Fig. 7-3.** A hypothetical pressure-volume relation for the left atrium is depicted.[32,33] At the low pressure end of the curve, inflow of blood (during ventricular systole), represented by the hatched bars, results in a relatively small increase in pressure, i.e., a small V wave; at the high pressure end of the curve, an identical inflow of blood results in a larger V wave.

## COMPLICATIONS

The flexibility of the flotation catheters and the protective function of the inflated balloon tend to minimize serious complications. However, the simplicity of the procedure itself has led on more than one occasion to underestimation of potential hazards of this invasive method and to unnecessary complications. Fortunately, several prospective studies that examined complications associated with the placement and maintenance of pulmonary catheters found the morbidity and mortality rate to be quite low and generally outweighed by the information obtained.[38–41]

***Rupture of Balloon.*** If rupture of the balloon occurs, the catheter's flotation properties are lost. Injection of 1 to 2 ml of air into the right heart chambers or the pulmonary artery has not been reported to have adverse consequences. This does not apply to children and patients with congenital heart disease in whom the possibility of a right-to-left shunt exists. In these patients, carbon dioxide must be used as the inflation medium. Rupture of the balloon is often recognized fluoroscopically in the catheterization laboratory and can be frequently confirmed by the appearance of blood at the inflation port following gentle aspiration.

***Arrhythmias.*** Although the protective effect of the inflated balloon and the flexibility of the catheter minimize the incidence of serious arrhythmias, sustained ventricular tachycardia was reported in 3% and ventricular fibrillation in 2% of 119 critically ill patients undergoing bedside pulmonary artery catheterization.[42] Ventricular ectopy was more frequent among patients predisposed to ectopy or with prolonged catheterization time. A new right bundle branch block developed in 5% of patients and persisted for a mean of 10 hours. Caution must be exercised therefore in the catheterization of patients with preexistent left bundle branch block. Prophylactic use of lidocaine appears effective in reducing the incidence of catheter-induced advanced ventricular arrhythmias.[43]

***Pulmonary Complications.*** An ideal position of the catheter is with its tip in the right or left main branches of the pulmonary artery. Flotation catheters, even when the balloon is deflated, have a tendency to advance into a distal branch. Inadvertent wedging in a small branch of the pulmonary artery

for prolonged periods may result in the development of segmental pulmonary infarction. This can be avoided by carefully monitoring the catheter tip pressure and, if necessary, by determining the position of the catheter by radiologic means. Whenever possible, the catheter should be kept in a position in which inflation of the balloon to full capacity (indicated on the catheter) is necessary to achieve a change from pulmonary artery to pulmonary wedge pressure. Supervising personnel should be instructed clearly as to the significance of an apparently damped pressure from the pulmonary artery.

***Perforation or Rupture of Pulmonary Artery.*** Inadvertent injection of a large amount of fluid under high pressure into the balloon inflation port may cause rupture of the pulmonary artery. Therefore, it is advisable to keep the syringe with air or $CO_2$ constantly attached to the inflation lumen.

An instance of pulmonary artery rupture has been reported in a patient with mitral stenosis and pulmonary hypertension.[44] In this case, the catheter was advanced more distally into a smaller branch. Upon inflation of the balloon to full capacity, the pulmonary arterial wall was exposed to significant distending forces, which together with the weakening of the arterial wall by long-standing pulmonary hypertension resulted in rupture of the artery. The pressure gradient between the pulmonary artery and pulmonary wedge pressure advancing the catheter tip may have been a contributory factor.

Several other cases of fatal pulmonary hemorrhage have been reported in association with use of the flow-directed balloon-tipped catheter in relation to balloon inflation or tip perforation.[45] As pointed out in Chapter 3, these complications can be avoided if the guidelines of technique described previously are observed strictly.

As a rule, we recommend that inflation of the balloon always be performed gradually and under visual inspection of the pulmonary arterial pressure tracing and that the inflation be *stopped immediately* when a change from pulmonary arterial to pulmonary wedge waveform is noted on the pressure tracing. Furthermore, the balloon should remain inflated only for the shortest possible time, particularly in patients with pulmonary hypertension.

***Knotting.*** Knotting due to coiling of the catheter is more frequent with smaller more flexible catheters. To minimize the likelihood of knotting in the absence of fluoroscopy, advancement of the catheter should be discontinued if the right ventricle is not reached within the expected distance from the insertion site or if the pulmonary artery is not reached within 15 cm from the right ventricle. Nonsurgical techniques for untying knots have been developed.[46,47]

***Thrombotic Complications.*** It has been demonstrated that a small thrombus may form on pulmonary artery catheters in most patients.[48] Coating of catheters by heparin appears to reduce greatly the incidence of such adherent thrombi.[48]

***Infections.*** Whenever a foreign body enters the vascular system, it may introduce infection. The likelihood of bacterial contamination increases with repeat catheter manipulations. A sterile protective sleeve has been introduced which allows for repositioning of the catheter with minimal bacteriologic risk.[49]

## SIGNIFICANCE

Balloon-tipped flow-directed cardiac catheters permit the measurement of many parameters of cardiovascular function at the bedside, without the requirement of fluoroscopy or a special facility for their placement, and at a low risk of significant arrhythmias. Variables that may be measured easily include: right atrial, right ventricular, pulmonary artery and pulmonary wedge pressures, right ventricular and right atrial cavity potentials, cardiac output by the thermodilution technique, and oxygen saturation of mixed venous blood.

Catheterization using the balloon-tipped catheters permits entry into chambers or vessels hardly accessible by conventional means in complex cardiac anomalies. Significantly, this easy and safe way of monitoring physiologic variables enables the physician to utilize direct data routinely in the management of his patient.

## REFERENCES

1. Swan HJC, et al: Catheterization of the heart in man with use of a flow-directed balloon-tipped catheter. N Engl J Med 283:447, 1970.
2. Buchbinder N, Ganz W: Hemodynamic monitoring: Invasive techniques. Anesthesiology 45:145, 1976.
3. Swan HJC, Ganz W: Measurement of right atrial and pulmonary arterial pressures and cardiac output: Clinical application of hemodynamic monitoring. Adv Intern Med 27:453, 1982.
4. Forrester JS, Diamond G, McHugh TJ, Swan HJC: Filling pressures in the right and left sides of the heart in acute myocardial infarction. A reappraisal of central-venous pressure monitoring. N Engl J Med 285:190, 1971.
5. Riley CP, Russell RO, Rackley CE: Left ventricular gallop sound and acute myocardial infarction. Am Heart J 86:598, 1973.
6. Carabello B, Cohn PF, Alpert JS: Hemodynamic monitoring in patients with hypotension after myocardial infarction. The role of the medical center in relation to the community hospital. Chest 74:5, 1978.
7. McHugh TJ, et al: Pulmonary vascular congestion in acute myocardial infarction: Hemodynamic and radiologic correlations. Ann Intern Med 76:29, 1972.
8. Kostuk W, Barr JW, Simon AL, Ross JR: Correlations between the chest film and hemodynamics in acute myocardial infarction. Circulation 48:624, 1973.
9. Connors AF, McCaffree DR, Gray BA: Evaluation of right-heart catheterization in the critically ill patient without acute myocardial infarction. N Engl J Med 308:263, 1983.
10. Eisenberg P, et al: Clinical evaluation compared to pulmonary artery catheterization in the hemodynamic assessment of critically ill patients. Crit Care Med 12:549, 1984.
11. Ganz W, et al: A new technique for measurement of cardiac output by thermodilution in man. Am J Cardiol 27:392, 1971.
12. Forrester JS, et al: Thermodilution cardiac output determination with a single flow-directed catheter. Am Heart J 83:306, 1972.
13. Zaidan JR, Freniere S: Use of a pacing pulmonary artery catheter during cardiac surgery. Ann Thorac Surg 35:633, 1983.
14. Lichtenthal PR, Collins JT: Multipurpose pulmonary artery catheter. Ann Thorac Surg 36:493, 1983.
15. Steele P, Davies H: The Swan-Ganz catheter in the cardiac laboratory. Br Heart J 35:647, 1973.
16. Kotoda K, Hasegawa T, Mizuno A, Saigusta M: Transseptal left-heart catheterization with Swan-Ganz flow-directed catheter. Am Heart J 105:436, 1983.
17. Sakurai T, et al: Balloon catheter test in patients

with atrial septal defect and patent ductus arteriosus. Jpn Heart J 21:779, 1980.

18. Forrester JS, et al: Medical therapy of acute myocardial infarction by application of hemodynamic subjects. N Engl J Med 2985:1356, 1404, 1976.

19. Meister SG, Helfant RH: Rapid bedside differentiation of ruptured interventricular septum from acute mitral insufficiency. N Engl J Med 287:1024, 1972.

20. Cohn JN, Guiha NH, Broder MI, Limas CJ. Right ventricular infarction: Clinical and hemodynamic features. Am J Cardiol 33:209, 1974.

21. Lorell B, et al: Right ventricular infarction: Clinical diagnosis and differentiation from cardiac tamponade and pericardial constriction. Am J Cardiol 43:465, 1979.

22. Reddy PS, Curtiss EI, O'Toole JD, Shaver JA: Cardiac tamponade: Hemodynamic observations in man. Circulation 58:265, 1978.

23. Unger KM, Shibel EM, Moser KM. Detection of left ventricular failure in patients with adult respiratory distress syndrome. Chest 67:8, 1975.

24. Gooding JM, Laws HL: Interpretation of pulmonary capillary wedge pressure during different modes of ventilation. Resp Care 22:161, 1977.

25. Berryhill RE, Benumof JL, Rauscher LA: Pulmonary vascular pressure reading at the end of exhalation. Anesthesiology 49:365, 1978.

26. Milic-Emili J, et al: Improved technique for estimating pleural pressure from esophageal balloons. J Appl Physiol 19:207, 1964.

27. Cohen JL, et al: Hemodynamic monitoring of patients undergoing abdominal aortic surgery. Am J Surg 146:174, 1983.

28. Kelly DT, Krovetz LJ, Rowe RD: Double-lumen flotation catheter for use in complex congenital cardiac anomalies. Circulation 44:910, 1971.

29. Stanger P, Heymann MA, Hoffman JIE, Rudolph AM: Use of Swan-Ganz catheter in cardiac catheterization of infants and children. Am Heart J 83:749, 1972.

30. Black JFS: Floating a catheter into the pulmonary artery in transposition of the great arteries. Am Heart J 84:761, 1972.

31. Jones SM, Miller GAH: Catheterization of the pulmonary artery in transposition of the great arteries using a Swan-Ganz flow-directed catheter. Br Heart J 35:298, 1973.

32. Fuchs RM, Heuser RR, Yin FCP, Brinker JA: Limitations of pulmonary wedge V waves in diagnosing mitral regurgitation. Am J Cardiol 49:849, 1982.

33. Pichard AD, et al: Large V waves in the pulmonary wedge pressure tracing in the absence of mitral regurgitation. Am J Cardiol 50:1044, 1982.

34. Rabinovitch M. et al: Quantitative analysis of the pulmonary wedge angiogram in congenital heart defects. Circulation 63:152, 1981.

35. Bell ALL, et al: Wedge pulmonary arteriography. Its application in congenital and acquired heart disease. Radiology 73:566, 1959.

36. Dougherty JE, LaSala AF, Fieldman A: Bedside pulmonary angiography utilizing an existing Swan-Ganz catheter. Chest 77:43, 1980.

37. LePage JR, Gracia RM: The value of bedside wedge pulmonary angiography in the detection of pulmonary emboli: A predictive and prospective evaluation. Radiology 144:67, 1982.

38. Boyd KD, et al: A prospective study of complications of pulmonary artery catheterizations in 500 consecutive patients. Chest 84:245, 1983.

39. Davies MJ, Cronin KD, Domaingue CM: Pulmonary artery catheterization. An assessment of risks and benefits in 220 surgical patients. Anaesth Intens Care 10:9, 1982.

40. Elliott CG, Zimmerman GA, Clemmer TP: Complications of pulmonary artery catheterization in the care of critically ill patients. Chest 76:647, 1979.

41. Sise MJ, et al: Complications of the flow-directed pulmonary artery catheter: A prospective analysis in 219 patients. Crit Care Med 9:315, 1981.

42. Sprung CL, et al: Advanced ventricular arrhythmias during bedside pulmonary artery catheterization. Am J Med 72:203, 1982.

43. Sprung CL, et al: Prophylactic use of lidocaine to prevent advanced ventricular arrhythmias during pulmonary artery catheterization. Prospective double-blind study. Am J Med 75:906, 1983.

44. Lapin ES, Murray JA: Hemoptysis with flow-directed cardiac catheterization. JAMA 29:1246, 1972.

45. Kelly TF Jr, et al: Perforation of the pulmonary artery with Swan-Ganz catheters: Diagnosis and surgical management. Ann Surg 193:686, 1981.

46. Cho SR, et al: Percutaneous unknotting of intravascular catheters and retrieval of catheter fragments. AJR 141:397, 1983.

47. Dumesnil JG, Proulx G: A new nonsurgical technique for untying tight knots in flow-directed balloon catheters. Am J Cardiol 15:395, 1984.

48. Hoar PF, et al: Heparin bonding reduces thrombogenicity of pulmonary-artery catheters. N Engl J Med 305:993, 1981.

49. Bessette MC, Quintin L, Whalley DG, Wynands JE: Swan-Ganz contamination: A protective sleeve for repositioning. Can Anaesth Soc J 28:86, 1981.

# PART III
## *Hemodynamic Principles*

*chapter eight*

# Blood Flow Measurement: The Cardiac Output

WILLIAM GROSSMAN

⬛⬛⬛

T HE MAINTENANCE of blood flow commensurate with the metabolic needs of the body is a fundamental requirement of human life. In the absence of major disease of the vascular tree (e.g., arterial obstruction), the maintenance of appropriate blood flow to the body depends largely upon the heart's ability to pump blood in the forward direction. The quantity of blood delivered to the systemic circulation per unit time is termed the *cardiac output*, generally expressed in liters/minute.

## ARTERIOVENOUS DIFFERENCE AND EXTRACTION RESERVE

Since the extraction of nutrients by metabolizing tissues is a function not only of the rate of delivery of those nutrients (the cardiac output) but also of the ability of each tissue to extract those nutrients from the circulation, tissue viability can be maintained despite a fall in cardiac output as long as there is increased extraction of required nutrients. The extraction of a given nutrient (or of any substance) from the circulation by a particular tissue is expressed as the *arteriovenous difference* across that tissue, and the

factor by which the arteriovenous difference can increase at constant flow (due to changes in metabolic demand) may be termed the *extraction reserve*. For example, arterial blood in man is normally 95% saturated with oxygen; that is, if 1 L of blood has the *capacity* to carry approximately 200 ml of oxygen when fully saturated, arterial blood will usually be found to contain 190 ml of oxygen per liter (190/200 = 95%). Venous blood returning from the body normally has an average oxygen saturation of 75%; that is, mixed venous blood generally contains 150 ml of oxygen per liter of blood (150/200 = 75%). Thus, the normal arteriovenous difference for oxygen is 40 ml/L (190 ml/L − 150 ml/L).

The normal extraction reserve for oxygen[1] is 3, which means that, given adequate metabolic demand, the body's tissues can extract 120 ml of oxygen (3 × 40 ml) from each liter of blood delivered. Thus, if arterial saturation remains constant at 95%, full utilization of the extraction reserve will result in a mixed venous oxygen content of 70 ml/L (190 ml/L − 120 ml/L), or a mixed venous oxygen saturation of 35% (70/200 = 35%). This is essentially the value found for mixed venous (i.e., pulmonary artery) oxygen saturation in normal men studied at maximal

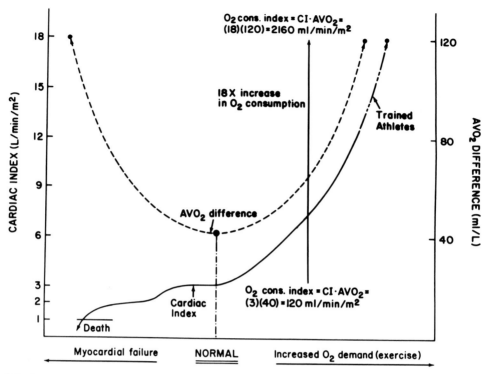

**Fig. 8-1.** Relationship between arteriovenous oxygen ($AVO_2$) difference (broken line) and cardiac index (solid curve) in normal subjects at rest (center) and during exercise (right), and in the patient with progressively worsening myocardial failure (left). See text for discussion.

exercise. The relation between cardiac output and arteriovenous $O_2$ difference is illustrated in Figure 8-1.

put to below one third of normal is incompatible with life.

## LOWER LIMIT OF CARDIAC OUTPUT

The value of 3 for the oxygen extraction reserve predicts that, in progressive cardiac decompensation, in order to meet the basal oxygen requirements of the body, oxygen extraction increases as cardiac output falls until arteriovenous oxygen difference has tripled and cardiac output has fallen to one third of its normal value (Fig. 8-1). Since the extraction reserve has now been fully utilized, further reduction of cardiac output will result in tissue hypoxia, anaerobic metabolism, acidosis, and eventually, circulatory collapse. This prediction seems quite accurate; clinical investigators have observed for many years that a fall in resting cardiac out-

## UPPER LIMIT OF CARDIAC OUTPUT

Several studies have indicated that the largest increase in cardiac output that can be achieved by a trained athlete at maximal exercise is 600% of the resting output. If a normal 70-kg man has a cardiac output of 5 L/min or 3.0 L/min/$M^2$, then his maximal cardiac output might be as high as 30 L/min (18/L/min/$M^2$). Since cardiac output increases approximately 600 ml for each 100 ml increase in oxygen requirements of the body, an increase in cardiac output of 25 L/min with maximal exercise would suggest an increase in total body oxygen requirements of 4167 ml/min, which is approximately an 18-fold increase over the normal resting value of 250 ml/min. The 18-fold increase in total body oxygen requirements is met by the combined sixfold increase in oxygen "delivery" (i.e., cardiac output), and threefold increase in oxygen extraction (oxygen reserve). These relations are illustrated in Figure 8-1.

## FACTORS INFLUENCING CARDIAC OUTPUT IN NORMAL SUBJECTS

The range of the "normal" cardiac output is difficult to define with precision, since it is influenced by several variables. Obviously, body size is important, and the ranges of normal values for cardiac output of 2-year-old children, 10-year-old children, and 50-year-old men will be so different that they will show only minimal overlap. For this reason, normalization of the cardiac output for differing body size is considered fundamental by all students of this subject, although there is disagreement about the best way to accomplish this normalization. Since cardiac output seems to be predominantly a function of the body's oxygen consumption or metabolic rate,[1,2] and since metabolic rate was thought to correlate best with body surface area,[3,4] it has become customary to express cardiac output in terms of the *cardiac index* (L/min)/(body surface area, $M^2$). Body surface area is not measured directly but is instead calculated from one of the experimentally developed formulae, such as that of Dubois:[4]

Body surface area ($M^2$) =
$$0.007184 \times \text{Weight}^{0.425} \times \text{Height}^{0.725}$$
$$\text{(kg)} \qquad \text{(cm)}$$

Despite the shortcomings and weaknesses of this approach to normalization of the cardiac output,[1,5] the method has gained nearly universal acceptance by clinicians over the past 25 years, and will be employed throughout this book. A chart to aid calculation of body surface area (if weight and height are known) appears in Figure 8-2.

Although expression of cardiac output as the *cardiac index* greatly narrows the range of normal values among our groups of 2-year-old children, 10-year-old children, and 50-year-old men, it does not completely abolish the differences in these ranges. In fact,

the normal cardiac output appears to vary with age, steadily decreasing from approximately 4.5 L/min/$M^2$ at age 7 years to 2.5 L/min/$M^2$ at age 70 years.[1,6] This is not surprising, since it is well known that the body's metabolic rate is affected greatly by age, being highest in childhood and progressively diminishing to old age.

In addition to age, cardiac output is affected by posture, decreasing approximately 10% when rising from lying to sitting position and approximately 20% when rising (or being tilted) from lying to standing position. Also, body temperature, anxiety, environmental heat and humidity, and a host of other factors influence the normal resting cardiac output,[1] and these must be considered in interpreting any value of cardiac output measured in the clinical setting.

## TECHNIQUES FOR DETERMINATION OF CARDIAC OUTPUT

Of the numerous techniques devised over the years to measure cardiac output, two have won general acceptance in cardiac catheterization laboratories: the Fick oxygen technique and the indicator dilution technique. Both techniques resemble each other in that they are based on the theoretic principle enunciated by Adolph Fick in 1870.[7] The principle, which was never actually applied by Fick, states that the total uptake or release of any substance by an organ is the product of blood flow to the organ and the arteriovenous concentration difference of the substance. For the lungs the substance released to the blood is oxygen, and the pulmonary blood flow can be determined by knowing the arteriovenous difference of oxygen across the lungs and the oxygen consumption per minute.

Fick's principle is illustrated in Figure 8-3. In this figure, a train is passing by a hopper that is delivering marbles to the boxcars at a rate of 20 marbles/min. If the boxcars each contain 16 marbles before passing under the hopper and 20 marbles after passing under the hopper, then each boxcar is picking up 4 marbles, and must be taking only ⅕ of a minute to pass under the hopper, since it would pick up 20 marbles in each full minute under

# BSA

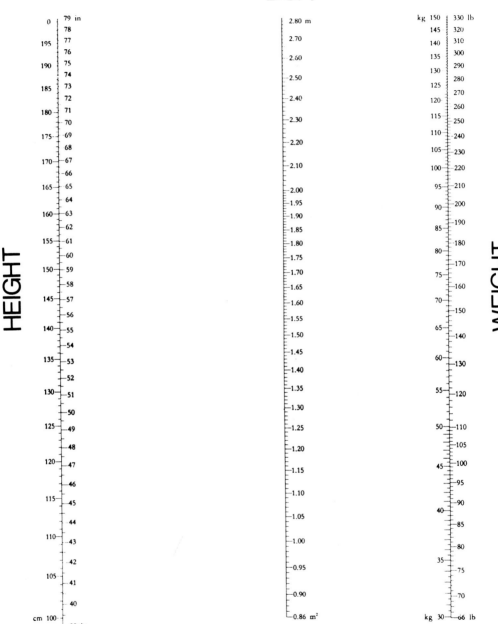

**Fig. 8-2.** Nomogram for calculation of body surface area, given the weight and height of the patient. From the formula of Dubois.[4]

the hopper. Now, if each boxcar takes ⅕ of a minute to pass by the hopper, then the train is moving at a speed sufficient to deliver 5 boxcars/min to any point down the line. This could have been calculated as shown on the facing page:

Train's speed
(boxcars/min)
= Marble delivery rate/"A-V" marble difference
   (marbles/min)       (marbles/boxcar)
= (20 marbles/min)/(4 marbles/boxcar)
= 5 boxcars/min

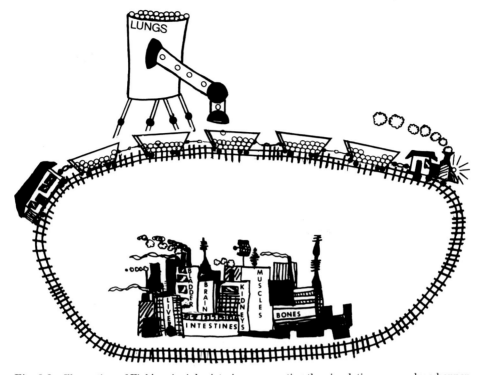

**Fig. 8-3.** Illustration of Fick's principle. A train, representing the circulation, passes by a hopper (the lungs) that delivers marbles (oxygen) to the train's boxcars at a rate of 20 marbles/min. Since the boxcars each contain 16 marbles before and 20 marbles after passing under the hopper, each boxcar is picking up 4 marbles, and must be taking only ⅕ minute to pass under the hopper, since it would pick up 20 marbles in each full minute under the hopper. Now, if each boxcar takes only ⅕ minute to pass by the hopper, then the train is moving at a speed sufficient to deliver 5 boxcars /min to any point down the line. This could have been calculated as

Train's speed  = Marble delivery rate/"A-V" marble difference
(boxcars/min)   (marbles/min)     (marbles/boxcar)

= (20 marbles/min)/(4 marbles/boxcar)

= 5 boxcars/min

If one boxcar is 1 L of blood and each marble is 10 ml oxygen, then we have an arteriovenous oxygen difference of 40 ml/L, an $O_2$ consumption of 200 ml/min, and a cardiac output of 5 L/min. (Illustration kindly provided by Jennifer Grossman, age 11.)

If each boxcar is 1 L of blood, and each marble is 10 ml of oxygen, then we have an arteriovenous $O_2$ difference of 40 ml/L, an oxygen consumption of 200 ml/min, and a cardiac output of 5 L/min.

## Fick Oxygen Method

In the Fick oxygen method, pulmonary blood flow should be determined by measuring the arteriovenous difference of oxygen across the lungs and the rate of oxygen uptake by blood from the lungs. If there is no intracardiac shunt and pulmonary blood flow is equal to systemic blood flow, then the Fick oxygen method also measures systemic blood flow. Thus, *cardiac output = oxygen consumption ÷ arteriovenous oxygen difference.*

In actual practice, the rate at which oxygen is taken up from the lungs by blood is not measured, but rather the uptake of oxygen from room air by the lungs is measured, because in a steady state, these two measurements are equal. Furthermore, arteriovenous oxygen difference across the lungs is not measured directly. Generally, pulmonary arterial blood (true mixed venous blood) is sampled, but pulmonary venous blood is not sampled. Instead, left ventricular or systemic arterial blood is sampled and assumed to have an oxygen content representative of mixed pulmonary venous blood. Actually, because of bronchial venous and thebesian venous drainage, the oxygen content of systemic arterial blood is commonly 2 to 5 ml/L of blood lower than pulmonary venous blood as it leaves the alveoli.

## Oxygen Consumption

Two different methods for measurement of oxygen consumption are widely used today: the polarographic method and the Douglas bag method.

***Polarographic $O_2$ Method.*** In our laboratory, oxygen consumption is currently measured using the metabolic rate meter (MRM) made by Waters Instruments (Rochester, Minnesota). The instrument contains a polarographic oxygen sensor cell (gold and silver/silver chloride electrodes), a hood or face mask and a blower of variable speed connected to a servocontrol loop with the oxygen sensor (Fig. 8-4). This device is convenient and accurate and represents a significant advance over the older, standard procedure of collecting expired air for 3 minutes in a Douglas bag and measuring volume (Tissot spirometer) and oxygen content. The principle of operation for the MRM involves using a variable-speed blower to maintain a unidirectional flow of air from the room through the hood and via a connecting hose to the polarographic oxygen-sensing cell. As illustrated in Figure 8-4, room air enters the hood at a rate, $\dot{V}_R$ (ml/min), which is determined by the blower's discharge rate, $\dot{V}_M$ (ml/min), as well as the patient's ventilatory rate ($\dot{V}_i$, inhaled air in ml/min; $\dot{V}_E$, exhaled air). The blower speed, $\dot{V}_M$, is controlled by a servoloop designed to maintain the oxygen content of air flowing past the polarographic cell constant at a predetermined value. In a steady state, the average value of $\dot{V}_M$ together with the oxygen content of room air and of air flowing past the polarographic cell can be used to calculate the patient's oxygen consumption, as follows:

The patient's oxygen consumption, $\dot{V}_{O_2}$ is given by:

$$\dot{V}_{O_2} = (F_R O_2 \cdot \dot{V}_R) - (F_M O_2 \cdot \dot{V}_M)$$

[Equation 1]

where $F_R O_2$ and $F_M O_2$ are the fractional contents of oxygen in room air and in air flowing past the polarographic cell, respectively.

As can be seen from Figure 8-3

$$\dot{V}_M = \dot{V}_R - \dot{V}_i + \dot{V}_E$$

which can be rewritten as

$$\dot{V}_R = \dot{V}_M + \dot{V}_i - \dot{V}_E$$

Substituting this in Equation 1 gives

$$\dot{V}_{O_2} = F_R O_2(\dot{V}_M + \dot{V}_i - \dot{V}_E) - F_M O_2 \cdot \dot{V}_M$$
$$= F_R O_2(\dot{V}_M) - F_M O_2(\dot{V}_M) + F_R O_2(\dot{V}_i) - F_R O_2(\dot{V}_E)$$
$$= \dot{V}_M(F_R O_2 - F_M O_2) + F_R O_2(\dot{V}_i - \dot{V}_E)$$

Since the fractional content of oxygen in room air ($F_R O_2$) is 0.209, oxygen consumption is given by:

$$\dot{V}_{O_2} = \dot{V}_M(0.209 - F_M O_2) + 0.209(\dot{V}_i - \dot{V}_E)$$

[Equation 2]

Thus, in a steady state (where $\dot{V}_i - \dot{V}_E$ is constant) oxygen consumption can be determined by measurement of the volume rate of air moved by the blower motor ($\dot{V}_M$) and the fractional $O_2$ content of air moving past the polarographic sensor. In the MRM, a servocontrolled system adjusts $\dot{V}_M$ to keep $F_M O_2$ at a constant predetermined value. In practice, $F_M O_2$ is set at 0.199, so that Equation 2 becomes

$$\dot{V}_{O_2} = \dot{V}_M(0.209 - 0.199) + 0.209(\dot{V}_i - \dot{V}_E)$$
$$\dot{V}_{O_2} = 0.01 \dot{V}_M + 0.209(\dot{V}_i - \dot{V}_E).$$

For practical purposes, the respiratory quotient (RQ) is assumed to be 1.0; accordingly, $\dot{V}_i = \dot{V}_E$ and $\dot{V}_{O_2} = 0.01 \dot{V}_M$. If the RQ is actually 0.9 (e.g., the patient releases 0.9 liters of $CO_2$ for each liter of $O_2$ consumed), the error in $\dot{V}_{O_2}$ resulting from the assumption of an RQ of 1.0 is 1.6%, and if RQ is 0.8 the error would be 3.2%. The MRM $O_2$ consumption monitor has a calibrated blower motor in addition to the servocontrol polarographic sensor, and gives a readout of oxygen consumption in liters/minute by digital scale (MRM-2) or by meter and paper (MRM-1). The MRM-2 model is calibrated to be highly accurate in the oxygen consumption range from 10 to 1000 ml $O_2$/min and is thus best suited for measurement of resting $O_2$ consumption in the catheterization laboratory. The MRM-1 model, which is calibrated in the 150 to 5000 ml $O_2$/min range, is best suited for exercise studies.

SERVO UNIT

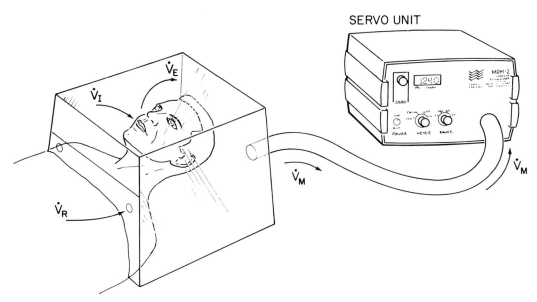

**Fig. 8-4.** Measurement of $O_2$ consumption by a polarographic cell technique using the Waters Instruments metabolic rate meter (MRM). A transparent hood fits snugly over the patient's head, resting on his pillow. Air enters the hood through holes in a plastic sheet at a flow rate $V_R$. The patient's inspiratory ($V_I$) and expiratory ($V_E$) flow rates subtract and add to $V_R$ to yield $V_M$, the flow rate leaving the hood and entering the servo-unit. A blower motor in the servo-unit adjusts $V_M$ to keep the $O_2$ sensed by a polarographic cell constant. See text for details.

***Douglas Bag Method.*** In addition to the MRM $O_2$ device, it is valuable to have as backup the older, standard volumetric technique for measuring $O_2$ consumption which involves the collection of expired air for subsequent analysis. In this method, a timed sample (usually 3 minutes) of the patient's expired air is collected in a Douglas bag.* In making this collection, the patient's nose is first firmly clipped† shut so that no air can escape through it. Once the clip is in place, the patient is asked to hold a special mouthpiece between his lips and breathe entirely through the mouthpiece, great care being taken that no air escapes around it. A technician holds the mouthpiece for the patient in a steady and comfortable position with one hand and may use the other hand to hold the patient's lips firmly around the mouthpiece. The mouthpiece is attached to the Douglas bag by a two-way valve‡ that has a sidearm open to room air. The valve and sidearm

function in such a way that the patient inspires air from the room but expires completely into the Douglas bag. The Douglas bag has a built-in three-way valve that allows the operator to open and then seal off the bag after the timed sample of expired air has been collected. An equilibration period of at least 30 seconds of breathing quietly through the mouthpiece should be allowed before beginning the timed air collection. This permits the patient to adjust to the technique and washes out the deadspace in the valve and connecting tubing interposed between the patient and the Douglas bag.

Contents of the bag should be analyzed as soon as possible following the collection, because some diffusion occurs through the walls of the bag. However, the bag may be placed aside until completing the cardiac catheterization, although it is helpful to know the oxygen consumption before the catheterization is completed and the catheters are removed from the patient's vascular system.

In calculating the oxygen consumption using the Douglas bag to collect expired air, it is helpful to have a flow sheet such as the one reproduced in Figure 8-5. Calculation of the oxygen consumption is done in two

*60-Liter Douglas type gas bag, Warren Collins, Inc., Boston, MA.

†Rubber-tipped nose clip, Warren Collins, Inc., Boston, MA.

‡Two-way valve with rubber fittings, Warren Collins, Inc., Boston, MA.

**TABLE 8-1.** *Millimeters to be Subtracted from Barometer Readings to Reduce Them to 0°C*

| Temp. °C. | Barometric pressure in mm Hg | | | | |
|---|---|---|---|---|---|
| | 740 | 750 | 760 | 770 | 780 |
| 11.0 | 1.33 | 1.35 | 1.36 | 1.38 | 1.40 |
| 11.5 | 1.39 | 1.41 | 1.42 | 1.44 | 1.46 |
| 12.0 | 1.45 | 1.47 | 1.49 | 1.51 | 1.53 |
| 12.5 | 1.51 | 1.53 | 1.55 | 1.57 | 1.59 |
| 13.0 | 1.57 | 1.59 | 1.61 | 1.63 | 1.65 |
| 13.5 | 1.63 | 1.65 | 1.67 | 1.69 | 1.71 |
| 14.0 | 1.69 | 1.71 | 1.73 | 1.76 | 1.78 |
| 14.5 | 1.75 | 1.77 | 1.79 | 1.82 | 1.84 |
| 15.0 | 1.81 | 1.83 | 1.86 | 1.88 | 1.91 |
| 15.5 | 1.87 | 1.89 | 1.92 | 1.94 | 1.97 |
| 16.0 | 1.93 | 1.96 | 1.98 | 2.01 | 2.03 |
| 16.5 | 1.99 | 2.02 | 2.04 | 2.07 | 2.09 |
| 17.0 | 2.05 | 2.08 | 2.10 | 2.13 | 2.16 |
| 17.5 | 2.11 | 2.14 | 2.16 | 2.19 | 2.22 |
| 18.0 | 2.17 | 2.20 | 2.23 | 2.26 | 2.29 |
| 18.5 | 2.23 | 2.26 | 2.29 | 2.32 | 2.35 |
| 19.0 | 2.29 | 2.32 | 2.35 | 2.38 | 2.41 |
| 19.5 | 2.35 | 2.38 | 2.41 | 2.45 | 2.48 |
| 20.0 | 2.41 | 2.44 | 2.47 | 2.51 | 2.54 |
| 20.5 | 2.47 | 2.50 | 2.54 | 2.57 | 2.61 |
| 21.0 | 2.53 | 2.56 | 2.60 | 2.63 | 2.67 |
| 21.5 | 2.59 | 2.63 | 2.66 | 2.70 | 2.73 |
| 22.0 | 2.65 | 2.69 | 2.72 | 2.76 | 2.79 |
| 22.5 | 2.71 | 2.75 | 2.78 | 2.82 | 2.86 |
| 23.0 | 2.77 | 2.81 | 2.84 | 2.88 | 2.92 |
| 23.5 | 2.83 | 2.87 | 2.91 | 2.95 | 2.99 |
| 24.0 | 2.89 | 2.93 | 2.97 | 3.01 | 3.05 |
| 24.5 | 2.95 | 2.99 | 3.03 | 3.07 | 3.11 |
| 25.0 | 3.01 | 3.05 | 3.09 | 3.13 | 3.17 |
| 25.5 | 3.07 | 3.11 | 3.15 | 3.20 | 3.24 |
| 26.0 | 3.13 | 3.17 | 3.21 | 3.26 | 3.30 |
| 26.5 | 3.19 | 3.23 | 3.28 | 3.32 | 3.36 |
| 27.0 | 3.25 | 3.29 | 3.34 | 3.38 | 3.42 |
| 27.5 | 3.31 | 3.35 | 3.40 | 3.45 | 3.49 |
| 28.0 | 3.37 | 3.41 | 3.46 | 3.51 | 3.55 |
| 28.5 | 3.43 | 3.48 | 3.52 | 3.57 | 3.62 |
| 29.0 | 3.49 | 3.54 | 3.58 | 3.63 | 3.68 |
| 29.5 | 3.55 | 3.60 | 3.65 | 3.69 | 3.74 |
| 30.0 | 3.61 | 3.66 | 3.71 | 3.75 | 3.80 |
| 30.5 | 3.67 | 3.72 | 3.77 | 3.82 | 3.87 |
| 31.0 | 3.73 | 3.78 | 3.83 | 3.88 | 3.93 |
| 31.5 | 3.79 | 3.84 | 3.89 | 3.94 | 3.99 |
| 32.0 | 3.85 | 3.90 | 3.95 | 4.00 | 4.05 |
| 32.5 | 3.91 | 3.96 | 4.01 | 4.07 | 4.12 |
| 33.0 | 3.97 | 4.02 | 4.07 | 4.13 | 4.18 |
| 33.5 | 4.03 | 4.08 | 4.14 | 4.19 | 4.25 |
| 34.0 | 4.09 | 4.14 | 4.20 | 4.25 | 4.31 |
| 34.5 | 4.15 | 4.20 | 4.26 | 4.31 | 4.37 |
| 35.0 | 4.21 | 4.26 | 4.32 | 4.38 | 4.43 |
| 35.5 | 4.26 | 4.32 | 4.38 | 4.44 | 4.50 |
| 36.0 | 4.32 | 4.38 | 4.44 | 4.50 | 4.56 |

steps. First, one measures the oxygen content of room air and that of the patient's expired air. This may be done with a Beckman oxygen analyzer,[*] which enables one to determine the oxygen content of a gas sample in millimeters of mercury partial pressure, or a Lex-$O_2$-Con[†] oxygen analyzer, which precisely measures oxygen content of air by a fuel-cell technique. Corrected barometric pressure is determined each day from a barometer and thermometer located in the catheterization laboratory. Barometric pressure is corrected for temperature with the aid of a standard table (Table 8-1). The values for barometric pressure, temperature, and corrected barometric pressure are entered at the top of the flow sheet (Fig. 8-5, a, b, and c).

The volume of expired air in the Douglas bag may be measured with a Tissot spirometer[‡] or gas meter,[¶] and this is corrected to standard temperature and pressure (STP) by means of standard tables. (Tables for correcting gas volumes to STP, "dry" or saturated, are available in a number of texts of standard tables, such as Documenta Geigy—Scientific Tables. Ardsley, NY, Geigy Pharmaceuticals, 1962, pp. 300–309). Some spirometers give volume readings directly; others require that the volume be calculated from the difference in height of the spirometer before and after the introduction of the expired air (steps 4 and 5, Fig. 8-5). The total volume originally present in the Douglas bag equals the Tissot spirometer volume plus the small volume of air removed for analysis in the Beckman oxygen analyzer (step 6, Fig. 8-5). The total volume of expired air is corrected to STP by standard tables (step 7, Fig. 8-5) and is divided by the number of minutes of collection time to obtain the minute ventilation (step 8, Fig. 8-5).

The oxygen difference, milliliters of oxygen consumed per liter of air (step 3, Fig. 8-5), is multiplied by the minute ventilation (step 8, Fig. 8-5) to obtain the oxygen consumption in milliliters/minute (step 9, Fig. 8-5). The latter is divided by the body surface

[*]Model C2 oxygen analyzer, Beckman Instruments, Fullerton, CA.

[†]Lexington Instruments, Lexington, MA.

[‡]Respiratory gasometer, Tissot type, Arthur Thomas & Co., Philadelphia, PA.

[¶]Wet test meter. Precision Scientific Company, Chicago, IL.

Name: _____ Date: _____

BSA: _____ Height: _____ Weight: _____ No.: _____

       (a)  Barometric pressure             _____ mm Hg

       (b)  Barometric temperature      _____ ° C

       (c)  Corrected barometric pressure _____ mm Hg (Table 8-1)

       (d)  $pO_2$ room air                 _____ mm Hg

       (e)  $pO_2$ expired air             _____ mm Hg

       (f)  Tissot: initial                 _____ cm

       (g)  Tissot: final                   _____ cm

       (h)  Sample volume              _____ L

       (i)  Correction factor           _____ (standard tables)

       (j)  Collection time              _____ min

## OXYGEN DIFFERENCE

Step 1.  $O_2$ content in room air:

$$\frac{pO_2 \text{ room air (d)} \times 100}{\text{corrected barometric pressure (c)}} = \underline{\hspace{2cm}} \text{ ml } O_2/100 \text{ ml air}$$

Step 2.  $O_2$ content of expired air:

$$\frac{pO_2 \text{ expired air (e)} \times 100}{\text{corrected barometric pressure (c)}} = \underline{\hspace{2cm}} \text{ ml } O_2/100 \text{ ml air}$$

Step 3.  $\begin{bmatrix} O_2 \text{ room air} - O_2 \text{ expired air} \end{bmatrix} \times 10 = \underline{\hspace{2cm}}$ ml $O_2$ consumed/L air
          (step 1)       (step 2)

## MINUTE VENTILATION

Step 4.  Tissot initial (f) − Tissot final (g) = _____ cm

Step 5.  Tissot volume:

Difference (step 4) × 1.329* = _____ L

Step 6.  Total volume:

Tissot volume (step 5) + sample (h) = _____ L

Step 7.  Total volume (step 6) × correction factor (i) = _____ L

Step 8.  $\dfrac{\text{Ventilation volume (step 7)}}{\text{Collection time (j)}} = \underline{\hspace{2cm}}$ L/min

Step 9.  Oxygen consumption:

$O_2$ difference × minute ventilation = _____ ml/min
   (step 3)          (step 8)

Step 10. Oxygen consumption index:

$\dfrac{O_2 \text{ consumption (step 9)}}{\text{Body surface area}} = \underline{\hspace{2cm}}$ ml/min/m²

---

*Correction factor for each instrument. In this case 1.0L of gas produces an excursion of 1.329 cm on the meter scale.

**Fig. 8-5.** Oxygen consumption calculation.

area (Fig. 8-2), yielding the oxygen consumption index in milliliters of oxygen consumed per minute per square meter of body surface area (step 10, Fig. 8-5). The normal basal oxygen consumption in man is usually between 110 and 150 ml $O_2$ per minute square meter of body surface area.[8]

### Arteriovenous Oxygen Difference

The arteriovenous oxygen difference across the lungs must be measured to calculate cardiac output by Fick's principle, and this can be accomplished by the following method. From appropriately positioned catheters, systemic arterial and mixed venous (pulmonary arterial) blood samples are obtained during the period when $O_2$ consumption is being measured. The samples are drawn into heparinized syringes and quickly capped. If the patient has received heparin systemically, the syringes for collection of these blood samples need not be heparinized. If the samples will be analyzed immediately by oximetry, plastic syringes may be used. However, $O_2$ may diffuse through the walls of plastic syringes, and glass syringes are considered preferable by some if there will be a delay in oximetric analysis of the blood. In a test in our laboratory, no appreciable increase in $O_2$ saturation of venous blood could be detected over 2 hours (capped plastic 15-ml syringe filled with venous blood sitting at room temperature was sampled every 15 minutes for oximetry). The samples should be drawn simultaneously and as close to the midpoint of the oxygen consumption determination as possible. Care must be taken to avoid contamination of the blood samples with air bubbles.

*Oxygen content* (in milliliters of oxygen per liter of blood) can be determined by a variety of methods, the most classic of which (and the one that serves as a standard for all others) is the manometric technique of Van Slyke and Neill.[9] The major drawback of the Van Slyke technique is that 15 to 30 minutes are required to run a single blood sample. Reflectance oximetry of heparinized blood samples is simple and quick and measures the percentage of hemoglobin present as oxyhemoglobin. This percentage, multiplied by the theoretic *oxygen carrying capacity* of the patient's blood, yields the calculated *oxygen content* of that sample. (See Fig. 8-6.) A

formula for approximating the theoretic oxygen carrying capacity in man is:

$$\text{Hemoglobin (gm/dl)} \times 1.36 \text{ (ml } O_2/\text{gm hemoglobin)} \\ \times 10 = \text{theoretic } O_2 \text{ carrying capacity} \\ \text{(ml } O_2/\text{L blood)}$$

In several textbooks, the constant is given as 1.34, but studies on crystalline human hemoglobin suggest that the correct number may be 1.36.[10,11] Whatever its correct value, the formula is only an approximation. To the extent that some hemoglobin may be bound to carbon monoxide (cigarette smokers) or that abnormal hemoglobins (e.g., HgbS) may be present, the approximation will be incorrect. Newer methods have been introduced that utilize an oxygen sensing cell for direct measurement of oxygen content.*

Figure 8-6 is a flow sheet that may be used to calculate oxygen content of blood samples and arteriovenous oxygen difference when the spectrophotometric oximeter method is used. Oxygen contents of arterial and mixed venous blood samples are calculated as the percentage of oxyhemoglobin saturation of these samples multiplied by the oxygen carrying capacity (steps 2 to 5, Fig. 8-6). The arteriovenous oxygen difference, (step 3 minus step 5, Fig. 8-6) may then be divided into the oxygen consumption to yield the cardiac output.

Arterial blood may be taken from a systemic artery, the left ventricle, the left atrium, or the pulmonary veins. Theoretically, pulmonary venous blood is preferable to peripheral arterial blood for the arteriovenous oxygen difference calculations. Except in the presence of a right-to-left intracardiac shunt, pulmonary venous oxygen content may be approximated by systemic arterial oxygen content, ignoring the small amount of venous admixture resulting from bronchial and thebesian venous drainage. If arterial desaturation (e.g., arterial blood oxygen saturation <95%) is present, a central right-to-left shunt should be excluded before accepting systemic arterial oxygen content as representative of that of pulmonary venous blood. Techniques for detecting and quantifying such shunts are described in Chapter 12.

The most reliable site for obtaining mixed venous blood is the pulmonary artery. Because of streaming and incomplete mixing,

---

*Lex-$O_2$-Con, Lexington Instruments, Waltham, MA.

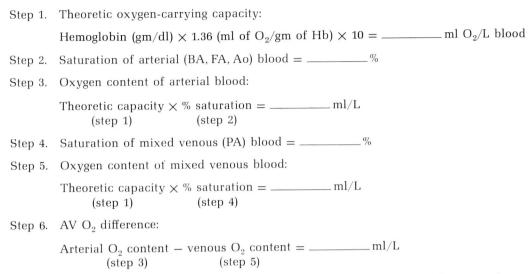

Step 1.  Theoretic oxygen-carrying capacity:

Hemoglobin (gm/dl) $\times$ 1.36 (ml of $O_2$/gm of Hb) $\times$ 10 = _____ ml $O_2$/L blood

Step 2.  Saturation of arterial (BA, FA, Ao) blood = _____ %

Step 3.  Oxygen content of arterial blood:

Theoretic capacity $\times$ % saturation = _____ ml/L
    (step 1)           (step 2)

Step 4.  Saturation of mixed venous (PA) blood = _____ %

Step 5.  Oxygen content of mixed venous blood:

Theoretic capacity $\times$ % saturation = _____ ml/L
    (step 1)           (step 4)

Step 6.  AV $O_2$ difference:

Arterial $O_2$ content − venous $O_2$ content = _____ ml/L
    (step 3)           (step 5)

**Fig. 8-6.**  Calculation of oxygen content and AV oxygen difference when using the reflectance oximetry method.

considering blood from more proximal sites such as the right atrium or vena cavae as representative of mixed venous blood is much less accurate.[12,13] Right ventricular blood is closer to true mixed venous blood, and may be substituted for pulmonary arterial blood if necessary.

***Sources of Error.*** The techniques described for cardiac output measurement by application of Fick's principle assume that a steady state exists; that is, that the cardiac output and oxygen consumption are constant during the period of measurement. Therefore, strict quiet, calm, and decorum must be maintained in the catheterization laboratory during this time, to encourage the achievement of a steady state condition. Potential errors in the determination of cardiac output by the Fick oxygen technique may come from a number of sources, among which are the following:

(1) *Incomplete collection of the expired air sample when the Douglas bag method is used* may result in underestimation of oxygen consumption and, therefore, of cardiac output. Malfunction of the rubber fittings within the unidirectional air-flow valves in the patient's mouthpiece is a common problem. The technician should observe these valves to see that they open freely and close snugly with inspiration and expiration, respectively. Having the patient take deep slow breaths will help proper function of the valves, whose inertia may not allow adequate response to rapid, shallow respirations.

Perforated ear drums, an air leak around the mouthpiece (e.g., from loose dentures), or incomplete clamping of the nostrils are also common causes of incomplete air collection. If the patient's ear drums are perforated, rubber ear plugs should be used. Careful attention given by the technician collecting the expired air sample to holding the patient's lips firmly around the mouthpiece and to proper placement of the nose clamp will obviate some of these problems.

These problems are obviated with the use of the MRM technique with either hood or face-mask method. However, with these methods it is essential that a tight seal be obtained with the hood or face mask, so that room air entering the hood or face mask must flow across the patient's face before exiting through the tube connected to the polarographic sensor (Fig. 8-4), and all the patient's expired air is evacuated towards the sensor.

(2) *Changes in mean pulmonary volume* can result in a major error in oxygen consumption and cardiac output calculations. It is clear from the foregoing descriptions that the Douglas bag expired air method, as well as the MRM method, do not measure the amount of oxygen entering the blood each

minute; instead, they measure (at best) the amount of oxygen entering the lungs each minute. Since the lungs could act as a reservoir, oxygen *consumption* by the body is not necessarily measured by these techniques. For example, if a patient progressively increases his pulmonary volume by 300 ml/min, by the end of a three-minute collection of expired air he will have taken into his lungs 900 ml of air (or 180 ml of oxygen) more than that necessary for his steady state metabolic oxygen requirements. This extra 180 ml of oxygen, which is now in his "pulmonary reservoir," will falsely elevate the estimate of his actual oxygen consumption and cardiac output. If his actual oxygen consumption is 250 ml/min, then his "measured" oxygen consumption will be 250 + (180/3) = 310 ml/min, and this will result in a 24% error in the cardiac output calculation. In practice, the error probably occurs more often in the opposite direction, since when patients first have their nose clamps placed and start breathing into the mouthpiece or when they are first placed in the MRM hood, they may become somewhat "claustrophobic" and tend to breathe faster and deeper (during the equilibration period) than they do later during the actual expired air collection. This obviously results in an *artifactual underestimation of oxygen consumption* and cardiac output.

(3) As can be seen from Figure 8-5, the Douglas bag method assumes that the patient's minute ventilation (step 8) can be calculated from the measurement of the volume of expired air, and this assumption in turn requires that the volume of air entering the lungs per minute equals the volume of air leaving the lungs per minute (in a steady state). However, this is not quite true, even in a steady state, since the ratio of carbon dioxide molecules produced to oxygen molecules consumed does not equal unity. In fact, this ratio (the respiratory quotient) varies depending on the diet and metabolic state of the patient. Thus, a small error is introduced into the measurement of the oxygen consumption as calculated here because *the volume of carbon dioxide expired is not exactly equal to the volume of oxygen taken up.* A correction for this, assuming a respiration quotient of 0.8, is performed in some catheterization laboratories.

An example of the error introduced by neglecting the respiratory quotient follows:

Suppose a patient breathes in 5.00 L of air/min, and that the inspired air contains 20% oxygen and 80% nitrogen. From the 5000 ml of air, the patient extracts 250 ml of oxygen (his oxygen consumption) but returns only 200 ml of carbon dioxide, as would be expected if his respiratory quotient is 0.8. The expired air collection will then contain 4000 ml nitrogen, 750 ml of oxygen, and 200 ml of carbon dioxide, for a total volume of 4950 ml expired air. If analyzed as indicated in Figure 8-5, the calculations will indicate that oxygen difference between inspired and expired air is 48.5 ml/L, since inspired air contained 20% oxygen while expired air contained 15.15% oxygen (750 ml $O_2$/4950 ml air). By neglecting the respiratory quotient, it will be assumed that minute ventilation was 4.950 L/min, and therefore the oxygen consumption was 4.950 L air/min $\times$ 48.5 ml $O_2$/L air = 240 ml $O_2$/min. Since the true oxygen consumption in this example was 250 ml/min, we can see that neglecting the respiratory quotient leads to an underestimation in both the oxygen consumption and cardiac output calculations.

(4) *Incorrect timing of the expired air collection* may be a problem when the Douglas bag technique is used, and it is best to use either a hand-held stop watch or some other precision timing device. Some laboratories use a five-minute period for collection of expired air to minimize errors related to inaccuracies of timing, or the problem of beginning and ending at different phases of the respiratory cycle.

(5) *The spectrophotometric determination of blood oxygen saturation* may introduce inaccuracies related to carboxyhemoglobin or other abnormal hemoglobins, as discussed previously. This method may also be inaccurate if indocyanine green dye is present in the circulation. Therefore, indicator dilution curves should be done only after all samples for spectrophotometric oximetry have been taken. Reflectance oximetry, as performed on whole blood (e.g., Ao oximeter) is accurate in the range of blood oxygen saturations from 45 to 98% but may not be reliable when blood $O_2$ saturation is less than 40%, as is the case in pulmonary artery blood from patients with very low cardiac output or during strenuous exercise.

(6) *Improper collection of the mixed venous blood sample* (e.g., air bubbles) is a common source of error. Partial contamina-

tion of pulmonary arterial blood with pulmonary capillary wedge blood may result in a falsely high mixed venous oxygen content. If the mixed venous blood sample is taken from the right atrium, inferior vena cava, coronary sinus, or similar sites, a falsely low or high value for arteriovenous difference may result. Also, care must be taken not to dilute the blood sample with too much heparinized saline solution.

The average error in determining oxygen consumption has been estimated to be approximately 6%.[13] The error for arteriovenous oxygen difference has been estimated at 5%.[14,15] Narrow arteriovenous oxygen differences are more prone to introduce error than wide arteriovenous oxygen differences. Thus, *the Fick oxygen method is most accurate in patients with low cardiac output,* in whom the arteriovenous oxygen difference is wide. The total error in determination of the cardiac output by the Fick oxygen method has been estimated to be about 10%.[16]

*Does oxygen consumption actually need to be measured?* To avoid the technical difficulties and expense associated with measurement of oxygen consumption, some laboratories *assume* that $O_2$ consumption can be predicted from the body surface area, with or without a correction for age and sex. Thus, some laboratories assume that resting $O_2$ consumption is $125 \, ml/M^2$, or $110 \, ml/M^2$ for older patients. The validity of such an assumption has been addressed in a study from the University of Texas at Dallas.[17] Cardiac output was determined by the indicator dilution technique, and $O_2$ consumption was calculated by dividing cardiac output by arteriovenous oxygen difference, which was measured directly. In the 108 patients studied, $O_2$ consumption index averaged $126 \pm 26 \, ml/min/M^2$ (mean $\pm$ standard deviation), but there was wide variability as indicated by the standard deviation, and the authors concluded that $O_2$ consumption varies greatly among adults at the time of cardiac catheterization, and the assumption that $O_2$ consumption can be estimated as $125 \, ml/min/M^2$ is fraught with major potential error.

## Indicator Dilution Methods

The indicator dilution method is merely a specific application of Fick's general princi-

ple. In the Fick oxygen method, the "indicator" is oxygen, the site of injection is the lungs, and the injection procedure is that of continuous infusion. Stewart was the first to use the so-called indicator dilution method for measuring cardiac output; he used the continuous infusion technique and reported his first studies in 1897.[18]

There are two general types of indicator dilution method: the continuous infusion method and the single injection method. The single injection method is the most widely used and is discussed here in detail. The fundamental requirements for this method include the following:

1. A bolus of nontoxic indicator substance, which mixes completely with blood and whose concentration can be measured accurately, is injected.
2. The indicator substance is neither added to nor subtracted from the blood during passage between injection and sampling site.
3. Most of the indicator must pass the site of sampling before recirculation begins.
4. The indicator substance must go through a portion of the central circulation where all the blood of the body becomes mixed.

For the single injection method, theoretical considerations may be summarized as follows. An injection of a specified amount of an indicator (I) into a proximal vessel or chamber (e.g., the vena cava or right atrium for the thermodilution method, and the pulmonary artery for the indocyanine green dye method) is followed by continuous measurement of the indicator concentration (C) in blood as a function of time (t) at a point downstream from the injection (e.g., pulmonary artery for thermodilution technique, radial or femoral artery for indocyanine green dye method). Since all of the injection indicator, I, must pass the downstream measurement site,

$$I = \dot{Q} \int_0^\infty C(t)dt$$

where $\dot{Q}$ is the volume flow (ml/min) between the sites of injection and measurement. Thus $\dot{Q}$ (which is the cardiac output in the methods to be described) may be calculated as:

$$\dot{Q} = \frac{I}{\int_0^\infty C(t)dt}$$

Numerous indicators have been successfully employed, and the history of this subject is reviewed thoroughly by Guyton.[1] Indocyanine green has enjoyed long-standing acceptance in clinical practice, although recently thermodilution (in which "cold" is the indicator) has become more widely used.

***Indocyanine Green Method.*** Typically, indocyanine green solution is prepared with a concentration of 5 mg/ml, and 1.0 ml is injected on the right side of the circulation as a bolus (commonly into the pulmonary artery). Samples are taken from a peripheral systemic artery (e.g., the brachial, radial, or femoral artery). Sampling is done by continuous withdrawal of arterial blood at a constant rate (at least 15 ml/min) through a densitometer cuvette capable of measuring the concentration of indocyanine green dye in the blood. Injection must be made as a precise bolus, and the catheter through which the injection is made must be flushed immediately to ensure that the total amount of indicator has been delivered into the circulation and is not partially sitting in the catheter, stopcocks, or connecting tubing. The densitometer records a concentration curve such as that in Figure 8-7, which is calibrated by passing known concentrations of dye in blood through the densitometer cuvette. Note the lag between injection (time zero) and the point of first appearance of green dye in the arterial blood (A), the steep rise to a peak (B), and the subsequent gradual decline of the indicator dilution curve which is interrupted by a secondary rise (C) due to recirculation of the indicator substance.

The problem of isolating data related only to the first pass of the indicator has been attacked by several investigators, but the method originally proposed by Kinsman, Moore, and Hamilton[19] is perhaps the best known. This method depends on replotting the curve on semilog paper, as shown in Figure 8-8. Note that the downslope of the curve to the point of recirculation is essentially a straight line. Kinsman et al. showed mathematically that the true or "first pass" curve will be obtained by plotting the concentration decline on a semilog scale and extrapolating the early linear part of the plot. Therefore, the dotted line of Figure 8-8 completes the true curve, which could then be replotted in Figure 8-7.

To calculate the cardiac output, we use a special application of Fick's principle: $\dot{Q} =$

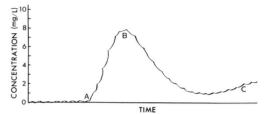

**Fig. 8-7.** Indicator dilution concentration curve in a patient with normal cardiac output: 1.0 ml of indocyanine green dye solution (5.0 mg/ml), was injected into the pulmonary artery at time zero. Blood was withdrawn continuously from the brachial artery through a densitometer cuvette, and the time-concentration curve from the densitometer was recorded. First appearance (A) is followed by a steep rise to peak concentration (B), and the subsequent gradual decline of the indicator curve, which is interrupted by a secondary rise (C) due to recirculation of the indicator substance.

$I/(\overline{C} \times t)$, where Q is the flow rate (in this case, the cardiac output), I is the amount of indicator injected, $\overline{C}$ is the average concentration of indicator during the first pass, and t is the total duration of the curve. The product $\overline{C} \times t$ is easily measured as the area under the first pass curve, determined by

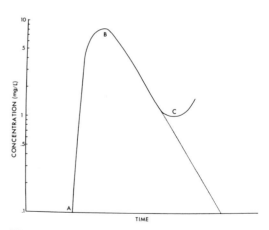

**Fig. 8-8.** Replotting of the indicator-dilution curve from Figure 8-6 on semilog paper. Note that the downslope of the curve to the point of recirculation is essentially a straight line. It can be shown mathematically[19] that the true or "first pass" curve is given by such a semilogarithmic replot of the concentration curve, and by extrapolating the early linear part of the concentration decline, as illustrated here by the dotted line. See text for details.

planimetry. This may be further simplified by the use of any number of available computer methods in which the semilog replotting, area computation, and cardiac output calculation are all accomplished electronically.

### Practical Aspects of Indocyanine Green Dye Curves.

A typical cardiac output determination may be accomplished as follows. Catheters are placed in the pulmonary artery and brachial or femoral artery, and hemodynamic measurements are recorded. The arterial catheter is connected by short stiff plastic tubing to a densitometer cuvette, which is then connected to a 30- to 50-ml syringe mounted in a constant withdrawal pump. A precise bolus of 1.0 ml of a solution containing 5.0 mg of indocyanine green/ml is loaded into the right heart catheter (if its capacity is greater than 1.5 ml, as is true for most 7 French and 8 French catheters) and the arterial withdrawal pump is turned on. As blood passes through the densitometer cuvette (e.g., at a withdrawal rate of 20 ml/min), the densitometer is carefully adjusted until a stable zero reading is obtained. At that moment, the green dye bolus is loaded in the right heart catheter and immediately flushed into the circulation with approximately 10 ml of heparinized saline solution. The densitometer concentration curve is recorded at a slow paper speed (e.g., 10 mm/sec) until the curve has been recorded through part or all of its recirculation phase.

The arterial blood in the withdrawal syringe may be returned to the patient if desired by utilizing strictly aseptic precautions. Alternatively, the contents of the syringe may be used in obtaining the calibration curve after the catheterization. This is obtained by adding indocyanine green dye to the patient's blood in varying amounts and plotting the known concentration *increments* (they are not necessarily absolute concentrations, since there may be some green dye in the blood used for making the calibration samples) against the densitometer deflections that result when each sample is passed through the densitometer. The slope of the resultant calibration line ($D_s$, which is mg green dye/L/mm deflection), the area of the first pass curve (A, which is mm deflection × sec), and the amount of injected indicator (I, which in this case was 5.0 mg) are then used to calculate cardiac output, as follows:

$$\text{Cardiac Output (L/min)} = \frac{I}{A \times D_s} \times 60 \text{ (sec/min)}$$

Sixty is inserted to convert the output from liters/second to liters/minute. As can be seen, this equation is obtained by substitution in the fundamental indicator dilution equation given earlier in this chapter.

One can see from this example that, since I and $D_s$ are likely to be constant from patient to patient, cardiac output will be an inverse function of the area of the indicator dilution curve. Low outputs are associated with curves of large area, and high outputs are associated with curves of small area.

### Sources of Error.

Firm adherence to certain principles and procedures will help one to obtain accurate cardiac output determinations with the indicator dilution technique. For the *indocyanine green dye technique*, these principles include:

1. The indocyanine green dye solution should be freshly prepared each day and shielded from the light until ready for use (it is unstable with time and exposure to light).

2. The indicator must be introduced into the circulation as a single bolus over as brief an injection interval as possible.

3. The exact amount of dye injected must be known, and loss of indicator in stopcocks or other parts of the injecting system should be prevented. For example, if 1.0 ml of indocyanine green dye solution (5.0 mg/ml) is to be injected, the inadvertent loss of only 0.1 ml will result in a 10% error in the cardiac output calculation.

4. To be certain that the indicator is completely mixed with the blood, there should be a "mixing chamber" (ventricle) between the sites of injection and sampling.

5. The dilution curve obtained must have an exponential downslope of sufficient length to allow accurate extrapolation of the first-pass curve. Guyton suggests that it is unreasonable to use the semilog plot method for extrapolating the downslope of an indicator dilution curve if recirculation of the indicator begins before the halfway mark on the recorded downslope.[1] With severe valvular regurgitation or very low output states, the first-pass curve may be so prolonged that recirculation begins before the downslope of the primary curve has been inscribed, making accurate determination of cardiac output impossible by this method. For this reason, the green dye technique is least accurate in

low-output states, and most accurate in high-output states, in contrast to the Fick oxygen method, for which the reverse is true.

In addition to low-output states, intracardiac shunts that lead to "early recirculation" (see Chapter 12) of indicator invalidate this method of calculating cardiac output.

6. The withdrawal rate of the arterial sample must be constant. Air bubbles in the withdrawal tubing or syringe alter the rate of blood withdrawal and may result in artifactual alteration in the shape of the dilution curve. All connections, therefore, must be airtight and well flushed with saline.

*Thermodilution Method.* A thermal indicator method for measuring cardiac output was first introduced by Fegler[20] in 1954, but was not applied to the clinical situation until the work of Branthwaite[21] and Ganz et al.[22,23] In the initial report by Ganz et al.,[22] two thermistors were used: one in the superior vena cava at the site at which the cold dextrose solution was injected into the bloodstream, and a second "downstream" thermistor in the pulmonary artery. These two thermistors allowed accurate measurement of the temperature of the injectate ($T_I$) as well as the temperature of blood ($T_B$) downstream from the injectate. Using the basic indicator dilution equation, the cardiac output by thermodilution ($CO_{TD}$) in ml is given as:

$$CO_{TD} = \frac{V_I(T_B - T_I)(S_I \cdot C_I/S_B \cdot C_B)60 \text{ (sec/min)}}{\int_0^\infty \Delta T_B(t)dt}$$

where $V_I$ = volume of injectate (ml); $S_B$, $S_I$, $C_B$, and $C_I$ are the specific gravity and specific heat of blood and injectate, respectively. When 5% dextrose is used as an indicator, $(S_I \cdot C_I/S_B \cdot C_B)$ equals 1.08. Most commercially used thermodilution systems employ a single thermistor only, placed at the downstream site, and assume that the temperature of the injectate (measured in a bowl prior to injection) increases by a predictable amount ("catheter warming") during injection. The calculated cardiac output by the thermodilution equation is multiplied by an empiric correction factor (0.825) to correct for the catheter warming.[23,24] The thermodilution method for measuring cardiac output has several advantages over the indocyanine green dye method, and these include:

1. It does not require withdrawal of blood.
2. It does not require an arterial puncture.
3. An inert and inexpensive indicator is used.
4. There is virtually no recirculation, making computer analysis of the primary curve simple.

*Sources of Error.* 1. The method will be unreliable in the presence of significant tricuspid regurgitation.

2. The baseline temperature of blood in the pulmonary artery usually shows distinct fluctuations associated with respiratory and cardiac cycles. If these fluctuations are large, they may approach the magnitude of the temperature change produced by the "cold" indicator injection.

3. Loss of injected indicator ("cold") between injection and measuring sites (vena cava and pulmonary artery) is not usually a problem, but in low-flow, low-output states loss of indicator may occur due to warming of blood by the walls of the cardiac chambers and surrounding tissues. This concern is supported by the study of Grondelle et al.[25] who found that thermodilution cardiac output measurements overestimated cardiac output consistently in patients with low output (<3.5 L/min) and this overestimation was greatest, averaging 35%, in patients whose cardiac outputs were <2.5 L/min. This is what might be expected from the equation for calculation of cardiac output by thermodilution, since the change in pulmonary artery blood temperature ($\Delta T_B$) will be reduced if cold is lost by warming of the injectate during slow passage through the vena cava, right atrium, and right ventricle. Because $\Delta T_B$ is the denominator in the equation for cardiac output calculation, reduction in $\Delta T_B$ will result in a rise in calculated cardiac output.

4. The empiric correction factor of 0.825 may be inadequate to correct for deviations in true injectate temperature from the temperature of the injectate bowl or reservoir, due to warming in the syringe, by the hand of the individual injecting the dextrose solution from the syringe, or by catheter warming.

In general, indicator dilution cardiac output determinations have an error of 5% to 10% when performed carefully. The values obtained correlate well with those calculated by the Fick oxygen method.

# REFERENCES

1. Guyton AC, Jones CE, Coleman TG: Circulatory Physiology: Cardiac Output and Its Regulation. Philadelphia, WB Saunders, 1973, pp 4–80.
2. Dexter L, et al: Effect of exercise on circulatory dynamics of normal individuals. J Appl Physiol 3:439, 1951.
3. Berkson J, Boothby WB: Studies of metabolism of normal individuals. Comparison of estimation of basal metabolism from linear formula and surface area. Am J Physiol 116:485, 1936.
4. Dubois EF: Basal Metabolism in Health and Disease. Philadelphia, Lea & Febiger, 1936.
5. Holt JP, Rhode EA, Kines H: Ventricular volumes and body weight in mammals. Am J Physiol 215:704, 1968.
6. Brandfonbrener M, Landowne M, Shock NW: Changes in cardiac output with age. Circulation 12:556, 1955.
7. Fick A: Uber die Messung des Blutquantums in den Herzventrikeln. Sitz der Physik-Med ges Wurtzberg 1870, p 16.
8. Shock NW, Norris AH: *In* Altman PL, Dittmer DS (eds): Respiration and Circulation. Biological Handbooks. Bethesda, Federation of American Societies for Experimental Biology, 1971, pp 322–324.
9. Van Slyke DD, Neill JM: The determination of gases in blood and other solutions by vacuum extraction and manometric measurements. J Biol Chem 61:523, 1924.
10. Bernhart FW, Skeggs L: The iron content of crystalline human hemoglobin. J Biol Chem 147:19, 1943.
11. Diem K, (ed): Documenta Geigy—Scientific Tables. 6th ed. Ardsley, NY, Geigy Pharmaceuticals, 1962, p 578.
12. Dexter L, et al: Studies of congenital heart disease. II: The pressure and oxygen content of blood in the right auricle, right ventricle, and pulmonary artery in control patients. J Clin Invest 26:554, 1947.
13. Barratt-Boyes BG, Wood EH: The oxygen saturation of blood in the venae cavae, right heart chambers, and pulmonary vessels of healthy subjects. J Lab Clin Med 50:93, 1957.
14. Selzer A, Sudrann RB: Reliability of the determination of cardiac output in man by means of the Fick principle. Circ Res 6:485, 1958.
15. Thomassen B: Cardiac output in normal subjects under standard conditions. The repeatability of measurements by the Fick method. Scand J Clin Lab Invest 9:365, 1957.
16. Visscher MB, Johnson JA: The Fick principle: analysis of potential errors in its conventional application. J Appl Physiol 5:635, 1953.
17. Dehmer GJ, Firth BG, Hillis LD: Oxygen consumption in adult patients during cardiac catheterization. Clin Cardiol 5:436, 1982.
18. Stewart GN: Researches on the circulation time and on the influences which affect it. IV: The output of the heart. J Physiol 22:159, 1897.
19. Kinsman JM, Moore JW, Hamilton WF: Human studies on the circulation. I: Injection method. Physical and mathematical considerations. Am J Physiol 89:322, 1929.
20. Fegler G: Measurement of cardiac output in anesthetized animals by a thermodilution method. Q. J Exp Physiol 39:153, 1954.
21. Branthwaite MA, Bradley RD: Measurement of cardiac output by thermal dilution in man. J Appl Physiol 24:434, 1968.
22. Ganz W, et al: A new technique for measurement of cardiac output by thermodilution in man. Am J Cardiol 27:392, 1971.
23. Forrester JS, et al: Thermodilution cardiac output determination with a single flow-directed catheter. Am Heart J 83:306, 1972.
24. Weisel RD, Berger RL, Hechtman HB: Measurement of cardiac output by thermodilution. N Engl J Med 292:682, 1975.
25. Grondelle AV, et al: Thermodilution method overestimates low cardiac output in humans. Am J Physiol 245 (Heart Circ Physiol 14):H690, 1983.

*chapter nine*

# Pressure Measurement

WILLIAM GROSSMAN

T HE MEASUREMENT of dynamic blood pressure has been of interest to physiologists and physicians since 1732, when Reverend Stephen Hales measured the blood pressure of a horse by using a vertical glass tube.[1] Methodology has advanced impressively since Reverend Hales' day, but with increased technical capability has come greater complexity of instrumentation, so that few physicians today have a firm understanding of the instruments on which they rely.

## THE INPUT SIGNAL: WHAT IS A PRESSURE WAVE?

Force is transmitted through a fluid medium as a pressure wave, and an important objective of the cardiac catheterization procedure is to assess accurately the forces and therefore the pressure waves generated by various cardiac chambers. For example, a ventricular pressure wave may be considered *a complex periodic fluctuation in force per unit area,* with one cycle consisting of the time interval from the onset of one systole to the onset of the subsequent systole. The number of times the cycle occurs in one second is termed the *fundamental frequency* of cardiac pressure generation. Thus, a fundamental frequency of two corresponds to a heart rate of 120 beats/minute. Definitions of terms relevant to the theory and practice of pressure measurement are listed in Table 9-1.

Considered as a complex periodic wave form, the pressure wave may be subjected to a type of analysis developed by the French physicist Fourier, whereby any complex wave form may be considered the mathematical summation of a series of simple sine waves of differing amplitude and frequency. As may be surmised from Figure 9-1, even the most complex wave form can be represented by its own Fourier series. The practical consequence of this analysis is that, in order to record pressure accurately, a system must respond with equal amplitude for a given input throughout the range of frequencies contained within the pressure wave. If components in a particular frequency range are either suppressed or exaggerated by the transducer system, the recorded signal will be a grossly distorted version of the original physiologic wave form. For example, the dicrotic notch of the aortic pressure wave contains frequencies above 10 cycles per second. If the pressure measurement system were unable to respond to frequencies greater than 10 cycles per second, the notch would be slurred or absent.

## PRESSURE MEASURING DEVICES

The manometer used by Starling, Wiggers, and others[2] was a modification of that devised by Hürthle[3] in 1888 and is illustrated in Figure 9-2. A rubber tambour was coupled with a writing lever that recorded change in pressure on a rotating smoked drum. The

**TABLE 9-1.** *Definitions of Terms Relevant to the Theory and Practice of Pressure Measurement*

| Term | Definition |
|---|---|
| Pressure wave | Complex periodic fluctuation in force per unit area. Units: *dynes/cm$^2$*: 1 dyne/cm$^2$ = 1 microbar = $10^{-1}$ N/M$^2$ = 7.5 × $10^{-4}$ mmHg<br>*mmHg:* 1 mmHg = 1 Torr = 1/760 atmospheric pressure |
| Fundamental frequency | Number of times the pressure wave cycles in 1 second |
| Fourier analysis | Resolution of any complex periodic wave into a series of single sine waves of differing frequency and amplitude |
| Sensitivity of pressure measurement system | Ratio of the amplitude of the recorded signal to the amplitude of the input signal |
| Frequency response of pressure measurement system | Ratio of output amplitude to input amplitude over a range of frequencies of the input pressure wave |
| Natural frequency | The frequency at which the pressure measurement system oscillates or responds when shock-excited; also, the frequency of an input pressure wave at which the ratio of output/input amplitude of an undamaged system is maximal. Units: cycles/sec, Hz. |
| Damping | Dissipation of the energy of oscillation of a pressure measurement system, due to friction. Units: Damping coefficient, D (see text) |
| Optimal damping | Damping that progressively blunts the increase in output/input ratio that occurs with increasing frequency of pressure wave input. Optimal damping can maintain frequency response "flat" (output/input ratio = 1) to 88% of the natural frequency of the system. |
| Strain gauge | Variable resistance transducer in which the strain ($\Delta$L/L) on a series of wires is determined by the pressure on the transducer's diaphragm. Over a wide range, electrical resistance (R) of the wire is directly proportional to $\Delta$L/L. |
| Wheatstone bridge | Arrangement of electrical connections in a strain gauge such that pressure-induced changes in resistance result in proportional changes in voltage across the bridge |
| Balancing a transducer | Interpolating a variable resistance across the output of a Wheatstone bridge/strain gauge transducer so that atmospheric pressure at the "zero level" (e.g., midchest) induces an arbitrary voltage output on the monitor/recording device (i.e., a voltage that positions the transducer output on the oscilloscopic pressure "baseline") |

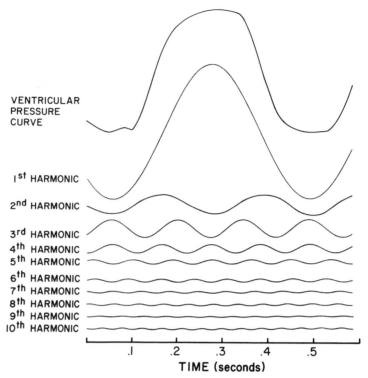

**Fig. 9-1.** Resolution of a normal ventricular pressure curve (top) into its first ten harmonics by Fourier analysis. If components in a particular frequency range (e.g., the third harmonic, which in this case is 7 cycles per second) were either suppressed or exaggerated by the transducer system, the recorded signal would be a grossly distorted version of the original physiologic signal. (Adapted from Wiggers.[2])

system had a high inertia and a low elasticity, giving it a narrow range of usefulness.

*Sensitivity.* The sensitivity of such a measurement system may be defined as the ratio of the amplitude of the recorded signal to the amplitude of the input signal. With the Hürthle manometer, the more rigid the sensing membrane, the lower the sensitivity; conversely, the more flaccid the membrane, the higher the sensitivity. This general principle applies to manometers currently employed.

*Frequency Response.* A second crucial property of any pressure measurement system is its frequency response. The frequency response of a pressure measurement system may be defined as the ratio of output amplitude/input amplitude over a range of frequencies of the input pressure wave. To accurately measure pressures, the frequency response (amplitude ratio) must be constant over a sufficient range of frequency varia-

tion. Otherwise, the amplitude of major frequency components of the pressure wave form may be attenuated while minor components are amplified, so that the recorded wave form becomes a distorted caricature of the physiologic event. Referring again to the Hürthle manometer, the range of good frequency response may be improved by stiffening the membrane, or it may be narrowed by making the membrane more flaccid, because the flaccid membrane cannot respond well to higher frequencies. Thus, it should be apparent that frequency response and sensitivity are related reciprocally, and one can be obtained only by sacrificing the other.

*Natural Frequency and Damping.* A third important concept is the natural frequency of a sensing membrane and the way it determines the degree of damping required for optimal recording. If the sensing membrane were shock-excited (like a gong), in

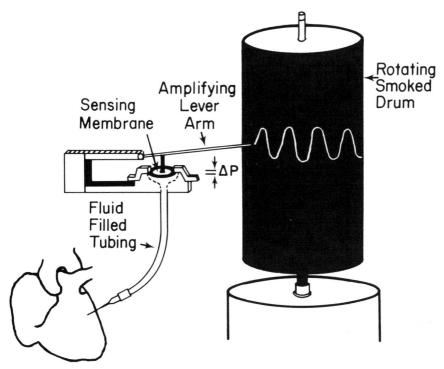

**Fig. 9-2.** Schematic illustration of the Hürthle manometer. A rubber tambour serves as the sensing membrane and is coupled with an amplifying lever arm that records changes in pressure ($\Delta$P) on a rotating smoked drum. Pressure is transmitted from the heart (lower left hand corner) to the sensing membrane by fluid-filled tubing.

the absence of friction it would oscillate for an indefinite period of time in simple harmonic motion. The frequency of this motion would be the natural frequency of the system. Any means of dissipating the energy of this system, such as friction, is called *damping*. The dynamic response characteristics of such a system are largely determined by the natural frequency and the degree of damping that the system possesses.[4]

The importance of proper damping is illustrated in Figure 9-3. Note that the amplitude of an input signal tends to be augmented as the frequency of that signal approaches the natural frequency of the sensing membrane. Optimal damping dissipates the energy of the oscillating sensing membrane gradually and thereby maintains the frequency response curve nearly flat (constant output/input ratio) as it approaches the region of the pressure measurement system's natural frequency.

As an analogy to further help the reader understand the significance of damping, con-sider the simple case of a weight suspended from a spring. If the weight is displaced and then released, the stretched spring will recoil so that the weight will move past its original position and will then oscillate up and down. In the absence of frictional forces *(damping)*, the oscillation would continue indefinitely at a frequency determined by the stiffness of the spring and an amplitude determined by the mass of the weight. In practice there is always some damping, and this has two effects: (1) the *amplitude* of the oscillations gradually dies away, and (2) the *frequency* of oscillation is reduced. This second important consequence of damping—to reduce the natural frequency of a system—is not widely appreciated. If we continue with our analogy, imagine that the spring and its weight are suspended in a jar of syrup or honey; it will clearly vibrate with lesser amplitude of vibration *and* lesser frequency. The effect of the viscous medium is to further damp the oscillations, and if its viscosity is high enough, it will prevent any overshoot

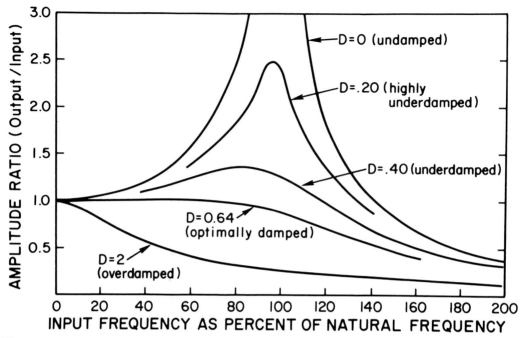

**Fig. 9-3.** Frequency response curves of a pressure measurement system, illustrating the importance of optimal damping. The amplitude of an input signal tends to be augmented as the frequency of that signal approaches the natural frequency of the sensing membrane. Optimal damping dissipates the energy of the oscillating sensing membrane gradually and thereby maintains a nearly flat natural frequency curve (constant output/input ratio) as it approaches the region of the pressure measurement system's natural frequency. D = damping coefficient. (See text.)

or oscillation: the weight will return to its original position regardless of its initial displacement. Further damping at this point will simply slow the return of the weight to its equilibrium position, thereby depressing the frequency response characteristics of the system. Thus, damping helps to prevent overshoot artifacts resulting from resonance of the system, but at the cost of frequency response.

## WHAT FREQUENCY RESPONSE IS DESIRABLE?

Wiggers suggested[2] that the shortest "significant" vibrations contained within physiologic pressure waves have one tenth the period of the entire pressure curve; that is, the essential physiologic information is contained within the first ten harmonics of the pressure wave's Fourier series. At a heart rate of 120 beats/minute, the fundamental

frequency is 2 cycles per second and the tenth harmonic is 20 cycles per second. Thus, a pressure measurement system with a frequency response range that is flat to 20 cycles per second should be adequate in such a circumstance, and support for this has come from experimental work comparing high frequency response systems with conventional catheter systems.[5]

The useful frequency response range of commonly used pressure measurement systems is generally less than 20 cycles per second unless special care is taken. Wood et al[6] and Gleason and Braunwald[7] found that frequency response was flat to less than 10 cycles per second with small-bore (6 French) catheters attached to standard strain gauge manometers.

To ensure a high frequency response range, the pressure measurement system must be set up in such a way that it has the highest possible *natural frequency* as well as *optimal damping*. The natural frequency is directly proportional to the lumen radius of the catheter system. It is inversely proportional to the length of the catheter and associated tubing and to the square root of the catheter and tubing compliance and the density of fluid filling the system. The highest natural frequency will thus be obtained by using a short, wide-bore, stiff catheter connected to its transducer without intervening tubing or stopcocks and filled with a low density liquid from which small air bubbles, which increase compliance, have been excluded (e.g., boiled saline solution). Such a system may well be impractical for routine use, but it is important to bear in mind that deviation from such a system occurs only at a significant sacrifice.

If such a system is constructed, it will be found to be grossly underdamped (see Fig. 9-3). Accordingly, it will be important to introduce damping into the system to keep the frequency response flat as the frequency of the input signal approaches the natural frequency of the pressure measurement system. With optimal damping, the frequency response can be maintained flat ($\pm 5\%$) to within 88% of the natural frequency according to Fry,[4] although it is unusual to achieve more than 50% in most laboratories. Damping may be introduced by interposing a "damping needle" between the catheter and manometer[6] and gradually shortening it until optimal damping is obtained, by filling the manometer or tubing with a viscous medium, such as Renografin (a radiographic contrast agent); or by any of several other methods.

## EVALUATION OF FREQUENCY RESPONSE CHARACTERISTICS

Ideally, the frequency response characteristics of a pressure measurement system should be evaluated using a sine wave pressure generator to construct curves similar to those seen in Figure 9-3. By altering the characteristics of the system discussed just previously, a reasonable compromise between frequency response, damping, and practicality can be achieved for each laboratory. Such a sine wave pressure generator has become commercially available.* An example of the use of this device in estimating frequency

response of a pressure measurement system is seen in Figure 9-4.

Another method, which does not require the use of such a pressure waveform generator, is described here. This technique may be used for measuring the dynamic response characteristics of a pressure measurement system.

The catheter to be studied is connected by means of a three-way stopcock with or without intervening tubing to one arm of a strain gauge transducer (Fig. 9-5). The transducer used should be of the low-volume-displacement type (small chamber capacity) to enhance frequency response. The tip of the catheter is snugly projected through a hole in a No. 6 rubber stopper, which is tightly inserted into the cut-off barrel of a 60-ml plastic syringe.* The syringe plunger has been removed, and the barrel is fixed in a vertical position, pointing downward, so that the catheter enters from below. The manometer and catheter are filled with saline solution, care being taken to avoid even small air bubbles, and the catheter is flushed until the catheter tip and holes are submerged in approximately 30 ml of saline solution. The plunger is slowly inserted into the syringe, producing an upward deflection of the pressure trace on the recording apparatus oscilloscope. When the trace comes to rest at the top of the oscilloscope, the recorder is turned on at rapid paper speed and the plunger is suddenly withdrawn. This method, modified from Hansen,[8] produces shock excitation vibrations of the type seen in Figure 9-6. The mathematical foundation for analysis of such a shock excitation has been described by Wiggers[2] and Fry,[4] and may be summarized as follows:

The frequency of the after-vibrations produced by shock excitation is the damped natural frequency of the system. This is obtained by measuring the time, t, between two successive vibrations and obtaining the damped natural frequency, $N_D$ as $1/t$. In the example in Figure 9-6, $N_D = 1/0.04 = 25$ cycles/sec. Next, the damping coefficient D is calculated as a function of the ratio by which successive single vibrations decrease. In Figure 9-6, this may be calculated from the ratio of $x_2$ to $x_1$, the percent overshoot, as

*Millar instruments, Houston, TX.

*60-ml disposable plastic syringe, Monoject. Sherwood Medical Industries, Inc., DeLand, FL.

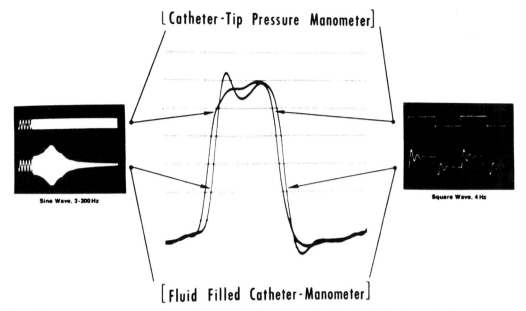

**Fig. 9-4.** Left ventricular pressure (center panel) measured using fluid-filled standard catheter and micromanometer (catheter-tip pressure manometer) in a patient undergoing cardiac catheterization. Left- and right-hand panels show in-vitro comparisons of frequency response for micromanometer (upper) and fluid-filled (lower) systems. The left-hand panel recordings were obtained by continuously increasing the input frequency of a sine-wave pressure waveform from 2 to 200 Hz. The fluid-filled system resonates (natural frequency) at 37 Hz, but was "flat" (±5%) only to 12 Hz. Therefore its useful range is only to ~12 Hz. The right-hand panel shows the response of each system to a square wave pressure-input signal. (From Nichols et al.: Percutaneous left ventricular catheterization with an ultraminiature catheter-tip pressure transducer. Cardiovasc. Res. 12:566, 1978, with permission.)

$D = \sqrt{\ln^2(x_2/x_1)/\{\pi^2 + \ln^2(x_2/x_1)\}}$, where $\ln(x_2/x_1)$ is the natural logarithm of the percent overshoot. In our example, $x_2/x_1 = 0.093$, $\ln(x_2/x_1) = -2.379$, and $D = 0.603$. From the damping coefficient D and the damped natural frequency $N_D$ we may determine the undamped natural frequency N as $N = N_D/\sqrt{1 - D^2}$. A simple practical goal is to try to regulate the damping of an actual pressure measurement system so that its damping coefficient is as close to 0.64 (so-called "optimal" damping) as possible. At this value, the pressure measurement system shows uniform frequency response (±5%) to about 88% of its natural frequency according to Fry.[2] If such optimal damping is achieved for the system illustrated in Figure 9-6, its frequency response could be considered flat to 0.88N = 27.5 cycles per second. Improperly damped systems with a low natural frequency (because of small air bubbles, excessively compliant tubing) may achieve uniform frequency response to less than 10 cycles per second.

## TRANSFORMING PRESSURE WAVES INTO ELECTRICAL SIGNALS: THE ELECTRICAL STRAIN GAUGE

Pressure measurement systems in use today are essentially all electrical strain gauges and employ the principle of the Wheatstone bridge. The strain gauge is a variable resistance transducer whose operation depends on a simple phenomenon: when a wire is stretched, its electrical resistance increases. As long as the strain remains well below the elastic limit of the wire, there is a wide range within which the increase in resistance is accurately proportional to the increase in length.

Figure 9-7 illustrates how the Wheatstone bridge employs this principle in converting a pressure signal into an electrical signal. In this schematic representation of a pressure transducer, pressure is transmitted through port P and acts on diaphragm D, which is

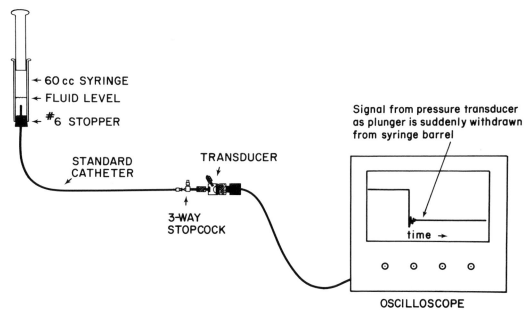

**Fig. 9-5.** Practical evaluation of dynamic response characteristics of catheter-transducer system. The catheter hub is connected by means of a three-way stopcock to one arm of a low-volume-displacement pressure transducer. The tip of the catheter is snugly projected through a hole in a No. 6 rubber stopper, which is tightly inserted into the cut-off barrel of a 60-ml plastic syringe. The manometer and catheter are filled with saline solution, care being taken to avoid even small air bubbles, and the catheter is flushed until the catheter tip and holes are submerged in approximately 30 ml of saline solution. Next, the plunger is slowly inserted into the syringe, producing an upward deflection of the pressure trace on the recording apparatus oscilloscope. When the pressure trace comes to rest at the top of the oscilloscope screen, the recorder is turned on and the plunger suddenly withdrawn from the syringe barrel. Dynamic response characteristics are then calculated as shown in Figure 9-6.

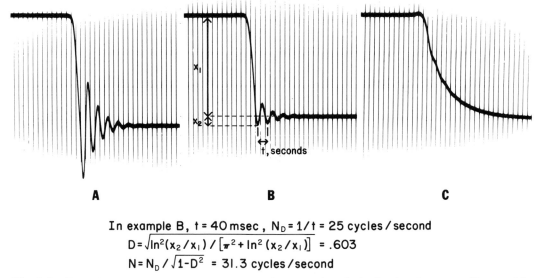

$$\text{In example B, } t = 40 \text{ msec}, \ N_D = 1/t = 25 \text{ cycles / second}$$
$$D = \sqrt{\ln^2(x_2/x_1) / [\pi^2 + \ln^2(x_2/x_1)]} = .603$$
$$N = N_D / \sqrt{1-D^2} = 31.3 \text{ cycles/second}$$

**Fig. 9-6.** Records of dynamic frequency response characteristics obtained using the system illustrated in Figure 9-5. Panels A, B, and C represent progressive increases in damping produced by introducing increasing amounts of a viscous radiographic contrast agent (Renografin-76) into the catheter-transducer system. The catheter was 80-cm long and its diameter was 8 French. Panel A is underdamped, Panel C overdamped, and Panel B nearly optimally damped. The percent overshoot $x_2/x_1$ is used in the calculation of the damping coefficient, D. The undamped natural frequency, $N$, is calculated from D and the damped natural frequency, $N_D$. Time lines are 20 msec. Using the curves illustrated in Figure 9-3 for various values of D, the frequency response of the system in Panel B can probably be considered flat ($\pm5\%$) to 0.88N = 27.5 cycles per second.

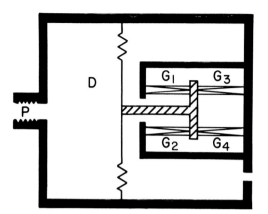

**Fig. 9-7.** Schematic representation of a strain-gauge pressure transducer. Pressure is transmitted through port P and acts on diaphragm D, which is vented to atmospheric pressure on its opposite side. Pressure on the diaphragm stretches and therefore increases the resistance of wires $G_1$ and $G_2$, while having the opposite effect on $G_3$ and $G_4$. The wires are electrically connected as shown in Figure 9-8.

vented to atmospheric pressure on its opposite side. The manner of attachment is such that increased pressure on the diaphragm stretches and therefore increases the electrical resistance of $G_1$ and $G_2$, while having the opposite effect on $G_3$ and $G_4$. In the Wheatstone bridge, $G_1$, $G_2$, $G_3$, and $G_4$ are electrically connected, as in Figure 9-8, and are attached to a voltage source, B. If all four resistances are equal, then exactly half the voltage of battery B will exist at the junction of $G_1$ and $G_4$, and also at the junction of $G_2$ and $G_3$, and therefore no current will flow between the output terminals. However, when pressure is applied to the diaphragm in Figure 9-7, the resistances are unbalanced, so that the junction of $G_1$ and $G_4$ becomes negative, and a current will flow across the output terminals.

Since movement of the diaphragm D in Figure 9-7 is necessary to produce current flow in the Wheatstone bridge, a certain volume of fluid must actually move through the catheter and connecting tubing to produce a recorded pressure. Therefore, the use of low-volume-displacement transducers with a small chamber volume will improve frequency response characteristics of the system.

*Balancing a transducer* is simply a process whereby a variable resistance (the R balance of most amplifiers) is interpolated into the circuit of Figure 9-8, so that at an arbitrary baseline pressure the voltage across the output terminal can be reduced to zero. Some currently employed amplifiers use an alternating current (A-C) signal in place of the DC current source in Figure 9-8. When these "carrier current" amplifiers are employed, it becomes necessary to utilize a variable capacitor (the C balance) as well as a variable resistor in balancing the bridge.

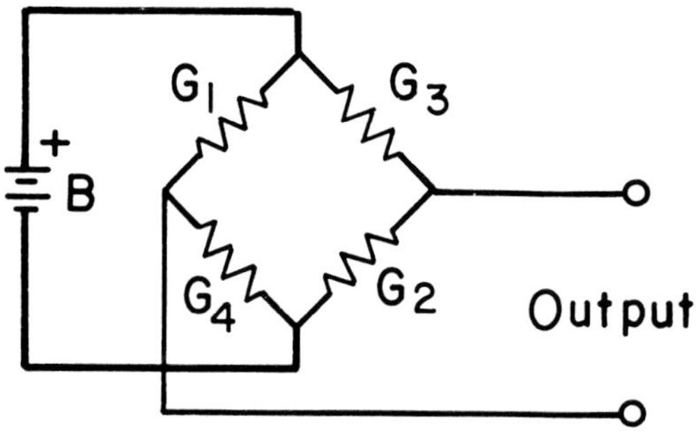

**Fig. 9-8.** Strain-gauge connection of the Wheatstone bridge. In this arrangement, if all resistances are equal, then exactly half the voltage of battery B will exist at the junction of $G_1$ and $G_4$ and also at the junction of $G_2$ and $G_3$, and therefore no current will flow between the output terminals. However, when pressure is applied to the diaphragm in Figure 9-7, the resistances are unbalanced, so that the junction of $G_1$ and $G_4$ becomes negative, and a current will flow across the output terminals.

## PRACTICAL PRESSURE TRANSDUCER SYSTEM FOR THE CATHETERIZATION LABORATORY

Trying to incorporate all of the principles discussed so far in this chapter, we have settled on a practical system in which a fluid-filled catheter is attached by means of a manifold to a small-volume-displacement strain-gauge type pressure transducer (Fig. 9-9). In the transducer we use (Gould Statham P50 transducer), the sensing element is a tiny silicon beam. When the diaphragm is deflected by positive or negative fluid pressure, the silicon beam is stressed, changing the resistance of the strain elements in a Wheatstone bridge circuit. The circuit delivers an electrical output proportional to the pressure being applied, as dis-

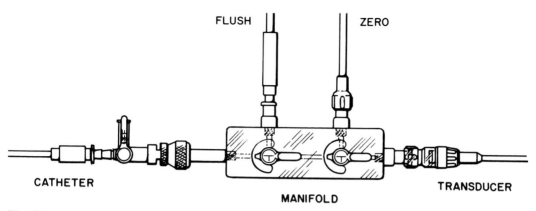

**Fig. 9-9.** A practical system for pressure measurement with excellent frequency response. The catheter is connected by a stopcock to a manifold, which is connected at its other end to a small volume fluid-filled pressure transducer. The manifold's two sidearms are connected by fluid-filled tubing to zero pressure level and to pressurized flush solution.

cussed previously. A small dome permits attachment to a two-stopcock manifold (Fig. 9-9). To the first sidearm of the manifold, a fluid-filled connecting tube is attached, the distal end of which is adjusted to midchest level (zero reference). The second sidearm is connected by a fluid-filled tube to a pressurized flush bag containing heparinized saline solution. The cardiac catheter is connected directly to the front of the manifold through a built-in rotating adaptor. By turning the stopcock attached to the flush solution, the catheter may be intermittently flushed clear of blood (e.g., every three minutes). Turning this stopcock the other way permits filling and flushing of the zero line or

the pressure transducer. With this system, a frequency response flat ±5% to >20 Hz can be achieved routinely. The transducers may be sterilized with gas or Cidex between uses.

## PHYSIOLOGIC CHARACTERISTICS OF PRESSURE WAVEFORMS

Recognizing the normal appearance of pressure waveforms is a prerequisite to identifying abnormalities that characterize certain cardiovascular disorders. As seen in Figure 9-10 *forward* pressure and flow waves as seen in the central aorta are intrinsically

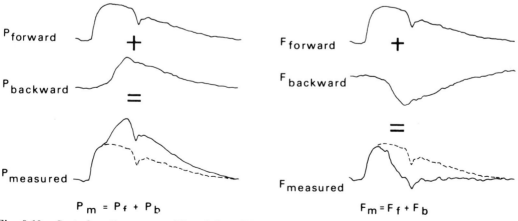

$$P_m = P_f + P_b$$

$$F_m = F_f + F_b$$

**Fig. 9-10.** Central aortic pressure (P) and flow (F) measured in a patient during cardiac catheterization. Computer-derived forward and backward pressure and flow components are shown individually: their sum results in the measured waves. See text for discussion. (From Murgo JP, et al., Circulation 63:122, 1981, with permission.)

identical in shape and timing. However, the pressure wave is modified by summation with a *reflected* pressure wave ($P_{backward}$), and the resultant *measured* central aortic pressure wave shows a steady increase throughout ejection.[9,10] The flow wave is also modified by summation with a reflected flow wave ($F_{backward}$), but since flow is directional, $F_{backward}$ reduces the magnitude of flow in late ejection, giving the characteristic $F_{measured}$ as is seen with aortic flow meters or doppler signals.

The reflections for pressure occur from many sites within the arterial tree, but the major effective reflection site in man appears to be the region of the terminal abdominal aorta.[10] As seen in Figure 9-11, ascending aortic pressure is substantially increased within 1 beat following bilateral occlusion of the femoral arteries by external manual compression (arrow, left). High speed recordings (right panel) show that the major part of the increase in pressure occurs late in systole, consistent with an increase in the magnitude of the reflected pressure.

Pressure reflections are diminished during the strain phase of the Valsalva maneuver,[9] with the result that pressure and flow waveforms become similar in appearance (Fig. 9-12). Following release of the Valsalva strain,

reflected waves return and are exaggerated. Thus the commonly noted late-peaking appearance of central aortic and left ventricular pressure tracings in man (Fig. 9-13), referred to as the type A waveform pattern,[9] is a result of strong pressure reflections in late systole. In addition to the Valsalva maneuver, pressure reflections are diminished during hypovolemia, hypotension, and in response to a variety of vasodilator agents. In these circumstances the left ventricular and central aortic pressure waves will exhibit a type C pattern (Fig. 9-13). On the other hand, vasoconstriction and hypertension may be expected to accentuate the normal type A waveform. Since the contribution of reflections to the arterial pressure waveform should move earlier in systole, it is not surprising that the closer one gets to the source of the reflections, the earlier the pressure peaks as the catheter is withdrawn from the central aorta to the periphery (Fig. 9-14).

## SOURCES OF ERROR AND ARTIFACT

Even when every effort has been made to design a pressure measurement system with

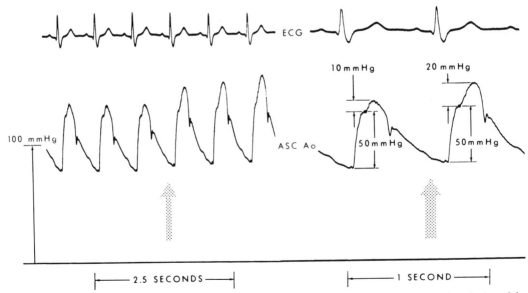

**Fig. 9-11.** Ascending aortic (ASC Ao) pressure waveform in a patient before and after bilateral occlusion of the femoral arteries by external manual compression (left, arrow). On the right, high speed recordings show that the major portion of the increase in pressure results from augmentation of the late (reflected) wave. (From Murgo JP, et al.: Circulation 62:105, 1980, with permission.)

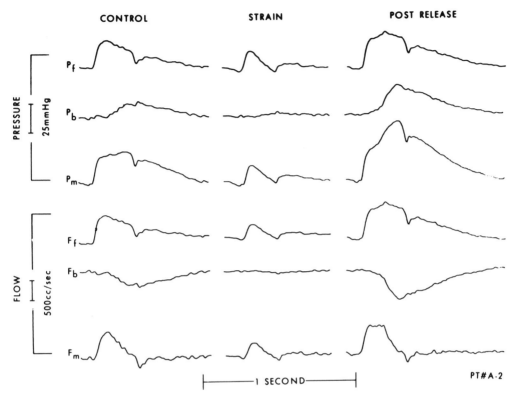

**Fig. 9-12.** Measurements of central aortic pressure ($P_m$) and flow ($F_m$) in a patient performing Valsalva maneuver during cardiac catheterization. Control, Valsalva strain, and post-Valsalva release tracings are shown. $P_m$ is the sum of forward ($P_f$) and backward or reflected ($P_b$) pressure waves, and $F_m$ is the sum of $F_f$ and $F_b$. See text for discussion. (Reproduced from Murgo JP, et al.: Circulation 63:122, 1981, with permission.)

high sensitivity, uniform frequency response, and optimal damping, distortions and inaccuracies in the pressure waveform may occur. Some of the common sources of error and artifact in clinical pressure measurement include deterioration in frequency response, catheter whip artifact, end-pressure artifact, catheter impact artifact, systolic pressure amplification in the periphery, and errors in zero level, balancing, and calibration.

***Deterioration in Frequency Response.*** Although frequency response may be high and damping optimal during setup of the transducers, substantial deterioration in the characteristics may develop in the course of a catheterization study. Air bubbles may be introduced into the catheters, stopcocks, or tubing during the catheterization procedure, or dissolved air may come out of the saline solution used to fill the transducer (just as dissolved air may come out of solution in a glass of water allowed to

stand unperturbed for a few hours). Even the smallest air bubbles have a drastic effect on pressure measurement as a result of lowering the natural frequency (by serving as an added compliance) as well as excessive damping. When the natural frequency of the pressure measurement system falls, rapid changes of pressure (such as those that occur with intraventricular pressure rise and fall) may set the system in oscillation producing the ventricular pressure "overshoot" commonly seen in early systole and diastole (Fig. 9-4 and 9-15).

***Catheter Whip Artifact.*** Motion of the tip of the catheter within the heart and great vessels accelerates the fluid contained within the catheter, and such catheter whip artifacts may produce superimposed waves of ±10 mmHg. Catheter whip artifacts are particularly common in tracings from the pulmonary arteries, and are difficult to avoid.

***End-Pressure Artifact.*** Flowing blood

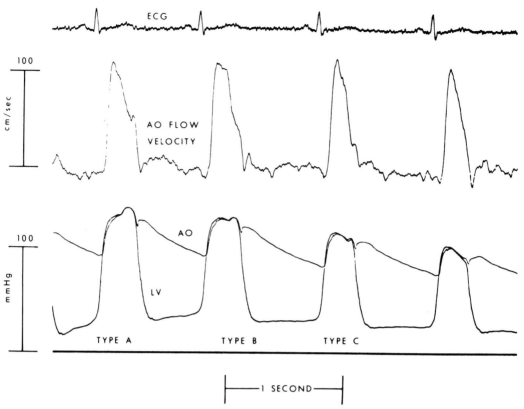

**Fig. 9-13.** Left ventricular (LV) and central aortic (AO) pressure and aortic flow velocity tracings in a patient at the initiation of the strain phase of a Valsalva maneuver. See text for details. (From Murgo JP et al: Circulation 63:122, 1981, with permission.)

has a kinetic energy by virtue of its motion, and when this flow suddenly comes to a halt the kinetic energy is converted in part into pressure. Therefore, if an end-hole catheter is pointing upstream, (e.g. radial or femoral arterial pressure monitoring line) it will record a pressure artifactually elevated by the converted kinetic energy. This added pressure may range from 2 to 10 mmHg.

*Catheter Impact Artifact.* This is similar but not identical to catheter whip artifact. When a fluid-filled catheter is "hit" (e.g., by valves in the act of opening or closing, or by the walls of the ventricular chambers), a pressure transient is created. Any frequency component of this transient that coincides with the natural frequency of the catheter-manometer system will cause a superimposed oscillation on the recorded pressure wave. Catheter impact artifacts are common with pigtail catheters in the left ventricular chamber, where the terminal "pigtail" is

often hit by the mitral valve leaflets as they open in early diastole.

*Systolic Pressure Amplification in the Periphery.* When radial, brachial, or femoral arterial pressures are measured and used to represent aortic pressure, it is important to recall that peak systolic pressure in these arteries may be considerably higher (e.g., by 20 to 50 mmHg) than peak systolic pressure in the central aorta (Fig. 9-16), although mean arterial pressure will be the same or slightly lower. There has been debate concerning the mechanism of this amplification of systolic pressure. McDonald[5] and Murgo[9,10] present convincing evidence that the change in waveform of arterial pressure as it travels away from the heart is largely a consequence of reflected waves. These waves, presumably reflected from the aortic bifurcation, arterial branch points, and small peripheral vessels, reinforce the peak and trough of the antegrade pressure waveform,

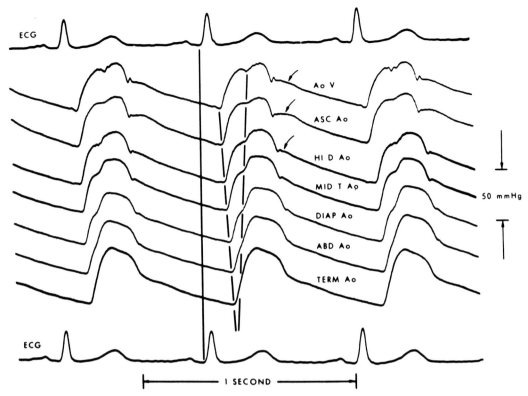

**Fig. 9-14.** Pressure waveforms in a patient undergoing cardiac catheterization as a function of distance from the aortic (Ao) valve (V). ASC, ascending; Hi D, high descending; MID T, midthoracic; DIAP, diaphragmatic; ABD, abdominal; TERM, just above aortic bifurcation. First vertical line marks onset of primary (forward) pressure wave, which occurs progressively later after the QRS complex with increasing distance from the aortic valve. Second vertical line marks onset of secondary pressure rise associated with the backward or reflected pressure wave. See text for discussion. (From Murgo JP et al.: Circulation 62:105, 1980, with permission.)

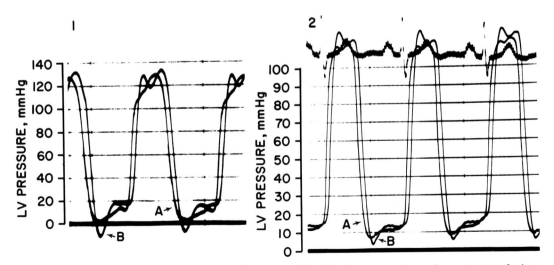

**Fig. 9-15.** Left ventricular (LV) pressure signals as recorded with micromanometer and a system employing long fluid-filled tubing and several interposed stopcocks between the pressure transducer and the 7F NIH catheter. The micromanometer tracing is labeled A and the fluid-filled catheter tracing is labeled B. Note both the early diastolic and early ejection phase overshoot seen with the fluid-filled catheter, indicating a poor frequency response, especially in panel 1.

131

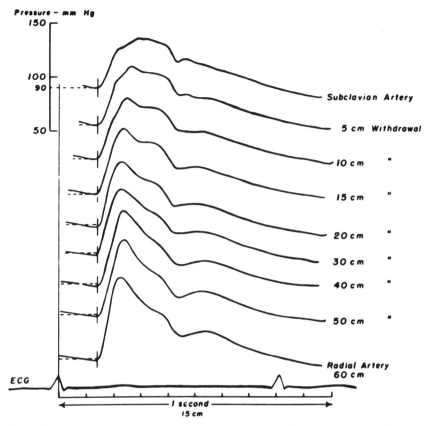

**Fig. 9-16.** Transformation of arterial pressure waveform with transmission to the periphery in a healthy 30-year-old man. Onset of pressures are aligned for purposes of comparison. As pulse wave moves peripherally, the upstroke steepens and increases in magnitude, giving the pressure a "spiky" appearance. Horizontal line intersecting onset of each pulse contour is calibration reference of 90 mmHg. (From Marshall, HW, et al.: Physiologic consequences of congenital heart disease. *In* Hamilton, WF, and Dow, P (eds.): Handbook of Physiology. Sect. 2. Circulation, Vol. 1. Washington, DC, American Physiological Society, 1962, p. 417.)

causing amplification of the peak systolic and pulse pressures (Fig. 9-14). This phenomenon may tend to mask and distort pressure gradients across the aortic valve or left ventricular outflow tract. The transseptal technique with a second catheter in the central aorta offers one way of avoiding this problem (see Chapter 5). Giving special attention to performing careful pull-back tracings may also help the operator to avoid this particular error.

We routinely record central aortic pressure together with peripheral arterial pressure immediately before entering the left ventricle during retrograde left heart catheterization. If this tracing shows a "reverse gradient" (peak systolic pressure in periphery higher than in central aorta), the amount of this pressure difference must be considered when subsequently comparing left ventricular and "systemic arterial" pressure for the detection of aortic or subaortic stenosis. The peripheral arterial systolic pressure may commonly appear to be 20 mmHg higher than left ventricular systolic pressure as a result of this phenomenon. This pressure amplification in the periphery is particularly marked in the radial artery (Fig. 9-16), especially if there is also some end-pressure artifact, and may mask the presence of aortic stenosis because of failure to appreciate a systolic gradient. If any doubt exists concerning the presence of a true pressure gradient, a full length catheter should be exchanged for the arterial pressure monitor and advanced to central aorta.

***Errors in Zero Level, Balancing, or Calibration.*** Error in the quantitation of pressures due to improper zero reference is common. In our laboratory, the zero reference point is taken at the midchest with the patient supine, although some laboratories use 10 cm vertically up from the back or 5 cm vertically down from the sternal angle. All manometers must be zeroed at the same point, and the zero reference point must be changed if the patient's position is changed during the course of the study (e.g., if pillows are placed to prop him up). Transducers should be calibrated frequently against a standard mercury reference, preferably prior to each period of use. Electrical calibration signals and "calibration factors" should not be relied upon as a substitute for mercury calibration. Linearity of response should be checked by using mercury inputs of 25 mmHg, 50 mmHg, and 100 mmHg. If possible, all transducers should be exposed to the calibrating system simultaneously to avoid false "gradients" due to unequal amplification of the same pressure signal. In our system (Fig. 9-9), a bubble in the zero-reference line can give a false zero level; therefore, in tracking down an unexpected pressure gradient, flushing of the zero line is an important initial step.

## MICROMANOMETERS

In order to reduce the mass and inertia of the pressure measurement system, improve the frequency response characteristics, and decrease artifacts associated with overdamping and catheter whip, miniaturized transducers have been developed that fit on the end of standard catheters and thus may be used as intracardiac manometers (Figs. 9-4, 9-15). Several models are commercially available, but many still have major technical shortcomings, such as fragility, electrical drift problems, temperature sensitivity, and inability to withstand the usual catheter sterilization techniques. After trying many varieties, we have settled on the Mikro-tip,* which

*Millar Instruments, Houston, TX.

has met all the foregoing objections in our experience. Commercially available modifications of this catheter have multiple side holes and thus permit angiography and high fidelity pressure measurement through the same catheter. A modification of this catheter has a pigtail tip. The catheter may be subjected to gas sterilization (ethylene oxide) along with other catheters and instruments, and it may be calibrated externally at room temperature because its response characteristics are not appreciably affected by temperature changes over a wide range. In our experience, it has proven remarkably stable and resistant to breakage over multiple periods of use. In addition, modifications are available with electromagnetic flow velocity sensors and other special capabilities for research applications.

For accurate measurement of the rate of ventricular pressure rise (dP/dt) and other parameters of myocardial performance occurring during the first 40 to 50 msec of ventricular systole, high frequency response characteristics are necessary. Although there is some debate on this subject,[11] micromanometer-tipped catheters are generally required in patient studies when myocardial mechanics are being examined. In this regard, Gersh and co-workers have published a careful study on the physical criteria for measurement of left ventricular pressure and its first derivative.[12] They showed that pressure measurement flat to ±5% of the first 20 harmonics of the left ventricular pressure curve is required for accurate reproduction of the amplitude of maximal dP/dt. In their study, accuracy to six harmonics led to only a 20% underestimation of peak dP/dt. At a heart rate of 80 beats/min, the fundamental frequency is $80/60 = 1.33 \sec^{-1}$, and the twentieth harmonic is 26.7 cycles/sec. As seen in Figure 9-6, this may be possible to achieve with a short, wide-bore catheter attached directly to the pressure transducer, with optimal damping. However, if the heart rate increases to 100 beats/min, the twentieth harmonic will now be $(100 \div 60) \times 20 = 33.3 \sec^{-1}$, which exceeds the capacity for even this optimal fluid-filled system. Thus, to minimize the chance of error, we use micromanometer catheters exclusively when dP/dt is being measured. Examples of pressure recordings taken with and without micromanometer-tipped catheters may be seen in Figures 9-4 and 9-15.

# REFERENCES

1. Hales S: *In* Willius FA, Keys TE (ed): Classics in Cardiology. New York, Dover Publications, 1961. pp 131–155.
2. Wiggers CJ: The Pressure Pulses in the Cardiovascular System. London, Longmans, Green and Co., 1928. pp 1–14.
3. Hürthle K: Beiträge zur Hämodynamik. Arch Ges Physiol 72:566, 1898.
4. Fry DL: Physiologic recording by modern instruments with particular reference to pressure recording. Physiol Rev 40:753, 1960.
5. McDonald DA: Blood Flow in Arteries, ed. 2. Baltimore, Williams & Wilkins, 1974.
6. Wood EH, Leusen IR, Warner HR, Wright JL: Measurement of pressures in man by cardiac catheters. Circ Res 2:294, 1954.
7. Gleason WL, Braunwald E: Studies on the first derivative of the ventricular pressure pulse in man. J Clin Invest 41:80, 1962.
8. Hansen AT: Pressure measurement in the human organism. Acta Physiol Scand 19(Suppl. 68):87, 1949–50.
9. Murgo JP, Westerhof N, Giolma JP, Altobelli SA: Manipulation of ascending aortic pressure and flow wave reflections with Valsalva maneuver: relationship to input impedance. Circulation 63:122, 1981.
10. Murgo JP, Westerhof N, Giolma JP, Altobelli SA: Aortic input impedance in normal man: relationship to pressure wave forms. Circulation 62:105, 1980.
11. Falsetti HL, Mates RE, Greene DG, Bunnell IL; $V_{max}$ as an index of contractile state in man. Circulation 43:467, 1971.
12. Gersh BJ, Hahn CEW, Prys-Roberts C: Physical criteria for measurement of left ventricular pressure and its first derivative. Cardiovasc Res 5:32, 1971.

*chapter ten*

# Clinical Measurement of Vascular Resistance and Assessment of Vasodilator Drugs

WILLIAM GROSSMAN

## POISEUILLE'S LAW

IN 1842 a French physician, Jean Léonard Marie Poiseuille, empirically derived a series of equations describing the flow of fluids through cylindrical tubes. Although Poiseuille was interested in blood flow, he substituted simpler liquids in his measurements of flow through rigid glass tubes.

Poiseuille's law may be stated as:

$$Q = \frac{\pi(Pi - Po)r^4}{8\eta l}$$

where:

$$
\begin{aligned}
Q &= \text{volume flow} \\
Pi - Po &= \text{inflow pressure} - \text{outflow pressure} \\
r &= \text{the radius of the tube} \\
l &= \text{the length of the tube} \\
\eta &= \text{viscosity of the fluid}
\end{aligned}
$$

This relationship is applicable in the specific circumstance of steady state laminar

Note: Some material in this chapter has been retained from the first and second editions, to which Dr. L. P. McLaurin had contributed.

flow of a homogeneous fluid through a rigid tube. Under these conditions, flow, Q, varies directly as the pressure difference, Pi − Po, and the *fourth power* of the tube's radius, r. It varies inversely as the length, l, of the tube and the viscosity, $\eta$, of the fluid.[1,2]

Hydraulic resistance, R, is defined by analogy to Ohm's law as the ratio of mean pressure drop, $\Delta P$, to flow, Q, across the vascular circuit. The various factors contributing to vascular resistance can be illustrated by rearranging Poiseuille's law as follows:

$$R = \frac{Pi - Po}{Q} = \frac{8\eta l}{\pi r^4}$$

It is apparent from this equation that, in the condition of steady laminar flow of a homogeneous fluid through a rigid cylindrical tube, resistance to flow depends only upon the dimensions of the tube and the viscosity of the fluid. In particular, the resistance is remarkably sensitive to changes in the radius of the tube, varying inversely with its fourth power.

135

## VASCULAR RESISTANCE AND PRESSURE-FLOW RELATIONSHIPS

The applicability of laws derived from steady-state fluid mechanics in assessing vascular resistance is somewhat ambiguous because blood flow is pulsatile, blood is a nonhomogeneous fluid, and the vascular bed is a nonlinear, elastic, frequency dependent system. In such a system, resistance varies continuously with pressure and flow and is influenced by many factors, such as inertia, reflected waves, and the phase angle between pulse and flow wave velocities.

To assess both vessel caliber and elasticity, the resistive and compliant characteristics of the vascular system, the concept of *vascular impedance* has been employed.[2] Vascular impedance has been defined as the instantaneous ratio of pulsatile pressure to pulsatile flow.[3] Since impedance may not be the same for all frequencies, its calculation requires resolution of the harmonic components of both pressure and flow pulsations. The *impedance modulus* so calculated is then expressed as a spectrum of impedance versus frequency.

As a consequence of the foregoing considerations and the many active and passive factors that influence pressure and flow in blood vessels, the concept of vascular resistance in its pure physical sense is limited in application. In the context of the clinical and physiologic setting, however, vascular resistance derived from hemodynamic measurements made during cardiac catheterization has acquired empiric pathophysiologic meaning and is often an important factor in clinical decision-making.

## ESTIMATION OF VASCULAR RESISTANCE

Calculations of *vascular resistance* are usually applied to both the pulmonary and systemic circulations. Although many authors refer to systemic or pulmonary *arteriolar* resistances, we prefer the term *vascular* resistance, since it is less committal concerning the anatomic site of the resistance. As will be discussed, arteriolar tone is only one determinant of vascular resistance to

blood flow. Knowledge of both the pressure differential across the pulmonary and systemic circuits and the respective blood flow through them is required.

The formulae generally used are:

1. Systemic Vascular Resistance $= \dfrac{\overline{Ao} - \overline{RA}}{Q_s}$

2. Total Pulmonary Resistance $= \dfrac{\overline{PA}}{Q_p}$

3. Pulmonary Vascular Resistance $= \dfrac{\overline{PA} - \overline{LA}}{Q_p}$

where: $\overline{Ao}$ = mean systemic arterial pressure, $\overline{RA}$ = mean right atrial pressure, $\overline{PA}$ = mean pulmonary arterial pressure, $\overline{LA}$ = mean left atrial pressure, $Q_s$ = systemic blood flow, $Q_p$ = pulmonary blood flow.

In many laboratories, the mean pulmonary artery wedge pressure is used as an approximation of mean left atrial pressure. This should cause no problem because there is ample evidence that pulmonary artery wedge pressure, properly obtained, closely approximates the level of left atrial pressure.[4,5] The flows are *volume* flows (as opposed to velocity flows), and are expressed in liters/minute, and pressures are in millimeters of mercury. These equations yield resistance in arbitrary resistance units (R units) expressed in mmHg/(L/min), also called "hybrid units." These units are sometimes referred to as Wood units, since they were first introduced by Dr. Paul Wood. They may be converted to metric resistance units expressed in dynes-seconds-cm$^{-5}$ by use of the conversion factor 80. In this system resistance is expressed as:

Resistance:

$$= \frac{\Delta P(\text{mm Hg}) \times 1332 \text{ dynes/cm}^2/\text{mm Hg}}{Q_s \text{ or } Q_p \text{ (L/min)} \times 1000 \text{ ml/L} \div 60 \text{ sec/min}}$$

$$= \frac{\Delta P}{Q_s \text{ or } Q_p} \times 80$$

$$= \text{dynes-sec-cm}^{-5}$$

There is no particular advantage to either system, since both express precisely the same ratio. Most pediatric cardiologists use hybrid units, whereas cardiologists with adult practices generally use metric units.

In pediatric practice it is conventional to normalize vascular resistances for body surface area (BSA), thus giving a resistance

**TABLE 10-1.** *Normal Values for Vascular Resistance*

| | |
|---|---|
| Systemic Vascular Resistance | $1170 \pm 270$ dynes-sec-cm$^{-5}$ |
| Systemic Vascular Resistance Index | $2130 \pm 450$ dynes-sec-cm$^{-5} \cdot$ M$^2$ |
| Pulmonary Vascular Resistance | $67 \pm 30$ dynes-sec-cm$^{-5}$ |
| Pulmonary Vascular Resistance Index | $123 \pm 54$ dynes-sec-cm$^{-5} \cdot$ M$^2$ |

Values are expressed as mean ± standard deviation, and are derived from 37 subjects without demonstrable cardiovascular disease (17 males, 20 females age 47 ± 9 years) who underwent diagnostic cardiac catheterization at the Peter Bent Brigham Hospital between July 1, 1975, and June 30, 1978.

index. Although this is not commonly done in adult cardiac catheterization laboratories, the practice makes sense, since normal cardiac output and therefore vascular resistance may be substantially different in a 260-pound man as compared to a 110-pound woman. However, the normalized resistance is *not* obtained by dividing resistance as calculated in equations 1 to 3 by body surface area. Rather, normalized resistance is calculated by substituting blood flow index for blood flow in the resistance formula. Thus systemic vascular resistance index (SVRI) is calculated as

$$SVRI = (\overline{Ao} - \overline{RA})80/CI$$

where CI is the cardiac (or systemic blood flow) index. Therefore, *SVRI equals SVR multiplied by BSA.*

Cardiac output, usually measured by either the Fick or the thermal dilution method, is used as mean blood flow. It is important to realize that in conditions of intracardiac shunts or shunts between the pulmonary and systemic circulations, *pulmonary blood flow and systemic flow may not be equal,* and the respective flow through each circuit must be measured and used in the appropriate resistance calculation.

Normal values for vascular resistance in adults are given in Table 10-1.

## CLINICAL USE OF VASCULAR RESISTANCE

As can be deduced from the Poiseuille equation, changes in systemic or pulmonary vascular resistance may theoretically result from one of three mechanisms. Since changes in *length* of the vascular beds are uncommon after growth has been com-

pleted, changes in vascular resistance reflect either altered *viscosity* of blood or a change in cross-sectional area *(radius)* of the vascular bed.

There is ample evidence that changes in blood viscosity alter measured vascular resistances. Nihill[6] has shown an approximate doubling of pulmonary vascular resistance with increases in hematocrit from 43% to 64%. Similarly, low values for measured vascular resistance are commonly seen in patients with severe chronic anemia, although the low vascular resistance in such cases probably represents more than a viscosity effect alone.

With regard to changes in cross-sectional area of the pulmonary or systemic vascular bed, such changes *do not invariably imply altered arteriolar tone.* In the normal systemic circulation, mean aortic pressure may be 100 mmHg while right atrial pressure is only 5 mmHg. Although the greatest part of this pressure drop occurs at the arteriolar level (approximately 60%), about 15% occurs in the capillaries, 15% in small veins, and 10% in the arterial system proximal to the arterioles.[2] Thus, although systemic vascular resistance is dominated by the caliber of the arterioles, the other components of the systemic vascular bed are by no means negligible. For example, Read and co-workers[7] studied systemic vascular resistance in dogs with constant (pump controlled) cardiac output, and found that a rise in venous pressure consistently caused a fall in resistance. The magnitude of the fall was proportional to the increment in venous pressure rise and was about 20% for an increase in venous pressure of 20 mmHg. Other studies show no change in resistance when arterial pressure is so manipulated (in the absence of baroreceptor control). These findings have been interpreted by McDonald[2] to suggest that the decline in systemic vascular resistance with increased venous pressure results from dilatation of small venous channels, whereas systemic arterioles do not distend passively with increased pressure. Therefore, measurement of vascular resistance is not a precise tool for assessing the dynamics of individual sections of the vascular bed.

The minute-to-minute control of vascular resistance, at least in the systemic bed, is an amalgam of autonomic nervous system influences and local metabolic factors. Hypotension or reduced cardiac output generally triggers increased systemic resistance by means of the baroreceptors, alpha-adrenergic neural pathways, and the release of humoral vasoconstrictor hormones, but these influences may be opposed by metabolic factors if the hypotension or low cardiac output results in decreased tissue perfusion with local hypoxia and acidosis. This latter circumstance is commonly seen in congestive heart failure or shock.

Knowledge of changes in systemic vascular resistance is also important in evaluating the hemodynamic response to stress tests, such as dynamic or isometric exercise.[8] In this regard, there is ample evidence that systemic vascular resistance normally falls in response to dynamic exercise, but pulmonary vascular resistance is unchanged (at least with supine bicycle exercise). Transient elevations in systemic vascular resistance have been provoked by infusions of vasopressor drugs in an effort to evaluate the left ventricular response to a sudden increase in afterload.[9] Such tests often provide useful information regarding left ventricular performance and reserve.

Low systemic vascular resistance may be seen in conditions in which blood flow is inappropriately increased, such as arteriovenous fistula, severe anemia, and other high-output states. It is important to realize that in these circumstances there may well be regional differences in vascular resistance, and calculations based on mean pressure and flow in the entire systemic circulation may lead to inaccurate conclusions.

***Total Pulmonary Resistance.*** Calculated as the ratio of mean pulmonary artery pressure to pulmonary blood flow, total pulmonary resistance expresses the resistance to flow in transporting a volume of blood from the pulmonary artery to the left ventricle in diastole, neglecting left ventricu-

lar diastolic pressure. This relationship is obviously influenced by alterations in left atrial pressure and will not consistently provide useful information about the condition of the pulmonary vasculature. Although widely used 25 years ago, it is rarely used today.

***Pulmonary Vascular Resistance.*** Sometimes called pulmonary arteriolar resistance, pulmonary vascular resistance expresses the pressure drop across the major pulmonary vessels, the precapillary arterioles, and the pulmonary capillary bed, and is more precise in assessing the presence and degree of pulmonary vascular disease. Simple calculation of pulmonary vascular resistance provides general information about the pulmonary circulation, but this must be interpreted in the context of the clinical situation and other hemodynamic data obtained during cardiac catheterization. The pulmonary vasculature is a dynamic system and is subject to many mechanical, neural, and biochemical influences. Some of these factors are listed in Table 10-2.

Several investigators have taken advantage of this responsiveness of the pulmonary circulation to various manipulations in the hope of assessing the reversibility of pulmonary hypertension. Oxygen inhalation,[10] infusions of acetylcholine,[11] and infusions of tolazoline[12] have all been utilized in attempts to relieve whatever reflex pulmonary vasoconstriction may be present.

The tolazoline test is generally performed in the following manner.[12,13] After a complete set of baseline data including pulmonary blood flow, pulmonary artery and pulmonary artery wedge pressures are measured, 1.0 mg/kg of tolazoline is infused over a one-minute period into the pulmonary artery. Patients frequently experience a sense of warmth accompanied by cutaneous flushing soon after injection. This rapidly passes and the pulmonary arterial and systemic arterial pressures are monitored at one-minute intervals. After ten minutes, pulmonary blood flow, pulmonary artery and pulmonary artery wedge pressures are again determined.

Utilizing this test, Brammel and his associates identified a small number of patients with the Eisenmenger syndrome and high pulmonary resistance who had a drop in total pulmonary resistance to less than 450 dynes-sec-cm$^{-5}$ m$^2$ in response to tolazo-

**TABLE 10-2.** *Factors That May be Related to Changes in Pulmonary Vascular Resistance*

I. Mechanical
   A. Changes in pulmonary venous pressure
   B. Changes in pulmonary blood flow
   C. Changes in pulmonary blood volume
   D. Changes in alveolar pressures
   E. Changes in intrathoracic pressure
   F. Pericapillary edema
   G. Changes in size of pulmonary vascular bed
II. Neural
   A. Autonomic nervous system
   B. Intravascular chemoreceptors
   C. Intravascular mechanoreceptors
   D. Changes in neuroregulation of ventilation
III. Biochemical and Hormonal
   A. Changes in oxygen tension
   B. Acute hypercapnia
   C. Acute acidosis
   D. Catecholamines (esp. isoproterenol)
   E. Acetylcholine
   F. Tolazoline
   G. Serotonin
   H. Histamine
   I. Prostaglandins

line.[13] Postoperative cardiac catheterization confirmed a substantial drop in pulmonary resistance and pulmonary artery pressure. These patients were considered to be "pulmonary vascular hyperreactors" who respond to increased pulmonary blood flow with pulmonary vasoconstriction. When pulmonary hypertension has been present for many years, permanent obliterative changes in the pulmonary vasculature occur, and reactive vasoconstriction is less significant. For this reason, the tolazoline test has its widest application in young children, and has less value in assessing adults with pulmonary hypertension.

The value of oxygen inhalation in assessing pulmonary vascular reactivity is substantial. Any patient with high pulmonary vascular resistance (i.e., $\geq 600$ dynes-sec-cm$^{-5}$) in association with a central shunt (e.g., ventricular septal defect) should be given 100% oxygen by face mask before concluding that the changes are fixed. Older patients with a combination of left heart failure and chronic obstructive lung disease may have considerable pulmonary vasoconstriction due to alveolar hypoventilation and its resultant hypoxia. Inhalation of 100% oxygen in such cases may result in a dramatic fall in pulmonary arterial pressure and vascular resistance.

The decision whether or not a patient with either congenital or valvular heart disease would profit from corrective surgery often hinges on the pulmonary vascular resistance. Although each case must be evaluated on its own characteristics, many criteria for operability have been proposed.[14-17] It has been suggested that the ratio between pulmonary vascular resistance and systemic vascular resistance (resistance ratio PVR/SVR) be used as a criteria for operability in dealing with congenital heart disease.[14] Normally this ratio is about 0.25 or less. Values of 0.25 to 0.50 indicate moderate pulmonary vascular disease, and values greater than 0.75 indicate severe pulmonary vascular disease. When the PVR/SVR resistance ratio equals 1.0 or more, surgical correction of the cardiac disease is considered contraindicated because of the severity of the disease.

We have been impressed with the clinical value of the resistance ratio. It has the value of factoring in miscellaneous neural, hormonal and blood viscosity influences that may be affecting *both* pulmonary and systemic vascular beds, and which may be primarily related to the patient's immediate clinical status rather than to intrinsic pulmonary vascular changes. Many patients with left ventricular failure and low systemic output (from whatever cause) have associated high systemic and pulmonary vascular resistance, but the resistance ratio will be normal in the absence of intrinsic vascular pathology.

DiSesa and co-workers[14] have reported three patients with congenital heart disease (2 with atrial septal defect and 1 with patent ductus arteriosus) with cyanosis and pulmonary arterial hypertension at near systemic levels, each of whom had progressive improvement in pulmonary vascular resistance toward normal following operative closure of the shunts. They point out that the increased blood viscosity associated with the polycythemia of cyanosis (hematocrits in the 56 to 66% range) contribute substantially to the measured increase in pulmonary and systemic vascular resistances. This influence, as well as the generalized vasoconstriction often seen in patients with advanced cardiac disease, will be factored out by the ratio of PVR/SVR. All of DiSesa's patients[14] had ratios of <0.50 and net left-to-right shunts despite severe pulmonary hypertension (e.g., pulmonary artery pressure 110/55 mmHg).

In his classic description of the Eisenmenger syndrome, Wood pointed out that attempted surgical repair of the shunt defect was a major source of death in these patients.[15] He stated that in patients with pulmonary blood flow less than 1.75 times systemic flow or with total pulmonary vascular resistance greater than 12 Wood or "hybrid" units (960 dynes-sec-cm$^{-5}$), ordinary surgical repair of the defect should not be attempted. Others have suggested similar criteria for special instances or conditions.[16,17] Briefly summarized, it can be stated that surgical repair should be limited to patients in whom the net shunt is left to right and the total pulmonary vascular resistance is less than systemic vascular resistance, preferably with a resistance ratio of <0.50.

Marked elevations in pulmonary vascular resistance may also be seen in acquired heart disease, notably in mitral stenosis. The effect of mitral valve replacement in patients with mitral stenosis and/or regurgitation associated with pulmonary hypertension has been evaluated.[18,19] Most patients experience significant reduction in pulmonary vascular resistance following successful repair of the mitral valve lesion. Although some degree of pulmonary hypertension may persist postoperatively, significant palliative benefit usually occurs, and the decision regarding surgery must be made in light of information regarding left and right ventricular function as well as the degree of pulmonary hypertension.

## ASSESSMENT OF VASODILATOR DRUGS

Cardiac catheterization provides an ideal opportunity for assessing the potential response of a patient to a change in medical regimen, particularly with regard to vasodilator drugs. In recent years, vasodilator drugs have assumed a major role in the treatment of patients with congestive heart failure. However, there is great variability among currently employed vasodilator agents, and the relative effects of a particular drug on resistance and capacitance vessels is of major importance in predicting its hemodynamic effects.[20-23] This problem may become complex in the circumstance in which a particular drug may have different effects depending on the level of resting tone in resistance and capacitance beds. For example, nitrate preparations are well known to influence venous capacitance; this is presumably responsible (at least in part) for the fact that ventricular filling pressures and pulmonary congestion are consistently improved when nitrate therapy is given to patients with congestive heart failure. Despite this consistent effect on preload, the effect of nitrates on forward cardiac output has been variable,[24-27] and studies have reported decreases, increases, or mixed effects on cardiac output in normal subjects and in patients with heart failure. Goldberg et al.[28] studied 15 patients with chronic congestive heart failure who were given an oral nitrate (erithrityl tetranitrate) at the time of cardiac catheterization in order to identify predictors of nitrate effect on cardiac output. There were significant reductions in right atrial, pulmonary capillary wedge, and mean arterial pressure in nearly all patients. Augmentation in cardiac output by ≥10% occurred in 8 patients (thereby defined as "responders"), but no change or decline occurred in 7 patients ("nonresponders"). The level of peripheral vasoconstriction, as reflected by resting systemic vascular resistance, was significantly higher for the "responders" than for the "nonresponders" (2602 ± 251 versus 1744 ± 193 dynes-sec-cm$^{-5}$, p <.02). Furthermore, a significant reduction in systemic vascular resistance occurred only in "responders," and the decline was a linear function of resting resistance (Fig. 10-1).

Thus, although reductions in arterial pressure and left and right ventricular filling pressures are a constant result of nitrate therapy, significant augmentation in forward cardiac output is likely only in those patients with the most intense resting peripheral vasoconstriction. The design of a catheterization protocol in a patient with congestive heart failure can include assessment of vasodilator therapy based on these principles. For example, if the resting cardiac output is

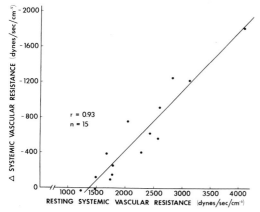

**Fig. 10-1.** The change ($\Delta$) in systemic vascular resistance following administration of erythrityl tetranitrate plotted as a function of resting systemic vascular resistance in 15 patients with congestive heart failure. Patients with the greatest degree of vasoconstriction at rest demonstrated the greatest fall in resistance in response to the nitrate. (From Goldberg et al: Nitrate therapy of heart failure in valvular heart disease. Am J Med 65:161, 1978.)

low and if right and left ventricular filling pressures as well as systemic vascular resistance are high, a long-acting nitrate or a balanced agent (such as captopril) might be expected to be particularly beneficial, and should be tested while the catheters are still in place. Alternatively, if the output is low, resistance is high, but filling pressures are near normal, a nitrate might not help, since the lowered resistance may be offset by the

fall of the already normal preload, with the result being no increase in output. In such a patient, a selective lowering of resistance would be desirable, and hydralazine could be tested before removing the catheters. If the cardiac output is low but resistance is normal, nitrate or captopril most likely will not increase output, and should only be tested if filling pressures are high and symptoms of congestion are a prominent part of the clinical picture. In such patients the combination of an inotropic agent and a nitrate may be particularly helpful and could be tested at the time of catheterization. Finally, if the output is low, but filling pressures and systemic vascular resistance are normal, vasodilator drugs will probably do more harm than good, and a therapeutic trial of preload elevation (administration of colloid) with or without an inotropic agent could be tested during the catheterization.

These examples are presented merely to illustrate the principle of using cardiac catheterization parameters (i.e., resistances, flows, and filling pressures) to design a therapeutic regimen and then, while the catheters are still in place, put it to the test. We have found this most useful with regard to the patient with heart failure, and we feel strongly that cardiac catheterization in such patients must include full right and left heart catheterization with measurement of cardiac output, left and right heart pressures, and systemic and pulmonary vascular resistances.

# REFERENCES

1. Burton AC: Physiology and Biophysics of the Circulation. 2nd ed. Chicago, Year Book Medical Publishers, 1972. p 40.
2. McDonald DA: Blood Flow in Arteries. 2nd ed. Baltimore, Williams & Wilkins, 1974.
3. Milnor WR: Pulsatile blood flow. N Engl J Med 287:27, 1972.
4. Connolly DC, Kirklin JW, Wood CH: The relationship between pulmonary artery pressure and left atrial pressure in man. Circ Res 2:434, 1954.
5. Rapaport E, Dexter L: Pulmonary "capillary" pressure. Meth Med Res 7:85, 1958.
6. Nihill MR, McNamara DG, Vick RL: The effects of increased blood viscosity on pulmonary vascular resistance. Am Heart J 92:65, 1976.
7. Read RC, Kuida H, Johnson JA: Venous pressure and total peripheral resistance in the dog. Am J Physiol 192:609, 1958.
8. Grossman W, et al: Changes in inotropic state of the left ventricle during isometric exercise. Br Heart J 35:697, 1973.
9. Ross J Jr, Braunwald E: The study of left ventricular function in man by increasing resistance to ventricular ejection with angiotensin. Circulation 29:739, 1964.
10. Fishman AP: Respiratory gases in the regulation of the pulmonary circulation. Physiol Rev 41:214, 1961.
11. Wood P, Besterman EM, Towers MK, McIlroy MB: The effect of acetylcholine on pulmonary vascular resistance and left atrial pressure in mitral stenosis. Br Heart J 19:279, 1957.

12. Grover RF, Reeves JT, and Blount SG Jr: Tolazoline hydrochloride (Priscoline): An effective pulmonary vasodilator. Am Heart J 61:5, 1961.

13. Brammel HL, Vogel JHK, Pryor R, Blount SG Jr: The Eisenmenger syndrome. Am J Cardiol 28:679, 1971.

14. DiSesa VJ, Cohn LH, Grossman W: Management of adults with congenital bidirectional shunts, cyanosis, and pulmonary vascular obstruction: successful operative repair in 3 patients. Am J Cardiol 51:1495, 1983.

15. Wood P: The Eisenmenger syndrome or pulmonary hypertension with reversal central shunt. Br Med J 2:701, 1958.

16. Kimball KG, McIlroy MB: Pulmonary hypertension in patients with congenital heart disease. Am J Med 41:883, 1966.

17. Ellis FH Jr, Kirklin JW, Callohan JA, Wood EH: Patent ductus arteriosus with pulmonary hypertension. J Thorac Surg 31:268, 1956.

18. Braunwald E, Braunwald NS, Ross J Jr, Morrow AG: Effects of mitral-valve replacement on the pulmonary vascular dynamics of patients with pulmonary hypertension. N Engl J Med 273:509, 1965.

19. Dalen JE et al: Early reduction of pulmonary vascular resistance after mitral valve replacement. N Engl J Med 277:387, 1967.

20. Chatterjee K: Vasodilator therapy for heart failure. Ann Intern Med 83:421, 1975.

21. Cohn JN: Vasodilator therapy for heart failure. The influence of impedance on left ventricular performance. Circulation 48:5, 1973.

22. Honig CR, Tenney SM, Gabel PV: The mechanism of cardiovascular action of nitroglycerin: an example of integrated response to unsteady state. Ann J Med 29:910, 1960.

23. Braunwald E, Colucci WS: Vasodilator therapy of heart failure. Has the promissory note been paid? N Engl J Med 310:459, 1984.

24. Ferrer MI et al: Some effects of nitroglycerin upon the splanchnic, pulmonary and systemic circulations. Circulation 33:357, 1966.

25. Williams JF, Glick G, Braunwald E: Studies on cardiac dimensions in intact unanesthetized man V. Effects of nitroglycerin. Circulation 32:767, 1965.

26. Gold HK, Leinbach RC, Sanders CA: Use of sublingual nitroglycerin in congestive failure following acute myocardial infarction. Circulation 46:389, 1972.

27. DeMaria AN et al: Effects of nitroglycerin on left ventricular cavitary size and cardiac performance determined by ultrasound in man. Am J Med 57:754, 1974.

28. Goldberg S, Mann T, Grossman W: Nitrate therapy of heart failure in valvular heart disease: importance of resting level of peripheral vascular resistance in determining cardiac output response. Am J Med 65:161, 1978.

## chapter eleven

# Calculation of Stenotic Valve Orifice Area

BLASE A. CARABELLO *and* WILLIAM GROSSMAN

T HE NORMAL cardiac valve offers little resistance to the flow of blood, even when blood flow velocity across it is high. As valvular stenosis develops, the valve orifice produces progressively greater resistance to flow, resulting in a fall in pressure (*pressure gradient*) across the valve. At any given stenotic orifice size, greater flow across the orifice yields a greater pressure gradient. Using this principle together with two fundamental hydraulic formulas, Dr. Richard Gorlin and his father developed a formula for the calculation of cardiac valvular orifices from flow and pressure-gradient data.[1]

## GORLIN FORMULA

The first basic equation the Gorlins used was Torricelli's law, which describes flow across a round orifice:

$$F = AVC_c \qquad (1)$$

where F = flow rate, A = orifice area, V = velocity of flow, and $C_c$ = coefficient of orifice contraction. The constant $C_c$ compensates for the physical phenomenon that, except for a perfect orifice, the area of a stream flowing through an orifice will be less than the true area of the orifice.

Rearranging the terms:

$$A = \frac{F}{VC_c} \qquad (2)$$

The second basic equation used in the derivation of Gorlin's formula relates pressure gradient and velocity of flow; $V^2 = (C_v)^2 \cdot 2gh$ or $V = (C_v) \sqrt{2gh}$ where V = velocity of flow, $C_v$ = coefficient of velocity, correcting for energy loss as pressure is converted to kinetic or velocity energy, g = acceleration due to gravity (980 cm/sec/sec) and h = pressure gradient.

Combining the two equations:

$$A = \frac{F}{C_v \sqrt{2gh} \cdot C_c} = \frac{F}{C_v C_c \sqrt{2 \cdot 980 \cdot h}}$$

$$A = \frac{F}{(C)(44.3) \sqrt{h}} \qquad (3)$$

where C is an empiric constant accounting for $C_v$ and $C_c$, and correcting calculated valve area to actual measured valve area at surgery or necropsy.

It is obvious that flow across the normal mitral and tricuspid valves occurs only in diastole and that flow across the semilunar valves occurs only in systole. Accordingly, the flow (F) for equation 3 is the total cardiac output expressed in terms of the seconds per minute during which there is actually flow across the valve. For the atrioventricular valves this is calculated by multiplying the diastolic filling period (sec/beat) times the heart rate (beats/min), yielding the number of seconds/minute during which there is diastolic flow. The cardiac output in ml/min (or cm³/min) is then divided by the seconds per minute during which there is flow, yielding diastolic flow in cm³/second. For the semilunar valves the systolic ejection period is substituted for diastolic filling period. The manner in which the diastolic filling period and systolic ejection period are measured is shown in Figure 11-1. The diastolic filling period begins at mitral valve opening and continues until end diastole. Systolic ejection period begins with aortic valve opening and proceeds to the dicrotic notch or other evidence of aortic valve closure.

Thus, the final equation for the calculation of valve orifice area (A, in cm²) is

$$A = \frac{CO/(DFP \text{ or } SEP)(HR)}{44.3 \, C \, \sqrt{\Delta P}} \quad (4)$$

where CO = cardiac output (cm³/min), DFP = diastolic filling period (sec/beat), SEP = systolic ejection period (sec/beat), HR = heart rate (beats/min), C = empiric constant, and P = pressure gradient. The empiric constant for the tricuspid, pulmonic,

and aortic valves, as well as for a patent ductus arteriosus or ventricular septal defect, is assumed to be 1.0. The empiric constant for the mitral valve was originally reported by Gorlin and Gorlin to be 0.7, but in their early studies DFP was derived from an arterial pressure tracing by subtracting the systolic ejection period from the RR interval.[1] This method overestimates DFP, because it neglects the isovolumic contraction and relaxation periods. When the DFP is measured directly from left ventricular versus pulmonary capillary wedge or left atrial pressure tracings, as in Figure 11-1, an empiric constant for the mitral valve of 0.85 should be used.[2]

In their initial correlations, Gorlin and Gorlin compared the calculated mitral valve area to actual measured area from autopsy or surgical specimens in eleven patients.[1] The maximum deviation of calculated valve area from measured valve area was 0.2 cm². To date there has been remarkably little validation of the empiric constant for the aortic, pulmonic, and tricuspid valves. However,

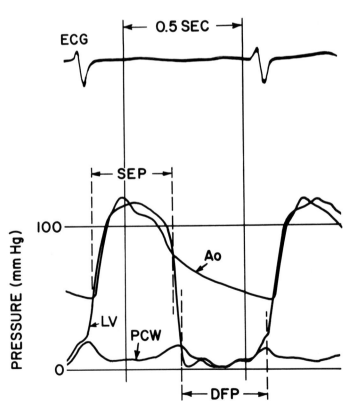

**Fig. 11-1.** Left ventricular (LV), aortic (Ao), and pulmonary capillary wedge (PCW) pressure tracings from a patient without valvular heart disease, illustrating the definition and measurement of diastolic filling period (DFP) and systolic ejection period (SEP). See text for discussion.

extensive clinical experience with the formula and its success in predicting severity of stenosis (particularly with aortic stenosis) continue to justify its usage.

## MITRAL VALVE AREA

By rearranging the terms of equation 4 one sees that for the mitral valve:

$$\Delta P = \left[ \frac{CO/(HR)(DFP)}{(MVA)(44.3)(0.85)} \right]^2 \quad (5)$$

where $\Delta P$ = mean transmitral pressure gradient, and MVA = mitral valve area. Thus, by doubling cardiac output one will quadruple the gradient across the valve, if heart rate and diastolic filling period remain constant. The normal mitral orifice in an adult has a cross-sectional area of $4.0 - 5.0$ cm$^2$ when the mitral valve is completely open in diastole. Considerable reduction in this orifice area can occur without symptomatic limitation, but when the area is $\leq 1.0$ cm$^2$, a substantial resting gradient will be present across the mitral valve, and any demand for increased cardiac output will be met by increases in left atrial and pulmonary capillary pressure that lead to pulmonary congestion and edema.

As can be seen in Figure 11-2, a cardiac output of 5 liters/min can be maintained with only a minimal mitral diastolic gradient as the mitral orifice area contracts from its normal $4.0 - 5.0$ cm$^2$ to a moderately stenotic area of 2.0 cm$^2$. After that, the gradient rises so that at an orifice area of 1.0 cm$^2$ a resting gradient of 8 to 10 mmHg is required to maintain cardiac output at 5 liters/minute, with a normal resting heart rate of 72 beats/min (Fig. 11-2A). Note that even at this level of cardiac output, substantial increases in gradient may occur in response to tachycardia (Fig. 11-2, B and C), which reduces the total time per minute available for diastolic filling. Thus 1.0 cm$^2$ is generally viewed as the "critical" mitral valve area, since only small increases in cardiac output will lead to pulmonary congestion and severe dyspnea. However, some allowance needs to be made for the patient's size in assessing critical valve area. Larger patients need greater flows to maintain tissue perfusion than smaller patients and will have higher gradi-

ents because of higher cardiac output for any given valvular area. Thus, 1.2 cm$^2$ could be a critical mitral valve area for a larger patient. Currently, no uniform agreement exists on indexing critical valve area to body size.

***Example of Valve Area Calculation in Mitral Stenosis.*** Figure 11-3 shows pulmonary capillary wedge (PCW) and left ventricular (LV) pressure tracings in a 40-year-old woman with rheumatic heart disease and severe mitral stenosis. This woman also had hypertension and significant elevation of her left ventricular diastolic pressure. The valve area is calculated with the aid of a form reproduced as Table 11-1. In this patient, five beats were chosen from the recordings taken closest in time to the Fick cardiac output determination. Planimetry of the area between PCW and LV pressure tracings (Fig. 11-3) was done for these 5 beats, and these areas were divided by the length of the diastolic filling periods for each beat, giving an average gradient deflection in millimeters (mm). The mean gradient in mmHg (Table 11-1, B) was calculated as the average gradient deflection in millimeters (mm) multiplied by the scale factor (mmHg/mm deflection). In this case, the mean gradient was 30 mmHg. Next, the average diastolic filling period is calculated (Table 11-1, C) using the average measured length between initial PCW-LV crossover in early diastole and end diastole (peak of the R wave by EKG). This average length in mm is divided by the paper speed (mm/sec) to give the average diastolic filling period, which in this case was 0.40 seconds. Heart rate and cardiac output (Table 11-1 D and E) are recorded, ideally from data collected simultaneously with the recording of the PCW-LV pressure gradient. Heart rate was 80 beats/min and cardiac output was 4680 cm$^3$/minute in the case illustrated in Figure 11-3. Note that cardiac output must be expressed in cm$^3$/min if valve area is expressed in cm$^2$ cross-sectional area.

Entering these values in the formula given in Table 11-1 F, and using a constant of $0.85(44.3) = 37.7$ for the mitral valve, we get:

Mitral Orifice Area =

$$\frac{(4680 \text{ cm}^3/\text{min})/(80 \text{ beats/min})(0.40 \text{ sec/beat})}{37.7 \sqrt{30} \text{ mmHg}}$$

Mitral Orifice Area = 0.71 cm$^2$

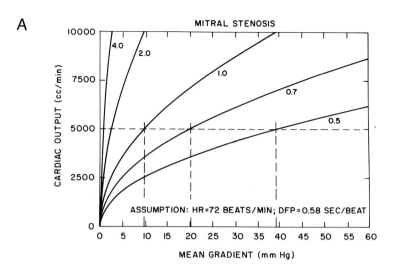

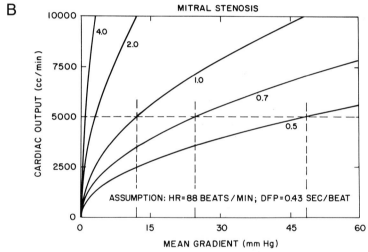

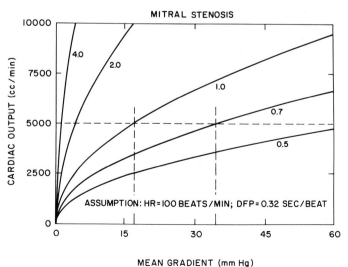

**Fig. 11-2.** Relationships between cardiac output and mean diastolic pressure gradient in patients with mitral stenosis, calculated using Equation 5 derived from the Gorlin formula. Individual curves represent orifice areas of 4.0, 2.0, 1.0, 0.7, and 0.5 cm². A, B, and C represent flow-gradient relations at differing heart rates and diastolic filling periods. See text for discussion. (Courtesy of Dr. James J. Ferguson, III.)

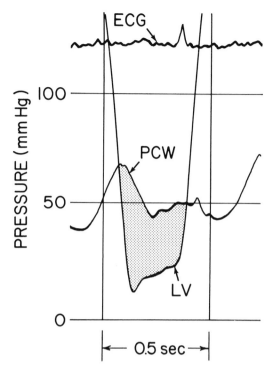

**Fig. 11-3.** Pulmonary capillary wedge (PCW) and left ventricular (LV) pressure tracings in a 40-year-old woman with mitral stenosis. This woman also had hypertension and significant elevation of her LV diastolic pressure. See text for discussion.

## Pitfalls

***Pulmonary Capillary Wedge Tracing.*** In most cases, pulmonary capillary wedge pressure is substituted for left atrial pressure under the assumption that a *properly confirmed wedge pressure* accurately reflects left atrial pressure. We believe that the weight of evidence and experience supports this assumption as correct, except in some patients with pulmonary veno-occlusive disease or cor triatriatum. However, failure to wedge the catheter properly may cause one to compare a damped pulmonary artery pressure to the left ventricular pressure, yielding a falsely high gradient. In order to insure that the right heart catheter is properly wedged one should verify that:

1. The mean wedge pressure is lower than the mean pulmonary artery pressure.
2. Blood withdrawn from the wedged catheter is ≧95% saturated with oxygen, or at least equal in saturation to arterial blood.

***Alignment Mismatch.*** Alignment of the pulmonary capillary wedge and left ventricular pressure tracings does not match alignment of simultaneous left atrial and left ventricular tracings because there is a time delay in the transmission of the left atrial pressure signal back through the pulmonary venous and capillary beds. The resulting pressure mismatch is small and largely inconsequential when pulmonary capillary wedge pressure is measured in the distal pulmonary arteries using a 7F or 8F Cournand or Goodale-Lubin catheter but may be larger when wedge pressure is measured more proximally in the pulmonary arterial tree, using a balloon-tipped flow-directed catheter. In such instances, the wedge pressure may need to be realigned with the left ventricular pressure (using tracing paper) by shifting it leftward.

The V wave, which is normally present in the left atrium (where it represents pulmonary venous return), peaks immediately prior to the downstroke of the left ventricular pressure tracing. With a wedge pressure measured distally using a 7F Goodale-Lubin catheter (Fig. 11-3) the peak of the V wave is bisected by the rapid downstroke of left ventricular pressure decline. Realignment of a wedge tracing so that the V wave peak is bisected by (or slightly to the left of) the downstroke of left ventricular pressure is a practical method for achieving more physiologic realignment.

***Calibration Errors.*** Failure to calibrate pressure transducers properly and to adjust them to the same zero reference point may yield an erroneous gradient. A quick way to check the validity of an unsuspected mitral gradient is to switch left and right heart catheters to opposite transducers, which if calibrated equally will yield the same gradient.

***Cardiac Output Determination.*** Cardiac output must be determined accurately, as described in Chapter 8. The cardiac output used in valve area calculation should be the value measured simultaneously with the gradient determination. The measurement used in the valve area formula is usually the *forward* cardiac output determined by Fick or indicator dilution methods. If mitral valvular regurgitation exists, the gradient across the valve will reflect not only forward flow but forward plus regurgitant or total transmitral diastolic flow. Thus, using only forward flow to calculate the valve area will

**TABLE 11-1.** *Valve Orifice Area Determination*

Patient _____ Age _____ Unit Number _____ Date _____

| A. Complex No. | Area of Gradient (mm²) | / | Length of Diastolic or Systolic Period (mm) | = | Average Gradient (deflection, mm) |
|---|---|---|---|---|---|
| 1. | _____ | / | _____ | = | _____ |
| 2. | _____ | / | _____ | = | _____ |
| 3. | _____ | / | _____ | = | _____ |
| 4. | _____ | / | _____ | = | _____ |
| 5. | _____ | / | _____ | = | _____ |

B. Mean Gradient = Average Gradient (mm deflection) × Scale Factor

(mmHg/mm deflection)

= _____ × _____ = _____ mmHg

C. Average Diastolic or Systolic Period = Average Length (mm)/Paper Speed (mm/sec)

= _____ / _____ = _____ sec/beat

D. Heart Rate = _____ beat/min

E. Cardiac Output (Fick or Indicator dilution) = _____ cc/min

F. Valve Area = $\dfrac{\text{Cardiac Ouput/(Heart Rate} \times \text{Avg. Diastolic or Systolic Period)}}{\text{Valve Constant* } \times \sqrt{\text{Mean Gradient}}}$

= $\dfrac{\underline{\hspace{1cm}}/(\underline{\hspace{1cm}} \times \underline{\hspace{1cm}})}{\underline{\hspace{1cm}} \times \sqrt{\underline{\hspace{1cm}}}}$ = _____ cm²

G. Valve Area Index = Valve Area/Body Surface Area = _____ cm²/M²

*Valve Constants: for mitral valve use 37.7; for aortic, tricuspid, and pulmonic valves use 44.3.

underestimate the actual anatomic valve area in cases where regurgitation coexists with stenosis.

***Early Diastasis.*** Even when left atrial and left ventricular pressures equalize (diastasis) prior to the end of diastole, there will generally still be flow through the mitral valve after diastasis. The *diastolic filling period thus includes all of nonisovolumic diastole,* not just the period during which the gradient is present.

## AORTIC VALVE AREA

An aortic valve area of 0.7 cm² or less is generally considered severe enough to account for the symptoms of angina, syncope, or heart failure in a patient with aortic stenosis.

Figure 11-4 illustrates the relationship between cardiac output and aortic pressure gradient over a range of values for aortic valve area and at three values for heart rate and systolic ejection period. For the aortic valve, equation 4 can be rearranged as:

$$\Delta P = \left[ \frac{\text{CO/(HR)(SEP)}}{44.3 \, \text{AVA}} \right]^2 \quad (6)$$

As can be seen in Figure 11-4A, at a normal resting cardiac output of 5.0 liters/min, an aortic orifice area of 0.7 cm² will result in a gradient of approximately 33 mmHg across the aortic valve. Doubling of the cardiac output, as might occur with exercise, would increase the gradient by a factor of 4 to 132 mmHg if the systolic time/minute did not change. This increase in gradient would require a peak left ventricular pressure in excess of 250 mmHg to maintain a central aortic pressure of 120 mmHg. Such a major increase in left ventricular pressure obviously increases myocardial oxygen demand and also limits ejection performance; these factors contribute to the symptoms of angina and congestive heart failure, respectively.[3,4]

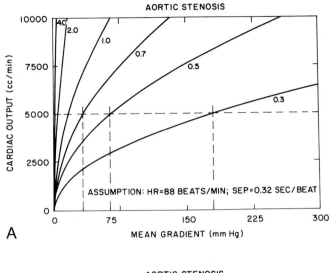

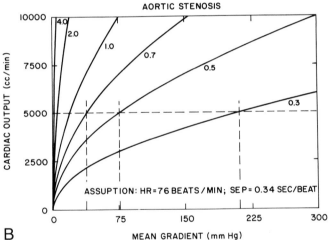

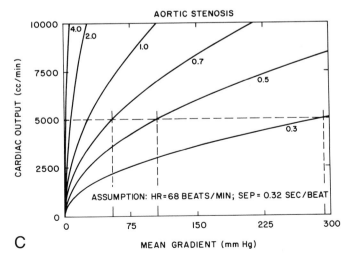

**Fig. 11-4.** Relationships between cardiac output and mean aortic systolic pressure gradient in patients with aortic stenosis, calculated using equation 6, derived from the Gorlin equation. Individual curves represent orifice areas of 4.0, 2.0, 1.0, 0.7, 0.5, and 0.3 cm$^2$. A, B, and C represent flow-gradient relations at differing heart rates and systolic ejection periods. (Courtesy of Dr. James J. Ferguson, III.)

The limitations in cardiac output imposed by high afterload may contribute to hypotension when peripheral vasodilation occurs during muscular exercise. Actually, the systolic time per minute *does not* remain constant during the increase in cardiac output associated with exercise. As heart rate increases during exercise, the systolic ejection period tends to become shorter, but the tendency is counteracted by both increased venous return and systemic arteriolar vasodilation, factors that normally help to maintain left ventricular stroke volume constant (or even increased) during exercise. Thus, heart rate is increasing, but systolic ejection period is diminishing only slightly, so that their product (systolic ejection time per minute) increases. This is the counterpart of the decreased diastolic filling time per minute during exercise, discussed above. Examining equation (6), it can be seen that the increase in cardiac output will be partially offset by the increase in (HR)(SEP), so that the gradient will not quadruple with a doubling of cardiac output during exercise.

Figure 11-4 B and C show that with *decreasing* heart rate, the gradient increases in aortic stenosis for any value of cardiac output. This is opposite to the effect of heart rate in mitral stenosis and reflects the oppo-

site effects of heart rate on systolic and diastolic time per minute. Viewed another way, as the heart rate slows in aortic stenosis, the stroke volume increases if cardiac output remains constant. Thus, the flow/beat across the aortic valve increases, and so does the pressure gradient.

As with mitral stenosis, some allowance must be made for body size in deciding what is a critical valve area in aortic stenosis: larger patients who require higher output may become symptomatic at somewhat larger valve areas. Thus, a very large man with a body surface area of 2.4 $M^2$ and a cardiac index of 3.0 L/min/$M^2$ would have a cardiac output of 7200 ml/min. At a heart rate of 68 beats/min (Fig. 11-4C), this man might have a 50 mmHg aortic valve gradient with an orifice area of 0.9–1.0 $cm^2$. Thus, for him, this might be a critical valve area.

***Example.*** Figure 11-5 demonstrates simultaneous pressure tracings from the left ventricle (LV) and right femoral artery (RFA) in a patient with exertional syncope. Since the pulse wave takes a finite period of time to travel from the left ventricle to the femoral artery, the femoral artery tracing is somewhat delayed (Fig. 11-5A). Figure 11-5B shows the LV and RFA tracings realigned to correct for the delay in transmission time.

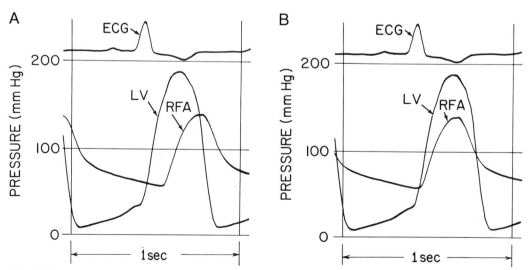

**Fig. 11-5.** Left ventricular (LV) and right femoral artery (RFA) pressure tracings in a patient who presented with exertional syncope due to aortic stenosis. A shows the tracings actually recorded, and demonstrates the signficant time delay for the pressure waveform to reach the RFA. B shows realignment using tracing paper. See text for discussion.

This is accomplished using tracing paper and aligning the arterial upstroke to coincide with the LV upstroke. After such alignment, the mean pressure gradient can now be obtained by planimetry, and the orifice area can be calculated using the form given in Table 11-1. For this example, the average aortic pressure gradient was 40 mmHg, the systolic ejection period 0.33 sec, the heart 74 beats/min, and the cardiac output 5000 cm$^3$/min. Using these values together with an aortic valve constant of (1)(44.3) = 44.3 in the equation in Table 11-1 gives:

Aortic valve area =

$$\frac{(5000 \text{ cm}^3/\text{min})/(74 \text{ beats/min}) \cdot (0.33 \text{ sec/beat})}{44.3 \sqrt{40 \text{ mmHg}}}$$

Aortic valve area = 0.73 cm$^2$

If a peripheral catheter is not employed to obtain simultaneous left ventricular and peripheral pressure, the gradient may be obtained by recording left ventricular pressure and superimposing it upon the aortic pressure obtained immediately after the left ventricular catheter is pulled back into the aorta.

## Pitfalls

***Transducer Calibration.*** As with calculation of mitral valve area, attention to cardiac output determination and transducer calibration is critical. Assurance that proper transducer calibration has been accomplished can be obtained by comparing the left heart catheter pressure to the peripheral arterial catheter pressure prior to insertion of the left heart catheter into the left ventricle. Since in the absence of peripheral stenosis mean arterial pressure will be the same throughout the arterial tree, the mean pressure recorded by both catheters should be identical, confirming identical transducer calibration. Further gradient verification is made by comparing the left ventricular pressure to aortic pressure obtained by the left heart catheter during catheter pullback. In this case, both left ventricular and aortic pressures are recorded by the same catheter and transducer, eliminating the second transducer as a source of error.

***Low Flow States.*** In low cardiac output states, only a small gradient may be present across a critically narrowed aortic valve. For instance, at a cardiac output of 3 liters/minute, a pressure gradient of 20 mmHg will yield an aortic valve area of 0.7 cm$^2$. In such cases, small errors in gradient or cardiac output measurement may substantially alter the hemodynamic assessment of stenosis severity and may lead to an incorrect conclusion concerning the need to replace the aortic valve. Furthermore, at low flows a valve that is sclerotic, but not truly stenotic, may fail to open fully. This results in a reduced effective valve area.[5,6] In such cases, the use of exercise or infusion of a positive inotropic agent allows for calculation of gradient and valve area at a higher and more reliable cardiac output.

***Substitution of Peripheral Arterial Pressure for Central Aortic Pressure.*** Many laboratories, including our own, use peripheral arterial pressure as a substitute for central aortic pressure for the measurement of gradients in patients with aortic stenosis. As mentioned, we correct for temporal delay by realignment (Fig. 11-5). However, as discussed in Chapter 9, peripheral arterial pressure waveforms are distorted in ways other than simply time delay. These distortions include systolic amplification and spreading out (widening) of the pressure waveform. To assess possible errors introduced by the use of peripheral arterial pressure as a substitute for ascending aortic pressure, Folland and co-workers compared the left ventricular-ascending aortic (LV-Ao) mean gradient in 26 patients with aortic stenosis with the left ventricular-femoral artery (LV-FA) systolic gradient, with and without realignment (Fig. 11-6).[7] Without realignment, the LV-FA gradient *overestimated* the LV-Ao gradient by ~9 mmHg. In contrast, aligned LV-FA gradients *underestimated* the LV-Ao gradient by ~10 mmHg, possibly representing the fact that peak systolic arterial pressure is higher in peripheral arterial pressure tracings than in central aortic tracings, so that the planimetered gradient will be smaller when using LV-FA. Without realignment, this effect is offset by the fact that much of the arterial systolic waveform is outside and to the right of the left ventricular pressure tracing (Fig. 11-6). Folland et al suggest averaging the results from aligned and unaligned gradients to most closely approximate true LV-Ao gradient.[7] We have generally

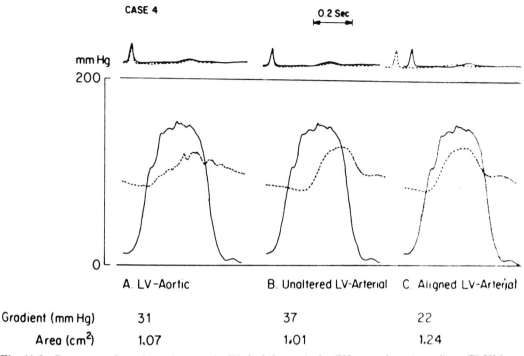

CASE 4                              0.2 Sec

| | A. LV-Aortic | B. Unaltered LV-Arterial | C. Aligned LV-Arterial |
|---|---|---|---|
| Gradient (mm Hg) | 31 | 37 | 22 |
| Area (cm²) | 1.07 | 1.01 | 1.24 |

**Fig. 11-6.** Pressure gradients in aortic stenosis. (A) the left ventricular (LV)-central aortic gradient; (B) LV-femoral artery gradient without alignment; and (C) LV-femoral artery gradient with alignment obtained by moving the femoral artery tracing leftward so that its upstroke coincides with the LV pressure upstroke. (Reproduced with permission from Folland ED, Parisi AF, Carbone C: Is peripheral arterial pressure a satisfactory substitute for ascending aortic pressure when measuring aortic valve gradients? J Am Coll Cardiol 4:1207, 1984.)

used the aligned gradients, but if there is a significant difference between central and peripheral arterial peak systolic pressures (as measured prior to entry into the left ventricle), we add this difference to the planimetered gradient.

***Pullback Hemodynamics.*** When the aortic valve area is diminished to 0.6 cm² or less, a 7F or 8F catheter placed retrograde across the valve takes up a significant amount of the residual orifice area, and the catheter may actually increase the severity of stenosis. Conversely, removal of the catheter will reduce the amount of stenosis. We have observed that a peripheral pressure rise occurs in severe aortic stenosis when the left ventricular catheter is removed from the aortic valve orifice.[8] In our experience, an augmentation in peripheral systolic pressure of >5 mmHg at the time of left ventricular catheter pullback indicates that significant aortic stenosis is present. This sign is present in

more than 80% of patients with an aortic valve area of 0.5 cm² or less, a point which is discussed further in Chapter 23.

## AREA OF TRICUSPID AND PULMONIC VALVES

Because of the rarity of tricuspid and pulmonic stenosis in adults, no general agreement exists as to what constitutes a critical orifice area for these valves. In general, a mean gradient of 5 mmHg across the tricuspid valve is sufficient to cause symptoms of systemic venous hypertension. Gradients across the pulmonic valve of less than 50 mmHg are usually well tolerated, but gradients of greater than 100 mmHg indicate a need for surgical correction. Between 50 mmHg and 100 mmHg, decisions regarding surgical correction will depend on the clinical features in each individual case.

## ALTERNATIVES TO THE GORLIN FORMULA

A simplified valve formula for the calculation of stenotic cardiac valve areas has been proposed by Hakki et al and tested in 100 consecutive patients with either aortic or mitral stenosis.[9] The simplified formula is simply:

$$\text{Valve area} = \frac{\text{Cardiac output (L/min)}}{\sqrt{\text{Pressure gradient}}}$$

and is based on their observation that the product of heart rate, SEP or DFP, and the Gorlin equation constant was nearly the same for all patients whose hemodynamics were measured in the resting state, and the value of this product was close to 1.0. For the examples given earlier in this chapter, the simplified formula works reasonably well. Thus, for the patient with mitral stenosis (Fig. 11-3) with a cardiac output of 4680 ml/min and a mitral diastolic gradient of 30 mmHg, mitral valve area = 4.68 ÷ $\sqrt{30}$ = 0.85 cm$^2$ using the simplified formula, as opposed to the value of 0.71 cm$^2$ calculated using the Gorlin formula. For the patient with aortic stenosis whose tracings are shown in Figure 11-5 (cardiac output 5 L/min, aortic gradient 40 mmHg) the aortic valve area by the simplified formula is 5 ÷ $\sqrt{40}$ = 0.79 cm$^2$, as opposed to 0.73 cm$^2$ by the Gorlin formula. Since the percentage of time per minute spent in diastole or systole changes substantially at higher heart rates, the simplified formula may be less useful in the presence of substantial tachycardia. However, this point has not been tested adequately.

Angel et al.[10] have introduced a modification of Hakki's simplified formula for calculation of valve areas. They added a correction for heart rate, dividing Hakki's equation by 1.35 when heart rate was <75 beats/min for patients with mitral stenosis and >90 beats/min for patients with aortic stenosis.[10] This empiric correction improved the predictive accuracy of Hakki's formula.

Another alternative to the Gorlin formula has been suggested recently by Cannon and co-workers who utilized an in-vitro pulsatile flow model which mimicked many of the characteristics of physiologic LV and aortic pressure and flow.[11] Using this model, they found that the Gorlin formula constant C was not constant at all, but was a linear function of the square root of the mean transvalvular gradient. Using data from this experimental model, Cannon et al derived a new orifice formula which was tested in the clinical setting.[11] The new orifice formula was

$$A = F/K' \, \Delta P + h$$

where F = transvalvular flow in ml/sec, $\Delta P$ = mean transvalvular gradient, and K' and h are constants which differ for different valves (e.g., porcine, native aortic valve). This formula reliably predicted actual valve areas in a group of patients with normally functioning porcine aortic valves. An interesting prediction of Cannon's formula is that for any given value of A, F is a linear function of $\Delta P$. Thus, Figures 11-2 and 11-4 would consist of a series of straight lines, if constructed by Cannon's formula.

**ACKNOWLEDGEMENT** The authors express their appreciation to Dr. James J. Ferguson, III, who supplied Figures 11-2 and 11-4, constructed by him from computer simulation.

## REFERENCES

1. Gorlin R, Gorlin G: Hydraulic formula for calculation of area of stenotic mitral valve, other cardiac values and central circulatory shunts. Am Heart J 41:1, 1951.
2. Cohen MV, Gorlin R: Modified orifice equation for the calculation of mitral valve area. Am Heart J 84:839, 1972.
3. Strauer BE, Burger SB: Systolic stress, coronary hemodynamics and metabolic reserve in experimental and clinical cardiac hypertrophy. Basic Res Cardiol 75:234, 1980.
4. Carabello BA, et al: Hemodynamic determinants of prognosis of aortic valve replacement in critical aortic stenosis and advanced congestive heart failure. Circulation 62:42, 1980.
5. Thubrikar M, Harry RR, Nolan SP: Normal aortic valve function in dogs. Am J Cardiol 40:563, 1977.
6. Gasper J, et al: Overestimation of aortic stenosis

with the Gorlin equation in low flow states. J Am Coll Cardiol 1:639, 1983.

7. Folland ED, Parisi AF, Carbone C: Is Peripheral arterial pressure a satisfactory substitute for ascending aortic pressure when measuring aortic valve gradients? J Am Coll Cardiol 4:1207, 1984.

8. Carabello BA, Barry WH, Grossman W: Changes in arterial pressure during left heart pullback in patients with aortic stenosis: A sign of severe aortic stenosis. Am J Cardiol 44:424, 1979.

9. Hakki AH, et al: A simplified valve formula for the

calculation of stenotic cardiac valve areas. Circulation 63:1050, 1981.

10. Angel, J., Soler-Soler, J., Anivarro, I., Domingo, E.: Hemodynamic evaluation of stenotic cardiac valves: II. Modification of the simplified formula for mitral and aortic valve area calculation. Cathet Cardiovasc Diagn 11:127, 1985.

11. Cannon SR, Richards KL, Crawford M: Hydraulic estimation of stenotic orifice area: A correction of the Gorlin formula. Circulation 71:1170, 1985.

## chapter twelve

# Shunt Detection and Measurement

WILLIAM GROSSMAN

DETECTION, localization, and quantification of intracardiac shunts are an integral part of the hemodynamic evaluation of patients with congenital heart disease. In most cases, an intracardiac shunt is suspected on the basis of the clinical evaluation of the patient prior to catheterization. However, there are several circumstances in which data obtained at catheterization should alert the cardiologist to look for a shunt that previously had not been suspected:

1. Unexplained arterial desaturation should immediately raise the suspicion of a right to left intracardiac shunt, which may then be assessed by the methods to be discussed. Most commonly, arterial desaturation (i.e., arterial blood oxygen saturation <95%) detected at the time of cardiac catheterization represents alveolar hypoventilation. The causes for this alveolar hypoventilation and its associated "physiologic" right to left shunt include (a) excessive sedation from the premedication, (b) chronic obstructive lung disease or other pulmonary parenchymal disease, and (c) pulmonary congestion/edema secondary to the patient's cardiac disease. Alveolar hypoventilation associated with each of these problems is exacerbated by the supine position of the patient during the catheterization procedure, and by excessively tight "chest straps" used in some laboratories to hold the patient firmly in the cradle-type x-ray table. Loosening the chest straps, helping the patient to assume a more upright posture (head-up tilt, or propping the patient up with a large wedge if tilt mechanism is not available), and encouraging the patient to take deep breaths and to cough will correct arterial hypoxemia, or substantially ameliorate it, in most cases. If arterial desaturation persists, oxygen should be administered by face mask both for therapeutic and diagnostic purposes. If full arterial blood oxygen saturation cannot be achieved by face-mask administration of oxygen (it is best in this regard to use a rebreathing mask that fits snugly), a right to left shunt must be presumed to be present, and its anatomic site and magnitude determined using the methods described later in this chapter.

2. Conversely, when the oxygen content of blood in the pulmonary artery is unexpectedly high, that is, if the pulmonary artery (PA) blood oxygen saturation is above 80% or if it is higher than expected, the possibility of a left to right intracardiac shunt should be considered. It is for these two reasons that arterial and pulmonary artery saturation should be measured routinely *during* the catheterization.

3. When the data obtained at catheterization do not confirm the presence of the suspected lesion, one should consider the pres-

Some material in this chapter has been retained from the first and second editions, to which Dr. James E. Dalen had contributed.

ence of an intracardiac shunt. For example, if left ventricular cineangiography fails to reveal mitral regurgitation in a patient in whom this was judged to be the cause of a systolic murmur, it is prudent to look for evidence of a ventricular septal defect (VSD) with left to right shunting.

## DETECTION OF LEFT TO RIGHT INTRACARDIAC SHUNTS

Many different techniques are available for the detection, localization, and quantification of left to right intracardiac shunts. They vary in their sensitivity, in the type of indicator they use, and in the equipment needed to sense and read out the presence of the indicator.

## Measurement of Oxygen Content in the Right Heart (Oximetry Run)

In this basic technique for detecting and quantifying left to right shunts, the oxygen content or percent saturation is measured in blood samples drawn sequentially from the pulmonary artery, right ventricle (RV), right atrium (RA), superior vena cava (SVC), and inferior vena cava (IVC). A left to right shunt may be detected and localized if a significant "step-up" in blood oxygen saturation or content is found in one of the right heart chambers. A significant step-up is defined as an increase in blood oxygen content or saturation that exceeds the normal variability that might be observed if multiple samples were drawn from that cardiac chamber.

The technique of the oximetry run is based upon the fundamental studies of Dexter and his associates in 1947.[1] They found that multiple samples drawn from the right atrium could vary in oxygen content by as much as 2 volumes percent (vol%).* This variability has been attributed to the fact that the right atrium receives its blood from three sources of varying oxygen content: the superior vena cava, the inferior vena cava, and the coronary sinus. The maximal normal variation within the right ventricle was found to be 1 vol%. Because of more adequate mixing, a maximal variation within the pulmonary artery of only ½ vol% was found by Dexter. Thus, using the Dexter criteria, a significant

step-up is present at the atrial level when the highest oxygen content in blood samples drawn from the right atrium exceeds the highest content in the venae cavae by ≥2 vol%. Similarly, a significant step-up at the ventricular level is present if the highest right ventricular sample is ≥1 vol% higher than the highest right atrial sample, and a significant step-up at the level of the pulmonary artery is present if the pulmonary artery oxygen content is more than ½ vol% greater than the highest right ventricular sample.

Dexter's classic study described normal variability and gave criteria for a significant oxygen step-up only for measurement of blood oxygen content. This in part reflects the methodology available to him, since reflectance oximetry was not widely used at that time. In recent years, most cardiac catheterization laboratories (especially those primarily involved in pediatric catheterization) have moved toward the measurement of percent saturation by reflectance oximetry as the routine method for oximetric analysis of blood samples. Oxygen content may then be calculated from knowledge of percent saturation, the patient's blood hemoglobin concentration, and an assumed constant relationship for oxygen carrying capacity of hemoglobin, as discussed in Chapter 8 (1.36 ml $O_2$/gm hemoglobin). When oxygen content is derived in this manner, rather than by measurement by the Van Slyke or other direct oximetric technique, it is no more accurate (and probably less so because of the potential presence of carboxyhemoglobin or hemoglobin variants with $O_2$ capacity other than 1.36) than the percent oxygen saturation values from which it is calculated.

To clarify this situation, Antman and coworkers at the Peter Bent Brigham Hospital studied prospectively the normal variation of both oxygen content and oxygen saturation of blood in the right heart chambers.[2] The study population consisted of patients without intracardiac shunts who were undergoing diagnostic cardiac catheterization for evaluation of coronary artery disease, valvular heart disease, cardiomyopathy, or possible pulmonary embolism. Each patient had a complete right heart oximetry run (see below) with sampling of multiple sites in each chamber. Oxygen content was measured directly by an electrochemical fuel-cell method (Lex-02-Con*), a method that had

---

*1 volume percent = 1 ml $O_2$/100 ml blood or 10 ml $O_2$/Liter of blood.

*Lexington Instruments, Lexington, MA.

been validated previously against the Van Slyke method at the Peter Bent Brigham Hospital. Oxygen saturation was calculated as blood oxygen content divided by oxygen carrying capacity. It is obvious that the relationship between oxygen content and oxygen saturation depends on the hemoglobin concentration of the patient's blood; e.g., 75% oxygen saturation of pulmonary artery blood will be associated with a substantially lower oxygen content in an anemic patient than in one with normal hemoglobin concentration. Also, systemic blood flow may be an important determinant of oxygen variability in the right heart chambers, since high systemic flow will tend to equalize the differences across various tissue beds. In the context of these considerations, I have listed in Table 12-1 criteria for a significant step-up in right heart oxygen content and percent oxygen saturation associated with various types of left to right shunt, based on the study of Antman and co-workers[2] and other investigators[1,3,4].

The blood samples needed to determine whether a step-up is present in the right heart are obtained by·performing what is called an oximetry run. The samples needed, and the order in which we recommend they be obtained, follow.

Obtain a 2-ml sample from each of the following locations:

1. Left and /or right pulmonary artery
*2. Main pulmonary artery
*3. Right ventricle, outflow tract
†4. Right ventricle, mid
*†5. Right ventricle, tricuspid valve or apex
*6. Right atrium, low or near tricuspid valve
7. Right atrium, mid
8. Right atrium, high
9. Superior vena cava, low (near junction with right atrium)
10. Superior vena cava, high (near junction with innominate vein)
11. Inferior vena cava, high (just below diaphragm)
12. Inferior vena cava, low (at L4–L5)
13. Left ventricle
14. Aorta (distal to insertion of ductus)

In performing the oximetry run, an end-hole catheter or one with side holes close to

*Confirm location by pressure measurement.

†If frequent extrasystoles occur, do not persist. Obtain samples from three different locations in right ventricle and right atrium.

its tip (e.g., a Goodale-Lubin catheter‡) is positioned in the right or left pulmonary artery. Cardiac output is measured by the Fick method. As soon as the determination of oxygen consumption is completed, the operator begins to obtain 2-ml blood samples from each of the locations indicated. This is done under fluoroscopic control, with catheter position further confirmed by pressure measurement at the sites noted. The entire procedure should take less than seven minutes. If a sample cannot be obtained from a specific site because of ventricular premature beats, that site should be skipped until the rest of the run has been completed.

Oxygen content and saturation in each of the samples is determined as discussed previously, and the presence of a significant step-up is determined by applying the criteria listed in Table 12-1.

An alternative method for performing the oximetry run is to withdraw a fiberoptic catheter from the pulmonary artery through the right heart chambers and the inferior and superior venae cavae. This permits a continuous readout of oxygen saturation that allows detection of a step-up in oxygen content.

If the oximetry run reveals that a significant step-up is present, the pulmonary blood flow, systemic blood flow, and the magnitude of left to right and right to left shunts may be calculated according to the following formulae.

### Calculation of Pulmonary Blood Flow ($Q_P$).
Pulmonary blood flow is calculated by the same formula used in the standard Fick equation:

$$Q_P \text{ (L/min)} = \frac{O_2 \text{ consumption (ml/min)}}{\left[\begin{array}{c}PV\,O_2 \\ \text{content} \\ \text{(ml/L)}\end{array}\right] - \left[\begin{array}{c}PA\,O_2 \\ \text{content} \\ \text{(ml/L)}\end{array}\right]}$$

If a pulmonary vein (PV) has not been entered, systemic arterial oxygen content may be used in the preceding formula, if systemic oxygen saturation is 95% or more. If systemic oxygen saturation is <95%, one must determine whether a right to left intracardiac shunt is present. If there is an intracardiac right to left shunt, an assumed value for pulmonary venous oxygen content of 98% × oxygen capacity should be used in calculating pulmonary blood flow. If arterial

‡United States Catheter and Instrument Corp., Billerica, MA.

**TABLE 12-1.** *Detection of Left to Right Shunt by Oximetry*

| Level of Shunt | Criteria For Significant Step | | | | Approximate Minimal $Q_p/Q_s$ Required for Detection (Assuming SBFI = 3L/min/M²) | Possible Causes of Step-Up |
|---|---|---|---|---|---|---|
| | $\begin{bmatrix}\text{Mean of}\\\text{Distal}\\\text{Chamber}\\\text{Samples}\end{bmatrix} - \begin{bmatrix}\text{Mean of}\\\text{Proximal}\\\text{Chamber}\\\text{Samples}\end{bmatrix}$ | | $\begin{bmatrix}\text{Highest}\\\text{Value in}\\\text{Distal}\\\text{Chamber}\end{bmatrix} - \begin{bmatrix}\text{Highest}\\\text{Value in}\\\text{Proximal}\\\text{Chamber}\end{bmatrix}$ | | | |
| | O₂ Vol% | O₂% Sat | O₂ Vol% | O₂% Sat | | |
| Atrial (SVC/IVC to RA) | ≥1.3 | ≥7 | ≥2.0 | ≥11 | 1.5–1.9 | Atrial septal defect; anomalous pulmonary venous drainage; ruptured sinus of Valsalva; VSD with TR; coronary fistula to RA |
| Ventricular (RA to RV) | ≥1.0 | ≥5 | ≥1.7 | ≥10 | 1.3–1.5 | VSD; PDA with PR; primum ASD; coronary fistula to RV |
| Great Vessel (RV to PA) | ≥1.0 | ≥5 | ≥1.0 | ≥5 | 1.3 | PDA; aorta-pulmonic window; aberrant coronary artery origin |

Abbreviations: SVC and IVC, superior and inferior vena cavae; RA, right atrium; RV, right ventricle; PA, pulmonary artery; VSD, ventricular septal defect; TR, Tricuspid regurgitation; PDA, patent ductus arteriosus; PR, pulmonic regurgitation; ASD, atrial septal defect; SBFI, systemic blood flow index; $Q_p/Q_s$, pulmonary to systemic flow ratio.

desaturation is present and is not due to a right to left intracardiac shunt, the observed systemic oxygen saturation should be used to calculate pulmonary blood flow.

For example, let us suppose that a patient is found to have an atrial septal defect with a left to right shunt clearly detected by oximetry run. Furthermore, the catheter crosses the defect and a pulmonary vein is entered, from which a blood sample shows $O_2$ saturation of 98%. However, let us further suppose that systemic arterial blood saturation is 90% and that this is due to chronic pulmonary disease. After ruling out a right to left shunt (e.g., inhalation of 100% oxygen, indocyanine green dye injection in inferior vena cava, echocardiogram-bubble study), should we use 98% or 90% for pulmonary venous blood $O_2$ saturation in the calculation of $Q_p$? As indicated above, since arterial desaturation is not due to a right to left intracardiac shunt, the observed systemic arterial $O_2$ saturation (90%) should be used, since this summates all the pulmonary veins draining both lungs, not just the one with 98% $O_2$ saturation.

### Calculation of Systemic Blood Flow ($Q_s$).

$$\frac{Q_s}{\text{(L/min)}} = \frac{O_2 \text{ consumption (ml/min)}}{\left[\begin{array}{c}\text{systemic arterial} \\ O_2 \text{ content, ml/L}\end{array}\right] - \left[\begin{array}{c}\text{mixed venous} \\ O_2 \text{ content, ml/L}\end{array}\right]}$$

The key to the measurement of systemic blood flow in the presence of an intracardiac shunt is that the mixed venous oxygen con-

tent must be measured in the chamber immediately proximal to the shunt, as shown in Table 12-2.

The formula to be used for the calculation of venous content in the presence of an atrial septal defect (ASD) was derived by Flamm et al.[5] They found that systemic blood flow calculated from mixed venous oxygen content as determined from the formula listed in Table 12-2 most closely approximates systemic blood flow as measured by left ventricular to brachial artery (BA) dye curves in patients with atrial septal defect studied at rest. It should be noted that Flamm's formula "weights" blood returning from the superior vena cava more heavily than might be expected on the basis of relative flows in the superior and inferior cavae. The success of this empirical weighting of the relatively desaturated superior vena cava blood ($O_2$ saturation is almost always less in blood from the superior as opposed to the inferior vena cava) probably reflects the fact that the third contributor to mixed venous blood—desaturated coronary sinus blood—is not sampled during the oximetry run and therefore cannot be included directly in the formula. It must also be pointed out that the formula $(3\,\text{SVC}\,O_2 + 1\,\text{IVC}\,O_2)/4$ was validated by Flamm and associates for mixed venous oxygen content at rest.[5] Thus, in 18 patients without shunt, this value agreed closely with pulmonary artery blood oxygen content at rest. However, during supine bicycle exercise, a different relationship was found to apply, in which mixed venous (pul-

**TABLE 12-2.** *Calculation of Systemic Blood Flow in the Presence of Left to Right Shunt*

| Location of Shunt as Determined by Site of $O_2$ Step-up | Mixed Venous Sample to Use in Calculating Systemic Blood Flow |
| --- | --- |
| 1. Pulmonary Artery (e.g., patent ductus arteriosus) | Right ventricle, average of samples obtained during oximetry run |
| 2. Right ventricle (e.g., ventricular septal defect) | Right atrium, average of all samples during oximetry run |
| 3. Right atrium (e.g., atrial septal defect) | $\dfrac{3(\text{SVC } O_2 \text{ content}) + 1(\text{IVC } O_2 \text{ content})}{4}$ |

monary artery) oxygen content in patients without shunts was best approximated as (1 SVC $O_2$ + 2 IVC $O_2$)/3. This formula was then used for patients with atrial septal defect *during exercise*, and it reliably predicted systemic blood flow measured by left ventricular to brachial artery dye-dilution curve. Therefore, for patients with left to right shunt at the atrial level, the formula in Table 12-2 should be used only for calculation of *resting* mixed venous $O_2$ content.

Obviously, calculations from the formula in Table 12-2 would be little changed in many cases by ignoring inferior vena cava blood altogether, and this is done in some laboratories (especially those involved in pediatric catheterization). However, Flamm and associates examined the effects of assuming that superior vena cava $O_2$ content equaled mixed venous $O_2$ content, and they concluded that this was somewhat less accurate (in both the 18 subjects without shunt and the 9 patients with atrial septal defect and left to right shunt) than the formula given in Table 12-2.[5]

***Calculation of Left to Right Shunt.*** If there is no evidence of an associated right to left shunt, the left to right shunt is calculated by:

$$L \rightarrow R \text{ Shunt} = Q_p - Q_s$$
$$(L/\text{min})$$

***Examples of Left to Right Shunt Detection and Quantification.*** Some examples of oximetry runs are presented to illustrate interpretation. As seen in Figure 12-1 there is a step-up in oxygen saturation in the mid-right atrium. The average or mean value for the vena caval samples in this patient is calculated as [3(SVC) + 1(IVC)] ÷ 4. SVC is the average of SVC samples (i.e., 67.5% in this example), and IVC is the value for the IVC sample taken at the level of the diaphragm only (i.e., 73%). Thus, the vena caval mean $O_2$ saturation for the patient in Figure 12-1 is [3(67.5) + 1(73)] ÷ 4 = 69%. The right atrial mean $O_2$ saturation for this patient is (74 + 84 + 79) ÷ 3 = 79%. The 10% step-up in mean $O_2$ saturation from vena cava to right atrium is higher than the 7% value listed in Table 12-1 as a criterion for a significant step-up at the atrial level. Note that for this example, the highest-to-highest approach (highest right atrial $O_2$ saturation − highest vena caval $O_2$ saturation) would barely meet criteria for a significant step-up, because of the high value for IVC saturation (73%) compared to SVC saturation. Thus, for the detection of a significant step-up at the atrial level using the highest-to-highest approach, it is best to use the highest SVC sample and compare it to the highest RA sample. In this case, the result would be (84% − 68%) = 16%, which is clearly above the 11% value listed in Table 12-1 for detection of a significant step-up.

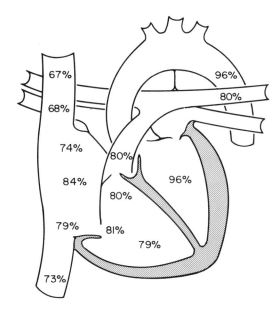

**Fig. 12-1.** Schematic representation of the results of an oximetry run in a patient with a small to moderate size atrial septal defect. Values represent % $O_2$ saturation of blood at multiple locations. See text for details.

To calculate pulmonary and systemic blood flows for the example given in Figure 12-1 we need to know $O_2$ consumption and blood $O_2$ capacity. If the patient's $O_2$ consumption determined by the methods described in Chapter 8 is 240 ml $O_2$/min and the blood hemoglobin concentration is 14 gm%, pulmonary and systemic blood flows may be calculated as follows:

$$Q_p = \frac{O_2 \text{ consumption (ml/min)}}{\begin{bmatrix} PV\ O_2 \\ \text{content} \\ \text{(ml/L)} \end{bmatrix} - \begin{bmatrix} PA\ O_2 \\ \text{content} \\ \text{(ml/L)} \end{bmatrix}}$$

PV $O_2$ content was not measured, but LV and arterial blood $O_2$ saturation was 96% (effectively ruling out a right to left shunt) and therefore it may be assumed that PV blood $O_2$ saturation was 96%. As described in Chapter 8, oxygen content for PV blood is calculated as:

$$0.96\left(\frac{14 \text{ gm Hgb}}{100 \text{ ml blood}}\right) \times \left(\frac{1.36 \text{ ml O}_2}{\text{gmHgb}}\right)$$

$$= 18.3 \text{ ml O}_2/100 \text{ ml blood}$$
$$= 183 \text{ ml O}_2/\text{L}$$

Similarly, PA $O_2$ content is calculated as:

$$0.80(14)1.36 \times 10 = 152 \text{ ml O}_2/\text{L}$$

Therefore,

$$Q_p = \frac{240 \text{ ml O}_2/\text{min}}{[183 - 152] \text{ ml O}_2/\text{L}} = 7.7 \text{ L/min}$$

Systemic blood flow for the patient in Figure 12-1 is calculated as

$$Q_s = \frac{240 \text{ ml O}_2/\text{min}}{\begin{bmatrix} \text{systemic} \\ \text{arterial} \\ O_2 \text{ content} \end{bmatrix} - \begin{bmatrix} \text{mixed} \\ \text{venous} \\ O_2 \text{ content} \end{bmatrix}}$$

$$= \frac{240}{(0.96 - 0.69)14(1.36)10}$$

$$= 4.7 \text{ Liters/min}$$

For this calculation, mixed venous $O_2$ saturation was derived from the formula given in Table 12-2, as 69%. Thus, the ratio of $Q_p/Q_s$ in this example is 7.7/4.7 = 1.6, and the magnitude of the left-to-right shunt is 7.7 − 4.7 = 3 liters/min. This patient has a small to moderate sized atrial septal defect.

Figure 12-2 shows another example of findings in an oximetry run. In this case the patient has a large $O_2$ step-up in the right ventricle, indicating the presence of a ventricular septal defect. If $O_2$ consumption is 260 ml/min and hemoglobin is 15 gm%,

$$Q_p = \frac{260}{(0.97 - 0.885)15(1.36)10} = 15 \text{ L/min}$$

$$Q_s = \frac{260}{(0.97 - 0.66)15(1.36)10} = 4.1 \text{ L/min}$$

$$Q_p/Q_s = 15/4.1 = 3.7$$

$$L \rightarrow \text{shunt} = 15 - 4.1 = 10.9 \text{ L/min}$$

In this case, the $O_2$ saturation of mixed venous blood is calculated by averaging the right atrial $O_2$ saturations, since the right atrium is the chamber immediately proximal to the $O_2$ step-up.

***Flow Ratio.*** The ratio $Q_p/Q_s$ gives important physiologic information about the magnitude of a left to right shunt. In addition, since it factors out other variables (e.g., $O_2$ consumption), it can be calculated from

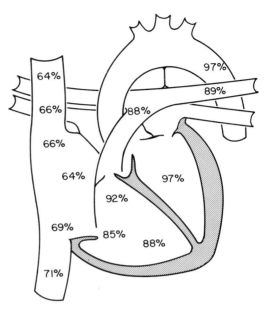

**Fig. 12-2.** Findings from an oximetry run performed in a patient with a large ventricular septal defect. See text for details.

knowledge of blood $O_2$ saturation alone. A $Q_p/Q_s$ ratio of <1.5 signifies a small left to right shunt and is often felt to argue against operative correction, particularly if the patient has an otherwise uncomplicated atrial or ventricular septal defect. A ratio of ≥2.0 indicates a large left to right shunt and is generally considered sufficient evidence to recommend surgical repair of the defect, in order to prevent late pulmonary vascular disease as well as other complications of prolonged circulatory overload. Flow ratios between 1.5 and 2.0 are obviously intermediate in magnitude: surgical correction is generally recommended if operative risk is low.

A flow ratio of <1.0 indicates a net right to left shunt, and is often a sign of the presence of irreversible pulmonary vascular disease.

A *simplified formula* for calculation of flow ratio can be derived by combining the equations for systemic and pulmonary blood flow to obtain:

$$\frac{Q_p}{Q_s} = \frac{(\text{ART O}_2 - \text{MV O}_2)}{(\text{PV O}_2 - \text{PA O}_2)}$$

where ART $O_2$, MVO$_2$, PVO$_2$, and PAO$_2$ are systemic arterial, mixed venous, pulmonary venous, and pulmonary arterial blood oxygen saturations, respectively. For the patient illustrated in Figure 12-1, $Q_p/Q_s$ = (96% − 69%)/(96% − 80%) = 1.68.

### Calculation of Bidirectional Shunts.

If there is evidence of a right to left shunt, as well as a left to right shunt, the following formulae[6] are used to calculate left to right and right to left shunts:

$$L \to R = \frac{Q_p \text{ (mixed venous } O_2 \text{ content} - PA\ O_2 \text{ content)}}{\text{(mixed venous } O_2 \text{ content} - PV^*\ O_2 \text{ content)}}$$

$$R \to L = \frac{Q_p \text{ (}PV^*\ O_2 \text{ content} - ART\ O_2 \text{ content)(}PA\ O_2 \text{ content} - PV^*\ O_2 \text{ content)}}{\text{(}ART\ O_2 \text{ content} - \text{mixed venous } O_2 \text{ content)}}$$
$$\times \text{(mixed venous } O_2 \text{ content} - PV^*\ O_2 \text{ content)}$$

### Limitations of Oximetry Method.

There are several limitations and potential sources of error in the calculations of blood flow using the data obtained from an oximetry run. A primary source of error may be the absence of a steady state during the collection of blood samples. That is, if the oximetry run is prolonged because of technical difficulties or if the patient is agitated or if arrhythmias occur during the oximetry run, the data may not be consistent.

An important limitation of the oxygen step-up method for detecting intracardiac shunts is that it lacks sensitivity. Most shunts of a magnitude that would lead to a recommendation for surgical closure of a ventricular septal defect or patent ductus arteriosus are detected by this method. However, small shunts are not consistently detected by this technique.

As pointed out by Antman and co-workers,[2] the normal variability of blood oxygen saturation in the right heart chambers is strongly influenced by the magnitude of systemic blood flow. High levels of systemic

flow tend to equalize the arterial and venous oxygen values across a given vascular bed. Therefore, elevated systemic blood flow will cause the mixed venous oxygen saturation to be higher than normal, and interchamber variability due to streaming will be blunted. Even a small increase in right heart oxygen saturation under such conditions might indicate the presence of a significant left to right shunt; larger increases would indicate voluminous left to right shunting of blood. For a patient with a systemic blood flow index of $\leq 3.0\ L/min/M^2$, minimum shunt sizes that could be detected reliably by oximetry are listed in Table 12-1.

Fundamental to the oximetric method of shunt detection is the fact that left to right shunting across an intracardiac defect will cause an increase in *blood $O_2$ saturation* in the chamber receiving the shunt proportional to the magnitude of the shunt. However, the increase in *blood $O_2$ content* in the chamber receiving the shunt will depend not only on the magnitude of the shunt, but on the $O_2$ carrying capacity of the blood (i.e., the hemoglobin concentration). As reported by Antman et al.,[2] the influence of blood hemoglobin concentration may be important when blood $O_2$ content (rather than $O_2$ saturation) is used to detect a shunt (Table 12-3).

Thus, the same shunt giving the same blood $O_2$ saturation step-up would give markedly different blood $O_2$ content step-

*If pulmonary vein is not entered, use 98% $\times\ O_2$ capacity.

**TABLE 12-3.** *Expected Value of $O_2$ Content (Volumes Percent) for Various Levels of $O_2$ Step-up and Blood Hemoglobin Concentration*

| Increase in $O_2$ Saturation | Hemoglobin Concentration (gm/100 ml) | | |
|:---:|:---:|:---:|:---:|
| | 10 | 12 | 15 |
| 5% | 0.68 vol% | 0.82 vol% | 1.02 vol% |
| 10% | 1.36 vol% | 1.63 vol% | 2.04 vol% |
| 15% | 2.04 vol% | 2.45 vol% | 3.06 vol% |
| 20% | 2.72 vol% | 3.26 vol% | 4.08 vol% |

*Modified from Antman et al[2] with permission.

ups if the blood hemoglobin concentration varied significantly. Accordingly, when evaluating oximetric data for shunt detection, it is more precise to exclude the potential influence of blood oxygen carrying capacity and utilize only $O_2$ saturation data. This is especially true in pediatric cases[4] where the normal blood $O_2$ carrying capacity may vary from 20 to 28 volumes percent in the neonate to 12 to 16 volumes percent in infancy.

To minimize errors and maximize the physiologic strengths of the oximetry method for shunt detection and quantification, the guidelines listed in Table 12-4 should be followed.

Many more sensitive techniques are available to detect smaller left to right shunts, and these are discussed in the following sections.

## Early Recirculation of an Indicator

In the presence of a left to right shunt, standard indicator dilution curves performed by injection of indocyanine green into the pulmonary artery with sampling in a systemic artery will demonstrate early recirculation on the downslope of the dye curve[7] (Fig. 12-3).

This technique is easily performed and can detect left to right shunts too small to be detected by the oxygen step-up method.[8] Thus,

**TABLE 12-4.** *Guidelines for Optimum Utilization of Oximetric Method for Shunt Detection and Quantification**

1. Multiple blood samples at multiple sites should be rapidly obtained.

2. Blood $O_2$ saturation data rather than $O_2$ content data are preferable to identify the presence of a shunt.

3. Comparison of the mean of all values obtained in the respective chambers is preferable to comparison of highest values in each chamber.

4. Because of the important influence of systemic blood flow on shunt detection, exercise should be used in equivocal cases where a low systemic blood flow is present at rest.

*Based on the data of Antman et al.[2]

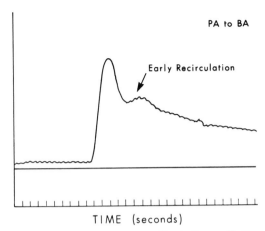

**Fig. 12-3.** Left to right shunt. This indicator dilution curve, performed by injecting indocyanine green into the pulmonary artery with sampling in the brachial artery, demonstrates early recirculation on the downslope, indicating a left to right shunt. Injection was at time zero. This technique does not localize the site of the left to right shunt.

if there is no evidence of a left to right shunt by this method, there is no need to perform an oximetry run. The studies of Castillo et al[9] suggest that left to right shunts as small as 25% of the systemic output can be detected by standard pulmonary artery to systemic artery dye curves.

Although a simple pulmonary to systemic artery dye curve may detect the presence of a shunt, it does not localize it. That is, a pulmonary artery to systemic artery dye curve will show evidence of early recirculation in the presence of a left to right shunt due to an atrial septal defect, ventricular septal defect, or patent ductus arteriosus.

Intracardiac defects with left to right shunts too small to cause detectable early recirculation on a standard pulmonary to systemic artery dye curve would rarely require surgical closure. However, when it is pertinent to detect shunts even smaller than those detected by this technique, a variety of more sensitive techniques are available.

## Early Appearance of an Indicator in the Right Heart

In this technique, an indicator such as indocyanine green[10] is injected into the left heart at the level of, or proximal to, the origin of a left to right shunt. Early appearance of the indicator is sought by measuring the appearance of the indicator in right heart blood.

If indocyanine green is used, blood is withdrawn from a standard catheter whose tip is positioned in the pulmonary artery; the blood is passed through a densitometer to determine the appearance time of the indocyanine green in the pulmonary artery. In the presence of a left to right shunt, the appearance time will be nearly instantaneous: <1 to 2 seconds. In the absence of a left to right shunt, the appearance time will be more than 4 to 6 seconds.

The site of the shunt may be localized by varying the injection site (e.g., left atrium, left ventricle, or aorta), or by varying the sampling site until early appearance is no longer present.

Figure 12-4 illustrates the use of this technique to detect and localize a left to right shunt. The top panel is a dye curve obtained by injecting 1 ml of indocyanine green into the left ventricle with sampling in the pulmonary artery. The appearance time of the dye,

when corrected for the time necessary to withdraw blood from the pulmonary artery catheter to the densitometer (4.2 seconds), is less than one second. This early appearance of dye is consistent with a left to right shunt at the level of the ventricle (ventricular septal defect) or the aorta (e.g., patent ductus arteriosus), or it could be due to an ostium primum defect with shunting from the left ventricle to the right atrium. The site of the shunt is further localized in the middle panel by sampling from the right ventricle. The appearance remains less than a second; thus the shunt is from the left heart to the right ventricle or to the right atrium. The lower panel shows that the appearance time from the left ventricle to the right atrium is normal. Thus the shunt is from the left ventricle or aorta to the right ventricle. A subsequent injection into the ascending aorta with sampling in the right ventricle demonstrated a normal appearance time. This series of dye curves thus demonstrated that the left to right shunt was due to a ventricular septal defect.

This method is very sensitive in detecting small left to right shunts across a ventricular septal defect or a patent ductus arteriosus. It is not as well adapted to detecting atrial septal defects because they require entry into the left atrium.

A variety of specialized indicators (e.g., hydrogen gas, krypton-85, nitrous oxide, ascorbic acid, freon, ether) have been used in shunt detection in the past and are still used by some laboratories. The interested reader is referred to the 2nd edition of this textbook, and to the literature.[11-18]

## Angiography

Selective angiography is effective in visualizing and localizing the site of left to right shunts. In fact, since angiographic demonstration of anatomy has become a routine part of the preoperative evaluation of patients with congenital or acquired shunts, the role of the indicator-dilution techniques just described in localizing the anatomic site of the shunt has been largely superseded. Actually, the use of angiography in this fashion should be considered an indicator-dilution method, with the radiographic contrast agent being the indicator and the cinefluoroscopy unit serving as the "densitometer."

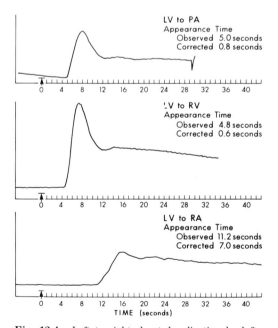

**Fig. 12-4.** Left to right shunt, localization by left-sided injection of indocyanine green dye into the left ventricular (LV) chamber with sampling in the pulmonary artery (PA), right ventricle (RV), and right atrium (RA), demonstrating a ventricular septal defect. See text for details.

In our laboratory, assessment of the patient with a left to right shunt virtually always includes a left ventriculogram. If this is performed in the left anterior oblique projection with cranial angulation (or done as a biplane study with both left and right anterior oblique views), excellent visualization of the interventricular septum, sinuses of Valsalva, and ascending and descending thoracic aorta will allow diagnosis and localization of essentially all the causes of left to right shunt other than atrial septal defect and anomalous pulmonary venous return.

Complicated lesions (e.g., endocardial cushion defects, coronary artery-right heart fistulae, ruptured aneuryms at the sinus of Valsalva) commonly require angiographic delineation before surgical intervention can be undertaken. Angiography also helps to assess the "routine" cases more completely. For instance, does the patient with secundum arterial septal defect have associated left ventricular dysfunction or mitral valve prolapse? Does the patient with ventricular septal defect have associated aortic regurgitation (due to prolapse of the medial aortic leaflet) or infundibular pulmonic stenosis?

However, angiography cannot replace the important physiologic measurements that allow quantitation of flow and vascular resistance. Without quantitative evaluation of pulmonary and systemic flows ($Q_p$ and $Q_s$) and their associated resistances (PVR and SVR), decisions regarding patient management cannot be made, nor can prognosis be assessed.

## Radionuclide Techniques

Radionuclide techniques have been developed that have proven to be of tremendous value in the detection and quantitation of intracardiac shunts. Since these are not methods that involve cardiac catheterization and angiography, they are discussed only briefly here, and the reader is referred elsewhere for details.[19] The radionuclide techniques rely on the indicator dilution theory. In one method, after oral administration of potassium perchlorate (to block uptake of radionuclide by the thyroid and speed its excretion), technetium 99m as sodium pertechnetate is injected intravenously as a bolus. The adequacy of the bolus should always be checked on a time-activity curve obtained over the superior vena cava. The duration of the bolus should be 2 sec or less. A pattern similar to a left to right shunt can be artificially created by a double peaked injection.

Calculation of a left to right shunt by this method assumes that there are no complicating conditions, such as valvular incompetence, large bronchial collaterals, congestive heart failure, or a right to left shunt. The technique employs quantitation of radioactivity from various regions of interest within the central circulation. The time activity curves closely resemble indicator dilution curves obtained with indocyanine green. In a patient with a left to right shunt, there will be a delay in the disappearance of radionuclide due to early pulmonary recirculation of the left to right shunt. Using computer techniques, the area (A) under the first pass curve is extrapolated, as is the area (B) under the early pulmonary recirculation component of the curve. Assuming that the areas are proportional to flows, the following equation is used:

$$\frac{\text{area A}}{\text{area A} - \text{area B}} = \frac{Q_p}{Q_s}$$

where $Q_p$ and $Q_s$ are the pulmonary and systemic flows. Thus, this technique yields a flow ratio but does not give values for the actual flows. The use of collimator techniques and angulated views has greatly increased the ability of this technique to distinguish radioactivity from different cardiac chambers and blood pools. Using such techniques, the *level* of the left to right shunt can be detected as the first chamber in which early recirculation is identified.

## DETECTION OF RIGHT TO LEFT INTRACARDIAC SHUNTS

The primary indication for the use of techniques to detect and localize right to left intracardiac shunts is the presence of cyanosis or, more commonly, hypoxemia. The presence of hypoxemia raises two specific questions: First, is the observed hypoxemia due to an intracardiac shunt, or is it due to a ventilation/perfusion imbalance secondary to a variety of forms of intrinsic pulmonary disease? This problem is particularly important in patients with coexistent congenital heart disease and pulmonary disease. Second, if hypoxemia is due to an intracardiac shunt, what is its site and what is its magnitude?

Attempts to measure right to left shunts in patients with cyanotic heart disease date back at least to 1941. Prinzmetal,[20] in a series of ingenious experiments, expanded the earlier observation of Benenson and Hitzig that ether injected intravenously in patients with cyanotic heart disease will cause a prickly, burning sensation of the face.[18] This sensation is due to the entrance of ether into the systemic circulation of patients with right to left shunts. In normal subjects without right to left shunts, the ether is eliminated by the lungs and thus does not reach the systemic circulation. Prinzmetal then measured the time necessary for an intravenous injection of a dilute solution of saccharin to be tasted. This time is equal to the transit time from a peripheral vein through the lungs, through the left heart, and then to the systemic circulation. By increasing the concentration of the saccharin he found that a second, much shorter appearance time occurred in patients with cyanotic heart disease due to the presence of a right to left shunt bypassing the pulmonary circulation. He then estimated the percent right to left shunt by the following formula:

$$\% \; R \rightarrow L \; \text{Shunt} = \frac{A}{A + C}$$

where A is the smallest concentration of saccharin to be tasted by way of the long circuit, and C is the smallest concentration of saccharin to be tasted by the short circuit. Our current methods of documenting and quantitating right to left shunts may not be as ingenious and certainly are not as sweet, but they are nonetheless effective.

## Angiography

With appropriate techniques, angiography may be utilized to demonstrate right to left intracardiac shunts. This method is particularly important in detecting right to left shunting due to a pulmonary arteriovenous fistula. In this circumstance, the shunt cannot be detected by indicator dilution curves on the basis of a shortened appearance time. That is, the difference in transit time when the pulmonary capillaries are bypassed is not perceptible by standard indicator dilution techniques. Although angiography may localize right to left shunts, it does not permit quantification.

## Oximetry

The site of right to left shunts may be localized if blood samples can be obtained from a pulmonary vein, the left atrium, left ventricle, and aorta. The pulmonary venous blood of patients with hypoxemia due to an intracardiac right to left shunt is fully saturated. Therefore, the site of a right to left shunt may be localized by noting which left heart chamber is the first to show desaturation; i.e., a step-down in oxygen concentration. That is, if left atrial saturation is normal, but desaturation is present in the left ventricle and in the systemic circulation, the right to left shunt is across a ventricular septal defect. The only disadvantage of this technique is that a pulmonary vein and the left atrium must be entered. This is not as often feasible in adults as it is in infants, in whom the left atrium may be entered by way of the foramen ovale.

## Early Appearance of an Indicator in the Systemic Circulation

A variety of techniques are based on the fact that, if an indicator is injected proximal to the site of a right to left shunt, its appearance time in the systemic circulation will be perceptibly shortened.

Swan and co-workers[21] demonstrated that injection of Evans blue proximal to the site of a right to left shunt with sampling in a systemic artery produces a distinctive indicator dilution curve. There is an early hump in the dye curve prior to the primary peak (Fig. 12-5). This technique, utilizing *indocyanine green*, can detect right to left shunts as small as 2.5% of the systemic output.[9] This method is simple and sensitive. Injection of indocyanine green into the inferior vena cava will detect right to left shunts at the level of the atrium, ventricle, and pulmonary artery. The site of the shunt is then localized by injecting more distally until the early appearance

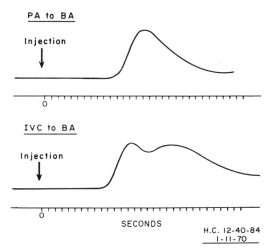

**Fig. 12-5.** Demonstration of a right to left shunt by indicator dilution curves. The top panel illustrated injection of indocyanine green into the pulmonary artery (PA) with sampling at the brachial artery (BA). There is a normal upstroke, with no early appearance of indicator in the systemic circulation. The lower panel shows a "double hump" contour, indicating early appearance of indicator in the systemic circulation when it is injected into the inferior vena cava (IVC). These two curves suggest the presence of a right to left shunt at either the atrial or ventricular level.

## Echocardiographic Methods

Finally, echocardiographic methods have proven to be quite sensitive for the detection and localization of left to right and right to left shunts. The so-called echocardiographic contrast or "bubble study" using agitated saline solution with microbubbles can detect small shunts, and the use of two-dimensional echocardiographic techniques can often localize the site of the shunt to the atrial or ventricular septum. Combined echocardiographic and cardiac catheterization studies allow injection of the echo contrast agent into the right or left heart chambers sequentially, thus permitting localization of the shunt and determination as to whether it is unidirectional or bidirectional. Echo-Doppler techniques can also be used to detect and localize intracardiac shunts. An example of the use of echo-contrast technique for the detection of an atrial septal defect with left to right shunting is shown in Figure 12-7. A full description of the use of echo/Doppler techniques in the detection of shunts is given in Dr. Patricia Come's textbook.[24]

hump is no longer noted in the dye curve. For example, if the right to left shunt is an atrial septal defect, early appearance of the dye will be noted with injection into the inferior vena cava, but not with injection into the right ventricle. It should be noted that right to left shunting across an atrial septal defect or patent foramen ovale is best detected by injection into the inferior vena cava, because of preferential streaming of blood from the inferior vena cava toward the region of the fossa ovalis.[22]

In the case of small right to left shunts at the atrial level, the magnitude of the shunt can be increased and thus more easily detected if dye is injected into the IVC while the patient performs a Valsalva maneuver (Fig. 12-6). This maneuver transiently increases right atrial pressure more than left atrial pressure, and thus increases the volume of the right to left shunt.[23]

The prime advantage of the indocyanine green method for detecting right to left shunts is that it is on-line and requires equipment that is available in most cardiac catheterization laboratories.

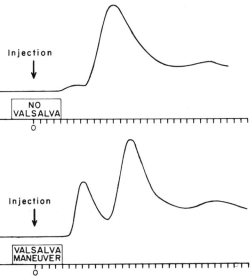

**Fig. 12-6.** Detection of right to left shunt by inferior vena cava (IVC) dye curves with and without Valsalva maneuver. A small right to left shunt is suggested by the early appearance in the upstroke of an IVC to brachial artery dye curve in the top panel. The early appearance becomes much more obvious when the dye curve is recorded during a Valsalva maneuver (bottom panel). The Valsalva maneuver transiently increases right atrial pressure with respect to left atrial pressure and thereby increases the magnitude of right to left shunts at the atrial level.

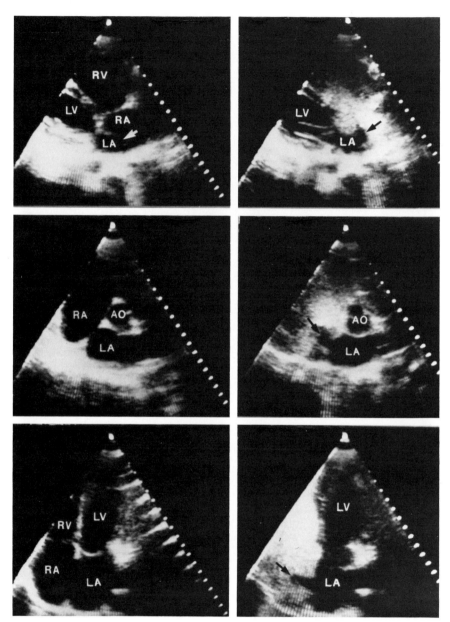

**Fig. 12-7.** Two-dimensional echo showing right ventricular (RV) inflow tract (upper panels), short axis views at the base (middle panels) and four chamber apical view (bottom panels) in a patient with an atrial septal defect (ASD) shown at cardiac catheterization to be associated with a $Q_P/Q_S$ of 3.0. The left side of each panel shows the anatomy before echo contrast injection. Following an intravenous injection of agitated saline solution (right side of each panel), a negative contrast effect (black arrow) is seen within the right atrium (RA), compatible with entry of unopacified blood from the left atrium (LA) across the ASD into the RA. The ASD is visualized (white arrow) as an area of septal drop out. (Reproduced from Come PC, Riley M: Contrast echocardiography. *In* Come PC, (ed.): Diagnostic Cardiology: Noninvasive Imaging Techniques. Philadelphia: JB Lippincott Co, 1984, p. 294, with permission.)

# REFERENCES

1. Dexter L et al: Studies of congenital heart disease. II. The pressure and oxygen content of blood in the right auricle, right ventricle, and pulmonary artery in control patients, with observations on the oxygen saturation and source of pulmonary capillary blood. J Clin Invest 26:554, 1947.

2. Antman EM, Marsh JD, Green LH, Grossman W: Blood oxygen measurements in the assessment of intracardiac left to right shunts: a critical appraisal of methodology. Am J Cardiol 46:265, 1980.

3. Barratt-Boyes BF, Wood EH: The oxygen saturation of blood in the vena cavae, right heart chambers, and pulmonary vessels of healthy subjects. J Lab Clin Med 50:93, 1957.

4. Freed MD, Miettinen OS, Nadas AS: Oximetric determination of intracardiac left to right shunts. Br Heart J 42:690, 1979.

5. Flamm MD, Cohn KE, Hancock EW: Measurement of systemic cardiac output at rest and exercise in patients with atrial septal defect. Am J Cardiol 23:258, 1969.

6. Dexter L et al: Studies of congenital heart disease. I. Technique of venous catheterization as a diagnostic procedure. J Clin Invest 26:547, 1947.

7. Swan HJC, Wood EH: Localization of cardiac defects by dye-dilution curves recorded after injection of T-1824 at multiple sites in the heart and great vessels during cardiac catheterization. Proc Staff Meet Mayo Clin 28:95, 1953.

8. Hyman AL et al: A comparative study of the detection of cardiovascular shunts by oxygen analysis and indicator dilution methods. Ann Intern Med 56:535, 1962.

9. Castillo CA, Kyle JC, Gilson WE, Rowe GG: Simulated shunt curves. Am J Cardiol 17:691, 1966.

10. Braunwald E, Tannenbaum HL, Morrow AG: Localization of left-to-right cardiac shunts by dye-dilution curves following injection into the left side of the heart and into the aorta. Am J Med 24:203, 1958.

11. Long RTL, Braunwald E, Morrow AG: Intracardiac injection of radioactive krypton: clinical applications of new methods for characterization of circulatory shunts. Circulation 21:1126, 1960.

12. Levy AM, Monroe RG, Hugenholtz PG, Nadas AS: Clinical use of ascorbic acid as an indicator of right-to-left shunt. Br Heart J 29:22, 1967.

13. Hugenholtz PG et al: The clinical usefulness of hydrogen gas as an indicator of left-to-right shunts. Circulation 28:542, 1963.

14. Amplatz K et al: The Freon test: a new sensitive technic for the detection of small cardiac shunts. Circulation 39:551, 1969.

15. Singleton RT, Dembo DH, Scherlis L: Krypton-85 in the detection of intracardiac left-to-right shunts. Circulation 32:134, 1965.

16. Morrow AG, Sanders RJ, Braunwald E: The nitrous oxide test: An improved method for the detection of left-to-right shunts. Circulation 17:284, 1958.

17. Long RT, Waldhausen JA, Cornell WP, Sanders RJ: Detection of right-to-left circulatory shunts: A new method utilizing injections of krypton-85. Proc Soc Exp Biol Med 102:456, 1959.

18. Benenson W, Hitzig WM: Diagnosis of venous arterial shunt by ether circulation time method. Proc Soc Exp Biol Med 38:256, 1938.

19. Parker JA, Treves S: Radionuclide detection, localization, and quantitation of intracardiac shunts and shunts between the great arteries. Prog Cardiovasc Dis 20 (No. 1–4):189, 1977–1978.

20. Prinzmetal M: Calculation of the venousarterial shunt in congenital heart disease. J Clin Invest 20:705, 1941.

21. Swan HJC, Zapata-Diaz J, Wood EH: Dye dilution curves in cyanotic congenital heart disease. Circulation 8:70, 1953.

22. Swan HJC, Burchell HB, Wood EH: The presence of venoarterial shunts in patients with interatrial communications. Circulation 10:705–713, 1954.

23. Banas JS et al: A simple technique for detecting small defects of the atrial septum. Am J Cardiol 28:467, 1971.

24. Come P. (ed.): Diagnostic Cardiology: Non-Invasive Imaging Techniques. Philadelphia, JB Lippincott Co., 1984, p 294.

# PART IV
## Angiographic Techniques

# chapter thirteen

# Coronary Angiography

DONALD S. BAIM *and* WILLIAM GROSSMAN

D UE TO progressive improvements in
catheter design, radiographic imaging, and contrast media, as well as
the development of effective options for the
treatment of coronary artery disease (bypass
surgery and angioplasty), diagnostic coronary angiography has grown into a safe and
widely practiced component of cardiac catheterization. It is estimated that more than
200,000 coronary angiographic procedures
are performed each year in the United States,
with a procedure-related mortality of 0.1%.[1,2]
In each procedure, the objective is to examine the entire coronary tree, recording details of coronary anatomy, including individual variations in arterial distribution,
anatomic or functional pathology (atherosclerosis, thrombosis, congenital anomalies,
or focal coronary spasm), and the presence
of inter- and intracoronary collateral connections. With repeat intracoronary contrast injections in a series of angulated views, a high
resolution image intensifier, and 35 mm cineangiographic film or other recording media,
it is possible to define all portions of the coronary arterial circulation down to vessels as
small as 0.2 mm, and to eliminate artifacts
due to vessel overlap or foreshortening.

## CURRENT INDICATIONS

There are a variety of current indications
for coronary angiography, based on the principle stated by F. Mason Sones that coronary

arteriography is indicated when a problem is
encountered which may be resolved by the
objective demonstration of the coronary
tree, provided competent personnel and adequate facilities are available and the potential risks are acceptable to the patient and
his physician. The most frequent such indication is the further evaluation of patients in
whom the diagnosis of coronary atherosclerosis is almost certain.[3] This includes patients with angina pectoris refractory to
medical therapy, in whom anatomic correction via coronary bypass surgery or transluminal coronary angioplasty is contemplated.
In such patients, angiographic evaluation of
coronary anatomy provides a crucial anatomic guide to the revascularization procedure. In patients with less severe anginal
symptoms, coronary angiography may still
be indicated if the clinical setting or noninvasive testing suggest a higher-than-usual probability of severe multivessel disease or left
main coronary stenosis.[3,4] Some cardiologists also favor angiographic evaluation of
patients with new onset, unstable, or postin-
farction angina, as well as younger patients
recovering from an uncomplicated myocardial infarction.[4] Moreover, while patients
with acute myocardial infarction were for-
merly subjected to coronary angiography
only when ongoing ischemic events or the
presence of a mechanical defect (papillary
muscle rupture, ventricular septal defect, or
large left ventricular aneurysm with shock)
compelled early surgical intervention, the
advent of thrombolytic therapy and coronary

angioplasty has made coronary angiography increasingly commonplace in this setting.[4]

A second group of indications for coronary angiography concerns patients in whom the presence or absence of coronary artery disease is unclear. This includes patients with troublesome chest pain syndromes but ambiguous noninvasive test results, patients with unexplained heart failure or ventricular arrhythmias, and patients with suspected or proven variant angina.[4] Finally, coronary angiography is widely employed in the preoperative evaluation of patients scheduled for the correction of congenital or valvular pathology. Patients with congenital defects such as tetralogy of Fallot frequently have anomalies of coronary distribution that may lead to surgical complications if unrecognized,[5] and older patients with valvular disease may have advanced coronary atherosclerosis. Although younger patients with valvular disease are commonly operated upon without prior coronary angiograms,[6] most surgical centers believe that it is critical to recognize and correct significant coronary lesions to provide the best and safest outcome during concurrent valve replacement.[7]

## TECHNIQUE

The initial attempts to perform coronary angiography utilized nonselective injections of contrast medium into the aortic root with simultaneous opacification of both the left and right coronary arteries and recording of the angiographic images on conventional sheet film.[8,9] To improve contrast delivery into the coronary ostia, some early investigators employed transient circulatory arrest induced by the administration of acetylcholine or by elevation of intrabronchial pressure, followed by occlusion of the ascending aorta by gas-filled balloon and injection of the contrast bolus. While nonselective aortic root injection is still employed today to evaluate ostial lesions, anomalous coronary ostia, or coronary bypass grafts, intentional circulatory arrest is no longer practiced, and the nonselective technique has largely been replaced by selective coronary injection using specially designed catheters advanced from either the brachial or the femoral approach.

Successful coronary angiography can be performed in most patients by either the brachial or femoral approach, leaving the choice up to physician and the patient. The brachial approach may offer a selective advantage in patients with severe peripheral vascular disease or known abdominal aortic aneurysm, but small elderly women are frequently more easily studied via the femoral approach. In either case, it is important for the catheterization team to meet the patient prior to the actual procedure to evaluate the best approach to catheterization, to gain an appreciation of the clinical questions to be answered by coronary angiography, to uncover any history of adverse reaction to medications or organic iodine compounds, and to explain the procedure in detail. Although coronary angiography has been widely performed as an in-patient procedure, some centers have adopted out-patient protocols for selected low-risk patients,[10,11] usually using the brachial approach to permit early postcatheterization ambulation. In either case, preparation for catheterization should include proscription of oral intake except for medications and limited quantities of clear liquids over the 6 to 8 hours before catheterization, a baseline 12 lead electrocardiogram, and a suitable sedative premedication (usually diazepam, 5 to 10 mg po, and diphenhydramine, 50 mg po) administered on call to the catheterization laboratory.

## The Femoral Approach

As described in Chapter 5, the femoral approach to left heart catheterization involves insertion of the catheter either directly over a guide wire, or through an introducing sheath. Systemic anticoagulation (heparin, 5000 units) is used by us and by most laboratories using this approach.[8] A series of preformed catheters are employed, usually a pigtail catheter for left ventriculography and separate catheters (either Judkins or Amplatz shapes) for cannulation of the left and right coronary arteries. Coronary catheters are available in either 7 or 8 Fr end-hole design, with a shaft that tapers to 5 Fr near the tip. They may be constructed of either polyethylene (Cook Inc, Bloomington, IN) or polyurethane (Cordis, Miami, FL, and

USCI, Billerica, MA) and contain either steel braid or nylon within the catheter wall to provide the excellent torque control needed for coronary cannulation. Although the 8 Fr catheters have traditionally permitted more rapid contrast delivery, recent improvements in the design of 7 Fr catheters (Cordis High Flow, USCI Nycore) allow a lumen comparable in diameter to that of standard 8 Fr catheter. Coronary catheters used for either femoral or brachial approach are shown in Figure 13-1.

The desired catheter is advanced to a point just above the diaphragm with the guide wire in place. The guide wire is then removed, and the catheter is attached to a specially designed manifold system which permits the maintenance of a "closed system" during pressure monitoring, catheter flushing, and contrast agent administration (Fig. 13-2). The catheter is immediately double flushed: blood is withdrawn and discarded, and heparinized saline flush is injected through the catheter lumen. Difficulty in blood withdrawal suggests apposition of the catheter tip to the aortic wall, which can be rectified by slight advancement or rotation of the catheter until free blood withdrawal is possible. If an introducing sheath is employed, its lumen should also be flushed immediately after each catheter insertion or removal and every 5 minutes thereafter to

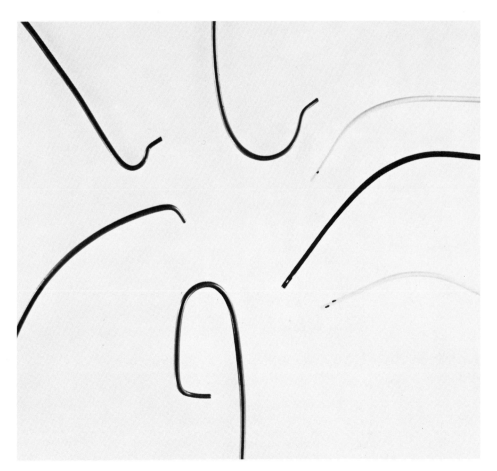

**Fig. 13-1.** Different types of catheters currently in wide use for selective coronary angiography. At the bottom, center, is the left coronary Judkins catheter. Proceeding clockwise from this catheter are the right coronary Judkins catheter, the right (R2) and left (L3) Amplatz catheters, the Schoonmaker multipurpose catheter, the Standard Sones catheter (woven dacron, USCI), the polyurethrane, Sones-type catheter (Cordis). (See text for discussion.)

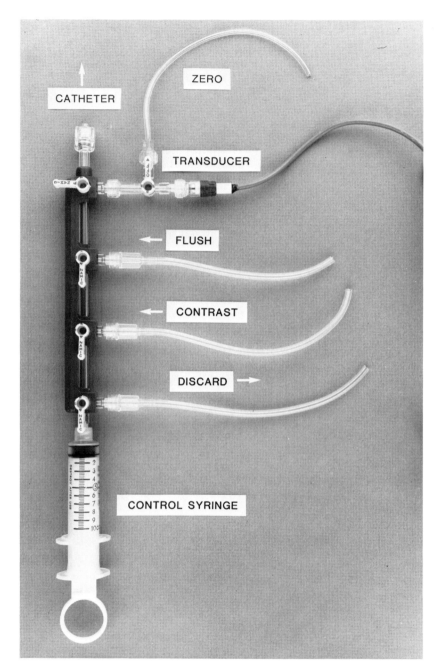

**Fig. 13-2.** Four-port coronary manifold (Namic). This manifold provides a closed system with which blood can be withdrawn from the catheter and discarded, the catheter can be filled with either flush solution or contrast medium, and catheter pressure can be observed, all under the control of a series of stopcocks. The fourth port is connected to an empty plastic bag and is used as a discard port (for blood from the double flush, air bubbles) so that the syringe need not be disconnected from the manifold at any time during the procedure. Attachment of the transducer directly to the manifold allows optimum pressure waveform fidelity (see Chapter 9), while the fluid-filled reference line allows zeroing of the transducer to midchest level.

prevent the encroachment of blood into the sheath. Once the catheter has been flushed with saline solution, tip pressure should be monitored at all times except during actual contrast injections. Next, the catheter lumen is gently filled with contrast agent under fluoroscopic visualization, avoiding selective contrast administration into small arterial vessels. Filling with contrast results in a slight reduction in high frequency components of the aortic pressure waveform, which should be noted carefully and compared continuously to the femoral sidearm pressure. Any change in waveform during coronary angiography (see damping and ventricularization, below) may signify an ostial coronary stenosis or an unfavorable catheter position within the coronary artery. The coronary angiographic catheter is then advanced around the arch into the ascending aorta under continuous pressure monitoring and fluoroscopic imaging in the left anterior oblique projection.

Cannulation of the left coronary ostium with the Judkins technique is usually quite easy to accomplish.[12] As Judkins himself has stated, "No points are earned for coronary catheterization—the catheters know where to go if not thwarted by the operator."[12] If a left Judkins catheter with a 4 cm curve (JL4) is simply allowed to remain en face as it is advanced down into the aortic root, it will engage the left coronary ostium without further manipulation in 80 to 90% of patients (Fig. 13-3). Engagement should take place with the arm of the catheter traversing the ascending aorta at an angle of approximately 45 degrees, the tip of the catheter in a more or less horizontal lie, and with no change in the pressure waveform recorded from the catheter tip.

### Damping and Ventricularization.

A fall in overall catheter tip pressure (damping) or a fall in diastolic pressure only (ventricularization) (Fig. 13-4) indicates restriction of coronary inflow due to insertion

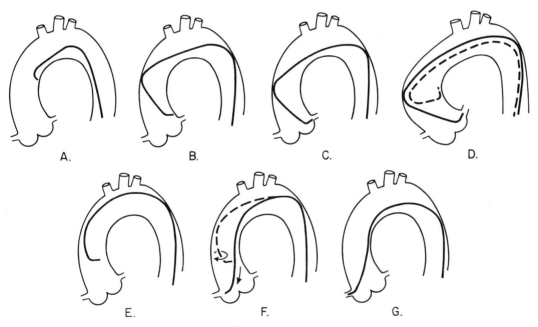

**Fig. 13-3.** Judkins technique for catheterization of the left and right coronary arteries as viewed in the LAO projection. In a patient with a normal sized aortic arch, simple advancement of the JL4 catheter leads to intubation of the left coronary ostium (A, B, and C). In a patient with an enlarged aortic root (D) the arm of the JL4 may be too short, causing the catheter tip to point upward or even flip back into its packaged shape (dotted catheter). A catheter with an appropriately longer arm (a JL5 or JL6) is required. To catheterize the right coronary ostium, the right Judkins catheter is advanced around the aortic arch with its tip directed leftward, as viewed in the LAO projection, until it reaches a position 2 to 3 cm above the level of the left coronary ostium (E). Clockwise rotation causes the catheter tip to drop into the aortic root and point anteriorly (F). Slight further rotation causes the catheter tip to enter the right coronary ostium (G).

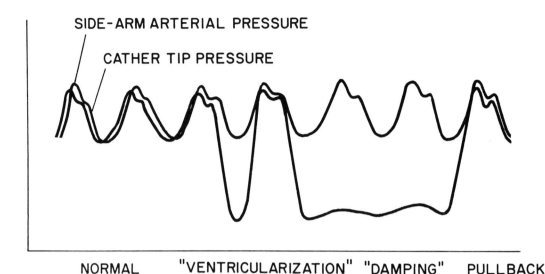

SIDE-ARM ARTERIAL PRESSURE

CATHER TIP PRESSURE

NORMAL          "VENTRICULARIZATION"  "DAMPING"   PULLBACK

**Fig. 13-4.**   Pressure tracings as recorded during coronary angiography. Except for its earlier phase and slightly lower systolic pressure, catheter tip pressure should resemble the pressure waveform simultaneously monitored via the femoral sidearm sheath or other arterial monitor (e.g., radial artery). In the presence of an ostial stenosis or an unfavorable catheter position against the vessel wall, the waveform will show either "ventricularization" (in which systolic pressure is preserved but diastolic pressure is reduced) or frank "damping" (in which both systolic and diastolic pressures are reduced. In either case, the best approach is to withdraw the catheter immediately until the waveform returns to normal and to attempt to define the cause of the problem by nonselective injections in the sinus of Valsalva.

of the catheter tip into a proximal coronary stenosis or to an adverse catheter lie against the coronary wall. If either of these phenomena is observed, the catheter should be withdrawn into the aortic root immediately until the operator can analyze the situation further using nonselective injections into the sinus of Valsalva or make very cautious small injections into the coronary artery followed immediately by catheter withdrawal. Vigorous injection despite a damped or ventricularized pressure waveform predisposes to dissection of the proximal coronary artery, and may lead to major ischemic complications.

In patients with a widened aortic root due to aortic valve disease or long-standing hypertension, the 4 cm left Judkins curve may be too short to allow successful engagement: the catheter arm may lie nearly horizontally across the aortic root with the tip pointing superiorly against the wall of the left main artery, or the catheter may even refold into its packaged shape during advancement into the aortic root. In this case, a left Judkins catheter with a larger (5 cm or even 6 cm) curve should be selected, rather than persevering in an effort to make an unsuitable

catheter work. On the other hand, even the 4 cm Judkins curve may be too long for occasional patients with short or narrow aortic roots: the catheter arm may lie nearly vertically with the tip pointing inferiorly. The left ostium may still be engaged by pushing the catheter down into the left sinus of Valsalva for approximately 10 seconds to tighten the angle on the catheter tip and then withdrawing the catheter slowly. Having the patient take a deep breath during this maneuver pulls the heart into a more vertical position and may also assist in engagement of the left ostium. The most satisfactory approach, however, is exchanging for a catheter with a 3.5 cm curve.

Occasionally, the operator may choose a left Amplatz catheter (Fig. 13-1) (available in progressively larger curves—I, II, III, IV) rather than a left Judkins catheter. The Amplatz family of catheters is more tolerant of rotational maneuvering during engagement of left coronary ostia which are positioned out of the conventional Judkins plane, and allows easy subselective engagement of the left anterior descending and circumflex coronary arteries in patients with short left main coronary segments or separate left coronary ostia.[13] The left Amplatz is advanced around the arch oriented toward the left coronary ostium (Fig. 13-5). The tip of the catheter usually passes by the coronary ostium and into the sinus of Valsalva below. As the catheter is advanced further, however, the Amplatz shape causes the tip of the catheter to ride up the wall of the sinus until it engages the ostium. At that point, slight withdrawal of the catheter will cause deeper engagement of the coronary ostium, whereas further slight advancement will cause paradoxical retraction of the catheter tip.

Cannulation of the right coronary ostium by the Judkins technique requires slightly more catheter manipulation than cannulation of the left coronary ostium.[8,12] The right Judkins catheter with a 4 cm curve (JR4) is typically brought around the aortic arch with its tip facing inward and thus comes to lie against the right side of the aortic root aimed at the left coronary ostium (Fig. 13-3). In a left anterior oblique projection, the operator must therefore slowly and carefully rotate the catheter clockwise by nearly 180 degrees to engage the right coronary artery. Because of its secondary curve, the tip of the right Judkins catheter tends to drop more deeply into the aortic root as the catheter is rotated towards the right ostium. To compensate for this effect, the operator must either begin the rotational maneuver with the tip 2 to 3 cm above the left coronary ostium or withdraw the catheter slowly during rotation. Catheters with smaller (3.5 cm) or larger (5 or 6 cm) Judkins curves or right Amplatz cathe-

ters (AR 1 or AR 2) may be of value if aortic root configuration and proximal right coronary anatomy make engagement difficult. Damping and ventricularization are far more common in the right coronary artery than in the left, and may be due to: (1) the generally smaller caliber of the vessel, (2) ostial spasm around the catheter tip, (3) subselective engagement of the conus branch, or (4) true ostial stenosis. These problems in right coronary engagement can usually be elucidated by nonselective injections into the right sinus of Valsalva or very cautious injections in a damped position with immediate post-injection withdrawal of the catheter.

***Bypass Graft Catheterization.*** While the Judkins and Amplatz catheters are the most widely used for the femoral approach, a variety of specialized catheters have been designed for engagement of internal mammary or saphenous vein bypass conduits. In general, however, the right Judkins catheter can be employed for both purposes, as well as for opacification of the native right coronary artery. If saphenous graft entry with the right Judkins catheter proves difficult, the right Amplatz shape may prove more satisfactory. In searching for the saphenous vein ostium, the catheter tip should be oriented against the desired aortic wall, and the catheter should be slowly advanced and withdrawn until it "catches" in a graft ostium. The process is repeated until all graft sites have been identified. Graft and native angiography may also be performed successfully using a single catheter such as a Schoon-

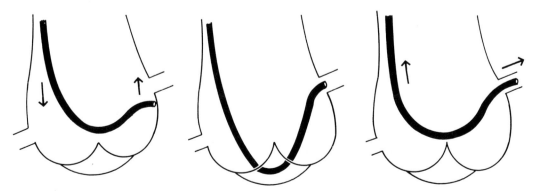

**Fig. 13-5.** Catheterization of the left coronary with an Amplatz catheter. The catheter should be advanced into the ascending aorta with its tip pointing downward, so that the terminal catheter configuration resembles a diving duck. As the Amplatz catheter is advanced into the left sinus of Valsalva, its tip initially lies below the left coronary ostium (left). Further advancement causes the tip to ride up the aortic wall and enter the ostium (center). Slight withdrawal of the catheter causes the tip to seat more deeply in the ostium (right).

maker,[14] which is manipulated much as the Sones catheter (see below). When femoral catheterization is not possible, many of the preformed coronary angiographic catheters described above can be used effectively via percutaneous axillary or brachial puncture.

## The Brachial Approach

The technique of brachial artery cutdown has been described previously in Chapter 4. The catheter designed by Dr. F. Mason Sones, Jr., is a thin-walled radiopaque woven Dacron catheter with a 2.67 mm (8 French) external diameter to its shaft.* The tip is open and in current models two side holes are arranged in opposed pairs within 7 mm of its distal end. The shaft tapers abruptly to 5 French external diameter at a point 5 cm from its tip. As Sones has stated, this provides a "flexible finger" which may be curved upward into the coronary orifices by pressure of the more rigid shaft against the aortic valve cusps. This standard catheter is available in lengths of 80, 100, and 125 cm and in 7 and 8 French sizes.

Some operators use a Sones type of coronary catheter constructed of polyurethane and made by Cordis Corporation.† This catheter has the same shape and taper as the woven Dacron catheter and has an end hole with four side holes within 7 mm of its tip. This catheter traverses a tortuous subclavian system with much greater facility and smoothness than does the woven Dacron catheter, and its enhanced torque control and reduced friction coefficient permit greater ease in engaging the coronary ostia. It is the first choice for coronary angiography of one of us (WG). It will pass an 0.035-inch guide wire, and is an excellent catheter for crossing a stenotic aortic valve. Figure 13-1 shows a variety of coronary catheters effective with the brachial approach.

When the Sones method is used, once the catheter enters the brachial artery, pressure should be monitored, and further passage of the catheter into the subclavian and innominate arteries should be accomplished with

pressure monitoring and fluoroscopic visualization. Occasionally, it will be difficult to pass the catheter from the subclavian artery to the aortic arch, but a simple maneuver by the patient, such as a deep inspiration, shrugging the shoulders, or turning his head to the left, often facilitates passage of the catheter into the ascending aorta. If passage of the catheter from the subclavian artery to the ascending aorta is not accomplished immediately and with complete ease, the operator should stop catheter manipulation and use a soft J tipped 0.035-inch guide wire. Once the catheter is in the ascending aorta, the guide wire is removed and the catheter is aspirated, flushed, and reconnected to the rotating adaptor of the manifold, either directly or by a short length of large bore flexible connecting tubing.

With the Sones technique, selective engagement of the *left coronary artery* is accomplished as follows (Fig. 13-6). In a shallow left anterior oblique position, the sinus of Valsalva containing the ostium of the left coronary artery lies to the left, and the sinus containing the ostium of the right coronary artery lies to the right. The noncoronary sinus lies posteriorly. The operator advances the catheter to the aortic valve and manipulates it in such a way that the tip bends cephalad and points toward the left coronary ostium. When the catheter is properly positioned with its tip bent cephalad, slightly advancing or rotating the catheter frequently results in selective engagement of the left coronary ostium, which is verified by a small injection of radiographic contrast agent. Occasionally, a deep breath taken by the patient will facilitate this selective engagement. Once the catheter tip is engaged, it commonly (but not always) appears to be fixed by the coronary orifice. There is more than one way to successfully engage the left coronary artery with the Sones catheter. Our usual approach, illustrated in the upper left panel of Figure 13-6, involves forming a smooth shallow loop and gradually "inching up" to the ostium from below. If the distal 2 to 3 mm of the catheter tip bends downward during this "inching up" process, the tip may enter the left coronary artery, giving a "cobra head" appearance (Fig. 13-6, upper right panel). This is a stable position that allows rotation of the patient in a cradle-type table top without disengaging the catheter. For the high take-off left coronary ostium, the cathe-

---

*United States Catheter and Instrument Co., Billerica, MA.

†80 cm Cordis brachial coronary A, Sones technique, type II.

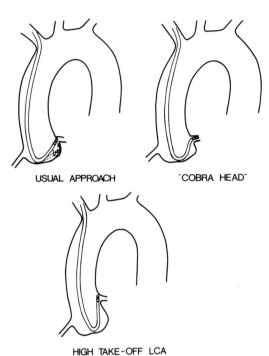

USUAL APPROACH          "COBRA HEAD"

HIGH TAKE-OFF LCA

**Fig. 13-6.** Selective catheterization of the left coronary artery using the Sones catheter. The standard approach involves forming a smooth shallow loop and gradually "inching up" to the ostium from below. If the distal 2 to 3 mm of the catheter tip bends downward during this inching up process, the tip may enter the left coronary artery, giving a "cobra-head" appearance (upper right). When the left coronary ostium originates high in the left sinus of Valsalva ("high take-off" left coronary artery), the catheter may have the appearance seen in the bottom panel, where the tip is lying across the ostium, at right angles to the course of the left main coronary artery. During coronary injection in this instance, coronary blood flow generally carries the contrast medium down the vessel, giving good opacification of the entire left coronary artery.

ter may have the appearance as in Figure 13-6, bottom, in which tip is lying across the ostium, at right angles to the course of the left main coronary artery. During coronary injection in this instance, coronary blood flow generally carries the contrast agent down the vessel, giving good opacification of the entire left coronary artery.

When the catheter tip has engaged the coronary ostium and no damping of pressure from the catheter tip is observed, cineangiography may be performed with selective injection of radiopaque material in a variety of views, as described below.

*Selective engagement of the right coronary orifice* may be accomplished as illustrated in steps 1 to 3 of Figure 13-7. In the shallow LAO projection, the catheter is curved up toward the left coronary artery (step 1) and clockwise torque is applied. While the operator is gradually applying clockwise torque, a gentle to-and-fro motion of the catheter (the to-and-fro excursions are not more than 5 to 10 mm in length) will help to translate the applied torque to the catheter tip. When the tip starts moving in its clockwise sweep of the anterior wall of the aorta, the operator maintains (but does not increase) a clockwise torque tension on the catheter and simultaneously pulls the catheter back slightly (step 2), since the right coronary ostium is lower than that of the left coronary artery. At this point, the catheter usually makes an abrupt turn into the right coronary ostium, at which time the operator must release all torque to prevent the catheter tip from continuing its sweep past the ostium. On occasion, the Sones catheter literally leaps into the right coronary artery and will be 4 to 5 cm down its lumen. If this occurs, the catheter should be gently withdrawn until its tip is stable just within the ostium. Another technique for catheterizing the right coronary artery involves a more direct approach by way of the right coronary cusp. With the catheter in the right sinus, the operator should make a small curve on the tip, directed rightward. A small dose of contrast material in the right sinus of Valsalva will allow visualization of the right coronary orifice and thus facilitate selective engagement. Occasionally, a deep inspiration by the patient accompanied by gentle advancement of the catheter to the right of the aortic root will result in selective engagement of the right coronary artery.

In addition to the Sones catheters, many other catheters may be used for coronary arteriography from the brachial approach, including the Amplatz, Schoonmaker, Bourassa, Judkins, and other specially designed catheters. Some of these catheters are illustrated in Figure 13-1. The Amplatz catheters* come in different shapes for the right and left coronary artery and basically incorporate a preformed Sones curvature. The left Amplatz comes in sizes L1, L2, L3, and L4; we have found the L2 adequate for most pa-

*Cook, Inc., Bloomington, Ind.

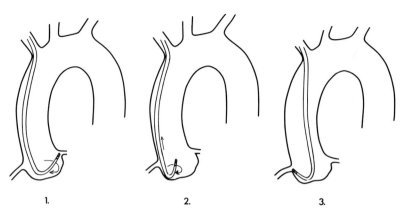

1.         2.         3.

**Fig. 13-7.** Selective catheterization of the right coronary artery using the Sones catheter. In the shallow LAO projection, the catheter is curved upward and to the left (1) and clockwise torque is applied. While the operator is gradually applying clockwise torque, a gentle to-and-fro motion of the catheter will help to translate the applied torque to the catheter tip. When the tip starts moving in its clockwise sweep of the anterior wall of the aorta, the operator maintains (but does not increase) a clockwise torque tension on the catheter and simultaneously pulls the catheter back slightly (2), since the right coronary ostium is lower than that of the left coronary artery. At this point the catheter will usually make an abrupt leap into the right coronary ostium (3), at which time the operator must release all torque to prevent the catheter tip from continuing its sweep and passing by the ostium. See text for details and alternative methods.

tients with normal aortic roots, whereas the L3 may be necessary for a dilated ascending aorta or in large men. Occasionally an L4 is needed for pronounced aortic dilatation or for a left coronary artery whose ostium originates very high in the left sinus of Valsalva ("high take-off" left coronary artery). The Amplatz right coronary catheter comes in R1 and R2 sizes; the R1 is usually adequate for patients with a normal aortic root. Although it was originally devised for use via the percutaneous femoral approach, we have found this catheter highly useful from the brachial approach in cases in which there was difficulty in seating the Sones catheter. The Amplatz catheter traverses the subclavian artery easily over a guide wire and is effective for bypass graft angiography. It cannot be used safely for ventriculography, however, as can the Sones catheter. We have also used the Judkins catheters from the brachial artery approach with success. We have not had experience with the Bourassa or Schoonmaker catheters from the brachial approach, but large published series attest to the effectiveness of these catheters from the femoral artery approach, and they should be effective from the brachial approach as well.

## MONITORING

During coronary angiography clinical, electrocardiographic, and catheter tip pressure should be monitored continuously. Monitoring is required for safe cannulation of the coronary arteries and prompt recognition and treatment of ischemia and arrhythmias precipitated by contrast injection and by inappropriate location of the catheter tip.

## RADIOGRAPHIC CONTRAST AGENTS

Renografin-76 (Squibb), an aqueous solution of the organic iodide diatrizoate as a mixture of methylglucamine (66%) and sodium (10%) salts with an iodine content of 0.37 mg/ml is the ionic contrast agent most commonly used for coronary angiography.[16] Angiovist 370 (Berlex Imaging, Inc.) has a similar formulation but different additives which reduce calcium binding.[17,18] Isopaque 370 contains methylglucamine, sodium, calcium, and magnesium salts, and a different organic iodide, metrizoic acid.[19]

***Hemodynamic Effects.*** When any of the radiographic contrast agents are injected into a coronary artery, transient *hemodynamic depression* occurs, marked by arterial hypotension and elevation of the left ventricular end-distolic pressure. This myocardial depression typically resolves within 10 to 20 seconds and appears to be due to lack of oxygen delivery to the myocardium, chelation of calcium, as well as direct myocardial toxicity of the hypertonic contrast agent.[17] While newer nonionic contrast agents such as iohexol, metrizamide, and iopamidol are being developed which may minimize this hemodynamic depression,[18,20] it is generally preferable to perform all hemodynamic measurements and left ventriculography prior to coronary angiography in clinically stable patients. On the other hand, we often perform coronary angiography *first* when catheterizing patients with severe unstable angina or suspected left main stenosis, so that the ability to define the coronary anatomy will not be compromised should adverse reactions occur during left ventriculography.

***Electrocardiographic Effects.*** In addition to its hemodynamic effects, intracoronary contrast injection also produces a variety of electrocardiographic changes. These include striking transient T-wave inversions in the inferior (II, III, AVF) leads,[21] following injection of the right coronary artery, and T-waves peaking following injection of the left coronary artery.

Marked sinus slowing, asystolic arrest, and prolongation of PR, QRS, and QT intervals are also common, particularly during injection of the arterial system which supplies the AV or SA node.[22,23] If bradycardia is prolonged or particularly severe, it may be terminated by having the patient cough vigorously (to raise aortic root pressure and speed the washout of contrast from the myocardium) or may be prevented by the administration of atropine or institution of demand ventricular pacing before subsequent injections. With the brachial approach, asystolic arrest can also be treated transiently by placing the Sones catheter into the left ventricle and "tapping" the myocardium repeatedly with its tip, a form of mechanical ventricular pacing.

Rarely, contrast injection into the coronary arteries produces ventricular tachycardia or fibrillation,[24,25] which should be treated by immediate DC countershock. In a well-functioning laboratory, the elapsed time between the onset of the arrhythmia and countershock should not exceed 15 to 20 seconds, during which time cerebral and coronary perfusion can usually be maintained by having the patient cough vigorously every 1 to 2 seconds. The coronary catheter should be removed from the ostium during the treatment of any severe arrhythmia, both to improve antegrade flow and to avoid coronary injury by the catheter tip.

***Myocardial Ischemia.*** Coronary injections may also precipitate myocardial ischemia, since the contrast medium replaces antegrade myocardial blood flow completely and reduces the arterial perfusion pressure following the injection. In addition, contrast injection induces a transient profound vasodilation of the coronary arterioles, which can lead to maldistribution of subsequent coronary blood flow (coronary "steal") from region to region or from endocardium to epicardium in the territory supplied by a stenotic lesion. These effects usually abate quickly unless transient ischemia is perpetuated by sympathetic stimulation with associated reflex tachycardia and hypertension. In this case, termination of angina may require the administration of nitroglycerin via the sublingual (400 mcg), intravenous (100 to 200 mcg), or intracoronary (100 mcg) routes. Sublingual administration of nifedipine (10 mg) may also be of value in control of prolonged angina precipitated by coronary angiography, particularly if marked hypertension is present. On rare occasions we have had to administer intravenous propranolol (1 mg every minute to a total dose of 0.1 to 0.15 mg/kg) to patients with prolonged angina and marked tachycardia. Failure of postinjection angina to resolve promptly, however, should make the operator think about possible complications including coronary dissection, air embolus, or thromboembolus, although the latter is uncommon when systemic heparinization is used routinely during coronary angiography. Review of the videotapes and careful reinjection of the coronary artery may disclose the problem and allow definitive treatment of the complication before irreversible myocardial damage occurs.

The adverse effects of coronary contrast injection listed above can be minimized by meticulous attention to technical detail and correct injection technique. While it is desirable to replace coronary blood flow and cause continuous reflux of contrast agent into the aortic root to obtain optimal visualization of the coronary anatomy, too vigorous or too prolonged an injection may contribute to complications. We train our fellows to monitor catheter tip pressure until the actual initiation of injection and then to build up the velocity of injection over 1 to 2 seconds until it is adequate to completely replace the antegrade flow of blood into the coronary ostium (Fig. 13-8). This injection rate is maintained until the entire vessel is opacified, following which the injection is culminated with a very brief extra push to augment reflux into the aorta and more clearly define any ostial pathologic condition. Injection is then terminated as cine filming is continued to allow completion of "paning" toward the distal vasculature and visualization of any late-filling branches supplied by collaterals. Depending upon the size of the involved vessel and coronary blood flow, opacification may be accomplished by the injection of as little as 1 ml, or as much as 10 ml of contrast agent. The operator should be careful to allow adequate time between repeat coronary injections to allow the arterial pressure and electrocardiographic morphology to return to baseline.

***Renal Toxicity.*** Other problems during coronary angiography are related to contrast administration in general, rather than to coronary angiography in particular, but should be kept in mind by the operator during each procedure. One such problem is renal toxicity, which may appear as a mild elevation of postprocedure creatinine or as frank acute renal failure.[26] Patients with prior renal insufficiency, diabetes mellitus, multiple myeloma, or impaired liver function are at increased risk, particularly if the angiographic procedure is performed with inadequate pre- or postprocedure hydration. While most patients with normal renal function will tolerate dye loads up to 3 ml/kg without problem, it is wise to keep the contrast load well below this limit in high-risk patients.

***Allergic Reaction.*** Another potential contrast-related problem is allergic reaction,[16] which may range from urticaria, to intense peripheral vasodilation, to frank anaphylactic reaction with mucosal edema, bronchospasm, and vascular collapse. These reactions are more common in patients with a history of shellfish allergy or prior adverse reactions to contrast studies. Severe reactions in such patients can be minimized by appropriate pretreatment with steroids (prednisone 20 to 40 mg q6h), conventional antihistamines (such as diphenhydramine

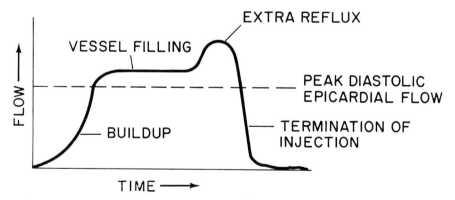

**Fig. 13-8.** Suggested injection pattern for coronary angiography. To appropriately replace antegrade coronary blood flow with contrast medium throughout the cardiac cycle, the operator should build up the velocity of injection over 1 to 2 seconds until no unopacified blood is seen to enter the ostium and there is reflux of contrast medium into the aorta during systole and diastole. This injection is maintained until the entire coronary artery is filled with contrast medium. If the ostium has not been well seen, a brief extra push should be given to cause adequate reflux into the aortic root, and the injection should be terminated. Prolonged held inspiration with some degree of Valsalva maneuver reduces coronary flow considerably and makes it much easier to replace blood flow by manual injection.

25 mg q6h), and $H_2$ antihistamines (cimetidine 300 mg q6h), starting 18 to 24 hours before the procedure.[27,28] We have seen a handful of patients who developed severe anaphylactoid reactions despite this pretreatment, but who responded promptly to the intravenous administration of epinephrine (0.1 mg = 1 ml of the 1:10,000 solution available on most emergency carts, repeated every 2 minutes until the blood pressure and/or wheezing improve).

## ANGIOGRAPHIC VIEWS AND QUANTITATION OF STENOSIS

*Coronary Anatomy.* The coronary angiographer must develop a detailed familiarity with normal coronary arterial anatomy and its common variations. The main coronary trunks can be considered to lie in one of two orthogonal planes (Fig. 13-9). The anterior descending and posterior descending coronary arteries lie in the plane of the interventricular septum, and the right and circumflex coronary trunks lie in the plane of the atrioventricular valves. In the 60-degree

left anterior oblique (LAO) projection, one is looking down the plane of the interventricular septum, with the plane of the AV valves seen en face; in the 30-degree right anterior oblique (RAO) projection, one is looking down the plane of the AV valves, with the plane of the interventricular septum seen en face.

RIGHT DOMINANT CIRCULATION. In 85% of patients, the coronary circulation is "right dominant"; that is, the right coronary artery supplies the inferior aspect of the interventricular septum by giving rise to the posterior descending artery and also supplies one or more posterior left ventricular branches after the origin of the posterior descending artery (Fig. 13-9). The left anterior descending artery has septal branches that curve down into the interventricular septum and diagonal branches that wrap over the anterolateral free wall of the left ventricle. In the right dominant coronary circulation the circumflex artery has one or more obtuse marginal branches that supply the lateral free wall of the left ventricle, as well as one or more left atrial branches. In some patients, a large intermedius branch (neither a diagonal nor a marginal) may originate directly from

**CORONARY ANGIOGRAPHIC ANATOMY: REPRESENTATION IN STANDARD PROJECTIONS**

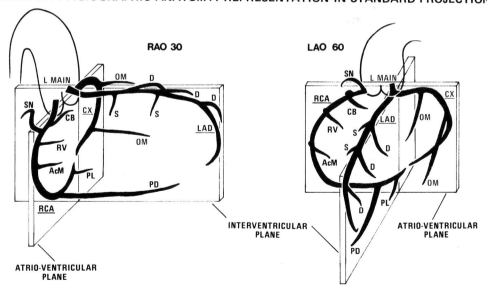

**Fig. 13-9.** Representation of coronary anatomy relative to the interventricular and atrioventricular valve planes. Coronary branches are as indicated—L Main (left main), LAD (left anterior descending), D (diagonal), S (septal), CX (circumflex), OM (obtuse marginal), RCA (right coronary), CB (conus branch) SN (sinus node), AcM (acute marginal), PD (posterior descending), PL (posterolateral left ventricular).

the left main trunk, bisecting the angle between the left anterior descending and circumflex arteries, so that there is a trifurcation of the left main coronary artery. The right coronary artery gives rise to the AV nodal artery in right dominant circulations and gives rise to a branch to the right ventricular outflow tract (conus branch), the sinus node (in 60% of patients), and the free wall of the right ventricle (acute marginal branches) whether the circulation is right dominant or not.

LEFT DOMINANT CIRCULATION. In 8% of patients the coronary circulation is "left dominant"; that is, the posterolateral left ventricular, posterior descending, and AV nodal arteries are supplied by the terminal portion of the left circumflex coronary artery, and the right coronary artery supplies only the right atrium and right ventricle.

Finally, about 7% of hearts exhibit a codominant or balanced system, with the right coronary artery giving rise to the posterior descending artery and then terminating, while the circumflex artery gives rise to all the posterior left ventricular branches and perhaps also a parallel posterior descending branch to the interventricular septum. Within this general description, it should be noted that there is considerable patient to patient variability in the size and position of different branches, and that 1 to 2% of patients may have more divergent coronary anatomic features (such as anomalous origin of the circumflex from the right coronary artery, separate ostia of the left anterior descending and left circumflex arteries, or separate ostia of the right coronary and its conus branch).

***Angiographic Views.*** To quantitate a coronary stenosis accurately, it must be seen in profile, free from artifact related to foreshortening or obfuscation by a crossing vessel. Multiple views are important, particularly in the evaluation of eccentric or slitlike stenoses, whose true severity may be underestimated if viewed only in a single projection.[29] These severely eccentric stenoses can often be recognized by their marked lucency in the major axis projection, due to thinning of the contrast column. It is important to confirm the presence of significant stenosis in an orthogonal projection, however, because similar lucency may be seen adjacent to areas of denser contrast due to tortuosity or overlapping vessels, as the result of a perceptual artifact (Mach effect) in the absence of any true abnormality at the site.[30]

The degree of stenosis (Fig. 13-10) is usually quantitated from the moving cineangiogram by visual evaluation of the percentage of diameter reduction relative to the caliber of the adjacent normal segments.[31] This is fairly accurate in very mild or very severe stenoses, but there is substantial inter-observer variability (frequently ±20%) in the visual quantitation of moderate stenoses between 40 and 80%.[32] This range of stenosis is particularly important, since a 50% diameter (75% cross-sectional area) stenosis is barely

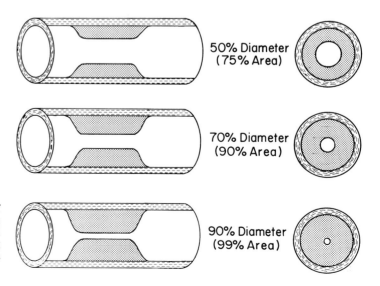

50% Diameter (75% Area)

70% Diameter (90% Area)

90% Diameter (99% Area)

**Fig. 13-10.** Coronary stenoses of 50, 70, and 90% diameter reduction are shown in longitudinal and cross section. The corresponding reductions in cross-sectional area are indicated in parentheses.

"hemodynamically significant" at peak coronary flows, but a 70% diameter (90% cross-sectional area) stenosis is quite severe at these same peak flows.[33,34] Direct measurement using a digital caliper[35] or optical reticule, video processing with visual[36] or automated edge detection[37] or densitometric analysis[38] offers the possibility of more consistent stenosis quantitation, but these techniques are not currently in wide use.

Accurate coronary diagnosis requires coronary injections in multiple views. When earlier cradle systems were used, these views were usually limited to different degrees of left or right anterior obliquity in the transverse plane, including the 60-degree LAO and 30-degree RAO projections (Fig. 13-11). Cradle systems have subsequently been modified to allow concurrent cranial angulation of the x-ray beam by propping the patient's shoulders up on a foam wedge—hence the name "sit-up" view for the LAO-cranial projection.[39] By mounting the x-ray tube and image intensifier on a parallelogram or a rigid U-arm supported by a rotating pedestal, however, modern gantries now allow for combination of any conventional transverse angulation with cranial or caudal angulation up to 45 degrees. While these views increase the demand on the generator and the scattered radiation (due to greater x-ray tube-intensifier separation and soft tissue depth), there is no doubt that they have improved our ability to define coronary anatomy.[40–42]

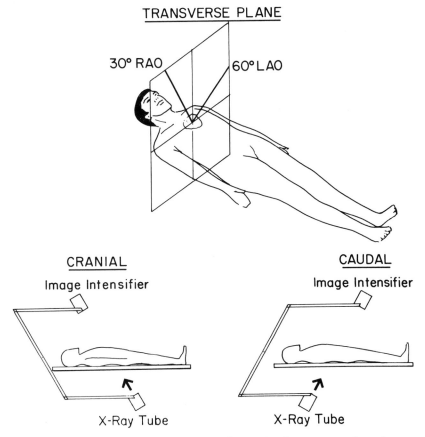

**Fig. 13-11.** Geometry of angulated views. Conventional coronary angiography was performed previously using angulation only in the transverse plane (top), as demonstrated by the 60 degree left anterior oblique (LAO) and 30 degree right anterior oblique (RAO) views. Currently, improved x-ray equipment permits simultaneous cranial or caudal angulation in the sagittal plane. Each view is named based on the location of the image intensifier, rather than the older nomenclature specifying the location of both the x-ray tube and intensifier (i.e., cranial = caudocranial).

It is important to point out that all potential views are not necessary in a given patient to constitute an adequate study. Rather, a series of "screening views" should be used as the foundation of the study, supplemented by one or more "special" views selected to define more completely suspicious areas observed on live fluoroscopy or on review of the videotape images that are recorded concurrently with cine film exposure. This requires the operator to interpret the coronary anatomy as each injection is made (rather than shooting a series of routine views and hoping that the study will prove adequate when the cine film is developed) and to understand the influence of angulation on the projected coronary anatomy. In respect to the latter issue, a coronary anatomic model is a valuable training tool (Fig. 13-12).[43]

RAO PROJECTION. For historic reasons, the screening views used in many laboratories are the conventional LAO-RAO angulations. In our laboratory, however, we have found that certain cranial and caudal angulated views may be preferable. The conventional 30-degree RAO projection suffers from overlap and foreshortening in both the left ante-

rior descending and circumflex territories (Fig. 13-12). The shallow RAO-cranial projection (5 to 15 degrees RAO and 25 to 35 degrees cranial) provides a superior view of the mid and distal left anterior descending artery, with clear visualization of the origins of the septal and diagonal branches. The shallow RAO cranial view is also quite good for examination of the distal right coronary artery, since it "unstacks" the posterior descending and posterolateral branches and projects them without foreshortening. Because of foreshortening and overlap, however, this view seldom provides useful information about the left main or circumflex coronary artery. In contrast, the shallow RAO-caudal projection (5 to 15 degrees RAO and 15 to 20 degrees caudal) provides an excellent view of the left main bifurcation, the proximal left anterior descending artery, and the proximal to mid circumflex artery and is our initial view of choice in studying unstable patients.

LAO PROJECTION. The conventional 60-degree LAO projection of the left coronary artery is limited by overlap and foreshortening, but is quite useful in the evaluation of the

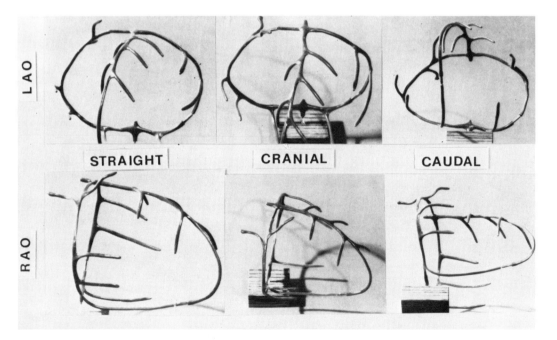

**Fig. 13-12.** Demonstration of angiographic projections using the author's coronary model. LAO and RAO projections are photographed straight (i.e., with no cranial or caudal angulation), as well as with moderate cranial and moderate caudal angulation (see text for details).

proximal and mid right coronary artery. The addition of 15 to 30 degrees of cranial angulation has the effect of elongating the left main and proximal left anterior descending arteries while projecting the intermedius or first diagonal branch downward off the proximal circumflex. If radiographic penetration in this view is difficult, reducing the LAO angulation to 30 to 40 degrees will usually allow the left anterior descending artery to fall into the lucent wedge between the right hemidiaphragm and the spine. The LAO-caudal view (40 to 60 degrees LAO and 10 to 20 degrees caudal) projects the left coronary artery in the appearance of a spider and offers improved visualization of the left main, proximal LAD, and proximal circumflex arteries. This view is particularly valuable in patients whose heart has a horizontal lie, i.e., the origin of the left main artery is located at or below the proximal left anterior descending artery in the standard LAO projection, but stresses the radiographic capacity of most older installations. This "spider view" (LAO-caudal) can often be enhanced by filming during forced maximal expiration, which accentuates a horizontal cardiac position and allows a better look from below.

AP AND LEFT LATERAL PROJECTIONS. Two underutilized views are the AP and left lateral projections. Since the left main coronary artery curves from a more leftward to an almost anterior direction along its length, the AP projection frequently provides the best view of the left main ostium, whereas the shallow RAO caudal view frequently provides a better look at the more distal left main artery. The left lateral projection is particularly useful in examining the proximal circumflex and the proximal and distal left anterior descending arteries, particularly if combined with slight (10 to 15 degrees) cranial angulation. It also provides an excellent look at the midportion of the right coronary artery and has the advantage of allowing easy radiographic penetration in most patients when performed with both of the patient's hands positioned behind his or her head.

***Coronary Collaterals.*** In reviewing the coronary angiogram, one basic principle is that there should be evident blood supply to all portions of the left ventricle. Previously occluded vessel branches are usually manifest as truncated stumps, but no stump may be evident if there has been a "flush-occlu-sion" at the origin of the involved vessel. These occluded or severely stenotic vessels will be seen frequently to fill late in the injection by antegrade (so-called bridging) collaterals or by collaterals that originate from the same ("intracoronary") or an adjacent ("intercoronary") vessel, which are reviewed in an excellent paper by Levin[44] and illustrated in Figures 13-13 through 13-15. Finally, coronary occlusion may present in some patients simply as an "angiographically arid" area to which there is no evidence of either antegrade or collateral flow and no evident vascular stump. If such an area fails to show regional hypokinesis on the left ventriculogram, the operator should search carefully for blood supply via anomalous vessels or unopacified collaterals (i.e., a separate-origin conus branch which was not opacified during the main right coronary injections), since myocardium cannot continue to function normally with no visible means of support.

## NONATHEROSCLEROTIC CORONARY ARTERY DISEASE

Although atherosclerotic stenosis is far and away the most common pathologic process identified on the coronary angiogram, the angiographer must be aware of a variety of other potential findings.[45] These include congenital anomalies of coronary origin, coronary fistulae (Fig. 13-16), and muscle bridges (Fig. 13-17).[5,45–48] The latter are sections of a coronary artery (almost always the left anterior descending) which run under a strip of left ventricular muscle and are compressed during ventricular systole but appear normal during diastole. These congenital anomalies are important to recognize, since they can be associated with ischemic symptoms in some patients in whom catheterization fails to demonstrate the expected finding of coronary atherosclerosis and can be surgically repaired if necessary. With regard to muscle bridges, there is evidence that they prevent a normal increase in coronary blood flow during tachycardia, when both systolic and diastolic coronary flow may be important. Surgical relief of such bridges has led to subjective and objective improvement in selected patients.

Finally, some patients who come to catheterization have *no* demonstrable coronary

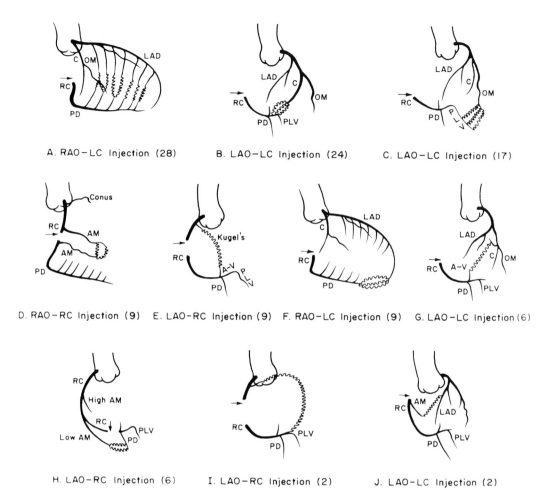

A. RAO–LC Injection (28)   B. LAO–LC Injection (24)   C. LAO–LC Injection (17)

D. RAO–RC Injection (9)   E. LAO–RC Injection (9)   F. RAO–LC Injection (9)   G. LAO–LC Injection (6)

H. LAO–RC Injection (6)   I. LAO–RC Injection (2)   J. LAO–LC Injection (2)

**Fig. 13-13.** Ten collateral pathways observed in patients with right coronary (RC) obstruction (total occlusion or >90% stenosis). Abbreviations for arteries: LAD, left anterior descending; C, circumflex; OM, obtuse marginal; PD, posterior descending; PLV, posterior left ventricular branch; AM, acute marginal branch of right coronary artery; A-V, atrioventricular nodal; LC, left coronary. Numbers in parentheses represent numbers of cases in this series. (From Levin DC: Pathways and functional significance of the coronary collateral circulation. Circulation 50:831, 1974. By permission of the American Heart Association, Inc.).

abnormality to account for their clinically suspected ischemic heart disease. Although angina-like pain can be seen in patients with noncoronary cardiac abnormality (mitral valve prolapse, hypertrophic cardiomyopathy, aortic stenosis, myocarditis) or extracardiac conditions (esophageal dysmotility,[49,50] cholecystitis), one must also consider the possibility of coronary vasospastic disease.[51] Coronary vasospasm is likely when a patient has episodes of rest pain, despite well preserved effort tolerance. An electrocardiogram recorded during an episode of sponta-

neous pain will usually show ST elevation in the territory supplied by the vasospastic artery, confirming the diagnosis of variant angina (Fig. 13-18). In these patients, the main purpose of coronary angiography is to look at the extent of underlying atherosclerosis;[52] we generally do not attempt to provoke spasm in patients with documented variant angina. In patients with no prior documented spontaneous ST elevation and insufficient coronary stenosis to explain chest pain, however, provocational testing for coronary spasm is frequently helpful.

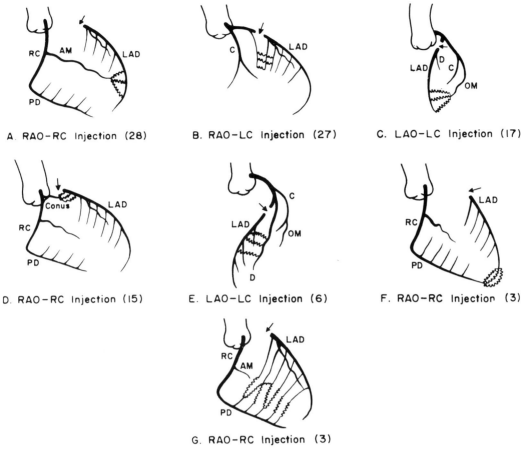

A. RAO-RC Injection (28)    B. RAO-LC Injection (27)    C. LAO-LC Injection (17)

D. RAO-RC Injection (15)    E. LAO-LC Injection (6)    F. RAO-RC Injection (3)

G. RAO-RC Injection (3)

**Fig. 13-14.** Seven collateral pathways observed in patients with left coronary artery obstruction. Abbreviations and format are the same as in Figure 13-13. (From Levin DC: Pathways and functional significance of the coronary collateral circulation. Circulation 50:831, 1973. By permission of the American Heart Association Inc.).

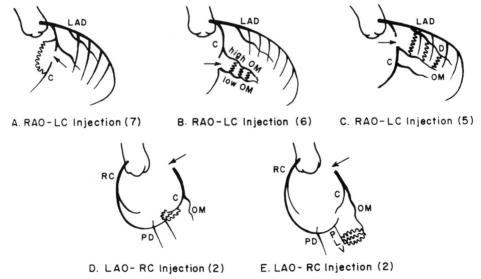

A. RAO-LC Injection (7)    B. RAO-LC Injection (6)    C. RAO-LC Injection (5)

D. LAO-RC Injection (2)    E. LAO-RC Injection (2)

**Fig. 13-15.** Five collateral pathways observed in patients with circumflex coronary artery obstruction. Abbreviations and format are the same as in Figure 13-13. (From Levin DC: Pathways and functional significance of the coronary collateral circulation. Circulation 50:831, 1974. By permission of the American Heart Association, Inc.).

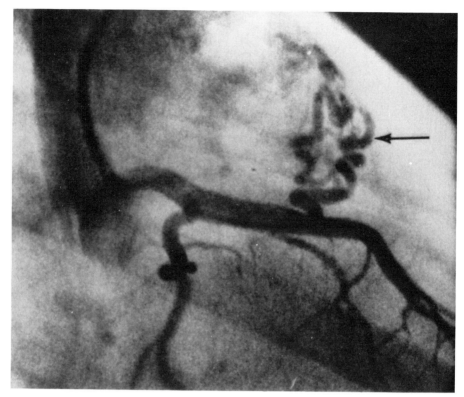

**Fig. 13-16.** Coronary artery fistula (arrow) between the midleft anterior descending coronary artery and the pulmonary artery, shown in the right anterior oblique view.

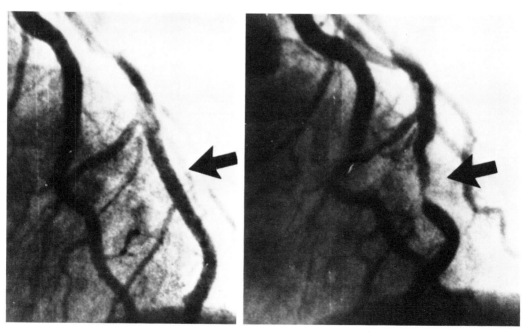

**Fig. 13-17.** Muscle bridge. Moderately severe muscle bridge of the left anterior descending coronary artery (arrow) as seen in diastole (left) and systole (right).

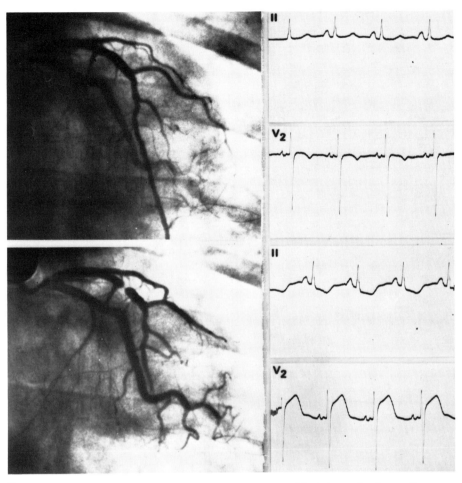

**Fig. 13-18.**   True coronary spasm. Intense focal vasospasm of the left anterior descending coronary artery is shown in the RAO projection in a patient with variant angina. Note the absence of a significant underlying atherosclerotic stenosis in the top panel, the absence of vasoconstriction of other vessel segments and the marked ST elevation in the anterior leads during the spontaneous vasospastic episode. (From Baim DS, Harrison DC: Nonatherosclerotic coronary heart disease. *In* Hurst JW (ed): The Heart, 5th ed. New York, McGraw-Hill Book Company, 1985, with permission.)

## DETECTION OF CORONARY VASOSPASM

If provocational testing for coronary spasm is contemplated, the patient should be withdrawn from calcium-channel blockers for at least 24 hours and long-acting nitrates for at least 12 hours prior to study and not be premedicated with either atropine or sublingual nitroglycerin. Ongoing therapy with any of these agents may render provocational tests falsely negative.[53] Although a variety of provocational tests have been employed (methacholine, epinephrine and propranolol, hyperventilation and tris-buffer, cold pressor) the most commonly used provocational agent is ergonovine maleate,[54–57] a stimulant of the alpha adrenergic and serotonin receptors in coronary vascular smooth muscle.

Testing for coronary spasm should be performed only following baseline angiographic evaluation of both the left and right coronary arteries. According to our protocol, a total of 0.4 mg (400 mcg = 2 ampules) of ergonovine maleate is diluted to a total volume of 8 ml in a 10-ml syringe which is appropriately labeled. The provocational test consists of intravenous administration of 1 ml (0.05 mg), 2 ml (0.10 mg), and 5 ml (0.25 mg) of this mixture at 3 to 5 minute intervals. *Parenteral nitroglycerin (100 to 200 mcg/ml) must be premixed and loaded in a labeled syringe before the testing is begun.* At one minute before each ergonovine dose, the patient is interrogated about symptoms similar to his clinical complaint and a 12-lead electrocardiogram is recorded. After each electrocardiogram, coronary angiography is performed, looking either at both arteries or only at the artery of highest clinical suspicion for vasospasm. In the absence of clinical symptoms, electrocardiographic changes, or focal coronary vasospasm exceeding 70% diameter reduction, the next ergonovine dose is administered and the cycle is repeated until the total dose of 0.4 mg has been given.

Clinical symptoms in the absence of electrocardiographic or angiographic evidence of vasospasm in either coronary artery suggest an alternative diagnosis such as esophageal dysmotility.[49,50] Even if there are no symptoms or electrocardiographic changes, both coronary arteries should be opacified at the end of the ergonovine test, and the generalized ergonovine vasoconstrictor effect should be terminated by administration of nitroglycerin. Coronary artery spasm may occur in two vessels simultaneously (Fig. 13-19), and visualization of only one vessel may fail to adequately assess the response to ergonovine. The provocational test should be considered positive only if focal spasm occurs and is associated with clinical symptoms and/or electrocardiographic changes. The patient is then treated immediately with parenteral nitroglycerin in the dose of 200 mcg administered either by vein or directly into the spastic coronary artery. The involved artery should then be re-opacified 1 minute following nitroglycerin administration, to document the resolution of spasm and the extent of underlying atherosclerotic stenosis. The operator should be prepared to use additional doses of parenteral nitroglycerin, sublingual nifedipine, or sodium nitroprusside to treat refractory spasm or the occasional severe hypertensive reaction that can occur following ergonovine administration. Temporary pacing and defibrillatory equipment should also be available to treat the brady- or tachyarrhythmias which sometimes accompany coronary spasm.

Several additional comments about ergonovine are in order. Our group does not perform ergonovine testing in patients with severe atherosclerotic stenosis (80% or greater) in whom spasm is not required to explain the clinical symptoms. In these patients, however, we frequently *do* repeat coronary angiography of the stenosed vessel after the intracoronary administration of 200 mcg of nitroglycerin, to exclude the possibility that spontaneous focal vasospasm is contributing to the appearance of severe atherosclerotic stenosis. Secondly, it is important to distinguish the intense focal spasm seen in patients with variant angina from the normal mild (15 to 20%) diffuse coronary narrowing seen as a pharmacologic response to ergonovine in normal patients[58,59] or from "catheter tip" spasm (Fig. 13-20).[60] The latter is most common in the right coronary artery, is not associated with clinical symptoms or electrocardiographic changes, and does not indicate variant angina. It should be recognized as such, however, and treated by withdrawal of the catheter, administration of nitroglycerin, and nonselective or cautious repeat selective opacification of the involved vessel, to avoid mistaking catheter-tip spasm for an atherosclerotic lesion. Finally, the operator should be aware that the positivity rate of ergonovine testing depends strongly on the patients studied; the test is almost always positive in patients with known variant angina (if their disorder is active and medications have been withheld), is positive in approximately one third of patients with clinically suspected variant angina, but is positive in fewer than 5% of patients whose symptoms do not suggest variant angina.[57,61]

## Abnormal Coronary Vasodilator Reserve

Evidence has been accumulating that the patient group with angina and angiographically normal coronary arteries may contain a subgroup of patients who have myocardial ischemia on the basis of abnormal vasodilator reserve.[62–64] In these patients, coronary sinus blood flow measured by thermodilution technique (as described in Chapter 21) fails to rise normally with pacing tachycardia or ergonovine, and the coronary vascular resistance is increased abnormally. Also,

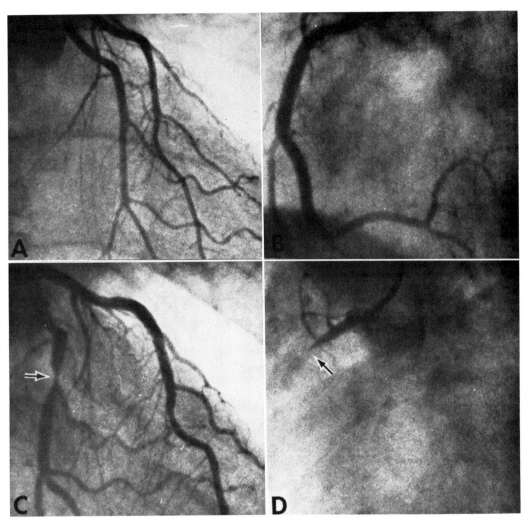

**Fig. 13-19.** Coronary angiograms before (A and B) and after (C and D) coronary artery spasm induced by ergonovine maleate in a patient with Prinzmetal's variant angina. Severe spasm occurred in both the circumflex and right coronary arteries. Catheterization was by Sones technique. (From Heupler FA, et al: Ergonovine maleate provocative test for coronary arterial spasm. Am J Cardiol 41:631, 1978.)

many of these patients show an abnormal rise in left ventricular end diastolic pressure following pacing tachycardia, and show less lactate consumption than normal subjects in response to pacing tachycardia. A failure of small vessel coronary vasodilation or an inappropriate vasoconstriction at the arteriolar level has been postulated to account for these findings, and a beneficial response to calcium antagonist therapy has been described. Coronary angiography in these patients is entirely normal.[62-64]

## MISTAKES IN INTERPRETATION

An inexperienced operator will often produce an incomplete, uninterpretable or misinterpreted study, especially if he is using poor equipment. The following discussion summarizes some of the more common pitfalls mentioned earlier that may lead the inexperienced coronary angiographer to mistaken conclusions.

***Inadequate Number of Projections.*** There is no standard number of projections

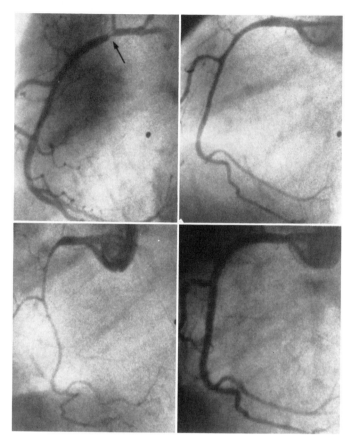

**Fig. 13-20.** Vasomotor changes *not* representing true coronary spasm. During right coronary catheterization with a Judkins catheter (upper left), this patient developed severe catheter-tip spasm. Re-catheterization 24 hours later with an Amplatz catheter (upper right) showed neither catheter-tip spasm nor an atherosclerotic stenosis. Following ergonovine 0.4 mg, marked diffuse coronary narrowing was observed (lower left), without angina or electrocardiographic changes. After the intracoronary administration of nitroglycerin 200 mcg (lower right), there is marked diffuse vasodilation.

that will always provide complete information. Each major vessel must be viewed in an isolated fashion as it stands apart from other vessels. Usually, the angulated views discussed earlier in this chapter will be necessary to visualize clearly the anatomy of the proximal left anterior descending and circumflex arteries.

***Pulsatile Injection of Contrast Material.*** The inexperienced operator or assistant has a tendency to hold back on the volume and force of injection into the coronary circulation. This results in inadequate opacification of the coronary arterial tree and pulsatile filling because the syringe pressure may exceed catheter tip pressure only during late diastole. Since there is inadequate mixing of contrast agent and blood, pockets of nonradiopaque blood may give the appearance of arterial narrowing.

***Superselective Injection.*** It is not uncommon to catheterize the left anterior descending or circumflex coronary artery superselectively, especially when the left main coronary artery is short and its bifurcation is early. To the inexperienced operator, this may give the impression of total occlusion of the nonvisualized vessel (e.g., if only the circumflex artery is opacified, the operator may conclude that the left anterior descending artery is occluded). With the right coronary artery, superselective injection may occur if the catheter tip is too far down the vessel, leading to failure to visualize the conus and sinus node arteries. Since these are important sources of collateralization of the left coronary system, important information may be missed. Adequate injection to give a continuous (nonpulsatile) reflux of contrast agent back into the sinus of Valsalva will help the operator to recognize vessels that originate proximally to the catheter tip and thus avoid the interpretation error of superselective injection.

***Catheter-Induced Coronary Spasm.***
Coronary artery spasm may be related to the
catheter itself, possibly caused by mechanical irritation and a myogenic reflex. It is seen
most commonly when the right coronary artery is engaged selectively, but it may occur
in the left anterior descending artery as well.
Although it can occur with either the brachial or femoral approaches, it is probably
more common with the right Judkins catheter, especially if the catheter tip enters the
right coronary ostium at an angle and produces tenting of the proximal vessel. If coronary narrowing suggests the occurrence of
spasm to the operator, sublingual, intravenous, or intracoronary nitroglycerin should
be given and the injection repeated.

***Congenital Variants of Coronary Origin and Distribution.*** This topic has been
discussed earlier in this chapter, but it bears
reemphasis. Variation in origin and distribution of the coronary artery branches may
confuse the operator and cause him to mistakenly diagnose coronary occlusion. For
example, a small right coronary artery that
terminates in the AV groove well before the
crux may be interpreted as an abnormal or
occluded artery, whereas it is a normal finding in 7 to 10% of human hearts. Double ostia
of the right coronary artery or origin of the
circumflex artery from the right coronary
artery may be similarly confusing and lead to
misdiagnosis.

***Myocardial Bridges.*** As discussed earlier, coronary arteries occasionally dip below
the epicardial surface under small areas of
myocardium. During systole the segment of
the artery surrounded by mocardium is narrowed and appears as a localized stenosis.
These "myocardial bridges" occur most commonly in the distribution of the left anterior
descending artery and its diagonal branches.
The key to the recognition of these bridges is
that the apparent localized stenosis returns
to normal during diastole. Although it is
likely that these bridges can cause true myocardial ischemia under certain circumstances, they may be seen in patients with
normal hearts and no evidence of ischemia.

***Total Occlusion.*** If a coronary artery or
branch is totally occluded at its origin, it may
not be visualized and the occlusion may be
missed. If the occlusion is "flush" with the
parent vessel, no stump will be seen. Such
occlusions are primarily recognized by visualization of the distal segment of the occluded vessel by means of collateral channels or by noting the absence of the usual
vascularity seen in a particular portion of the
heart.

# REFERENCES

1. Kennedy RH, et al: Cardiac-catheterization and cardiac-surgical facilities. Use, trends and future requirements. N Engl J Med 307:986, 1982.
2. Kennedy JW, et al: Complications associated with cardiac catheterization and angiography. Cathet Cardiovasc Diagn 8:5, 1982.
3. Silverman K, Grossman W: Angina pectoris: Natural history and strategies for evaluation and management. N Engl J Med 310:1712, 1984.
4. Ambrose JA: Unsettled indications for coronary angiography. J Am Coll Cardiol 3:1575, 1984.
5. Neufeld HN, Blieden LC: Coronary artery disease in children. Prog Cardiol 4:119, 1975.
6. St. John Sutton MG, et al: Valve replacement without preoperative catheterization. N Engl J Med 305:1233, 1981.
7. Roberts WC: No cardiac catheterization before cardiac valve replacement—a mistake. Am Heart J 103:930, 1982.
8. Conti CR: Coronary arteriography. Circulation 55:227, 1977.
9. Abrams HL, Adams DF: The coronary arteriogram. N Engl J Med 281:1277, 1969.
10. Mahrer PR, Eschoo N: Outpatient cardiac catheterization and coronary angiography. Cathet Cardiovasc Diagn 7:355, 1981.
11. Fierens E. Outpatient coronary arteriography. Cathet Cardiovasc Diagn 10:27, 1984.
12. Judkins MP: Selective coronary arteriography, a percutaneous transfemoral technic. Radiology 89:815, 1967.
13. Amplatz K, Formanek G, Stanger P, Wilson W: Mechanics of selective coronary artery catheterization via femoral approach. Radiology 89:1040, 1967.
14. Schoonmaker FW, King SB: Coronary arteriography by the single catheter percutaneous femoral technique, experience in 6,800 cases. Circulation 50:735, 1974.
15. Sones FM, Shirey EK: Cine coronary arteriography. Mod Concepts Cardiovasc Dis 31:735, 1962.
16. Grainger RG: intravascular contrast media—the

past, the present and the future. Br J Radiol 55:1, 1982.

17. Murdock DK, et al: Inotropic effects of ionic contrast media: the role of calcium binding additives. Cathet Cardiovasc Diagn 10:455, 1984.

18. Bourdillon PD, et al: Effects of a new non-ionic and a conventional ionic contrast agent on coronary sinus ionized calcium and left ventricular hemodynamics in dogs. J Am Coll Cardiol (in press).

19. Nitter-Hauge S, Enge I: Metrizoic acid (Isopaque Coronar) used in man for cardiac angiography. Radiology 121:537, 1976.

20. Gertz EW, Wisneski JA, Chiu D, Akin JR, Hu C: Clinical superiority of a new nonionic contrast agent (Iopamidol) for cardiac angiography. J Am Coll Cardiol 5:250, 1985.

21. Ovitt T, et al: Electrocardiographic changes in selective coronary arteriography: the importance of ions. Radiology 102:705, 1972.

22. Tragardh B, Bove AA, Lynch PR: Mechanism of production of cardiac conduction abnormalities due to coronary arteriography in dogs. Invest Radiol 11:563, 1976.

23. Higgins CB: Effect of contrast media on the conduction system of the heart: Mechanism of action and identification of toxic component. Radiology 124:599, 1977.

24. Paulin S, Adams DF: Increased ventricular fibrillation during coronary arteriography with a new contrast medium preparation. Radiology 101:45, 1971.

25. Snyder CF, Formanek A, Frech RS, Amplatz K: The role of sodium in promoting ventricular arrhythmia during coronary arteriography. Am J Roentgen 113:567, 1971.

26. Schwarz RD, et al: Renal failure following major angiography. Ann Intern Med 65:31, 1978.

27. Zweiman B, Mishkin MM, Hildreth EA: An approach to the performance of contrast studies in contrast material-reactive persons. Ann Intern Med 83:159, 1975.

28. Myers GE, Bloom FL: Cimetidine (tagamet) combined with steroids and H-1 antihistamines for the prevention of serious radiographic contrast material reactions. Cathet Cardiovasc Diagn. 7:65, 1981.

29. Spears JR, Sandor T, Baim DS, Paulin S: The minimum error in estimating coronary luminal cross-sectional area from cineangiographic diameter measurements. Cathet Cardiovasc Diagn 9:119, 1983.

30. Randall PA. Mach bands in cine coronary arteriography. Radiology 129:65, 1978.

31. Arnett EN, et al: Coronary artery narrowing in coronary heart disease: comparison of cineangiographic and necropsy findings. Ann Intern Med 91:350, 1979.

32. Zir LM, et al: Interobserver variability in coronary angiography. Circulation 54:627, 1976.

33. McMahon MM, et al: Quantitative coronary angiography: measurement of the "critical" stenosis in patients with unstable angina and single vessel disease without collaterals. Circulation 60:106, 1979.

34. Kirkeeide RL, Gould KL: Cardiovascular imaging: coronary artery stenosis. Hosp Pract 1984 (April) 160.

35. Rafflenbeul W, et al. Quantitative coronary arteriography—coronary anatomy of patients with unstable angina pectoris reexamined 1 year after optimal medical therapy. Am J Cardiol 43:699, 1979.

36. Brown BG, Bolson E, Frimer M, Dodge HT: Quantitative coronary arteriography—estimation of dimensions, hemodynamic resistance, and atheroma mass of coronary artery lesions using the arteriogram and digital computation. Circulation 55:329, 1977.

37. Spears JR, et al: Computerized image analysis for quantitative measurement of vessel diameter from cineangiograms. Circulation 68:453, 1983.

38. Crawford DW, Brooks SH, Barndt R, Blankenhorn DH: Measurement of atherosclerotic luminal irregularity by radiographic densitometry. Invest Radiol 12:307, 1977.

39. Vetrovec GW, Strash AM: Modification of cradle angiographic tables to more easily obtain axial coronary views. Cathet Cardiovasc Diagn 10:607, 1984.

40. Aldridge HE: A decade or more of cranial and caudal angled projections in coronary arteriography—another look. Cathet Cardiovasc Diagn 10:539, 1984.

41. Elliott LP, et al: Advantage of the cranial-right anterior oblique view in diagnosing mid left anterior descending and distal right coronary artery disease. Am J Cardiol 48:754, 1981.

42. Grover M, Slutsky R, Higgins C, Atwood JE. Terminology and anatomy of angulated coronary arteriography. Clin Cardiol 7:37, 1984.

43. Taylor CR, Wilde P: An easily constructed model of the coronary arteries. Am J Radiol 142:389, 1984.

44. Levin DC: Pathways and functional significance of the coronary collateral circulation. Circulation 50:831, 1974.

45. Baim DS, Harrison DC: Nonatherosclerotic coronary heart disease. *In* Hurst JW (ed): The Heart. 6th ed. New York, McGraw-Hill Book Company (in press).

46. Razavi M: Unusual forms of coronary artery disease. Cardiovasc Clin 7:25, 1975.

47. Engel HJ, Torres C, Page HL: Major variations in anatomical origin of the coronary arteries: angiographic observations in 4,250 patients without

associated congenital heart disease. Cathet Cardiovasc Diagn 1:157, 1975.

48. Levin DC, Fellows KE, Abrams HL: Hemodynamically significant primary anomalies of the coronary arteries, angiographic aspects. Circulation 58:25, 1978.

49. Cohen S: Motor disorders of the esophagus. N Engl J Med 301:183, 1979.

50. Kaye MD: Recognizing and managing esophageal spasm. Drug Therapy 1982 (March) 137.

51. Maseri A, Chierchia S: Coronary artery spasm: demonstration, definition, diagnosis, and consequences. Prog Cardiovasc Dis 25:169, 1982.

52. Mark DB, et al: Clinical characteristics and long-term survival of patients with variant angina. Circulation 69:880, 1984.

53. Waters DD, Theroux P, Szlachcic J, Dauwe F: Provocative testing with ergonovine to assess the efficacy of treatment with nifedipine, diltiazem and verapamil in variant angina. Am J Cardiol 48:123, 1981.

54. Schroeder JS, et al: Provocation of coronary spasm with ergonovine maleate. Am J Cardiol 40:487, 1977.

55. Heupler FA, et al: Ergonovine maleate provocative test for coronary arterial spasm. Am J Cardiol 41:631, 1978.

56. Raizner AE, et al: Provocation of coronary artery spasm by the cold pressor test. Circulation 62:925, 1980.

57. Meyers DG: Ergonovine provocation of coronary artery spasm. Cardiovasc Rev Reports 3:855, 1982.

58. Cipriano PR, et al: The effects of ergonovine maleate on coronary arterial size. Circulation 59:82, 1979.

59. Curry RC, et al: Effects of ergonovine in patients with and without coronary artery disease. Circulation 56:803, 1977.

60. Friedman AC, Spindola-Franco H, Nivatpumin T: Coronary spasm: Prinzmetal's variant angina vs. catheter-induced spasm; refractory spasm vs. fixed stenosis. Am J Radiol 132:897, 1979.

61. Bertrand ME, et al: Frequency of provoked coronary arterial spasm in 1089 consecutive patients undergoing coronary arteriography. Circulation 65:1299, 1982.

62. Cannon RO III, Watson RM, Rosing DR, Epstein SE: Angina caused by reduced vasodilator reserve of the small coronary arteries. J Am Coll Cardiol 1:1359–1373, 1983.

63. Cannon RO III, et al: Chest pain and "normal" coronary arteries—role of small coronary arteries. Am J Cardiol 55:50B–60B, 1985.

64. Cannon RO III, et al: Left ventricular dysfunction in patients with angina pectoris, normal epicardial coronary arteries, and abnormal vasodilator reserve. Circulation 72:218–226, 1985.

*chapter fourteen*

# Cardiac Ventriculography

L. DAVID HILLIS *and* WILLIAM GROSSMAN

CARDIAC ventriculography has been used extensively to define the anatomy of the ventricles and related structures in patients with congenital, valvular, coronary, and cardiomyopathic heart disease.[1-5] Specifically, *left ventriculography* may provide valuable information about global and segmental left ventricular function, mitral valvular incompetence, and the presence, location, and severity of a number of other abnormalities, including ventricular septal defect and hypertrophic cardiomyopathy. As a result, it should be a routine part of catheterization in patients being evaluated for coronary artery disease, aortic or mitral valvular disease, unexplained left ventricular failure, or congenital heart disease. Similarly, *right ventriculography* may provide information about global and segmental right ventricular function and can be especially helpful in patients with congenital heart disease.

## INJECTION CATHETERS

To achieve adequate opacification of the left or right ventricles, it is necessary to deliver a relatively large amount of contrast material in a relatively short time. In adults, a 7 or 8 French catheter with multiple side-holes is required, keeping in mind that the ease of delivery of contrast material is related to catheter lumen size. For left and right ventriculography at Parkland Memorial Hospital, every attempt is made to use a catheter in which the lumen is equivalent to that of a standard 8 French catheter, unless, of course, the size of the artery through which it is advanced mandates that it be smaller. For adult ventriculography, a 6 French (or smaller) catheter is usually unsatisfactory.

The ideal catheter for ventriculography should offer minimal resistance to the rapid delivery of contrast material, so that it remains in a stable position during injection and, therefore, produces no disturbance of cardiac rhythm. A catheter with only an end-hole, such as the *Cournand* or *multipurpose*, is unsatisfactory for ventriculography, since it often recoils during contrast delivery, causing ventricular ectopic beats and inadequate ventricular opacification, and may produce myocardial penetration (so-called endocardial staining) or even perforation. Similarly, straight catheters with an end-hole and several side-holes, such as the *Gensini* or *Sones*, have a propensity to recoil during contrast injection and may cause endocardial staining. Although the Sones catheter is used for left ventriculography in many catheterization laboratories, its tapered tip and end-hole design make it less than ideal for achieving optimal opacification of the left ventricle.

***NIH and Eppendorf Catheters.*** The NIH and Eppendorf catheters have multiple side-holes and no end-hole (Fig. 14-1). They are easily inserted through an arteriotomy (via the brachial approach) or a percutaneously introduced femoral arterial sheath. The 7F and 8F NIH catheters prepared by USCI are made of woven dacron with nylon rein-

Some of the material in this chapter has been retained from the first and second editions, to which Drs. Charles E. Rackley and William P. Hood, Jr. contributed.

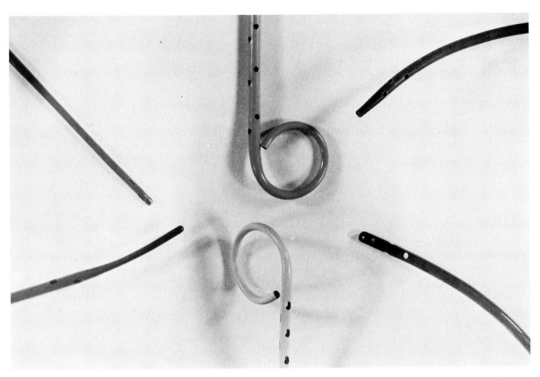

**Fig. 14-1.**   Examples of ventriculographic catheters in current use. Beginning at the top and moving clockwise: pigtail, 8.2 French (Cook); Gensini, 7 French; NIH, 8 French; pigtail, 8 French (Cordis); Lehman ventriculographic, 8 French; Sones, 7.5 French, tapering to a 5.5 French tip. The advantages and disadvantages of each catheter are discussed in the text. The Gensini and Sones catheters may cause endocardial staining because of the high pressure jet of contrast material exiting the end-hole; therefore, ventriculography with them should be performed with special attention to catheter position and rate of contrast injection.

forcement and are especially stiff. The Cordis NIH catheter (polyurethane) and Cook NIH torcon blue catheter (polyethylene) are much softer and less likely to cause dissection or perforation. The Eppendorf catheter (USCI, woven Dacron construction) is less stiff as well, and the tips of both the Cordis NIH and the USCI Eppendorf catheters are usually sufficiently soft that they can be gently prolapsed across the aortic valve. In our catheterization laboratories, the Eppendorf catheter (USCI) and polyurethane or polyethylene NIH catheters (Cordis, Cook Inc.) are used commonly for left ventriculography by the brachial approach. In addition, the Eppendorf catheter is almost always used for right ventriculography irrespective of whether access to the right ventricle is gained from the arm or leg. In some patients, especially those whose left ventricles are

small, left ventriculography with an NIH or Eppendorf catheter induces frequent ventricular premature beats. Despite the absence of an end-hole, endocardial staining occasionally occurs with these catheters, usually in patients in whom the end of the catheter is wedged within the ventricular trabeculae.

***Lehman Catheter***   The Lehman ventriculographic catheter has a tapered closed tip which extends beyond multiple side-holes (Fig. 14-1). The tapered tip may assist the operator in manipulating the catheter through tortuous arteries and across a stenotic aortic valve. Once in the left ventricle, the tip lessens the likelihood of endocardial staining, but, in our experience, it increases the chance of ventricular ectopy during the injection of contrast material.

***Pigtail Catheter.***   The pigtail catheter has several advantages for left and right ventriculography (Fig. 14-1). First, its end-hole permits its insertion and manipulation with a J-tipped guide wire, so that it can be advanced safely to the left ventricle from the arm or leg even in the patient with brachiocephalic or iliac arterial tortuosity. Second, the design of the catheter virtually eliminates the possibility of endocardial staining, since the end-hole usually is not positioned adjacent to ventricular trabeculae. Third, the catheter's shape substantially reduces the occurrence of ventricular ectopic beats. As noted, the pigtail can be used with the femoral or brachial approach. Its introduction through a brachial arteriotomy is made easier if a guide wire is used to straighten the curved end of the catheter. In many catheterization laboratories, the pigtail is the preferred catheter for left ventriculography via the brachial as well as the femoral approach. In our experience, the pigtail catheter can easily be passed across a porcine aortic valve bioprosthesis—more easily, in fact, than straight catheters, such as the NIH or Eppendorf. In such a situation, the pigtail configuration seems to prevent the catheter from glancing off the large valve cusps and sliding down into the lateral sinuses.

Recently, several catheter manufacturers have made available pigtail catheters of a "thinwall" variety. These polyurethane catheters are produced with little or no metal reinforcement in the wall. As a result, the wall is distinctly thinner, yielding a larger lumen for a given outer French size. Thus, a thinwall pigtail 7 French in outer size has a lumen similar in diameter to a conventional 8 French catheter. Because of the larger lumen, these thinwall catheters allow a greater delivery of contrast material without recoil or catheter movement. At the same time, the removal of metal reinforcement from the wall renders these catheters less stiff and, therefore, somewhat more likely to cause ventricular ectopy by moving within the ventricle during systole. We have found the thinwall pigtail catheter to be of particular advantage in patients in whom, for some reason, an unusually large amount of contrast material must be given quickly (i.e., a patient with a very high cardiac output or an individual whose left ventricle is greatly enlarged).

For right ventriculography, the NIH and Eppendorf catheters are practical and effective, as mentioned above. In addition, the

Grollman catheter (which has a pigtail tip and an angulated shaft) is often used for right ventriculography and pulmonary angiography.

## INJECTION SITE

The adequate opacification of either ventricle is accomplished only if a large amount of contrast material is delivered to it. Satisfactory opacification of the left ventricle usually can be achieved by the injection of contrast material into the left atrium, with cineangiographic acquisition as the left ventricle is filled. Such a left atrial injection is advantageous because it seldom causes atrial or ventricular ectopic activity. However, it introduces the hazard of transseptal catheterization; it does not allow an evaluation of mitral valvular incompetence; and it may obscure the basal portion of the left ventricle and the aortic valve. If the patient has aortic regurgitation, the left ventricle may be opacified adequately by aortography, but opacification is usually accomplished only in patients whose regurgitation is severe. Similarly, the right ventricle may be opacified satisfactorily by injecting contrast material into the vena cavae or right atrium. However, these peripheral injections do not allow an assessment of tricuspid valvular incompetence, and it is often difficult to film the injection in an obliquity that eliminates overlap of the vena cavae, right atrium, and right ventricle.

Ventriculography in the adult is best accomplished by injecting contrast material directly into the ventricle. In the left ventricle, the optimal catheter position is the midcavity, provided that ventricular ectopy is not a problem (Fig. 14-2). Such a midcavity position insures (1) that adequate contrast material is delivered to the chamber's body and apex; (2) that the catheter does not interfere with mitral valvular function, thereby producing factitious mitral regurgitation; and (3) that the holes through which the contrast material is injected are not wedged within the ventricular trabeculae (possibly causing endocardial staining). In some patients, a midcavity position induces repetitive ventricular ectopy, especially with an NIH or Eppendorf catheter. In these individuals, the tip of the catheter is best positioned in the left ventricular *inflow tract*, immediately in

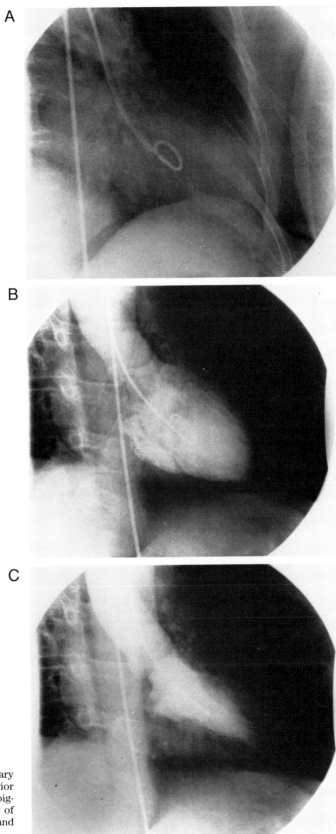

**Fig. 14-2.** An example of midcavitary catheter position for 30° right anterior oblique left ventriculography using a pigtail catheter: (A) before the injection of contrast material. (B) at end-diastole; and (C) end-systole.

front of the posterior leaflet of the mitral valve (Figs. 14-3 and 14-4). This position usually does not cause ventricular ectopy, but mitral regurgitation may be produced if the catheter is too close to the mitral valve.

In the right ventricle, the optimal catheter position is the midcavity, provided, of course, that repetitive ventricular ectopy does not occur. If ectopy is uncontrollable, the catheter may be positioned in the outflow tract, below the pulmonic valve. Even here, however, repetitive ventricular ectopy may present a difficult problem. In our experience, right ventriculography is often accompanied by frequent ventricular premature beats irrespective of catheter position.

## INJECTION RATE AND VOLUME

The rapid delivery of an adequate amount of contrast material requires the use of a power injector. There are two types of power injectors. The *pressure injector* allows one to select the volume of contrast material and its delivery pressure, but the rate of delivery is determined by the lumen size and length of the catheter, the viscosity of the contrast material, and the size of the injector syringe. The rapid delivery of contrast material is facilitated by a large-bore and short catheter, prewarmed contrast material, and an injector syringe of small diameter. The pressure injector is now outmoded and does not have the versatility of the flow injector.

The *flow injector* allows one to select both the volume and rate of delivery of contrast material. These injectors develop automatically a pressure sufficient to deliver a selected volume of injectate in a selected time. However, they are designed to shut down immediately if the pressure required exceeds a preset maximum. In most catheterization laboratories, the maximal pressure cutoff is set at 1000 psi. This high pressure is not actually delivered to the catheter tip; instead, most of it is dissipated by frictional losses in the shaft of the catheter.

Some injectors permit synchronization of the injection of contrast material with the R-wave of the electrocardiogram, so that a set flow rate is delivered in each of several successive diastolic intervals.[6,7] Although this technique has been said to lessen the incidence of ventricular ectopic beats and to

minimize the volume of contrast material required for adequate ventricular opacification, our impression is that it offers no clear advantage over nonsynchronized methods.

Cine left ventriculography is accomplished using an injection rate and volume that depend on (1) the type and size of catheter, (2) the size of the ventricular chamber to be opacified, (3) the approximate ventricular stroke volume, and (4) the preventriculography hemodynamics. We have asked our colleagues in several laboratories to tell us their usual parameters for left ventricular injection using various catheters and either femoral or brachial techniques, and these parameters are listed in Table 14-1. As can be seen, there is a fairly wide spectrum of injection rates and volumes for the pigtail catheter for either femoral or brachial approach. For the pigtail, Eppendorf, and NIH catheters, an injection rate of from 10 to 16 ml/sec (higher for high cardiac output and large ventricular chamber) and a total volume of 30 to 55 ml (depending on ventricular size) represent average values from Table 14-1. If a Sones catheter is used for left ventriculography, the rate of injection of contrast material should not exceed 8 to 12 ml/sec, thus lessening the chance of recoil and staining.

In the patient with hemodynamic evidence of severe left ventricular dysfunction (mean pulmonary capillary wedge pressure > 30 mmHg), the total volume of contrast material used for left ventriculography should be limited, if possible (i.e., 12 to 16 ml/sec for only 2 seconds, giving a total volume of 24 to 32 ml), and the ventriculogram should be performed during the administration of an acutely imposed "protective regimen." In the patient whose abnormal filling pressures are attributable to coronary artery disease, cardiomyopathy, or severe aortic or mitral regurgitation, left ventriculography is best performed after the administration of sublingual nitroglycerin or during the intravenous infusion of nitroglycerin or sodium nitroprusside. If the pulmonary capillary wedge pressure is greatly elevated because of mitral stenosis, left ventriculography should be preceded by the intravenous administration of morphine sulfate and furosemide. *Failure to take a highly elevated preventriculography pulmonary capillary wedge pressure seriously can lead to disastrous consequences, such as intractable pulmonary edema and even death.* In our experience, the left ven-

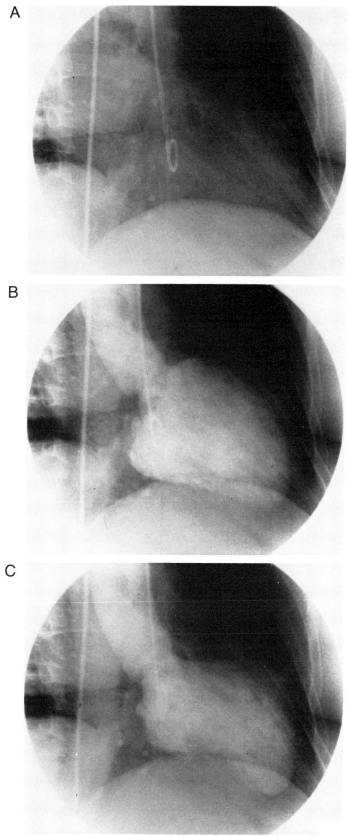

**Fig. 14-3.** An example of left ventricular inflow tract catheter position for 30° right anterior oblique left ventriculography using a pigtail catheter: (A) before the introduction of contrast material; (B) at end-diastole; and (C) end-systole. Note that this patient has a large anteroapical aneurysm.

**TABLE 14-1.** *Catheter Type, Injection Rate, and Volume of Contrast Material Used for Left Ventriculography*

| Institution & City | Femoral Approach | | | Brachial Approach | | |
|---|---|---|---|---|---|---|
| | Catheter Used | Injection Rate (ml/sec) | Volume (ml) | Catheter Used | Injection Rate (ml/sec) | Volume (ml) |
| Parkland Hospital Dallas, TX | pigtail | 12–16 | 40–55 | Eppendorf, pigtail | 12–16 | 40–55 |
| Beth Israel Hospital Boston, MA | pigtail | 12–15 | 36–45 | Eppendorf, NIH, Sones | 12–15 8–10 | 36–45 30–45 |
| U of Pennsylvania Philadelphia, PA | pigtail | 10–14 | 40–50 | pigtail, Sones | 10–14 8–10 | 40–50 40–45 |
| Barnes Hospital St. Louis, MO | pigtail | 10–14 | 30–40 | NIH | 10–14 | 30–40 |
| Temple University Philadelphia, PA | pigtail | 13–17 | 40–50 | Sones | 10–12 | 40–48 |
| Nat'l Inst. Health Bethesda, MD | pigtail | 10–15 | 30–45 | NIH | 10–15 | 30–45 |
| U of Washington Seattle, WA | pigtail | 15–20 | 40–50 | few catheter-izations by this approach | | |
| Baylor University Houston, TX | pigtail | 12–15 | 36–45 | Sones | 8–10 | 32–40 |
| Brown University Providence, RI | pigtail | 15–20 | 35–50 | pigtail, NIH | 15–20 | 35–50 |
| Yale University New Haven, CT | pigtail | 12–16 | 36–48 | pigtail, NIH | 12 | 36 |
| Mayo Clinic Rochester, MN | pigtail | 12–18 | 40–55 | NIH, Rodriguez | 12–18 | 40–55 |
| Columbia-Presbyterian New York, NY | pigtail | 15 | 45 | pigtail | 15 | 45 |
| U of Florida Gainesville, FL | pigtail | 8–12 | 25–36 | Sones | 8–12 | 25–36 |
| New York Hospital | pigtail | 8–12 | 30–45 | Sones | 8–12 | 30–45 |

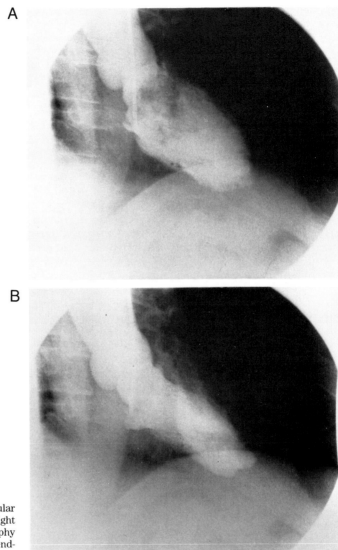

**Fig. 14-4.** An example of left ventricular inflow tract catheter position for 30° right anterior oblique left ventriculography using an Eppendorf catheter: (A) at end-diastole; and (B) end-systole.

tricular end-diastolic pressure is not as reliable a predictor of impending pulmonary edema as the wedge pressure, since (as discussed elsewhere) the left ventricular end-diastolic and mean pulmonary capillary wedge pressures may be widely disparate.

Newer nonionic contrast agents and contrast agents without calcium-binding additives may improve the safety of cardiac ventriculography in patients with depressed myocardial function. These newer agents have been discussed in Chapter 13.

Before the power injection of contrast material, one should (1) do a test injection of 3 to 5 ml to confirm proper catheter and patient position and (2) take appropriate precautions in filling and firing the power injector to prevent air embolism. In our catheterization laboratories, a Medrad Mark IV power injector with a 130 m translucent syringe is used. These syringes are made of siliconized plastic so that the contrast medium and any air may be easily seen. The injector is loaded with contrast material through roentgenography tubing 30 inches long while the syringe barrel is pointed upward. With the injector in the vertical position, air is expelled from the syringe and tubing by holding the load switch in the forward position as the operator taps the syringe and its Luer Lock connector to discharge all air bubbles. Subsequently, the injector is inverted, and a "running connection" is made between the roentgenography tubing and the catheter. Specifically, the connection is accomplished while blood is spurting from the hub of the catheter as the operator of the injector depresses the forward position of the load switch. After the connection is made, the injector operator presses the reverse position of the load switch, withdrawing gradually until the "interface" between contrast material and blood in the roentgenography tubing is easily visible and is noted to be free of air bubbles. A test injection of contrast material can then be done under fluoroscopic visualization, enabling the physician to assess catheter and patient position.

The physician performing the catheterization should look closely at the injector syringe to be sure that it is filled with contrast medium and free of air. This physician should also plan to hold the catheter at the point of its insertion into the body during the power injection of contrast, so that he may pull the catheter back instantaneously if ventricular extrasystoles, myocardial staining, or other untoward events develop during injection. Thus, the physician operator must have good visualization of the fluoroscopic screen during ventriculography. The technician or other individual firing the injector should be prepared to abort the injection upon command from the physician operator in the event of an untoward occurrence. In many laboratories the physician performing the catheterization holds the connection between catheter and roentgenography tubing tightly in one hand during the power injection to prevent a leak of contrast material at this point.

Proper catheter positioning is important to avoid extrasystoles during ventriculography, as discussed earlier in this chapter. If extrasystoles develop, it is our policy to withdraw the ventriculographic catheter immediately after the first extrasystole a distance of approximately 2 to 3 cm. This usually results in a quiet position for the remainder of the 3 to 4 second contrast injection, and is particu-larly effective when the Sones catheter is being used for left ventriculography: this technique has not resulted in ventricular staining in a very large experience.

Instructions to the patient with regard to respiration during contrast ventriculography vary from laboratory to laboratory. Previously, imaging systems were often inadequate to give good definition of the left ventricular silhouette unless ventriculography was performed during deep inspiration to move the diaphragm out of the radiographic field. With modern imaging systems excellent definition of the ventricular silhouette can be achieved without performing ventriculography during held deep inspiration. Left ventriculography done during normal quiet breathing allows physiologic interpretation of left ventricular volumes, angiographic stroke volume, and calculated left ventricular regurgitant fraction in cases of valvular regurgitation.

## FILMING PROJECTION AND TECHNIQUE

As a general rule, *biplane* ventriculography is preferable to *single plane* ventriculography, since it allows one to obtain more information at essentially no additional risk to the patient. For example, in the patient with coronary artery disease, biplane left ventriculography is superior to single plane left ventriculography in providing information on the location and severity of segmental wall motion abnormalities. In the patient with congenital heart disease, biplane right ventriculography allows one to assess accurately the anatomy of the right ventricular outflow tract, the pulmonic valve, and the proximal portions of the pulmonary artery. However, biplane ventriculography has several disadvantages, including (1) the increased expense of biplane cineangiographic equipment; (2) the reduced quality of cineangiographic imaging in each plane that results from the radiation scatter caused by the opposite plane; (3) the additional time required to position the biplane equipment appropriately, especially when the brachial approach is used; and (4) the additional radiation exposure to personnel in the room.

Whether doing biplane or single plane ventriculography, one should use the projection(s) that provide(s) maximal delineation of the structure(s) of interest and minimal overlapping of other structures. Most laboratories doing biplane left ventriculography prefer a 30° right anterior oblique (RAO) and a 60° left anterior oblique (LAO) view. The 30° RAO projection eliminates overlap of the left ventricle and the vertebral column, allows one to assess anterior, apical, and inferior segmental wall motion, and places the mitral valve in profile, thus providing a reliable assessment of the presence and angiographic severity of mitral regurgitation. As seen in Figure 14-5, the 30° RAO projection allows excellent visualization of the extent of an anterior wall aneurysm of the left ventricle in a patient with isolated proximal occlusion of the left anterior descending artery. The 60° LAO view allows one to assess ventricular septal integrity and motion, posterior

segmental function, and aortic valvular anatomy. *Cranial angulation* of the 60° LAO view may prevent the foreshortening of the left ventricle that commonly occurs with LAO views and places the entire length of the interventricular septum in profile.

If biplane cineangiographic equipment is not available, the single plane projection that provides the best delineation of structures of interest should be used. For example, the 30° RAO projection allows a reliable assessment of mitral regurgitation, whereas a 45° to 60° LAO view (with cranial angulation of 15° if possible) provides the opportunity to visualize a ventricular septal defect and the associated left-to-right shunting.

Almost all cineangiographic systems in use today employ a 35-mm camera. For routine left or right ventriculography, we perform cineangiography at 50 to 60 frames/sec-

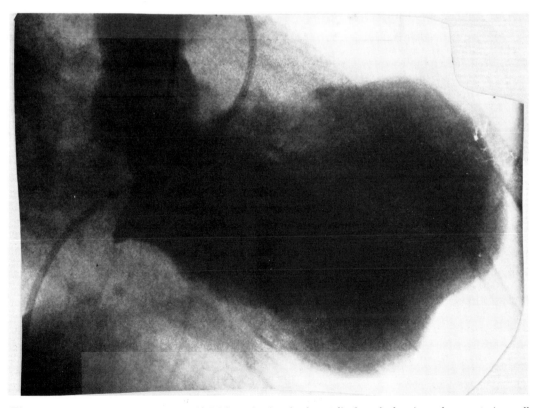

**Fig. 14-5.** Left ventriculogram in a 30° RAO projection (end systolic frame) showing a large anterior wall aneurysm. The patient was a 65-year-old man who had a massive myocardial infarction (peak CK 4460 units) and showed subsequently a progressively enlarged cardiac silhouette on a roentgenogram. Catheterization 4 weeks following infarction demonstrated a large anterior wall LV aneurysm, with LV pressure 95/40 mmHg, PCW pressure 34 mmHg, and occlusion of the left anterior descending artery proximal to the first septal perforator. Ejection fraction was 18%, and the other coronary arteries were normal.

ond and use a 9-inch image intensifier, thus allowing us to visualize the entire ventricle within the field. In many patients, ventriculography performed with a greater degree of magnification (e.g., 6-inch intensifier) will not be adequate for assessment of the entire ventricular silhouette together with the left atrium and ascending aorta.

## INTERVENTION VENTRICULOGRAPHY

Segmental dysfunction of the left ventricular wall can be caused by ischemia or infarction. Over the past 10 to 15 years, several techniques have been described that allow one to determine during left ventriculography if an asynergic segment of the left ventricle is ischemic or infarcted. With each of these techniques, segments whose abnormal wall motion is due to *ischemia* show improvement in systolic motion, whereas segments whose abnormal wall motion is due to *infarction* fail to improve.

First, left ventricular segmental wall motion can be improved substantially by the administration of catecholamines.[8] Two left ventriculograms are performed—the first in the resting (baseline) state, the second during a steady-state infusion of epinephrine (1 to 4 $\mu$/min). Segments that are ischemic and, as a result, hypokinetic or akinetic on baseline ventriculography improve their contractile pattern during epinephrine infusion; in contrast; segments that are asynergic due to infarction show no alteration in contractility when stimulated by epinephrine.

Second, left ventricular segmental wall motion can be influenced by nitroglycerin.[9] Here, also, two left ventriculograms are performed, one before and the other after sublingual administration of nitroglycerin, when there is evidence of a nitroglycerin-induced fall in systemic arterial pressure. Segments of the left ventricle in which contraction is abnormal on the baseline ventriculogram but which improve after nitroglycerin are reversibly injured (that is, ischemic), whereas those in which asynergy is present before nitroglycerin and is not altered by it are most likely irreversibly damaged (that is, infarcted). Segments in which motion improves with nitroglycerin generally maintain

this level of improvement after successful surgical revascularization; in contrast, segments in which contractile function is not influenced by nitroglycerin are not improved by revascularization.

Third, left ventricular segmental wall motion can be influenced by postextrasystolic potentiation.[10] A single ventricular premature beat is introduced during left ventriculography and is followed by a compensatory pause and then a potentiated beat. Segmental wall motion during one of the preceding sinus beats is compared to that of the postextrasystolic beat. Left ventricles with asynergic wall motion during a preceding sinus beat which improves on the potentiated beat are ischemic, whereas those in which asynergy is similar on the preceding sinus beat and on the postextrasystolic beat are infarcted. Augmentation ventriculography by this technique offers the advantage that both baseline and potentiated left ventricular wall motion can be characterized on a single ventriculogram. Postextrasystolic potentiation may be provided by introducing a timed stimulus (delivered through a right ventricular pacing catheter) or by pullback of a right ventricular catheter during left ventriculography. It is probably unwise to attempt to induce the ventricular extrasystole by manipulating the left ventriculographic catheter during the injection of contrast material, since such manipulation may cause endocardial staining.

Other types of intervention ventriculography may be of use in the patient with chronic left ventricular volume overload due to aortic or mitral regurgitation. In the patient with aortic regurgitation and well-preserved left ventricular function, angiotensin in a dose sufficient to increase left ventricular systolic pressure by 20 to 50 mmHg causes no change in left ventricular ejection fraction.[11] In the patient whose aortic regurgitation has caused a loss of left ventricular contractile reserve, a similar amount of angiotensin causes a fall in left ventricular ejection fraction > 0.10. Thus, left ventriculography during "afterload stress" may provide additional information about left ventricular functional capability. Alternatively, intervention ventriculography using sodium nitroprusside may be used in patients with mitral regurgitation, aortic regurgitation, or congestive cardiomyopathy to assess the potential benefit of chronic vasodilator therapy.

## COMPLICATIONS AND HAZARDS

Although complications of cardiac catheterization and angiography are discussed in detail in Chapter 3, certain specific points relevant to ventriculography are presented here.

### Complications of Injection

*Arrhythmias.* Ventricular extrasystoles occur frequently during ventriculography and are usually caused by mechanical stimulation of the ventricular endocardium by the catheter or a jet of contrast agent. Such extrasystoles can usually be eliminated or at least minimized by repositioning the catheter. Although short runs of ventricular tachycardia occur during an occasional ventriculogram, they almost always cease promptly when the catheter is removed from the ventricle. Rarely, the ventricular tachycardia caused by ventriculography is sustained even after catheter removal. It should be treated quickly with a bolus of intravenous lidocaine and, if necessary, direct current countershock. Ventricular fibrillation has been reported to be induced by an improperly grounded power injector.[12]

*Intramyocardial Injection (So-called Endocardial Staining).* The deposition of contrast material within the endocardium and myocardium is usually caused by improper positioning of the ventriculographic catheter. Although a small endocardial stain usually causes no problem, a large stain may lead to medically refractory ventricular tachyarrhythmias, including ventricular tachycardia or fibrillation. Very rarely, the power injection of contrast material causes myocardial perforation, with the resultant leakage of blood and contrast material into the pericardial space and the development of cardiac tamponade. This must be treated by emergency pericardiocentesis, and immediate consultation obtained from a cardiothoracic surgeon.

*Embolism.* The inadvertent injection of air or thrombus probably poses the greatest risk associated with ventriculography. The presence of thrombi on the ventriculographic catheter is minimized by (1) frequent flushing of the catheter with a solution containing heparin and (2) systemic heparinization of the patient when the ventriculographic catheter is first introduced.[13] For all adult patients, we administer 5000 units of heparin intravenously when the first arterial catheter (brachial or femoral) is introduced into the aorta.

An occasional patient is referred for catheterization in whom there is suspicion (from noninvasive testing) of a thrombus in the left ventricular apex. If left ventriculography is required in such a patient, great care should be taken to position the ventriculographic catheter in the left ventricular inflow tract, avoiding the apical portion completely. Partially organized thrombi may be dislodged from the left ventricular cavity by the catheter tip or the force of a power injection. Accordingly, the ventricular angiographic catheter should not be advanced to the left ventricular apex except under exceptional circumstances (e.g., suspicion of IHSS).

### Complications of Contrast Material

For 20 to 30 seconds after ventriculography, the patient has a "hot flash," due to the powerful vasodilation caused by the contrast material. Transient nausea and vomiting used to occur in 20 to 30% of patients, but with current formulations of contrast agent this is uncommon. The immediate but short-lived hemodynamic effects of ventriculography include a modest fall in systemic arterial pressure, a reflex increase in heart rate, and a transient depression of left ventricular contractility. Within 1 to 2 minutes, these effects usually resolve.

## REFERENCES

1. Pattison JN: Angiocardiography. Radiography 35:131, 1969.
2. Forwand SA, Schatzki SC, Nordberg ED: Cardiac catheterization and angiocardiography. Cardiovasc Clin 3:81, 1971.
3. Herman MV, Gorlin R: Implication of left ventricular asynergy. Am J Cardiol 23:538, 1969.
4. Bruschke AVG, Proudfit WL, Sones FM Jr: Progress study of 590 consecutive nonsurgical cases of coronary disease followed 5–9 years.

II. Ventriculographic and other correlations. Circulation 47:1154, 1973.

5. Rackley CE, Hood WP Jr: Quantitative angiographic evaluation and pathophysiologic mechanisms in valvular heart disease. Prog Cardiovasc Dis 15:427, 1973.

6. Schad N, et al: The intermittent phased injection of contrast material into the heart. Am J Roentgenol 104:464, 1968.

7. Viamonte M Jr: Innovations in angiography. Radiol Clin North Am 9:361, 1971.

8. Horn HR, et al: Augmentation of left ventricular contraction pattern in coronary artery disease by an inotropic catecholamine. The epinephrine ventriculogram. Circulation 49:1063, 1974.

9. Helfant RH, et al: Nitroglycerin to unmask reversible asynergy. Correlation with post coronary bypass ventriculography. Circulation 50:108, 1974.

10. Dyke SH, Cohn PF, Gorlin R, Sonnenblick EH: Detection of residual myocardial function in coronary artery disease using postextrasystolic potentiation. Circulation 50:694, 1974.

11. Bolen JL, et al: Evaluation of left ventricular function in patients with aortic regurgitation using afterload stress. Circulation 53:132, 1976.

12. Rowe GG, Zarnstorff WC: Ventricular fibrillation during selective angiocardiography. JAMA 192:947, 1965.

13. Walker WJ, et al: Systemic heparinization for femoral percutaneous coronary arteriography. N Engl J Med 288:826, 1973.

*chapter fifteen*

# Pulmonary Angiography

JOSEPH R. BENOTTI *and* WILLIAM GROSSMAN

## INDICATIONS

Pulmonary angiography is most frequently required to confirm or exclude the diagnosis of pulmonary embolism.[1,2] Other cardiovascular conditions where pulmonary angiography is indicated for diagnosis in anticipation of corrective surgery include branch pulmonary artery stenosis (Fig. 15-1) and pulmonary arteriovenous malformation (Fig. 15-2).[2,3] The effect of occluding the arteriovenous malformation (by inflating the balloon on the tip of a flotation catheter) on the magnitude of right-to-left shunt can be determined. Pulmonary arteriovenous malformations have been closed successfully by embolizing the communication with thrombogenic material. This is particularly advantageous in a patient with multiple pulmonary arteriovenous malformations that, by the diffuse nature of the process, preclude successful surgical management with segmental pulmonary resection. Pulmonary angiography is also sometimes indicated in the evaluation of bullous lung disease where resection of one or more blebs is being considered. Selective pulmonary angiography may be important in the evaluation of patients with suspected primary pulmonary hypertension to exclude large unresolved pulmonary embolism,[4] particularly when there are segmental or lobar perfusion abnormalities detected by the lung scan.[5] Wedge or balloon occlusion pulmonary angiography has been utilized in evaluating the severity of hypertrophic changes in the small pulmonary arteries. This informa-

tion may be useful in assessing the morphology and reversibility of reactive pulmonary vascular changes in congenital heart disease, particularly when there is a long-standing left-to-right shunt that has become bidirectional as a result of reactive pulmonary hypertension. Levo-phase pulmonary angiography may be useful in confirming or excluding a left atrial myxoma when echocardiographic findings are equivocal.

Pulmonary angiography is also occasionally utilized to identify the insertion site(s) of anomalous pulmonary vein(s). However, because of high pulmonary blood flow from the left-to-right shunt, a very large volume of contrast medium must be injected rapidly to opacify an anomolous vein with sufficient resolution. Hand-powered contrast injection through the distal lumen of a balloon-tipped catheter with the balloon inflated may be a useful technique for such a study. The inflated balloon stops antegrade pulmonary flow into the lobar artery from which the anomalous vein originates. Filming as contrast medium is injected and again later as the balloon is deflated allows the contrast medium to enter and satisfactorily opacify the anomalous vein. This technique may facilitate identification of anomalous pulmonary veins with much greater resolution and with a much lower cumulative contrast load.

***Role of the Lung Scan.*** Pulmonary arteriography is certainly not indicated in every patient whenever pulmonary embolism is suspected; rather, its performance is predicated on logical interpretation of all rel-

213

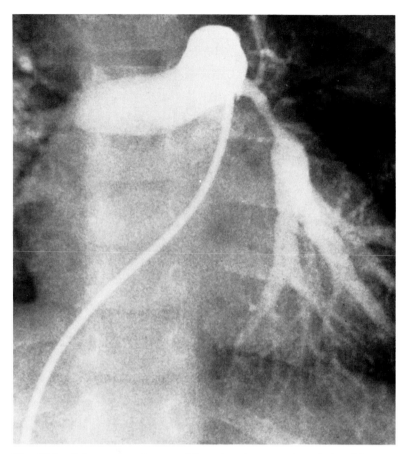

**Fig. 15-1.** Pulmonary angiogram of branch pulmonary stenosis in adolescent male. The catheter tip is positioned 1 to 2 cm beyond the origin of the right pulmonary artery so that with the powered injection of contrast agent the catheter tip recoils into the main pulmonary trunk to optimally opacify the left pulmonary artery and its ramifications.

evant clinical data including the ventilation-perfusion lung scan. Except in the patient with cardiogenic shock and cor pulmonale, where emergency pulmonary angiography is required for diagnostic confirmation prior to embolectomy, it is advisable to obtain a ventilation perfusion lung scan in all patients with suspected pulmonary embolism. A normal perfusion lung scan reliably excludes pulmonary embolism, sparing the patient the needless morbidity and expense of pulmonary angiography. Similarly, in a patient in shock a small unilateral regional perfusion abnormality on the lung scan would make it highly unlikely that massive pulmonary embolism could account for this hemodynamic derangement. Recognizing that pulmonary

embolism of such a small magnitude could not account for the clinical signs, the clinician should look for other causes of circulatory inadequacy (e.g., hemorrhage, sepsis, myocardial infarction).

Pulmonary angiography is most commonly indicated when there is a strong clinical suspicion of pulmonary embolism, but the ventilation-perfusion lung scan reveals one or more "matched" defects where perfusion and ventilation abnormalities coincide. Though the chest roentgenogram may be helpful in identifying localized pulmonary parenchymal findings (pneumonia, atelectasis, bullous disease) that satisfactorily account for the perfusion lung scan abnormalities in the absence of pulmonary embolism, angiography is usually required to confirm or exclude pulmonary embolism if, in the appropriate clinical setting, such findings cannot be explained otherwise. Even when the lung scan findings would not obviate the need for pulmonary angiography, it is often helpful to have obtained a lung scan prior to pulmonary angiography, since location of the perfusion defect(s) directs the angiographer in his choice of lung regions for selective study. A strategy for deciding when to perform pulmonary angiography based on the combined findings of lung scan and chest roentgenogram is presented in Table 15-1.

## CONTRAINDICATIONS

A relative contraindication to pulmonary arteriography is a history of allergic reaction to contrast material. However, with proper premedication with corticosteroids and antihistaminic agents (see Chapter 13) angiographic procedures can almost always be performed safely in such patients.

Pulmonary angiography is remarkably safe even in critically ill patients when performed by an experienced physician. Certainly, a carefully performed pulmonary angiogram that establishes the diagnosis and aids in selection of therapy carries less risk than treating a patient with anticoagulants empirically when there really is no pulmonary embolism or withholding anticoagulant therapy from a patient who has actually sustained pulmonary embolism.

## COMPLICATIONS

Pulmonary angiography may be associated with complications related to right heart catheterization (cardiac perforation, arrhythmia) or to administration of radiographic contrast agent (allergic reactions, intimal injection, hypotension, pulmonary edema). Iodinated angiographic contrast medium causes an immediate acute depression in myocardial contractility and associated peripheral vasodilation. Minutes to hours later it causes osmotic diuresis, thereby reducing afterload and preload. A clinical correlate in patients with normal underlying cardiovascular function is postural hypotension with warm, flushed, and well-perfused extremities

one to several hours following the angiographic procedure. Pulmonary edema may develop in patients with severe myocardial depression within a few minutes to one hour following angiography. This is usually a result of myocardial depression and acute volume expansion resulting from the osmotic load of contrast medium. To the extent that the pulmonary angiogram requires a rather large total contrast volume and is performed in patients with underlying heart disease, these problems can be anticipated and managed effectively.

Serious underlying cardiopulmonary disease increases the risk of pulmonary angiography, particularly when multiple contrast injections into the main and proximal pulmonary arteries subject the patient to a cumulative contrast dose exceeding 200 ml. Mainstream pulmonary angiography has been associated with acute myocardial depression and death in patients with primary pulmonary hypertension.[6,7] The risk is greatest when the pulmonary artery pressure approaches that in the systemic arterial circuit. Through preload augmentation and antecedent hypertrophy, the chronically pressure overloaded right ventricle may already be functioning at the limit of its preload reserve. The abrupt increase in right ventricular afterload and depression in contractility engendered by rapid contrast injection exceeding 25 to 30 ml into a major pulmonary artery acutely exceeds the limits of right ventricular compensation, sometimes with a fatal outcome. In reviewing 15 series involving over 400 pulmonary arteriograms, Goodman found a mortality rate of 0.2%, a cardiac perforation rate of 0.4% and a risk of cardiac arrhythmia of 0.7%.[8]

## HEMODYNAMIC EVALUATION AS PART OF PULMONARY ANGIOGRAPHY

Though the most common reason for requesting pulmonary angiography is to confirm or exclude the presence of pulmonary embolism with the highest degree of certainty, a carefully performed angiographic study that includes complete hemodynamic evaluation provides much additional information of clinical value. Hemodynamic as-

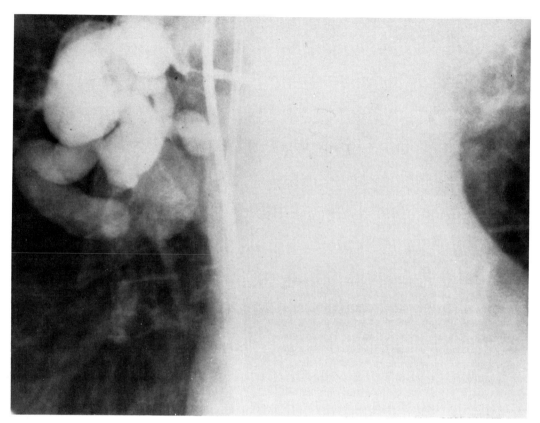

**Fig. 15-2.** Pulmonary angiogram of pulmonary arteriovenous malformation involving the right upper lobe pulmonary artery and vein in 48-year-old woman. Contrast agent is injected by hand through a balloon-tipped pulmonary artery catheter with the tip positioned at the origin of the right upper lobe vessel. The balloon is inflated so that the fistula is occluded, and it is adequately opacified with less than 10 ml of contrast agent.

**TABLE 15-1.** *Clinically Suspicious Pulmonary Embolism: Role of Pulmonary Angiography*

|  | Lung Scan | Chest Roentgenogram | Fraction of Patients with Documented Embolism |
|---|---|---|---|
| Angiography not ordinarily required | Normal |  | 1/8[*] |
|  | Low probability | No signs of embolism[†] | 0/18 |
|  | High probability | 2 or more signs | 17/17 |
| Angiography may be required | High probability | No signs of embolism | 4/8 |
|  | High probability | Only one sign | 16/21 |
|  | Low probability | At least one sign | 7/32 |
| Angiography normally required | Any abnormality | Cardiomegaly or left heart failure | 7/15 |

[*]Single small embolus in affected patient.

[†]Signs include infiltrate, effusion, atelectasis, elevated hemidiaphragm, and segmental oligemia (Westermark's sign).

(Adapted from Moses DC, et al: The complementary roles of chest radiography, lung scanning, and selective pulmonary angiography in the diagnosis of pulmonary embolism. Circulation 49:179, 1974.)

sessment preceding an angiographic evaluation that demonstrates pulmonary embolism allows rational selection of appropriate supportive, therapeutic, and prophylactic measures. For example, the patient with a depressed cardiac output and end-organ hypoperfusion in conjunction with massive pulmonary embolism and right ventricular failure requires supportive measures dictated by the hemodynamic findings. These might include colloid infusion to elevate right ventricular filling pressure and inotropic drugs to improve the force of right ventricular contraction, thereby overcoming the acute increase in right ventricular afterload imposed by the obstructing emboli. If prompt correction of the circulatory inadequacy cannot be achieved, definitive therapeutic measures to remove the obstructing emboli (e.g., surgical pulmonary embolectomy, catheter removal of pulmonary embolism, or administration of a thrombolytic agent) must be undertaken. Management of the patient with pulmonary embolism is predicated upon careful hemodynamic assessment, which can be accomplished at the time of pulmonary angiography. Conversely, hemodynamic assessment in conjunction with an angiogram that is negative or nondiagnostic for pulmonary embolism may enable the cardiologist to diagnose *other cardiopulmonary conditions* that may be responsible for the patient's clinical presentation and then to proceed with specific therapy. Careful hemodynamic evaluation may point to left ventricular failure, cardiac tamponade, occult constrictive pericardial disease, or cor pulmonale as a result of chronic obstructive lung disease as the underlying problem. In a patient with suspected pulmonary embolism referred for pulmonary angiography, one of us (JB) has observed cardiac tamponade resulting from right atrial perforation by the fine wire stylet of a central venous pressure catheter, hardly visible by image intensification fluoroscopy. This diagnosis was suggested initially by a continuously monitored femoral artery pressure demonstrating pulsus paradox of a magnitude insufficient to be detected by a sphygmomanometric pressure measurement, and by a right atrial pressure elevation not evident by visual inspection of the jugular meniscus because of the patient's obesity.

Hemodynamic evaluation prior to angiography also provides important information that facilitates technical performance of an optimal study at minimal risk to the patient. Pulmonary blood flow, either measured by the Fick or thermodilution technique or estimated from measurements of pulmonary artery and systemic arterial oxygen saturation will influence, in part, selection of the injection parameters (contrast volume and flow rate) required for adequate vascular opacification. The pulmonary artery wedge pressure, if elevated, restricts the total allowable contrast volume and directs the operator to treat the patient with diuretics or vasodilators. These interventions may permit administration of a sufficient total volume of contrast for performance of an adequate study. If *paradoxic embolism* is suspected, it is appropriate to perform indicator-dilution studies with injection of indocyanine green dye into the inferior vena cava to verify the potential for right-to-left shunting.

## VASCULAR ACCESS

Pulmonary angiography has been performed traditionally using a catheter advanced via a brachial vein by exposed cutdown in the antecubital fossa. This approach facilitates catheter manipulation between right and left pulmonary arteries, so that more selective views can be obtained in either lung. The percutaneous subclavian, internal jugular, and femoral venous approaches carry the potentially serious risk of delayed bleeding with anticoagulant and particularly with thrombolytic therapy. Also, there is always concern over the potential for dislodging loosely adherent iliofemoral or vena caval thrombi when a catheter is advanced from the femoral vein. If the thrombus has become organized in the iliofemoral venous system, it may not be possible to advance the catheter through this region. It is also usually more difficult to manipulate a catheter from the left to the right pulmonary artery or vice versa, when it has been introduced from the femoral vein. For these reasons we favor the brachial venous approach.

## TECHNIQUES

The standard technique of pulmonary angiography involves the powered injection of radiographic contrast medium at a high flow rate (10 to 30 ml/sec) and at high pressure through a suitable 5 to 8 French angiographic catheter positioned in a first or second order pulmonary artery.[6,9] The 7F or 8F Eppendorf catheter,[*] a woven Dacron catheter, which has four side holes and lacks an end hole, is an excellent catheter for pulmonary angiography. The end-hole occluded design minimizes catheter tip recoil that usually accompanies forceful contrast injection. A disadvantage of this catheter is that a soft-tipped guide wire cannot be extruded from the tip of the catheter for guiding purposes to facilitate safe catheter passage. End-hole catheters allow use of a guide wire to facilitate safe catheter passage through difficult-to-traverse right heart chambers. However, end-hole catheters have a much greater propensity to recoil proximally during angiography. The Grollman catheter[†] (a pigtail catheter with an acute angle on the terminal shaft, near the tip) has a natural shape that facilitates right heart catheterization and an end hole so that it can be advanced over a guide wire. It does not recoil because of its pigtail configuration and because contrast medium exits from side holes positioned opposite to one another. The result is that the forces responsible for catheter tip recoil cancel one another out. However, because of its preformed permanent shape and looped tip, the Grollman catheter usually cannot be advanced beyond the main right or left pulmonary artery into lobar vessels and is not ideal for more selective injections. The Berman angiographic catheter[‡] is a balloon-flotation catheter with multiple side holes designed especially for pulmonary angiography and is the preferred catheter for this procedure in some laboratories.

In patients with left bundle branch block one should have a pacing catheter prepared and ready to be advanced to the right ventricle in case right bundle branch block and asystole develop during placement of the angiographic catheter in the pulmonary artery.

For mainstream pulmonary angiography, the catheter is usually positioned in the right pulmonary artery with its tip 1 to 2 cm proximal to the takeoff of the upper lobe pulmonary artery branch and 1 to 2 cm distal to the origin of the right pulmonary artery. A wide or open loop is placed in the proximal catheter segment as it traverses the right ventricle to support the catheter in order to minimize recoil. Mainstream angiography usually requires 40 to 50 ml radiographic contrast medium injected at a rate of 20 to 30 ml/sec. Selective studies of lobar vessels usually require a total volume of 20 to 40 ml injected at a rate of 15 to 20 ml/sec. Subselective injections may be done at lower volumes and injection rates. Technical factors influencing selection of injection parameters (total contrast dose and injection rate) include the quality of the imaging equipment, the size of the vascular region of interest, pulmonary blood flow, the French size of the angiographic catheter, and the strong suspicion of major proximal emboli as evidenced by the perfusion scan or by a previous test injection. Low pulmonary blood flow or major proximal emboli reduce the total contrast volume required for an adequate study, and smaller catheter sizes limit the maximal injection rate. Selective views require a slower delivery rate and lower contrast dose relative to mainstream studies.

## RADIOGRAPHIC FILMING

Filming is accomplished during a maximal inspiration either by the large film or the cineangiographic technique. Each method has advantages and disadvantages, and the laboratory performing pulmonary angiography should be equipped to use both methods.

***Large Film Method.*** Prior to large film study, one or more scout films of the chest are obtained to select the kilovoltage that optimizes a gray-scale contrast between bone, vasculature, other soft-tissue structures and the pulmonary parenchyma. Large film, either roll or cutfilm, is exposed serially by a programmed automatic film changer, activated at the start of the powered contrast injection. Usually, peak opacification of the pulmonary arterial phase occurs 2 to 4 sec after injection, and when large film is used an exposure rate of 2 to 4 films/sec is utilized for this phase. The pulmonary venous-left heart phase occurs 5 to 7 sec after starting the injection and should be filmed at 1 to 2 films/sec. The systemic arterial phase peaks

*USCI, Billerica, MA.
†Cook, Inc., Bloomington, IN.
‡Elecath, Rahway, NJ.

7 to 10 sec after injection and may be recorded at 1 film/sec, so that for a complete run 14 to 20 films are obtained over 10 sec. If the cardiac output is reduced and the circulation time is prolonged, filming should continue for a total of 12 to 14 sec. Filming beyond the first 6 to 8 sec is usually performed at a frequency of 1 sec to minimize radiation and conserve film. As exemplified in Figure 15-3, the advantages of large film include quality of resolution, the clarity of vascular detail, and versatility in field size (from the entire thorax to a single lobe depending upon how the tube is positioned and how the field is coned). Large film views enable the angiographer to study the entire thorax, a whole lung, or a single lobe with the excellent demonstration of the detailed anatomy of each and every vascular branch. Filming during the levophase of a mainstream injection gives reasonably detailed anatomic information about left heart structures and the thoracic aorta.

The mainstream pulmonary angiogram recorded on large film provides information from which *the percentage of pulmonary vascular obstruction* resulting from pulmonary embolism can be estimated. In patients with no underlying cardiopulmonary disease this correlates directly with the severity of pulmonary hypertension and hypoxemia.[10]

An unequivocal angiographic diagnosis of pulmonary embolism requires demonstration of intralumenal filling defects and abrupt total or near-total cutoff of vessels resulting from embolic obstruction, as illustrated in Figure 15-3. Such findings are specific for pulmonary embolism. A disadvantage of the large film method is that vessels overlapping or crossing one another, viewed as consecutive static images, may mimic pulmonary embolism. Also it is tedious and time consuming to repetitively reposition the patient between the fluoroscopic image intensifier and the large filmchanger for catheter repositioning prior to selective studies. Indeed, if the patient is very ill, repositioning may not be possible and may limit the adequacy of the study. Even though the catheter is carefully positioned under fluoroscopic guidance, there is always concern that it may migrate during the interval required to position the patient between the x-ray generator and large film changer. Proximal catheter dislodgement usually results in a subselective and less than adequate study.

Migration of the catheter tip more distally may result in an injection at excessive pressure and flow that may damage or even disrupt a smaller pulmonary artery branch.

***Cineangiographic Method.*** Pulmonary cineangiography, though not useful for mainstream studies because of the smaller field size, may confer advantages over the large film method for visualizing lobar arteries under certain circumstances.[11] In an acutely ill patient, the catheter can be positioned rapidly for selective study of the right and left pulmonary arteries. Figure 15-4 illustrates a frame from a right main pulmonary cineangiogram and depicts the technical advantages and limitations of this technique. The quality of current cineangiographic and videotape equipment is sufficiently good that large proximal emboli are usually evident immediately to the angiographer during the actual performance of the angiogram or on immediate replay of the study recorded on videotape. This advantage may shorten the procedure considerably and allow more rapid therapeutic intervention. Thrombi in second or third order vessels are sometimes diagnosed more readily as the interface between thrombus and flowing blood moves to and fro in the pulsatile stream. Indeed, what often appears on the static large film study as an oligemic area, suggestive but not diagnostic of pulmonary embolism, may be easily appreciated on the cineangiogram to represent a subtotally occluded vessel as some contrast agent flows slowly around the occluding thrombus.

Recently, a relatively new and complimentary technique using a soft flexible balloon-tipped double-lumen catheter has been developed for pulmonary angiography.[12-15] In this method either a standard 7 French Swan-Ganz double-lumen catheter with a balloon capacity of 1.8 ml or a specially designed catheter with a balloon capacity of 3 ml (Edwards Laboratories, Santa Ana, CA) may be used. Both balloons may be filled with room air, although carbon dioxide is a safer inflation medium.

The catheter is positioned proximally in the lobar vessel perfusing the area suspected of harboring pulmonary embolism, as identified by regional perfusion defects on the lung scan. The balloon is then slowly inflated with air to its maximum volume according to the manufacturer's specifications, or until it occludes the lobar vessel in its most proximal

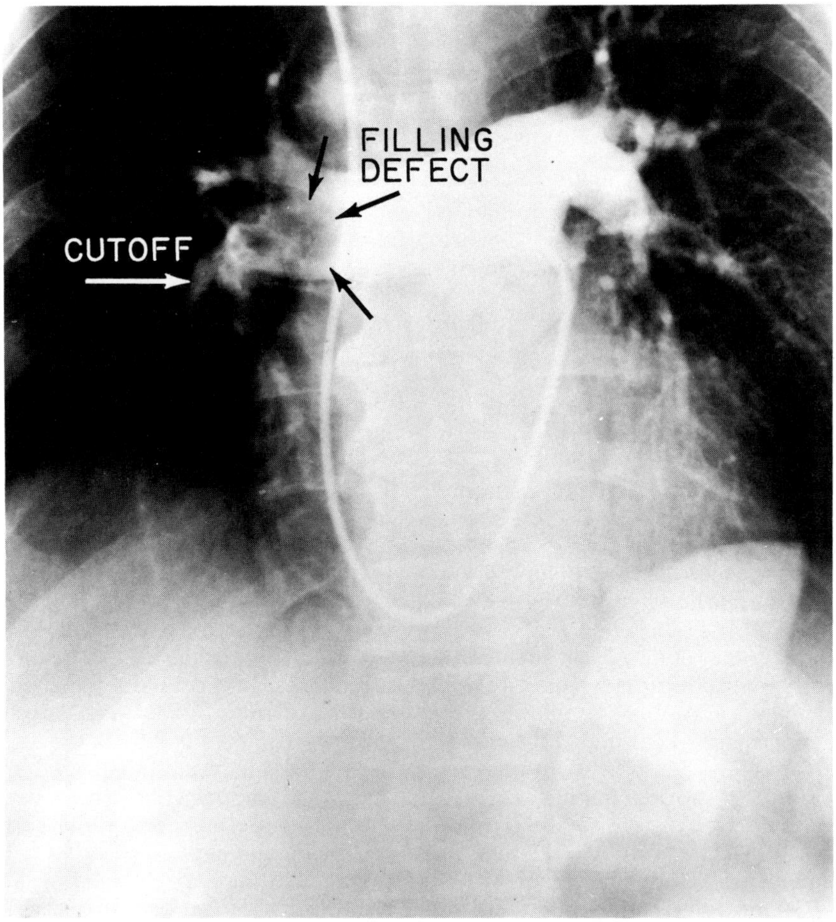

**Fig. 15-3.** Mainstream pulmonary angiogram of bilateral pulmonary embolism (PE) in 48-year-old man. The tip of an Eppendorf catheter is positioned in the proximal right pulmonary artery 1 to 2 cm beyond its takeoff from the main pulmonary trunk. There are intralumenal filling defects and vessel cutoffs involving the right and left pulmonary arteries and their branches. Regional oligemia and asymmetry of flow are also evident; these are nonspecific findings but not diagnostic of PE. (From Benotti JR, Ockene IS, Alpert JL, Dalen JE: The clinical profile of unresolved pulmonary problems. Chest 84:670, 1984.)

segment. Under fluoroscopic guidance 5 to 10 ml of contrast agent is then delivered by a hand-powered injection into the distal lumen of the catheter, so that the pulmonary arterial segment downstream from the inflated balloon is opacified. Because the inflow of blood into the lobe has been temporarily arrested by the inflated balloon, this small volume of contrast delivered by hand injection opacifies the regional pulmonary vasculature completely and permits identification of pulmonary emboli in third to fifth order vessels with great specificity. Filming may be either the cineangiographic or large film methods, but cine is usually quite adequate.

Figures 15-5 through 15-8 illustrate the technique, results, and advantages of balloon-occlusion pulmonary angiography in selected patients. A major advantage of the cineangiogram method is that it can be performed very rapidly. The balloon occlusion guarantees prompt identification of pulmonary emboli as intralumenal filling defects that readily stand out as contrast agent slowly flows around them to fill out the regional pulmonary vasculature; usually the

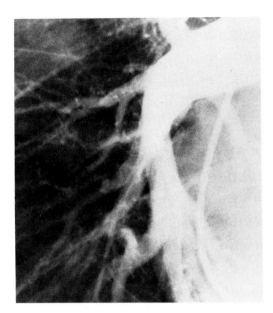

**Fig. 15-4.** Frame from a right main pulmonary cineangiogram where contrast agent was power injected through an Eppendorf catheter with its tip positioned in the midportion of the right main pulmonary artery. This technique allows prompt, unequivocal identification of emboli to the right or left pulmonary arteries and to the most proximal segments of the lobar branches. However, the obvious disadvantage is a small field precluding adequate study of the entire pulmonary vasculature. (From Benotti JR, Ockene IS, Alpert JS, Dalen JE: Balloon occlusion pulmonary cineangiography to diagnosing pulmonary embolism. Cathet Cardiovasc Diagn 10:524, 1984.)

diagnosis is readily evident even on the test injection performed under fluoroscopy and filming is required only to generate a permanent record, rather than for critical diagnostic scrutiny. Small emboli to fifth order vessels and beyond, which may be detected only as nonspecific multiple regions of oligemia on large film study, are particularly obvious on balloon-occlusion cineangiography. As depicted in Figure 15-6, when the balloon is deflated, unopacified blood enters the regional vessels and streams around the blood-thrombus interface. Radiographic contrast agent then selectively hangs up around the emboli and highlights their perimeter as it is washed out of the lobe. Balloon occlusion pulmonary angiography permits excellent regional opacification of more distal pulmonary arteries with a very small injection of contrast agent (5 to 10 ml) delivered by a hand-powered injection. This also minimizes

the motion artifact that may result from the uncontrollable coughing often induced by standard angiographic technique that requires rapid injection of a large volume of contrast agent. With the aid of a guide wire the balloon-tipped catheter can usually be manipulated selectively into every lobar vessel implicated by the perfusion lung scan. All five pulmonary lobes can usually be studied selectively using a cumulative contrast dose rarely exceeding 75 ml. As illustrated in Figure 15-7, this may be particularly advantageous in patients with congestive heart failure or pulmonary hypertension, where administration of large cumulative contrast volume will aggravate heart failure. The occlusion technique prevents catheter recoil and retrograde reflux of contrast agent back out of the vessel of interest. This prevents simultaneous opacification of multiple vessels and minimizes artifacts due to vessel overlap and crossing changes. Thus, in addition to speed, advantages of balloon-occlusion pulmonary cineangiography include its resolving power and the minimal contrast requirement for identifying pulmonary embolism in lobar vessels and beyond. This latter point is particularly important if the perfusion abnormalities on the lung scan are less than segmental in distribution. If perfusion defects are lobar or involve an entire lung, this finding suggests large proximal pulmonary embolism to the right or left pulmonary arteries, as illustrated in Figure 15-3. In this case it is advisable to confirm or exclude their presence by the injection of a large contrast volume at high pressure into the proximal vessel(s) in question through a standard angiographic catheter (e.g., Eppendorf catheter). If this study is negative, consideration should then be given to proceeding with balloon-occlusion pulmonary cineangiography of the lobar vessels.

Although we have not had any complications using the balloon-occlusion technique just described, a word of caution is in order. Previous investigators have reported on pulmonary angiography using temporary unilateral pulmonary artery occlusion.[15a–15d] Some authors have reported that prolonged exposure of the pulmonary vasculature to radiographic contrast may be harmful.[15b,15d] In addition, high injection pressures (injection pressures exceeding pulmonary capillary wedge pressure by $\geq$ 20 mmHg) may cause extravasation of contrast into the pulmonary

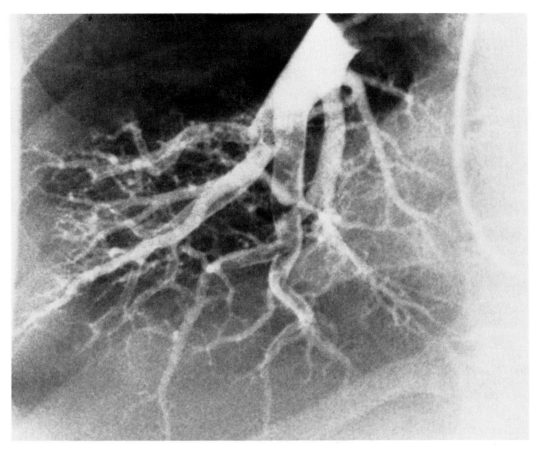

**Fig. 15-5.** Frame from a right lower lobe balloon-occlusion pulmonary cineangiogram in a 38-year-old woman who developed chest pain and dyspnea 1 week after an abdominal operation. The tip of the pulmonary artery catheter was positioned in the most proximal segment of the right lower lobe artery, the balloon was inflated with air to a volume of 1.5 ml (which occluded flow in this vessel), and the study was performed with a hand injection of 7 ml radiographic contrast medium. Intralumenal filling defects diagnostic of pulmonary embolism occupy almost the entire visualized segment of the artery to the right lower lobe. (From Benotti JR, Ockene IS, Alpert JS, Dalen JE: Balloon occlusion pulmonary cineangiography to diagnosing pulmonary embolsim. Cathet Cardiovasc Daign 10:525, 1984.)

parenchyma with a resultant pulmonary infiltrate.[15b] Accordingly, to reduce risks of pulmonary vascular damage, balloon-occlusion pulmonary angiography should be performed with small amounts of radiographic contrast injected under low pressures, with a minimal time of intravascular stasis.

## ANGIOGRAPHIC DIAGNOSIS OF PULMONARY EMBOLISM

A normal pulmonary arteriogram is relatively easy to recognize. Contrast flows sym-metrically from its site of proximal entry to uniformly fill second, third, and fourth order vessels that become progressively smaller in caliber. Similarly, as unopacified blood washes contrast from the pulmonary arterial to the pulmonary venous circulation, vascular definition is lost in a symmetrical fashion.

As discussed earlier in this chapter, the angiographic features specific for pulmonary embolism include *intralumenal filling defects* and *abrupt vessel cutoffs* (Fig. 15-8). Intralumenal filling defects result from flow of contrast around pulmonary emboli. Vessel cutoffs result from lobar or segmental vessels that have been totally occluded by em-

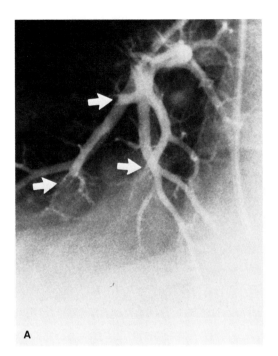
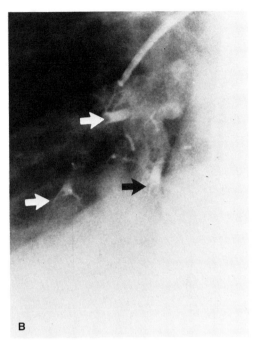

**Fig. 15-6.** Frame from a right lower lobe balloon-occlusion pulmonary cineangiogram filmed during contrast injection (A) and during contrast washout following balloon deflation (B). The tip of the catheter is positioned in the most proximal segment of the right lower lobe artery and the balloon is inflated to occlude arterial inflow. Occluded fifth order vessels show sudden interruption of the contrast filled vessel (vessel cutoff) during the injection phase (white arrows). These stand out clearly as intralumenal filling defects (pulmonary emboli) during the washout phase (black arrow) as contrast flows around the perimeter of the embolus.

bolic material. The pulmonary vascular anatomy is somewhat variable from patient to patient, and the angiographer frequently cannot be certain of the "normal" location and course of the smaller pulmonary arterial branches in an individual patient. Therefore, it may be very difficult to identify cutoff of vessels when third order (segmental) or smaller vessels are flush-occluded at their point of origin. In this circumstance, as demonstrated in Figure 15-8, when contrast flows slowly about the perimeter of a nearly totally occlusive embolus in a lobar or segmental artery giving rise to the so-called "railroad track" sign, the diagnosis of pulmonary embolism is unequivocal. When intralumenal filling defects, vessel cutoff, or "railroad tracking" are present, the diagnosis of pulmonary embolism can be made with a high degree of confidence.

Nonspecific angiographic findings in pulmonary embolism include localized asymmetry of flow and regional oligemia, defined as impaired local pulmonary artery flow. These findings are nonspecific because they can be due to conditions other than pulmonary embolism including pneumonia, asthma, bullous lung disease, atelectasis, or emphysema. However, when there is regional oligemia or asymmetry of flow without any corresponding abnormality on the chest roentgenogram or ventilation lung scan, it is advisable to regard the patient as having probable pulmonary embolism, in order that he or she receives the potential benefit of anticoagulant therapy.

## HEMODYNAMIC FINDINGS ASSOCIATED WITH PULMONARY EMBOLISM

The hemodynamic impact of pulmonary embolism is determined by the extent of pul-

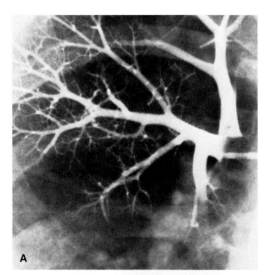

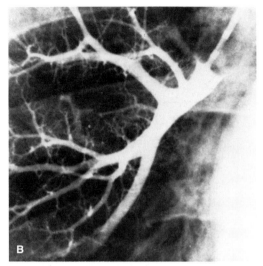

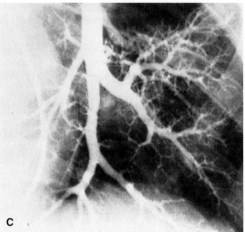

**Fig. 15-7.** Frames from balloon occlusion cineangiograms of the right upper lobe (A), right lower lobe (B), and left lower lobe (C) in a 52-year-old man with congestive heart failure where pulmonary embolism was considered as a cause for the patient's acute deterioration and a perfusion lung scan revealed multiple subsegmental defects. There is attenuation of vascularity compatible with lung disease, but no pulmonary emboli are identified. In each study the catheter tip is positioned in the most proximal segment of the artery in question and the balloon is inflated to occlude inflow of unopacified blood. Such a study, performed with less than 10 ml of contrast agent to opacify the vasculature of each lobe carries little increase in risk compared to bedside right heart catheterization, a procedure now frequently performed for hemodynamic monitoring in critically ill patients.

monary vascular cross-sectional compromise by embolic material and the patient's underlying cardiopulmonary status.[10,16,17] Acute pulmonary arterial obstruction augments the afterload opposing right ventricular ejection. This increases the wall tension the right ventricle must generate to eject its stroke volume. In the patient free of underlying cardiopulmonary disease, pulmonary artery hypertension (mean pressure >25 mmHg) develops as the magnitude of embolic obstruction exceeds 30 to 50% of the pulmonary arterial bed. As pulmonary arterial obstruction approaches 75%, mean pulmonary artery pressure approaches 35 to 45 mmHg. At this point, the previously un-

stressed right ventricle can no longer generate sufficient systolic tension to eject its stroke volume against such an extreme elevation in impedance. The consequence is a reduction in stroke volume and cardiac output, an increase in end systolic and end diastolic volumes, acute right ventricular dilation, and an increase in right atrial pressure.[16,17] The reduction in cardiac output usually evokes reflex sympathetic nervous system activation with a resultant increase in systemic vascular resistance and heart rate, and these adjustments tend to preserve blood pressure and cardiac output. The reflex increase in venous tone reduces vascular capacitance and translocates blood

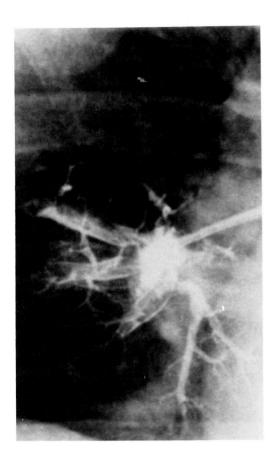

**Fig. 15-8.** Frame from a balloon-occlusion cineangiogram of the right lower lobe in a 72-year-old man with pulmonary embolism. The tip of the catheter is positioned very proximally in the artery to the right lower lobe and the balloon is inflated to prevent contrast dilution and washout by inflow of unopacified blood during the injection of contrast agent. This study, performed with 8 ml of radiographic contrast agent injected through the distal lumen of the balloon-tipped catheter, demonstrates a "railroad track" sign, as contrast streams about partially occlusive thrombi. Intralumenal filling defects and abrupt vessel cutoffs, diagnostic of pulmonary embolism, are also evident.

from the peripheral systemic venous reservoir to the central circulation, resulting in an elevation in right atrial pressure. Thus, in the patient with no underlying cardiopulmonary disease, pulmonary hypertension requires at least 30 to 50% obstruction of the pulmonary circulation, whereas acute cor pulmonale and right ventricular failure usually occur when at least 75% of the pulmonary arterial tree has been obstructed by embolism. If pulmonary vascular compliance has been reduced and pulmonary vascular resistance increased by preexisting heart or lung disease, the increase in pulmonary artery pressure in response to pulmonary embolism will be greater. However, a chronically pressure-overloaded right ventricle, having undergone hypertrophy, can often tolerate acute pulmonary hypertension of a more severe degree as a result of embolic pulmonary artery obstruction before the ventricle fails and the right atrial pressure rises. Specific hemodynamic and clinical profiles in pulmonary embolism are discussed in Chapter 25.

# REFERENCES

1. Robbins E: Overdiagnosis and overtreatment of pulmonary embolism: the emperor may have no clothes. Ann Int Med 87:775, 1977.
2. Menzioan JO, Williams JF: Is pulmonary angiography essential for the diagnosis of acute pulmonary embolism? Am Surg 137:543, 1979.
3. Dines DE, Arms RA, Bernatz PE, Gomes MR: Pulmonary arteriovenous fistulas. Mayo Clin Proc 49:460, 1974.
4. Benotti JR, Ockene IS, Alpert JS, Dalen JE: The clinical profile of unresolved pulmonary embolism. Chest 84:661, 1983.

5. Fishman AJ, Moser KM, Fedullo PF: Perfusion lung scans vs. pulmonary angiography in evaluation of suspected primary pulmonary hypertension. Chest 54:671, 1983.

6. Dalen JE, et al: Pulmonary angiography in acute pulmonary embolism: Indications, techniques and results in 367 patients. Am Heart 81:175, 1971.

7. Marsh JD, Glynn M, Torman HA: Pulmonary angiography. Application in a new spectrum of patients. Am J Med 75:763, 1983.

8. Goodman PG: Pulmonary angiography. *In* Symposium of Pulmonary Embolism and Hypertension: Clinics in Chest Medicine. Hyers TM (ed): Philadelphia, W.B. Saunders Co., 1984, pp. 465–477.

9. Bookstein JJ: Segmental arteriography in pulmonary embolism. Radiology 93:1007, 1969.

10. McIntyre KM, Sasahara AA: The hemodynamic response to pulmonary embolism in patients without prior cardiopulmonary disease. Am J Cardiol 78:288, 1971.

11. Meister SG, et al: Pulmonary cineangiography in acute pulmonary embolism. Am Heart J 84:33, 1972.

12. Bynum LJ, et al: Radiographic techniques for balloon-occlusion pulmonary angiography. Radiology 133:518, 1979.

13. LePage JR, Garcia RM: The value of bedside wedge pulmonary angiography in the detection of pulmonary emboli: A predictive and prospective evaluation. Radiology 144:67, 1982.

14. Ferris EJ, et al: Angiography of pulmonary emboli: digital studies and balloon-occlusion cineangiography. Am J Radiol 142:369, 1984.

15. Benotti JR, Ockene IS, Alpert JS, Dalen JS: Balloon occlusion pulmonary cineangiography to diagnosing pulmonary embolism. Cathet Cardiovass Diagn 10:519, 1984.

15a. Nordenstrom B: Temporary unilateral occlusion of the pulmonary artery. Acta Radiol, Suppl 108:1–141, 1954.

15b. Becu L, Paulin S, Varnauskas E: Pulmonary wedge angiography. Acta Radiol 57:209, 1962.

15c. Bell ALV, et al: Wedge pulmonary arteriography. Applications in congenital and acquired heart disease. Radiology 73:566, 1959.

15d. Dotter CT, Rosch J: Pulmonary arteriography: Technique. *In* Abrams Angiography, 3rd ed. Abrams HL (ed): Boston, Little Brown, 1983, pp. 707–708.

16. Dalen JS, et al: Resolution rate of acute pulmonary embolsim in man. N Engl J Med 280:1184, 1961.

17. McIntyre KM, Sasahara AA: Pulmonary angiography, scanning and hemodynamics in pulmonary embolism: Critical review and correlations. Crit Rev Radiol Sci 3:489, 1972.

## chapter sixteen

# Aortography

SVEN PAULIN

A ORTOGRAPHY, the radiographic demonstration of the contrast filled central large vessel from which all organ systems of the human body derive their arterial blood supply, has a long history. In 1929, the very year when W. Forssmann[1] reported that he had passed a catheter from an arm vein into his own right atrium, dos Santos and his colleagues[2] reported the successful performance of abdominal aortography following direct puncture of this vessel with a needle. The more daring approach to inject the ascending aorta in similar fashion resulting in angiographic visualization of the thoracic aorta was described by Nuvoli in 1936.[3] Since that time contrast angiography of the aorta has undergone many modifications aiming at greater patient safety, higher image quality, and optimal diagnostic yield. Angiographic study of the aorta may be performed in order to quantitate the degree of aortic valve incompetence, to delineate the topography of abnormal vascular pathways related to congenital malformations, or to search for congenital or acquired vascular lesions that might be the cause of systemic hypertension. These procedures may be performed for reasons of different urgency, reaching from the emergency condition of a traumatic aortic perforation, dissection, or rupture to the screening examination of an asymptomatic patient with an unexplained bruit. It should not be surprising, therefore, that a great variety of different technical and procedural approaches to aortography are available.

## TECHNICAL ASPECTS

The relatively large size of the aorta—the thoracic portion alone under normal conditions has a volume of several hundred milliliters—poses special demands on the technical performance of its successful angiographic demonstration. These requirements differ drastically from those applicable to selective arteriography of different organ systems. The angiography-performing cardiologist needs only be reminded about the disappointing results of contrast medium injections made during selective coronary arteriography when the catheter is not engaged selectively. Under such conditions a relatively small volume is delivered by manual injection at slow rate in a single jet through the catheter's end hole in a large vascular compartment, illustrating diametrically the opposite of what is needed; namely, a rapid delivery of a concentrated bolus of contrast medium properly mixed in the local blood pool. In addition, the phasically occurring rapid movement of the blood column, most marked in the ascending portion of the aorta and related to the vigorous ejection of the left ventricular stroke volume, requires proper timing and duration of the radiographic exposures and their sequence. Unrelated to the mode by which the central aorta has been filled with contrast medium, an unavoidable consequence is that all arterial compartments of the systemic circulation will be exposed to a temporary flow of contrast agent in proportion to their share of blood supply. This fact opens on one hand the possibility to extend the angiographic examination to include additional views by using special equipment, such as automatic stepwise table transport, so useful, for example, to follow the "runoff" of contrast medium completely through both lower extremities. On the other hand, the same fact reminds us that the contrast medium reaches all organ systems to be taken into consideration with regard to side effects and potential complications.

## Patient Preparation

Although the rapid injection of contrast medium in the amount necessary for an aortogram will be recognized by the patient in the form of a profound "heat wave" through the entire body, the intensity of this phenomenon when using modern tri-iodinated water-soluble compounds is not excessive. It is prudent practice for the operator to explain fully to the patient the purpose of the procedure, describe the side effects to be expected, and disclose the potential hazards. The latter may differ from one examination to the other and relate to a number of factors such as the technique chosen for the examination, the risk factor profile of the patient population under study, and the individual patient's condition at the time of the examination. The operator also must ask the patient if there is any previous history of adverse reaction to radiographic contrast media or of allergy to iodine-containing foods, which otherwise would call for special precautions such as premedication with steroids and/or cimetidine. Since aortography, particularly when including the proximal ascending aorta, may result in the contrast medium contacting the heart and the coronary circulation, precautions similar to those for coronary angiography are recommended (see Chapter 13). These should include EKG monitoring, review of cardiotropic medication, and pacemaker and

defibrillator standby. Finally, the establishment of a good patient-operator relationship cannot be overemphasized.

## Injection Techniques

Although injection of contrast medium in sufficient amount into the circulation at any site proximal to the aortic valve would eventually outline the aortic lumen, the general principle prevails that increased selectivity of delivery of contrast medium increases the quality of angiographic information. This influences strongly the choice of technique.

### *Catheter Aortography*

Retrograde advancement of the arterial catheter to the central portion of the arterial circulation can be accomplished from different sites using puncture and/or surgical exposure of an artery.

***Percutaneous Puncture of Femoral Artery.*** By far the most popular is the percutaneous puncture of a femoral artery by Seldinger's technique for catheter replacement of a needle using a flexible guide wire.[4] This procedure is described in detail in Chapter 5. Since the length of the catheter determines to a high degree the resistance to injection, thoracic aortography requires a larger catheter ($\geq$7 French) than abdominal aortography (5 or 6 French). Guide wire and catheter manipulations, as well as advancement, are performed under fluoroscopic control. J-shaped ends of the guide wires and similar catheter end configurations or deflector instruments are helpful to avoid aberrations into small side branches, to negotiate arterial tortuosity and wall irregularities, and to prevent perforations or entrances into false channels, e.g., dissections. So-called pigtail ends with a diameter approaching the expected caliber of the vessel will stabilize the catheter position during the phase of rapid injection, decrease catheter whipping, and accomplish good mixing of radiographic contrast medium with blood due to the multiple jets of contrast agent emerging from the appropriately placed multiple side holes. These catheters are similar to those used for selective left ventricular angiography (Chapter 14). For aortography, we prefer thin-walled catheters since they allow higher injection rates.

Throughout the procedure, the catheter is flushed meticulously and frequently (every 3 to 5 minutes) with isotonic saline solution containing a small amount of heparin. Alternatively, a pressure-bag infusion set may be used for continuous catheter irrigation. Temporary total-body heparinization is not used widely for aortography alone but should be considered when the procedure involves more time-consuming catheter manipulations in the thoracic aorta, potentially affecting the coronary and carotid circulation.

In spite of the known higher incidence of atherosclerotic changes in the arteries of the lower extremities and tortuosity of iliac vessels, particularly in the older population, the femoral approach has a high success rate when appropriate technique is used. Certain conditions, however, such as thoracic or abdominal coarctation, threatening abdominal aortic aneurysm, or complete occlusion may preclude this retrograde approach.

### Percutaneous Puncture of Axillary Artery.

An alternative approach is the percutaneous puncture of the axillary artery.[5,6,7] In general, catheter approach to the descending aorta is accomplished from the left and to the ascending aorta from the right axillary artery, but no greater difficulty exists to advance the catheter to both aortic territories from either side. As the axillary and higher brachial arteries can be quite mobile, they need to be fixed by the operator's hand while the needle puncture is performed, similar to the approach to the femoral artery. The procedure is not more difficult, but reluctance to its more frequent use arises from a higher complication rate.[8,9] This seems to be related mostly to local formation of hematomas affecting the brachial nerve plexus; therefore, meticulous post-procedure compression and observation are mandatory. If delayed bleeding occurs, early surgical exploration and axillary sheath decompression are advisable. Catheter shape and side holes are similar to those used for the femoral approach, but in general a smaller catheter caliber (5 or 6 French) will permit a sufficient injection rate of contrast medium because the catheter can be kept shorter.

*Surgical cutdown* on the brachial artery, as in cardiac catheterization from the brachial approach (Chapter 4), can also be used when a percutaneous femoral approach cannot be employed.

### Translumbar Aortography.

Another percutaneous approach still used is translumbar aortography, which was described as early as 1929 by dos Santos.[2] This procedure, performed with the patient in prone position, is done with an #18 gauge needle which is advanced through the skin below the inferior margin of the lowest left rib, some 10 cm to the left of the midline. This procedure can be performed with surprising ease and rapidity and finds its use mostly for delineation of the abdominal aorta and its branches to the lower extremities. More recently, this technique has been modified using catheter replacement and retrograde advancement into the thoracic aorta, and successful selective coronary arteriograms have even been reported when all other arterial approaches were blocked.[10]

### Transseptal Angiocardiography.

Percutaneous direct approaches to the thoracic aorta have historical importance only and are not practiced anymore because of the obvious risk of uncontrollable hemorrhage. Transseptal angiocardiography offers a reasonable alternative for aortography in special cases.[11]

### Antegrade Angiography and Venous Injections.

Less selective approaches resulting in angiographic delineation of the aorta and its branches are the rapid bolus injection of contrast medium in the right side of the circulation, either selectively in the pulmonary artery—so-called antegrade angiography of the left heart—injections close to the right atrium via catheters, or even venous injections through one or two wide bore needles simultaneously. These approaches require, however, a larger total dose of contrast medium in order to compensate for the unavoidable dilution effect. These less selective approaches are frequently enhanced by using conventional subtraction radiography and have received more importance with the recent introduction of computerized *digital subtraction techniques.*

### Contrast Agent

In the interest of obtaining a good aortographic result, the contrast medium injected into the thoracic aorta should have a relatively high concentration of iodine. Preparations containing 350 to 400 mg iodine per ml (76% contrast agent solution) seem to satisfy these requirements and are marketed by a number of companies: the solutions contain either diatrizoate, metrizoate, or iothalamate as anions. These compounds are all similar in chemical structure, contain 3 iodine atoms per molecule and belong to the so-called ionic conventional contrast agents that over many years have proven to be well tolerated clinically in all forms of intravascular use. Higher concentrations, advocated by some, do not really improve the angiogram, and the increased viscosity may reduce the injection rate. Increased side effects and more intense sensation of heat by the patient are good arguments against their use. Lower concentration levels of 280 to 300 mg iodine per ml (60% contrast agent solution) can be used in the interest of lesser patient discomfort, particularly in situations of favorable radiographic conditions such as small object size and nondilated aorta. More important than the absolute concentration (which will undergo an unavoidable significant dilution in the aortic blood pool) is the mode of injection; i.e., a sufficiently high injection rate and delivery through multiple catheter holes to assure rapid and homogeneous mixing.

With regard to side effects, one has to pay attention to the cation concentration. In particular, the content of free sodium ion should be close to the normal serum level (approximately 140 meq/ml), since both experimental and clinical studies have shown clearly that unphysiologic sodium content increases the risk of arrhythmias in selective coronary arteriography.[12,13] The cardiac angiographer is most familiar with Renografin-76 (Squibb), which fulfills such requirements; however, there are other preparations on the market that match it closely in chemical composition and clinical safety. Mention has to be made of the new nonionic contrast agents that offer equal radiographic density at lesser osmolarity, but their intravascular use still awaits Federal Drug Administration (FDA) approval. They hold great promise with regard to fewer side effects and better patient tolerance.[12,14]

The recommended contrast dose for a thoracic aortogram lies between 40 and 60 ml; slightly lesser amounts will suffice for an abdominal aortogram. More than one injection is frequently required and is usually well tolerated. Individual injections should be separated by a time interval of at least 5 to 10 minutes, and attention should be paid that the temporary hemodynamic reaction (such as increased heart rate and/or decreased blood pressure) has abated prior to delivery of another contrast injection. A general recommendation not to exceed 300 ml of contrast agent for the average adult patient during one examination is prudent, and lower limits may be set in particular patients such as those with heart failure or marginal renal function.

## Radiographic Techniques

The most widely used radiographic technique is the direct large film series. Indirect methods are cinefluorography and spot-film fluorography, both using an image intensifier. Ongoing development in electronic image recording can be expected to benefit both methods, and it may be possible that in the future film recording will be replaced by video display in analog or digital form. Presently, it may be concluded that for the purpose of aortography direct film series are preferred when the indications for the examination require greatest anatomic detail, whereas cinematography is more suitable for the detection of abnormal dynamic events, i.e., valve motion and incompetence, abnormal contrast flow in shunts, AV fistulae, arterial bleeding sites or extravasations.

*Large Film Series.* Optimal radiographic detail important for precise anatomic definition is classically achieved with large film series, and this is still the most widely used method. An important inherent advantage is the field size, covering up to 14 × 14 inches. This implies that in one projection the image may easily encompass the entire thoracic aorta, including the proximal portions of the large aortic arch branches, intercostal arteries, bronchial arteries, and internal mammary arteries. Modern large-film changers, less bulky than those of the past, allow varying film sequence up to a rate of 3 to 4 exposures per second, sufficient for the purpose of accurate sequential delineation of arterial filling and runoff. Powerful x-ray tubes with high speed rotating anodes (10,000 RPM) and optimal heat dissipation characteristics and small focal spot anode target (0.6 to 1.0 mm) fed by high output (80 to 100 kW) 12-pulse generators guarantee the production of high contrast and high resolution images on the films.

Biplane equipment, essentially an independent duplication of the equipment, increases the cost of the installation and may, therefore, not be available except in larger institutions. Two x-ray tubes placed slightly offset from each other and firing alternately on the same film changer are less expensive than a biplane system and provide stereoscopic pairs of images that enhance the information derived from one injection.[14] Similar to biplane examinations, these studies allow viewing of the same object in different projections. Single plane technique more frequently will require a second injection following appropriate repositioning of the patient. Film subtraction for enhancement of contrast medium and magnification techniques to depict greater detail can easily be applied.

*Cinefluorography.* In contrast to direct radiography, cinefluorography implies an indirect radiographic method. After having penetrated and being attenuated by the object, the x-ray photons activate the input phosphor of an image intensifier which by means of electron acceleration generates an image of considerably increased brightness on the smaller output phosphor. (See Chapter 2 for a full discussion of radiographic principles). Via an appropriate optical lens system, this image is photographed by a movie camera, usually employing 35 mm film at a frame rate of 24 to 60 per second. Smaller 16-mm cameras will allow even higher frame speed and may find use in imaging for physiologic research but are not recommended for practical clinical use. Technical improvements, in particular the introduction of cesium iodide screens, have led to near perfection of this cine technique, which is widely preferred in cardiac angiography. Its main advantage is the continuous imaging of the angiographic events, whereas the main disadvantage is the limited field size determined by the input aperture of the electron intensifier. Another disadvantage lies in the lesser resolution of details compared to direct radiography. This can be compensated for in part by electronic magnification, but as a general rule, it has to be recognized that the higher the definition the

smaller the field size and vice versa. The high film rate of cinematography reduces the time available for exposure of each individual frame (3 to 10 msec); correspondingly, each individual pulse x-ray burst is of lesser intensity (25 to 35 microroentgen). However, total patient dose per film run is similar to that of a direct film series.

*Spot-film Fluorography.* This technique takes an intermediate position and delivers 100 mm cut film or 105 mm roll film images at a rate of 6 per second. Using also an image intensifier and a larger x-ray dose per frame at the input plane (150 microroentgen), a resolution of significantly greater detail can be achieved compared to cinematography. This technique is not as popular and widely available but has found advocates for certain indications such as examination of congenital abnormalities in children.

## ANATOMY AND ANGIOGRAPHIC APPEARANCE OF THE NORMAL THORACIC AORTA

The thoracic portion of the aorta (Fig. 16-1) reaches from the aortic valve to its exit from the thoracic cavity into the abdomen at the level of the diaphragm. In frontal presentation the aortic root projects in the midline superimposed by the dense shadow of the spine. Because the aortic valve apparatus is directed cranially with a slight inclination to the right and posteriorly, the ascending aorta assumes a gentle curve with convexity to the right, however, it does not normally exceed the border of the right upper mediastinal shadow which is usually represented by the superior vena cava. The ascending aorta has a rather constant caliber varying between 22 and 38 mm in adults and is related to individual body dimensions and probably also to general physical activity. A slight increase in dimensions occurs with age. Approximately at the origin of its first large branch, the brachiocephalic trunk, the thoracic aorta curves to the left and posteriorly in front of the trachea and gives off the left carotid and left subclavian arteries in sequence before it assumes a caudal direction at the site of the aortic isthmus to continue in the descending

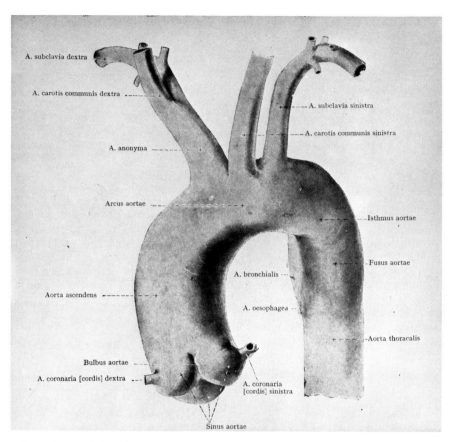

A. subclavia dextra

A. carotis communis dextra

A. subclavia sinistra

A. carotis communis sinistra

A. anonyma

Arcus aortae

Isthmus aortae

Fusus aortae

A. bronchialis

Aorta ascendens

A. oesophagea

Aorta thoracalis

Bulbus aortae

A. coronaria [cordis] dextra

A. coronaria [cordis] sinistra

Sinus aortae

**Fig. 16-1.** Thoracic aorta in LAO position according to Spalteholz. (From Paulin, S.: Coronary Angiography: A technical anatomic and clinical study. Acta Radiol., Suppl. 233, 1964, with permission.)

portion of the thoracic aorta slightly to the left and in front of the vertebral column.

At the site of the isthmus and the fetal ductus arteriosus, a slight anteriorly directed bulge in the contour may be seen. Likewise, a slightly more distally located fusiform dilatation may occur, the so-called aortic spindle. Both findings are probably related to slight distortions affected by the ligamentum arteriosum and are more marked in the young, but can persist in adult life.

Important vessels deriving from the descending portion of the thoracic aorta are the anteriorly directed bronchial arteries and the intercostal arteries with corresponding ramifications. Commensurate with the branching of the large arch arteries, the descending aorta has a slightly smaller caliber than the ascending aorta.

*Left Anterior Oblique (LAO) Projection.* The left anterior oblique (or right pos-

terior oblique) projection (Figs. 16-1 and 16-2) delineates the aortic arch optimally as it opens its curvature to the greatest extent. In most instances this projection also offers the tangential depiction of the large vessel orifices and may disclose variations in their relative position, which are frequent. This view also discloses most favorably the increased elongation and tortuosity of the aortic arch as it occurs in the elderly (Fig. 16-2).

*Right Anterior Oblique (RAO) Projection.* In the right anterior oblique (or left posterior oblique) projection, the ascending and descending aorta are more or less superimposed, and the aortic arch is markedly foreshortened. Consequently, this view is less favorable to delineate the takeoff of the large branches of the arch, but both oblique views may be useful to illustrate the proximal portions of the corresponding intercostal arteries.

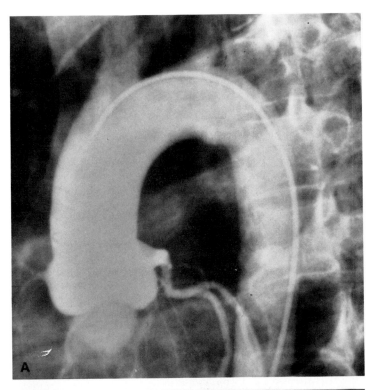

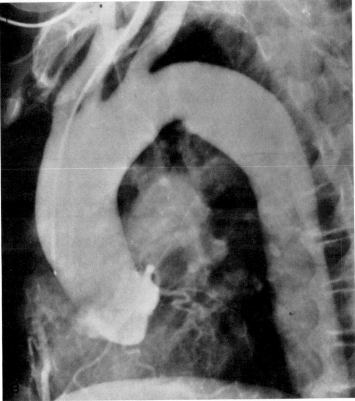

**Fig. 16-2.** Normal thoracic aortography in LAO projection: (A) young adult; (B) elderly person. Note the increased elongation of the aortic arch, resulting in a more proximal origin of the large vessels in the older individual. A small shallow bulge at the inner curvature of the arch just distally to the origin of the left subclavian artery corresponds to the obliterated ductus arteriosis, which is a common normal finding. The diameter of the descending aorta is slightly diminished compared to that of the ascending aorta.

***Cranial and Caudal Tilts.*** As in coronary angiography, cranial and caudal tilts may be added to achieve optimal visualization of specific anatomic details, e.g., a (LAO) projection with cranial tilt will result in a tangential depiction of the three aortic valve cusps (Fig. 16-3). A steep RAO projection with cranial tilt can demonstrate the aortic ostium en face.

## COMMON INDICATIONS FOR AORTOGRAPHY

Indications for thoracic aortography vary widely. They may extend from the evaluation of congenital vascular abnormalities in asymptomatic patients to the preoperative study of tumor vessel supply to assess operability. Since aortography when performed

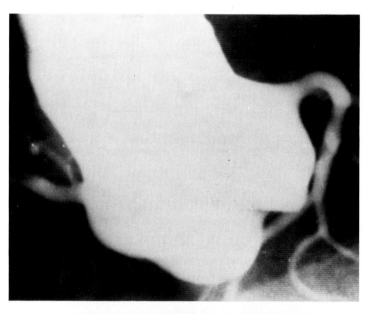

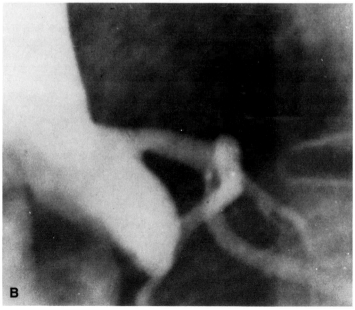

**Fig. 16-3.** Detail of aortic valve apparatus as seen in thoracic aortography. (A) Presentation of aortic bulb during diastole in LAO projection with cranial tilt. Both coronary cusps are identified by the orifices of the corresponding coronary arteries. The noncoronary cusp is located in the middle and slightly below. (B) Detail of left coronary cusp during systole. Note the straight border of the contrast-filled cusp leaflet against the nonopacified blood ejected from the left ventricle.

selectively presents an invasive procedure that includes a certain risk, the question should always be asked whether the information gained is important for the patient's management or whether the situation can be sufficiently assessed by less invasive diagnostic procedures or examinations. The most common conditions in which aortography is likely to render important information are aortic valve disease, aortic valve incompetence, aortic aneurysms, aortic coarctation, patent ductus arteriosus, and coronary bypass grafts.

## Aortic Valve Disease

*Aortic Valve Stenosis.* Although it is indisputable that the degree of functional impairment requires hemodynamic evaluation, angiographic examination contributes significantly to an optimal assessment of the condition. Anatomic delineation of the site and degree of abnormality is particularly important for the cardiovascular surgeon, as it might influence the technical operative approach, including choice of vessel substitutes or valve prosthesis. Obviously, angiography is the optimal method to distinguish between supravalvular, valvular, and subvalvular position of the lesion. In most instances such lesions are studied selectively by injections into the left ventricle (Fig. 16-4), but the supravalvular aortogram may render important, albeit partially inferential, information. In the presence of a valvular lesion a cineangiographic study in conjunction with a supravalvular injection in the proximal portion of the ascending aorta is considered optimal. Catheter position close to the valve apparatus improves image quality; however, care has to be taken that catheter and contrast jets, particularly through an open end hole, will not interfere with valve function and thus generate artifactual findings. The optimal position to separate clearly the aorta from the left ventricle and allow assessment of the interpositional relationship of the aortic cusps is approximately 45 degrees LAO, which when added to 10 to 15 degrees of cranial tilt will result in a practically true tangential depiction of the valve plane.

Cineangiography permits study of the motion of the three aortic valve leaflets, which normally move upwards rapidly during systole. The normal cusps are so thin that they will be seen only if the projection demonstrates them on edge. In diastole the closed valve is represented by the three semilunar cusps in LAO projection, the right and left coronary cusp side by side with their free edges adapting against each other in the center, and the noncoronary cusp slightly below posteriorly and seen en face.

An important aortographic sign of valvular aortic stenosis is the presence of poststenotic dilatation, a finding that is readily made and quantified by comparing the width of the midascending aorta and that of the aortic root. The cause of this finding is the flow turbulence that ensues immediately distally to the increased flow velocity through the significantly narrowed ostium and may assume asymmetric accentuation with a bulge to the right in cases of a narrow forceful blood jet.

The degree of poststenotic dilatation relates poorly to the tightness of the stenosis and to the existing systolic gradient between the left ventricle and the aorta. However, it has been shown that it is consistently greater in patients with congenital than in those with acquired types of aortic valve stenosis.

A characteristic finding for congenital aortic valve stenosis, at least in the early stages of life, is that the frequently fused, but still pliable leaflets assume an *upward-directed dome* (Fig. 16-4). As congenital aortic stenosis frequently includes developmental abnormalities of the cusps, an asymmetric appearance of the closed valve with the point of leaflet adaptation in a markedly eccentric position should be looked for, as it is typical for a bicuspid aortic valve. The angiographic appearance of the valve apparatus in acquired aortic stenosis is characterized by decreased mobility of the leaflets, frequently associated with marked thickening and irregular contours. It is advisable to begin filming the area of interest one or two heartbeats prior to the start of the contrast injection, so that the presence of calcification can be assessed. This is also helpful in differentiating calcium located in the free aortic valve, the proximal coronary arteries, the atrioventricular ring, and the upper portion of the interventricular septum. In advanced stages of acquired aortic stenosis extensive calcification is often present, and a dense, rather fixed, irregularly contoured plate is the counterpart of the so-called fish-mouth ap-

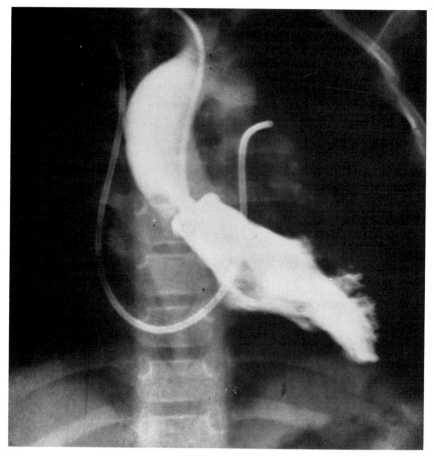

**Fig. 16-4.** Anteroposterior view of congenital aortic valve stenosis illustrating typical dome shape of pliable but fused aortic valve leaflets with centrally located narrowed opening. In this instance a selective left ventricular injection was performed. A supravalvular aortogram would show the findings with reversed contrast. The left heart catheter was passed retrograde from the right brachial artery. A right heart catheter is also seen, positioned in the pulmonary artery.

pearance of the valve as seen by the cardiac surgeon or pathologist.

Although the supravalvular aortogram contributes little in the situation of subvalvular narrowings, either congenital subvalvular membrane or muscular outflow tract stenosis in IHSS, this procedure is optimal for the evaluation of *supravalvular aortic stenosis*, a condition characterized by the presence of an aortic narrowing just above the aortic valve. This lesion may produce a tubular narrowing of the entire ascending aorta (Fig. 16-5), so-called ascending aorta hypoplasia, a thin membranous diaphragm, or an internally protruding circumferential ridge just above the sinuses of Valsalva. Although in these situations the aortic valve apparatus

itself may be normal, concomitant valve abnormalities such as bicuspid anatomy are frequently encountered. Supravalvular aortic stenosis may be part of a congenital syndrome that also includes peripheral pulmonary artery stenosis, physical and mental retardation, hypocalcemia, and facial abnormalities.[15,16]

***Aortic Valve Incompetence.*** Supravalvular injection of radiographic contrast during cineangiography constitutes the most definitive diagnostic technique to assess aortic valve insufficiency. The sensitivity to detect even small amounts escaping from the aorta to the left ventricle on the projected movie is high, and the possibility of erroneous overdiagnosis is a possibility. It has been

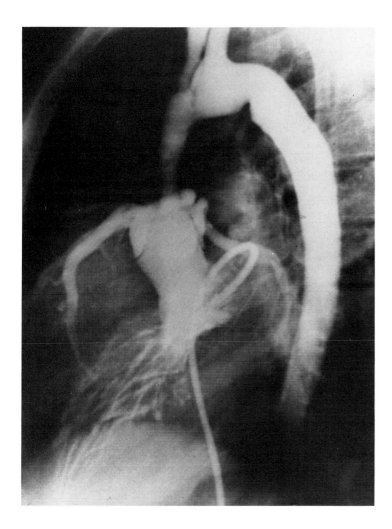

**Fig. 16-5.** Left lateral view of congenital supravalvular aortic stenosis. A transseptal catheter has been placed in the left ventricle. Contrast injection opacifies the left ventricular outflow tract, the coronary arteries, and the ascending and descending aorta. Note the long significant narrowing of the entire ascending aorta, so-called hypoplasia, and the significant dilation of the coronary arteries arising proximally to the narrowing.

shown that inappropriate technique, such as excessive injection volume and speed, catheter end-hole jet, mechanical catheter interference with the valve apparatus, simultaneous Valsalva maneuver, and transient bradycardia or premature beats may cause factitious angiographic appearance of aortic valve incompetence. On the other hand, an injection site too high in the upper portion of the ascending aorta so that the root of the aorta is not filled completely is inadequate for assessing aortic insufficiency. The optimal technique is to inject through a closed-end straight catheter with multiple side holes[17,18] or a pigtail catheter placed approximately 1 to 2 inches above the aortic valve. Our own practice is to inject 40 to 50 ml of contrast media at a rate of 20 to 25 ml/sec. If

significant displacement of the catheter detracts from the quality of the examination, a repeat injection following adjustment of the catheter position must be considered.

The concept of grading aortic insufficiency has to take several factors into consideration. Among these, the size and volume of the aorta, the concentration of contrast medium achieved by the injection, and the degree of dilatation and emptying capacity of the left ventricle rank highly. Technical factors of importance are the shape of the regurgitant jet of contrast medium which may be more impressive when seen tangentially in a particular projection, the type of exposure chosen, and the object density and the latitude of the film. It is advisable, therefore, that a particular laboratory develop a standard examination technique to achieve the greatest possible uniformity.

A common practice is to express the subjectively made observation of aortic valve incompetence in four degrees of severity (1 to 4 + ). Minor variations in definition exist at the lower end of the scale because some authors tend to include findings that are most likely factitious. A 1 + grading signifies a minor degree of radiopaque reflux throughout diastole dissipating in the left ventricular volume without resulting in a perceptible overall contrast increment of this chamber. A 4 + grading will denote rapid and massive reflux within one diastole resulting in fairly uniform opacification of the left ventricular chamber reaching a radiodensity similar to that of the ascending aorta. Grades 2 and 3 + are used to identify intermediate degrees of severity between these two extremes.

Comparison with clinical evidence of aortic valve incompetence has found good agreement in the majority of cases.[18] The radiologic contrast study was found to resolve clinical uncertainty in situations where combined valve lesions made the clinical assessment difficult.

Comparison with observations at operation has also demonstrated the predictive value of cineaortography to be very reliable. Patients without evidence of regurgitation on cineaortography were subsequently found to have no more than mild regurgitation at operation, whereas all those identified as 3 or 4 + had indeed severe incompetence.[18] The same angiographic approach can be used in the evaluation of a malfunctioning aortic valve prosthesis. Here, the possibility to differentiate on the cine films between valvular incompetence and paravalvular leak (Fig. 16-6) has to be emphasized, and the difference can be distinguished on the angiographic study.

## Aortic Aneurysms

Because a great proportion of the thoracic aorta's outer contours are seen on plain chest x-ray films, an aortic aneurysm is frequently suspected or diagnosed with this noninvasive test. Fluoroscopy, kymography, two-dimensional ultrasound, nuclear imaging, and CT scanning may be used for confirmation of the diagnosis. Thoracic aortography is, however, the most conclusive procedure because it renders the necessary details for potential surgical intervention. It is widely practiced both as an elective and an emergency procedure.

Both true and false aneurysms can occur in the thoracic aorta. The term *true aneurysm* implies that the outer wall of the aneurysm is composed of at least one of the three arterial wall layers, (intima, media, and adventitia) and the term *false* denotes that the wall actually has been perforated and the extravasating blood is contained by adjacent tissue and clot formation. The most common true aneurysms are arteriosclerotic, luetic, or congenital in nature, whereas traumatic rupture and perforation are typical causes for false aneurysms.

Important information that can be gained from the angiographic procedure includes location and size of the aneurysm, relationship to origins of other vessels, proximity to other adjacent structures such as superior vena cava, trachea, or esophagus, and the characteristics of the aortic wall at the border of the aneurysm. These factors are all of importance in guiding the surgeon to choose the proper site for resection and to exclude the presence of unrecognized additional vascular pathology.

***Arteriosclerotic Aneurysms.*** In the adult, particularly in the elderly, the most common type of thoracic aortic aneurysm by far is the arteriosclerotic type. The site of predilection is the distal arch or the descending aorta. The aneurysms are usually *fusiform* but may be *saccular*. As they are the result of wall weakening in the deeper portion of an atheromatous ulcer, one can expect the remaining wall of the aorta to show the typical changes of plaques and craters, and the aneurysms are frequently multiple.[19] The angiographic examination often demonstrates an increased distance between the inner contour and the outer wall (Fig. 16-7), which is related to the frequent occurrence of laminated clots and adventitial fibrosis.

***Arteria Magna.*** An interesting and extreme form of this condition is the so-called arteria magna,[20] observed predominantly in the elderly and apparently due to a profound diffuse loss of elastic tissue in the aortic media. In such cases the thoracic aorta becomes enormously widened and elongated. The risk of rupture is high, an event which in

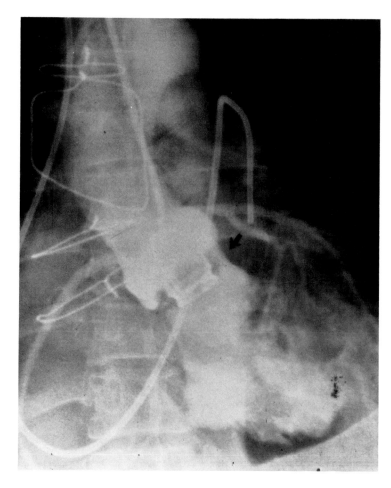

**Fig. 16-6.** Supravalvular aortogram in anteroposterior projection in a patient with an aortic valve prosthesis. Significant aortic regurgitation to the left ventricle occurred in paravalvular aortic position (arrow).

the thoracic region is most often fatal because of poor hemorrhage containment by adjacent organs. Fusiform and saccular aneurysms of the ascending aorta are less likely to be atherosclerotic. In the past, such aneurysms were most likely to be luetic, representing most often the late manifestation of syphilis. Typical and almost pathognomonic for these were linear calcifications in the ascending aortic wall, usually detectable on chest radiographs. This is a rare diagnosis today when other organisms are the cause of vascular abnormality. These infectious aneurysms are also located most frequently in the ascending aorta or in the sinuses of Valsalva, where they rarely calcify. They are frequently saccular.

*Other Types.* A subclass of thoracic aortic aneurysms involves the sinuses of Valsalva. Commonly, the origin is congenital or idiopathic, and the aneurysm may involve all three sinuses. The underlying abnormality is medial necrosis and aortic wall weakness. Specific examples include Marfan's syndrome, Ehlers-Danlos, and other connective tissue disorders. Incompetence of the aortic valve is frequently an associated finding. Less commonly, their origin may be due to acquired conditions such as bacterial endocarditis (e.g., occurring after cardiac surgical procedures such as aortic valve replacement[21]). Aneurysms of the sinus of Valsalva commonly rupture, resulting in fistulae with connections to other cardiac chambers, especially the right atrium and ventricle (Fig. 16-8).

Because many of the disease processes causing aortic aneurysms may also involve the major intrathoracic branches of the aorta, it is prudent to extend the angio-

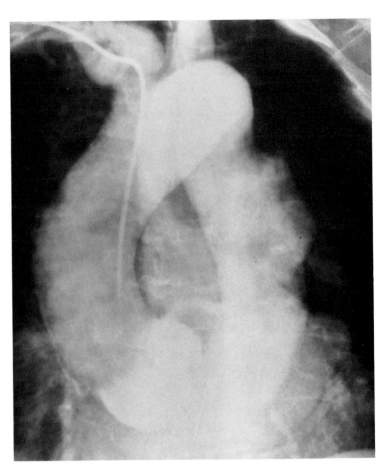

**Fig. 16-7.** Thoracic aortogram in anteroposterior projection illustrating general widening of the entire thoracic aorta. In the proximal portion of the descending aorta a large local contour bulge is noted, and the distance between the contrast-filled lumen and the outer contour of the distal descending aorta is increased. Operative findings confirmed the diagnosis of atherosclerotic aneurysm with marked wall thickening.

graphic examination to these vascular areas as well. In particular, the innominate and left subclavian arteries may be involved. However, aneursysms of the left common carotid, intercostal, and brachial arteries have also been described either as isolated findings or in combination with lesions in the aorta.

*Traumatic Aneurysms.* Post-traumatic aneurysms have increased in frequency. Rapid deceleration in conjunction with motor vehicle accidents explains their most frequent occurrence in the young and their localization to the isthmus of the aorta (Fig. 16-9), i.e., the border between the arch and the descending aorta where the inertia of the large column of blood exerts local wall stresses that may exceed elastic tolerance. Frequently the diagnosis of an aortic aneurysm is made after the acute phase, when during recovery of the severely injured victims a chest roentgenogram shows a bulge in

the aortic contour. The underlying abnormality consists of a wall rupture with contained hematoma, thus representing a false aneurysm. Although the patient may be asymptomatic at the time when the diagnosis is made on chest roentgenogram, aortography and subsequent surgical repair are indicated because of the high risk of late rupture.[22]

*Dissecting Aneurysm.* Dissection of the aortic wall involves the thoracic aorta most frequently. Its high incidence in the male population between the ages of 50 and 70, particularly in patients with a history of systemic hypertension, makes it an important differential diagnosis to acute myocardial infarction. The initiating cause is an intimal tear with formation of intramural hematoma that extends along the weakened media, which histologically shows signs of necrosis. Localization of the initial tear is

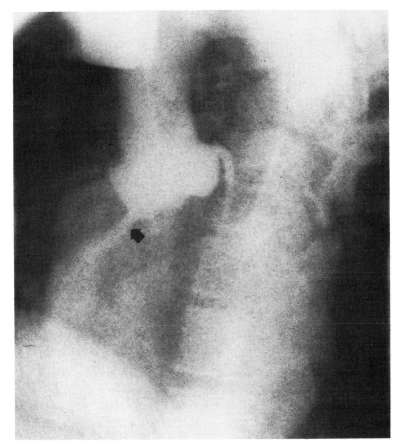

**Fig. 16-8.** Cineaortogram in LAO projection, demonstrating ruptured aortic sinus (sinus of Valsalva) aneurysm. The aneurysm formed from the wall of the right aortic sinus, just below the origin of the right coronary artery. Rupture (arrow) is into the right atrium.

important to determine patient risk and management. Application of the classification according to DeBakey is most useful in this respect. In this classification, type I describes a dissection whose initial tear is localized to the proximal portion of the ascending aorta, just above the aortic valve, with the false lumen extending around the arch (Fig. 16-10) to the descending aorta, not infrequently continuing to the abdominal portion of the aorta and the large pelvic arteries. A type II dissection is similar; however, the dissection terminates proximal to the first large arch vessel orifice. Type III dissection denotes a dissection that begins distal to the aortic arch (Fig. 16-11). Type III dissections generally involve less hazard, as they do not directly affect the circulation to

the most vital organs, the heart and the brain. Although less invasive approaches such as sequential chest roentgenograms, thoracic fluoroscopy, ultrasound, and computerized tomography (CT) may render important clues, a thoracic aortogram is the most definitive procedure in making an accurate diagnosis.

The optimal technical approach for a thoracic aortogram is retrograde from the femoral artery, preferably from the artery with the best pulsations. A nontraumatic catheter must be carefully guided by fluoroscopy and test injections. An increased distance between catheter and outer contour will alert the experienced angiographer to the presence of a dissection. Approach from brachial or axillary arteries is not necessary and

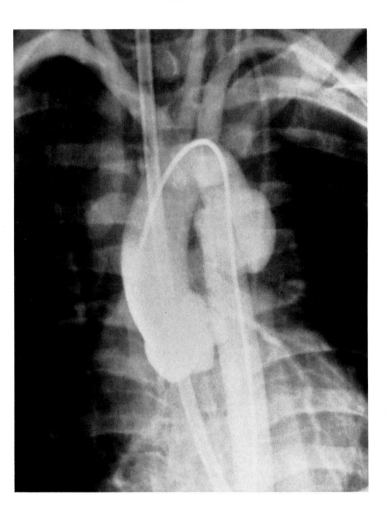

**Fig. 16-9.** Total rupture of the aorta at its isthmus by a rapid-deceleration vehicle accident. Note aortic wall contour defects and local bulbous accumulation of contrast medium, representing the false aneurysm contained by adjacent tissue. Surgical repair immediately following the angiogram was successful.

probably inadvisable when intermittent or persistent pulse deficits exist. Whereas the angiographic identification of the false lumen itself, filling rapidly or slowly, is relatively easy on rapid film series, the precise localization of the tear and dislodged intimal flaps may be very challenging. Additional injections at different sites within the aorta and using cineangiography for better identification of contrast flow pathways may be necessary. The same holds true for evaluation of complicating events such as aortic valve incompetence, compromise of coronary orifices, and perforations, e.g., bleeding into the pericardial space. These considerations are strong arguments for a direct arterial approach as opposed to the less invasive intravenous injections. The same holds true for those dissecting aneurysms that might be

found in Marfan's syndrome or be the result of iatrogenic trauma such as arterial catheterization, aortic valve replacement, or vascular surgery.

## Aortic Coarctation

The diagnosis of aortic coarctation can be made by careful clinical examination in most cases. Signs of coarctation are a late systolic murmur in the typical location over the spine, a pulse delay in the lower extremities, and a gradient of blood pressure readings between the upper and lower extremities. Not infrequently, however, the radiologist makes the diagnosis of aortic coarctation on chest roentgenograms by virtue of the im-

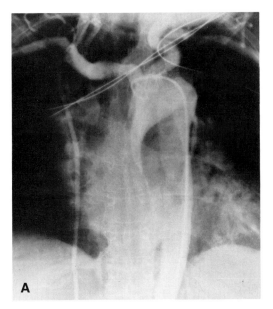
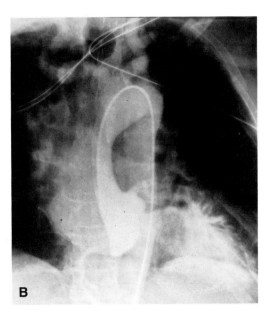

**Fig. 16-10.** Type I dissecting aortic aneurysm in a middle-aged patient with a history of hypertension. (A) Injection through a pigtail catheter was done at the aortic arch because further catheter advancement met resistance. Observe the marked narrowing of the ascending aorta, which is compromised by a large blood-distended and nonopacified false lumen. Large arch vessels are not compromised. (B) The aortic root was injected following careful advancement of the pigtail catheter. The injection demonstrates the large diameter of the false lumen. The dissection involves the aortic cusps, causing valve incompetence with contrast medium filling the left ventricle. Immediately after angiography the dissecting aneurysm and the regurgitant aortic valve were repaired surgically.

pressively abnormal contour of the aortic arch and large vessels in the upper mediastinum, as well as rib notching and a hypertrophic rounded appearance of the left ventricular contour. Prominence of the ascending aorta is noted frequently, and is usually unrelated to the degree of hypertension. However, it suggests the association of aortic valve abnormalities, such as bicuspid leaflets, present in up to a third of the cases of aortic coarctation.

Aortography again assumes an important diagnostic role and can differentiate the great variety of abnormal patterns (Fig. 16-12) which include complete aortic interruption, hypoplastic aortic segment, and the most common type, a stenosis of varying degrees at the site of the isthmus distal to the left subclavian artery. An interesting associated finding in some cases is an aberrant right subclavian artery arising from the descending thoracic aorta distal to the coarcta-

tion and with lower pulse pressure in the right than in the left arm. Coarctation of the aorta sometimes may be seen in association with right-sided aortic arch.[23]

The retrograde catheter approach through the site of narrowing is not advised. Not infrequently, collateral pathways entering into thin-walled poststenotic segments may be difficult to negotiate and definitely pose a hazard for inadvertent perforation. A brachial or axillary artery approach should be preferred for entrance to the prestenotic aorta. In some situations the indirect angiographic approach, with injections into the central venous system or the pulmonary artery may be a less hazardous alternative and may render sufficient information, particularly when image enhancement and subtraction techniques are used. If, however, the need for precise evaluation of hemodynamic changes exists, such as the exclusion of an aortic valve gradient or assessment of left

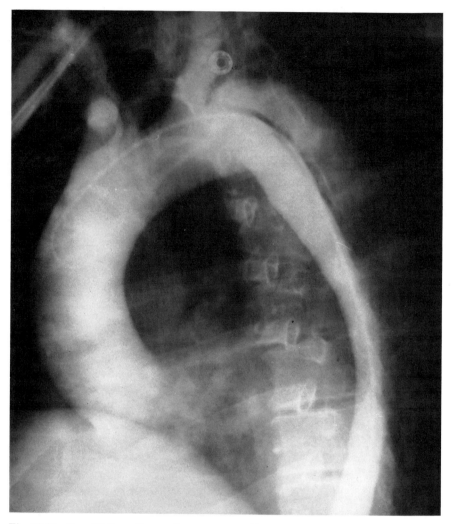

**Fig. 16-11.** Type III dissecting aortic anurysm in a 62-year-old man with previous hypertension. Aortogram in LAO projection shows faint opacification of the false lumen, which begins just after the origin of the left subclavian artery. A pigtail catheter was placed in the ascending aorta from the right groin and is in the true lumen. An intimal flap can be seen clearly dividing the true and false lumens in the descending thoracic aorta. The true lumen is compressed because of hematoma in the false lumen.

ventricular function, the unavoidable selective cardiac catheterization is conveniently combined with selective angiography.

## Patent Ductus Arteriosus

Thoracic aortography is a powerful diagnostic tool for identifying and evaluating a persistent ductus arteriosus. This lesion ranks high among congenital cardiovascular abnormalities with a prevalance of 1/5500 in the young population up to 14 years. If isolated, a patent ductus arteriosus carries a good prognosis, more than 95% of the patients reaching 18 years or older. In the child, typical symptoms and noninvasive findings may suffice to recommend surgical repair without the need for angiography. In the adult, subtle symptoms or combinations with other malformations make the need for angiographic confirmation more likely. Further-

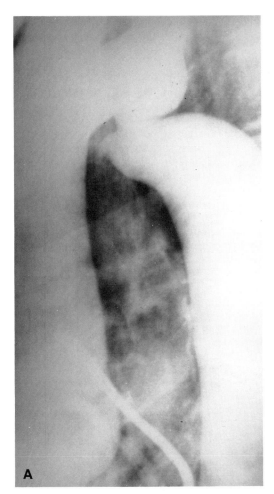 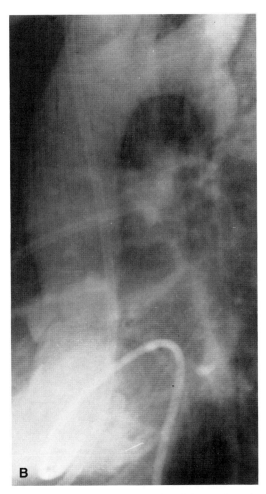

**Fig. 16-12.** Two cases of aortic coarctation in LAO projection. (A) Note marked distortion of the aortic arch with significant narrowing at the isthmus and poststenotic dilatation of the descending aorta. (B) The coarctation resulted in complete occlusion of the lumen.

more, differential diagnostic considerations in the presence of a continuous murmur in an adult have to include conditions that have a longer natural history to full development, such as shunts via aberrant coronary arteries connecting with the pulmonary circulation, coronary artery fistulae or arteriovenous connections in the thoracic wall (e.g., laceration of the internal mammary artery following penetrating trauma). Selective aortic cineangiography with injection near the site of the expected arterial entrance is very sensitive in demonstrating small shunts and surpasses the sensitivity of right heart catheterization with stepwise oximetry. Radionuclide tracer flow studies may match angiography in this respect; however, they are less conclusive with regard to topographic localization. Large shunts result in the typical appearance of increased pulmonary vascularity on the chest roentgenogram, and in such cases the aortogram may demonstrate a difference in caliber between the ascending and descending aorta. An aortogram is also able to establish the rare diagnosis of an aortopulmonary window, which has similar hemodynamic consequences to patent ductus arteriosus. In the event of secondary pulmonary hypertension with equilibrated resistance the shunt may be reversed, resulting in a corresponding negative contrast defect by the unopacified blood in the contrast column.

## Coronary Bypass Grafts

Following the initial demands to assess the longevity of aortocoronary venous bypass grafts, the current need for postoperative demonstration of these grafts exists primarily in patients with recurrence of angina pectoris. Selective injections into the individual grafts are generally performed in conjunction with a repeat selective coronary arteriogram of the native circulation. Although this selective approach is successful in most cases, difficulties may be encountered when the proximal graft anastomosis is in an unusual position or when a "flush" proximal occlusion has to be documented. As a last resort, a nonselective, large bolus of contrast medium is injected into the ascending aorta. The results of such injections are frequently disappointing. However, complete absence of filling following rapid injection (20 ml/sec or more) of 40 to 50 ml of contrast agent into the ascending aorta is reasonably good evidence for graft occlusion. If filling of the graft in question is noted, the diagnosis of a stenosis or impaired flow must be made cautiously. Digital subtraction technique enhances contrast and is, therefore, recommended.[24]

Frequently the results of the selective angiogram of the native coronary arteries give indirect, but important clues, such as retrograde filling of the distal graft and/or persistence or recurrence of collaterals directed to the bypassed coronary artery branch. Intravenous digital angiography has been advocated for the demonstration of coronary artery bypass grafts, but is even less likely to cope with the above mentioned difficulties. (Fig. 6-13). The same holds for the use of CT scanning advocated by some to identify the proximal grafts in transsectional fashion without demonstrating localized narrowing unless by serendipity. Modern high speed dynamic CT scanners presently being developed offer some promise because they may be used to determine the rate of contrast turnover possibly reflecting regional flow impairment.

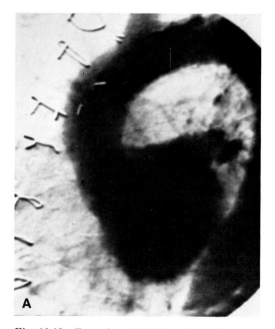
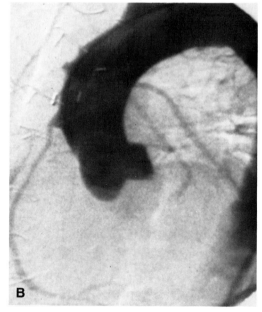

**Fig. 16-13.** Examples of digital angiography in patient with triple bypass surgery. (A) Following intravenous injection, contrast medium is seen in left ventricle and thoracic aorta, both viewed in LAO projection. Faint opacification of saphenous vein bypass graft segments can be seen between inner contour of ascending aorta and contrast-filled left ventricle. (B) Following direct injection of the aortic root, the three grafts can be clearly identified. Motion artifacts at distal grafts due to cardiac activity and overlapping with contrast medium in ascending aorta of proximal graft portions limit significantly the diagnostic information. (Courtesy of D. Kim, M.D.)

# REFERENCES

1. Forssmann W: Die Sondierung des rechten Herzens. Klin Wochenschr 8:2085, 1929.
2. dos Santos R, Lamas AC, Pereira-Caldas J: Arteriografia da aorta e dos vasos abdominalis. Med Contemp 47:93, 1929.
3. Nuvoli I: Arteriografia dell' aorta ascendente o del ventricolo. Policlinico (Prat) 43:227, 1936.
4. Seldinger SI: Catheter replacement of the needle in percutaneous arteriography: A new technique. Acta Radiol (Stockh) 39:368, 1953.
5. Hanafee W: Axillary artery approach to carotid, vertebral abdominal aorta, and coronary angiography. Radiology 81:559, 1963.
6. Roy P: Percutaneous catheterization by the axillary artery. AJR 94:1, 1965.
7. Boijsen E: Selective visceral angiography using a percutaneous axillary technique. Br J Radiol 39:414, 1966.
8. Dudrick S, Masland W, Mishkin M: Brachial plexus injury following axillary artery puncture. Radiology 88:271, 1967.
9. Molnar W, Paul DJ: Complication of axillary arteriotomies: Analysis of 1762 consecutive studies. Radiology 104:269, 1972.
10. Maxwell DD, March HB, Mispireta LA: Translumbar selective coronary arteriography. Cardiovasc Intervent Radiol 5:157, 1982.
11. Gishen P, Lakier JB: The ascending aorta in aortic stenosis. Cardiovasc Radiol 2:85, 1979.
12. Paulin S: Contrast agents for selective coronary arteriography. Cathet Cardiovasc Diagn 10:425, 1984.
13. Contrast Material Symposium, San Francisco, CA, October 22–23, 1983. Investigative Radiol 19:Suppl 4, 1984.
14. Nordenstrom B, Ovenfors CO, Westberg G: Experimental stereoangiography of the coronary and bronchial arteries. Acta Chir Scand Suppl 245, 1959.
15. Beuren AJ, et al: The syndrome of supravalvular aortic stenosis, peripheral pulmonary stenosis, mental retardation and similar facial appearance, Am J Cardiol 13:471, 1964.
16. Williams JCP, Barratt-Boyes BG, Lowe JB: Supravalvular aortic stenosis. Circulation 24:1311, 1961.
17. Taubman JO, Goodman DJ, Steiner RE: The value of contrast studies in the investigation of aortic valve disease. Clin Radiol 17:23, 1966.
18. Cohn LH, et al: Preoperative assessment of aortic regurgitation in patients with mitral valve disease. Am J Cardiol 19:177–182, 1967.
19. Sprayregen S: Radiologic spectrum of arteriosclerotic aneurysms of aortic arch. NY State J Med 78:2198, 1978.
20. Randall PA, et al: Arteria magna revisited. Radiology 132:295, 1979.
21. Holmes EC, Bredenberg CE, Brawley RK: Aneurysm of the sinus of Valsalva resulting from bacterial endocarditis. Ann Thorac Surg 15:1628, 1973.
22. Bennett DE, Cherry JK: The natural history of traumatic aneurysms of the aorta. Surgery 6:15, 1967.
23. Edelman RR, Weintraub R, Paulin S: Coarctation of the aorta with right aortic arch of the mirror-image type. AJR 140:1135, 1983.
24. Guthaner D, et al: A comparison of digital subtraction techniques in the evaluation of coronary graft patency. (Abstract) Presented at the American College of Cardiology Meeting, March 1984, Dallas, Texas.

# PART V
## *Evaluation of Cardiac Function*

## chapter seventeen

# Dynamic and Isometric Exercise during Cardiac Catheterization

BEVERLY H. LORELL *and* WILLIAM GROSSMAN

PATIENTS known to have significant heart disease may have entirely normal hemodynamics measured in the resting state during cardiac catheterization. However, since most cardiac symptoms are precipitated by exertion or some other stress, it is often important that hemodynamic performance be assessed both at rest and during some form of stress such as muscular exercise, pharmacologic intervention, or pacing-induced tachycardia. Such an evaluation enables the physician to assess both the level of cardiovascular reserve and the relation (if any) of specific symptoms to hemodynamic impairment. Physiologic information so obtained is often valuable in prescribing specific medical therapy, selecting patients for corrective cardiac surgery, and in predicting the likelihood of improvement following medical or surgical treatment.

Muscular exercise, both dynamic and isometric, has been studied extensively, and the normal hemodynamic responses are reasonably well understood. In the cardiac catheterization laboratory, muscular exercise is commonly employed in the hemodynamic evaluation of patients with heart disease. There are differences between the hemodynamic responses to dynamic supine, or erect

exercise and static, isometric exercise, and each will be discussed separately.

Dynamic muscular exercise is particularly useful in the assessment of valvular heart disease and cardiomyopathic heart disease and may be employed to assess the integrated physiologic response of the cardiovascular system to stress. Isometric exercise is particularly useful when it is desirable to produce a transient stress upon the left ventricle in order to assess left ventricular performance. Properly designed exercise studies can provide specific hemodynamic information enabling the cardiologist to make a more precise assessment of the significance, prognosis, and therapy of heart disease.

## DYNAMIC EXERCISE

Dynamic exertion is the major form of exertion in everyday activity. During dynamic exertion, skeletal muscles are actively contracting and developing force that is translated into motion and work. This is accompanied by an increase in the amount of oxygen taken up by pulmonary capillary

251

blood in the lungs and transported by arterial blood to working skeletal muscles. In normal sedentary individuals, the level of oxygen consumption during maximal exercise ($\dot{V}O_2$ max) can increase about 12-fold compared to that during the resting state.[1] Additional factors influencing $\dot{V}O_2$ max include gender, oxygen tension of inspired air, ambient and body temperature, and the hemoglobin content. Age and fitness also modify $\dot{V}O_2$ max, since there is about a 5% decrease in $\dot{V}O_2$ max per decade during aging. During athletic training, $\dot{V}O_2$ max increases due to both cardiovascular adaptation and skeletal muscle changes. In marathon runners and Olympic class athletes, $\dot{V}O_2$ max may represent an 18-fold increase in oxygen consumption above the resting state. In any individual, the maximal oxygen consumption depends on the integration of cardiac, metabolic, vascular, and pulmonary responses. The increased oxygen requirements of muscular exercise are met both by an increase in the cardiac output and by an increased extraction of oxygen from arterial blood by skeletal muscle, which causes widening of the arteriovenous oxygen difference. The ability of the heart to increase its output appropriately for the increase in oxygen consumption at any level of exercise is met predominantly by an increase in heart rate and by a lesser increase in stroke volume in response to enhanced sympathetic stimulation. The increased metabolic needs of exercising muscle are accompanied by a switch from utilization of free fatty acids at rest to an accelerated breakdown of muscle glycogen stores and enhanced uptake of blood-borne glucose which is supplied by increased hepatic gluconeogenesis. Because carbohydrate metabolism produces more carbon dioxide than fat metabolism, the respiratory quotient (ratio of $CO_2$ production to $O_2$ consumption) rises from a resting value of about 0.7 toward 1.0.[2] The delivery of blood-borne oxygen and glucose to working skeletal muscle is enhanced in the presence of normal vasculature by a reduction in skeletal muscle vascular resistance mediated by metabolic by-products and by sympathetically mediated vasoconstriction elsewhere which cause a redistribution of blood away from the renal and splanchnic beds to exercising muscle.

In addition to cardiovascular adaptation, exercise depends on the ability of the respiratory mechanism to increase oxygen supply. During progressive exercise, there is a linear increase in minute ventilation relative to the increase in oxygen consumption. When a level of exercise is reached such that insufficient oxygen is delivered to exercising muscle, anaerobic metabolism of glycogen and glucose develops which causes metabolic acidosis and an increase in respiratory quotient $\geq 1.0$ such that minute ventilation increases out of proportion to oxygen consumption.[3] At this level the accumulation of hydrogen ions usually causes skeletal muscle weakness, pain, and severe breathlessness, followed by exhaustion and cessation of exercise.

As will be discussed below, we usually structure exercise studies in the catheterization laboratory so that the patient reaches a *steady state level of submaximal exercise* below the anaerobic threshold, so that exercise can be sustained for several minutes. This approach permits a critical examination of cardiovascular reserve; that is, is the increase in cardiac output appropriate for the increase in oxygen consumption occurring at that particular level of exercise?

## Oxygen Uptake and Cardiac Output

Oxygen uptake as measured from expired air collections increases promptly during exercise[4,5] and within several minutes reaches a new steady state that is directly related to the level of exercise. Data illustrating these changes are shown in Figure 17-1. Simultaneously, the mixed venous blood oxygen saturation decreases to a lower steady level related to the intensity of exercise, producing an increase in the arteriovenous oxygen difference.

The cardiac output also increases with exercise. Dexter and his colleagues,[4] who studied the effect of exercise on circulatory dynamics in seven normal individuals, found that a strong linear correlation characterizes the relationship between cardiac output and oxygen consumption (Fig. 17-2). As can be seen from the regression equation for this relationship, for each increment of 100 ml/min/m$^2$ of oxygen consumption during exercise, there is an increase in cardiac output of 590 ml/min/m$^2$.

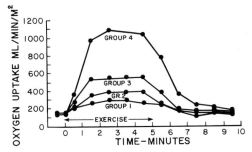

**Fig. 17-1.** Oxygen consumption in normal subjects during exercise. Each group represents a different level of exercise, with the most intense exercise being performed by Group 4. Note the prompt increase and establishment of a new steady state in oxygen uptake that is directly related to the intensity of the exercise. (From Donald KW. et al: The effect of exercise on the cardiac output and circulatory dynamics of normal subjects. Clin Sci 14:37, 1955. Used with permission of the publisher.)

indicates a normal cardiac output response to exercise.

Another way of using this same relationship between cardiac output and oxygen consumption involves calculation of the "exercise factor," which is the increase in cardiac output with exercise divided by the corresponding increase in oxygen consumption. A normal exercise factor would be an increase of $\geq 600$ ml/min in cardiac output per 100 ml/min increase in oxygen consumption.[5,6] An exercise factor less than

$$\frac{600 \text{ ml/min cardiac output}}{100 \text{ ml/min } O_2 \text{ consumption}}$$

indicates a subnormal response in cardiac output; similar to an exercise index of $\geq 0.8$, it suggests some pathologic process limiting the heart's ability to respond to exercise with an appropriate increase in cardiac output.

The linear relationship between oxygen uptake and cardiac output response during exercise, illustrated in Figure 17-2, may be used to assess whether the cardiac output response measured in an individual patient is appropriate to the level of exercise and increased oxygen uptake. The regression formula: cardiac index (L/min/m$^2$) = 0.0059X + 2.99 where X = $O_2$ consumption in ml/min/ m$^2$, may be used to calculate the *predicted cardiac index* for a given level of $O_2$ consumption (x), and the predicted cardiac index may then be compared to the measured cardiac index. This relationship is useful in assessing whether the patient's cardiac output response is appropriate to the level of exercise and oxygen consumption. Note that this assessment can be performed at any steady-state level of exercise, and does not depend on achieving any specific "target" level of exertion. This equation can be used to calculate a predicted cardiac index by measuring oxygen consumption during dynamic exercise. The patient's actual or measured cardiac index during exercise is then divided by the predicted cardiac index to determine the deviation from normal. We have termed this ratio the "exercise index," since it allows expression of exercise capacity as a percentage of the normal response. An exercise index of:

$$\frac{\text{measured cardiac index}}{\text{predicted cardiac index}} \geq 0.8$$

## Arterial Pressure and Heart Rate

Systemic arterial pressure increases during dynamic exercise in the supine or upright position in the normal subject, although the response is somewhat variable.[7-10] In spite of this increase in pressure, systemic vascu-

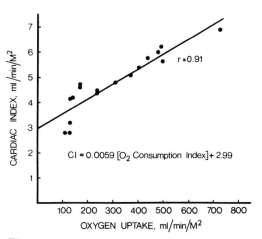

**Fig. 17-2.** The relationship between cardiac output and oxygen consumption (both indexed for body surface area) during supine dynamic exercise of varying intensity in normal subjects, based on the data of Dexter.[1] As can be seen from the regression equation for this relationship, for each increment of 100 ml/min/M$^2$ of oxygen consumption, there is an increase in cardiac output of 0.59 liters/min/M$^2$ or 590 ml/min/M$^2$.

lar resistance decreases,[4] indicating that the elevated arterial pressure is secondary to increased cardiac output. Patients who are unable to generate an adequate response in cardiac output may also increase their arterial pressure, but in this circumstance systemic vascular resistance may actually increase.

Heart rate increases consistently during dynamic exercise, and during mild exercise, it is likely that tachycardia is a prominent factor in increasing cardiac output. This is supported by the observation that stroke volume shows only minor (if any) increase during vigorous exercise.[4,5] Ross and co-workers compared the response of cardiac output, stroke volume, and heart rate to a given level of bicycle exercise in normal subjects and also found that the increase in cardiac output was due to an increase in heart rate with a negligible contribution by change in stroke volume.[9] However, during repeat exercise when heart rate was held constant, there was a comparable increase in cardiac output due to a marked increase in stroke volume. Furthermore, when heart rate is artificially increased by electrical pacing in the absence of dynamic exercise, a major fall in stroke volume occurs,[9] indicating that further cardiovascular adjustments are required for an adequate hemodynamic response to dynamic exercise.

## Left Ventricular Systolic Performance

Augmented left ventricular systolic performance during dynamic exercise results from the interaction of several factors. Tachycardia exerts a positive inotropic effect (the so-called Treppe phenomenon), but increased sympathetic nervous system activity appears to be the most significant factor leading to enhanced myocardial contractility.[6] In some circumstances, an increase in end-diastolic fiber tension (preload) may also occur, leading to improved cardiac performance by means of the Frank-Starling mechanism. The fact that left ventricular end-diastolic volume may not change, or more commonly decreases during dynamic exercise, has been taken as evidence that the Frank-Starling mechanism does not usually contribute to the cardiac response to exercise. However,

the effects of dynamic exercise on left ventricular end-diastolic volume in normal subjects are complex and are influenced by contractile state (end-systolic volume), posture, heart rate (length of the diastolic filling period), and age. End-diastolic volume at rest is near maximum when a normal subject is supine, smaller when he is sitting, and smallest when he is standing.[11,12] Thus, in most normal subjects, supine bicycle exercise is accompanied by an increase in ejection fraction and other ejection indices of left ventricular systolic function, a decrease in left ventricular end-systolic volume, and a decrease or no change in end-diastolic volume.[8,13,14] In the occasional normal subject in whom an increase in left ventricular end diastolic volume occurs during supine bicycle exercise, an increase in stroke volume is likely to contribute to the rise in cardiac output.[8] In the upright position, left ventricular end-diastolic volume, cardiac output, and stroke volume are lower than in the supine position.[10,15,16] During erect bicycle exercise, most normal subjects demonstrate an increase in ejection fraction and reduction in end-systolic volume, some enhancement of left ventricular end-diastolic volume, and an increase in stroke volume as well as heart rate.[10–12,17] Furthermore, it has been shown that left ventricular end-diastolic volume, end-systolic volume, and stroke volume are larger during exercise than during comparable heart rates induced by electrical pacing.[6] Thus, it seems likely that the Frank-Starling mechanism is active during dynamic exercise, but may be masked by the salutary effects of tachycardia and increased myocardial contractility, both of which tend to decrease left ventricular volume.

Left ventricular end-diastolic pressure is measured more readily during exercise than left ventricular volume, and it is often used as an approximation of end-diastolic myocardial fiber tension.[18] Exercise-induced changes in some parameter of left ventricular systolic performance (such as stroke volume or stroke work) may be compared to the change in left ventricular end-diastolic pressure to obtain a modified left ventricular function curve.[19] Typical normal and abnormal responses are illustrated in Figure 17-3. These data may be used to evaluate the relative contributions of increased contractility and increased preload to augmented left ventricular performance.

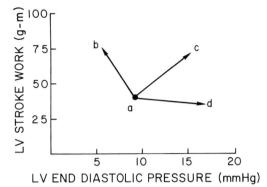

**Fig. 17-3.** A modified ventricular function curve constructed by comparing the change in left ventricular stroke work to the change in left ventricular end-diastolic pressure during dynamic exercise. The dot represents the resting values, the arrow-heads the exercise values. Change "a" to "b" indicates a normal response with increased left ventricular performance at a decreased filling pressure. Change "a" to "c" indicates an ability to increase left ventricular performance by utilization of the Frank-Starling mechanism, the situation that might exist with abnormal left ventricular hemodynamics and some limitation in "inotropic reserve." Change "a" to "d" indicates poor left ventricular performance with no increase or an actual decrease in left ventricular performance in spite of a significant increase in left ventricular filling pressure.

However, caution must be used in interpreting left ventricular function curves obtained during a dynamic exercise study. The effects of advancing age on the exercise response are pertinent to this evaluation of left ventricular performance. In healthy subjects, there appear to be no age-related changes in resting cardiac output, ejection fraction, end-systolic or end-diastolic volumes.[20] However, with advancing age there is a reduction in the heart rate and contractility response during exercise, such that the increase in cardiac output during exercise is accomplished by a significant increase in end-diastolic volume and in stroke volume.[20,21] The diminished heart rate and contractility responses and resultant increased dependence on the Frank-Starling mechanism during exercise in the elderly may reflect an age-related decrease in responsiveness to beta-adrenergic stimulation.[22,23]

The interpretation of normal versus abnormal left ventricular systolic performance during dynamic exercise may also be complicated by the effects of chronic beta-adrener-

gic blockade. Studies of the hemodynamic effects of chronic beta-adrenergic blockade on graded exercise in hypertensive but otherwise healthy young adults have shown that no impairment of maximal exercise capacity (maximal oxygen consumption) occurs during chronic beta-adrenergic blockade.[24] However, beta-blockade causes a reduction in heart rate at any level of exercise, and this relative reduction in heart rate is compensated for by both a widening of the arteriovenous $O_2$ difference and an increase in stroke volume, associated with an increased left ventricular preload and a reduced arterial blood pressure (impedance to ejection).[24] Other workers have also shown that in normal subjects during supine and upright bicycle exercise, heart rate and arterial pressure are lower, whereas left ventricular volumes are larger and the extent of shortening is reduced in the presence of beta-adrenergic blockade.[25-27] Thus, in a patient on chronic beta-adrenergic blocking therapy, dynamic exercise may be associated with an "inappropriately" low increase in cardiac output relative to oxygen consumption accompanied by excessive widening of the arteriovenous oxygen difference. Furthermore, utilizing a classic ventricular function curve, the increase in cardiac output would appear to be dependent on an increase in left ventricular end-diastolic volume (and pressure) which could be due either to beta-adrenergic blockade per se or to intrinsic impairment of left ventricular systolic function. For these reasons, strong consideration should be given to discontinuation of beta-adrenergic blocking drugs at least 24 hours prior to catheterization if the hemodynamic response to dynamic exercise is planned to assess the presence or absence of impaired cardiovascular reserve.

## Left Ventricular Diastolic Function

The interpretation of modified left ventricular function curves is keenly dependent on an appreciation of the determinants of left ventricular end-diastolic pressure during exercise, when this measurement is used as an approximation of end-diastolic myocardial fiber length and tension.[18] In normal subjects, there is little change in the left ventricular diastolic pressure-volume relation during exercise,[13] and it is reasonable to assume that changes in left ventricular end-diastolic pressure reflect changes in left ventricular end-diastolic fiber stretch. Thus, studies of the effects of dynamic supine bicycle exercise in young adults have generally shown no change or a fall in left ventricular end-diastolic pressure and volume during exercise.[7,8] Studies of older normal subjects or patients with atypical chest pain and normal coronary arteries have generally shown that dynamic supine and upright bicycle exercise is associated with a slight increase in left ventricular end-diastolic pressure,[10,13,28,29] which is probably related in part to the age-dependent reliance on an increase in preload during exercise, previously discussed. For example, in a group of 10 sedentary men whose average age was 46 years, there was a rise in left ventricular end-diastolic pressure from $8 \pm 1$ to $16 \pm 2$ mmHg during supine bicycle exercise, and a rise from $4 \pm 1$ to $11 \pm 1$ mmHg during upright bicycle exercise.[10]

Under certain circumstances, however, exercise may provoke an upward shift in the left ventricular pressure-volume relationship, such that any level of left ventricular end-diastolic volume is associated with a much higher left ventricular end-diastolic pressure (LVEDP). In such patients, the left ventricle may be regarded as exhibiting increased chamber stiffness (decreased distensibility) during exercise. In patients with coronary artery disease, a transient but striking upward shift in the left ventricular pressure-volume relation is common during episodes of ischemia.[30] Such patients with coronary artery disease who develop angina during dynamic exercise in the catheterization laboratory commonly show a marked rise in left ventricular end-diastolic pressure during exercise, such as the rise in LVEDP from $9.8 \pm 2.5$ to $31.2 \pm 6.5$ mmHg reported by Parker et al in a group of 24 patients who developed angina during supine bicycle exercise,[28] and seen by others during supine[29] and upright bicycle exercise.[31] Therefore, interpretation of an exercise-induced rise in left ventricular end-diastolic pressure in patients with coronary artery disease is complex and may be related both to a decrease in left ventricular chamber distensibility and to an increase in left ventricular end-diastolic volume secondary to a reduction in

ejection fraction and increase in left ventricular end-diastolic volume.[13,14,17]

A careful study of the dynamics of left ventricular diastolic filling during exercise in patients with coronary artery disease has been reported by Carroll and co-workers.[32] These authors studied left ventricular diastolic pressure-volume relations in 34 patients with coronary disease who developed ischemia during exercise and compared the findings to those in 5 patients with minimal cardiovascular disease (control) and 5 patients with an akinetic area at rest (scar group) from a prior infarction, but no active ischemia during exercise. There was an upward shift in the left ventricular diastolic pressure-volume relationship during exercise-induced ischemia, which was not seen in either the scar or the control group (Fig. 17-4). Actually, the left ventricular diastolic pressure-volume curve shifted downward in the control group, indicating improved diastolic distensibility. These findings with exercise-induced tachycardia are remarkably similar to changes in diastolic function seen during pacing tachycardia in similar patients, as described in Chapter 18.

## Evaluation of Left Ventricular Failure

Examples of the hemodynamic changes that can occur during supine bicycle exercise are shown in Tables 17-1 and 17-2. Table 17-1 illustrates the response to 6 minutes of supine bicycle exercise of a 36-year-old woman with an idiopathic dilated cardiomyopathy (ejection fraction 40%) whose major symptom was exertional dyspnea. Because her ejection fraction was only moderately depressed and her hemodynamics were nearly normal at rest, resting hemodynamic data alone did not clarify whether her cardiovascular reserve was impaired and whether her exertional dyspnea was likely to be cardiac in origin. During exercise, the cardiac index increased appropriately relative to the increase in oxygen consumption, yielding an exercise index of 1.1 and an exercise factor of

$$\frac{3300 \text{ ml/min/M}^2, \Delta \text{ cardiac index}}{387 \text{ ml/min/M}^2, \Delta O_2 \text{ cons. index}} = 8.5$$

However, the increase in cardiac output was

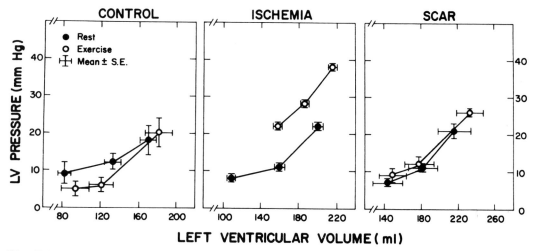

**Fig. 17-4.** Left ventricular (LV) diastolic pressure-volume relations at rest and during exercise in patients without heart disease (control), compared to patients with coronary disease who developed ischemia during exercise (ischemia) and patients with akinetic areas due to previous infarction but no active ischemia during exercise (scar). Pressure and volume are averaged at three diastolic points: early diastolic pressure nadir, mid-diastole, and end diastole. The control group had a downward shift of the early diastolic pressure-volume relation, but the ischemia group showed an upward and rightward shift. (Reproduced with permission from Carroll J.D., Hess OM, Hirzel HO, Krayenbuehl HP: Dynamics of left ventricular filling at rest and during exercise. Circulation 68:59, 1983.)

accomplished at the cost of a substantial increase in mean pulmonary capillary wedge pressure, which rose from 11 to 27 mmHg. These data suggest she had some limitation of inotropic reserve and that her ability to increase cardiac output was heavily dependent on utilization of the Frank-Starling mechanism. Thus, her dyspnea can be considered to be of cardiac origin.

A patient with more severe impairment of cardiovascular reserve is illustrated in Table 17-2, which shows the response to 6 minutes of supine bicycle exercise of a 60-year-old man with idiopathic dilated cardiomyopathy and symptoms of marked fatigue and dyspnea with minimal exertion. His chest roentgenogram showed cardiomegaly with no evidence of pulmonary edema, and his rest hemodynamics were nearly normal. However, supine bicycle exercise was associated with a marked rise in both left and right heart filling pressures, and a marginal ability to increase cardiac output appropriately relative to his increase in oxygen consumption. His exercise index was 0.85 with an exercise factor quite low at

$$\frac{1700 \text{ ml/min/M}^2, \Delta \text{ cardiac index}}{341 \text{ ml/min/M}^2, \Delta O_2 \text{ cons. index}} = 4.9$$

The exercise responses of patients with severe congestive heart failure have been well studied. The cause of exercise intolerance in some patients is diminished cardiovascular reserve so that inadequate oxygen is delivered to working skeletal muscle, maximal oxygen consumption is reduced, and the anaerobic threshold occurs prematurely at a low work load.[33] However, the relative contributions of the inability of the heart to augment cardiac output and an exercise-induced rise in pulmonary capillary wedge pressure which could impair gas exchange, as illustrated in the above examples, are controversial.

Recently, the hemodynamic and ventilatory responses to upright graded bicycle exercise were studied in 28 patients with severe left ventricular failure.[34] In these patients, oxygen consumption, heart rate, cardiac index, and stroke volume increased linearly with increments in work load. However, the maximal oxygen uptake and the work load at which anaerobic metabolism occurred were about 50% below normal capacity. For the group at peak exercise, cardiac index rose from $2.5 \pm 0.7$ to $4.5 \pm 1.6$ L/min/m$^2$ associated with a rise in mean pulmonary capillary wedge pressure from $20 \pm$

**TABLE 17-1.**  *Response to Supine Bicycle Exercise in a 36-Year-Old Woman with Dilated Cardiomyopathy*

|  | Resting | Exercise (6 minutes) |
|---|---|---|
| $O_2$ consumption index (ml/min/m$^2$) | 117 | 504 |
| AV $O_2$ difference (ml/L) | 34 | 75 |
| Cardiac index (L/min/m$^2$) | 3.4 | 6.7 |
| Heart rate (beats/min) | 80 | 140 |
| Systemic arterial pressure (mmHg), systolic/diastolic (mean) | 130/70 (95) | 142/83 (110) |
| Right atrial mean pressure (mmHg) | 6 | 7 |
| Pulmonary capillary wedge mean pressure (mmHg) | 11 | 27 |
| Left ventricular pressure (mmHg) | 130/17 | 142/28 |
| Exercise index | — | 1.1 |
| Exercise factor | — | 8.5 |

**TABLE 17-2.**  *Response to Supine Bicycle Exercise in a 60-Year-Old Man with Dilated Cardiomyopathy*

|  | Resting | Exercise (6 minutes) |
|---|---|---|
| $O_2$ consumption index (ml/min/m$^2$) | 128 | 469 |
| AV $O_2$ difference (ml/L) | 40 | 96 |
| Cardiac index (L/min/m$^2$) | 3.2 | 4.9 |
| Heart rate (beats/min) | 90 | 141 |
| Systemic arterial pressure (mmHg), systolic/diastolic (mean) | 91/62 (73) | 107/67 (88) |
| Right atrial mean pressure (mmHg) | 5 | 20 |
| Pulmonary capillary wedge mean pressure (mmHg) | 12 | 34 |
| Left ventricular pressure (mmHg) | 91/16 | 107/34 |
| Exercise index | — | 0.85 |
| Exercise factor | — | 4.9 |

10 to 38 ± 9 mmHg. Despite the striking and sustained rise in pulmonary capillary wedge pressure, arterial carbon dioxide tension was unchanged and systemic arterial oxygen content increased during exercise. These observations suggest that in many patients with chronic left ventricular failure exercise intolerance is *not* caused by arterial hypoxemia secondary to the marked elevation of pulmonary capillary wedge pressure, but rather by the inability of the heart to increase cardiac output and oxygen delivery to working tissues adequately. These observations contrast with the effects of an abrupt elevation of pulmonary capillary wedge pressure in patients with previously normal pressures, who develop acute myocardial ischemia or acute valvular insufficiency and transient pulmonary venous hypertension which often result in pulmonary edema and systemic arterial hypoxemia.

## Evaluation of Valvular Heart Disease

Exercise may also be used in the cardiac catheterization laboratory to evaluate valvular heart disease. Gradients across the atrioventricular and semilunar valves may become apparent during exercise and may reach levels that account for the clinical symptoms of the patient. This is especially useful when the transvalvular gradient or estimated valve area has borderline significance; exercise may elicit hemodynamic changes that clearly establish the pathophysiologic significance of the valve stenosis.

An example of the hemodynamic changes in moderate mitral stenosis during supine dynamic exercise is shown in Figure 17-5. As the result of increased mitral valve flow and decreased diastolic filling period, the pressure gradient has to increase significantly, producing left atrial pressures of sufficient magnitude to cause clinical symptoms. Cardiac output increased significantly, yielding an exercise index of 1.2 and an exercise factor of

$$\frac{2800 \text{ ml/min, } \Delta \text{ cardiac output}}{481 \text{ ml/min, } \Delta O_2 \text{ consumption}} = 5.8$$

These data are compatible with mild mitral stenosis and illustrate the changes in the diastolic pressure gradient across the mitral valve required to produce an increase in cardiac output appropriate to the increased oxygen requirements of strenuous exercise.

In evaluating hemodynamic changes across *stenotic valves* during exercise, it is often found that the calculated valve area during exercise may vary somewhat (it is usually slightly larger) from that calculated on the basis of resting data. This variance is generally small and may be related to actual changes in the degree of valvular obstruction (a higher gradient and greater flow may force the stenotic leaflets to open farther), deficient data, or computational errors inherent in the assumptions applied to the equation for calculating of valve orifice size.[35,36]

The hemodynamic consequences of *valvular insufficiency* with ventricular volume overload may be subtle at rest. Dynamic exercise, by calling upon the heart to signifi-

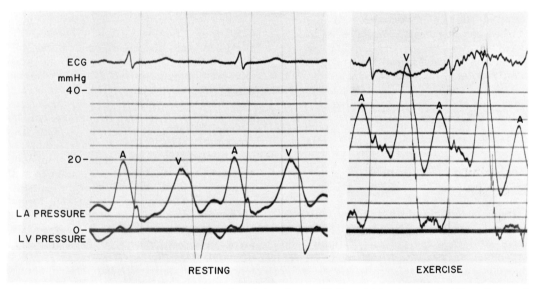

**Fig. 17-5.** Simultaneous pressure recordings from left atrium and left ventricle at rest and at five minutes of bicycle ergometer exercise in a patient with mitral stenosis. The following hemodynamic data were obtained:

| | Resting | Exercise |
|---|---|---|
| Left atrium pressure (mm Hg) | | |
| A | 20 | 34 |
| V | 18 | 46 |
| mean diastolic | 10 | 26 |
| Left ventricle mean diastolic pressure (mm Hg) | 1 | 4 |
| $O_2$ consumption (ml/min) | 207 | 688 |
| AV $O_2$ difference (ml/min) | 31 | 74 |
| Cardiac output (L/min) | 6.5 | 9.3 |
| Heart rate (beat/min) | 72 | 108 |
| Mitral valve area (cm²) | 1.6 | 1.8 |
| Exercise index | | 1.2 |
| Exercise factor | | 5.9 |

cantly augment its forward cardiac output, may elicit changes in left ventricular end-diastolic pressure and volume (preload) and in systemic vascular resistance (afterload) that are useful in assessing the cardiovascular limitations imposed by the valve lesion. Of particular importance here is the inability of many of these patients to increase forward cardiac output in an appropriate manner, resulting in a low exercise index and an abnormal exercise factor. Dynamic exercise is especially valuable in such patients because the qualitative assessment of valvular insufficiency from angiograms may be unreliable and does not correlate well with the extent of functional impairment.

Figure 17-6 shows the effects of dynamic bicycle exercise in a 55-year-old man with rheumatic heart disease and mitral regurgitation. His main symptom was dyspnea on exertion, but he did not have easy fatigability, a symptom commonly present in mitral regurgitation. The patient was able to increase cardiac output normally, but as seen in Figure 17-6, mean pulmonary capillary wedge pressure increased from 18 mmHg to 30 mmHg, with V waves to 60 mmHg, during 6 minutes of supine bicycle exercise. This patient had successful mitral valve replacement, with relief of symptoms.

## Performing a Dynamic Exercise Test

Dynamic exercise during cardiac catheterization is easily performed with a bicycle ergometer while the patient is supine. The ergometer we use[*] is constructed so that an appropriate work load can be selected; the rate of pedaling should be monitored and maintained as constant as feasible. Some coaching of the patient is useful in this regard. A protocol detailing the exercise test should be prepared prior to the test to insure that all essential data are obtained. Pressures should be obtained so that the appropriate valve gradients can be evaluated, and left ventricular pressure should be monitored if left ventricular performance is in question.

Supine bicycle exercise tests are performed most easily when catheterization is

[*]Monark Model 880, Quinton Instrument Co., Seattle, WA.

by the arm approach. However, supine bicycle exercise tests can also be done with safety when catheterization is by the femoral approach if care is taken to place the right and left heart manifolds and transducers in a stable and accessible position on the chest away from leg motion artifact and if the femoral venous and arterial sheaths are visualized and secured in place by the hand of one operator during exercise to insure that catheters and sheaths are not displaced during leg movement.

We usually plan to carry out a supine bicycle exercise test immediately after baseline hemodynamics and cardiac output have been measured, prior to contrast angiography. The patient's feet are secured in the bicycle stirrups, and the right heart, left heart, and systemic arterial catheters and attached manifolds are positioned so that they are not kinked or under tension and will not be disturbed during the exercise. Next, the system for measuring oxygen consumption is put in place (see Chapter 8): we have used the MRM-2 (Waters Instruments, Inc., Rochester, NY), which gives oxygen consumption readings continuously during dynamic exercise and allows assessment of whether a steady state has been achieved (Fig. 17-1). The patient is instructed that he or she will be coached to achieve a certain level of submaximal exercise over the first minute of exercise which can be sustained for an additional 4 to 6 minutes. This detailed patient instruction is useful, since some patients may be accustomed to the different format of progressively graded exercise aimed at achieving a transient level of maximal exhaustion-limited exercise utilized in upright treadmill tests. Syringes for measuring systemic arterial and mixed venous (pulmonary artery) oxygen content should be at hand.

With the patient resting quietly and feet positioned on the bicycle, all pressures are zeroed, phasic and mean pressures are recorded at 25 or 50 mm/sec paper speed, and at the gain to be used in exercise, and cardiac output measurements are repeated to obtain an accurate pre-exercise baseline with legs elevated in the stirrups. Pressures are zeroed once again, *all* pressures are then redisplayed, and paper speed is slowed (5 to 10 mm/sec). Exercise is then begun, with *all pressures continuously displayed on the monitor and recorded at slow speed.* We generally record LV phasic pressure, sys-

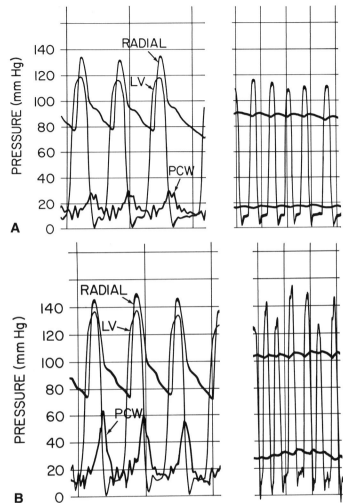

**Fig. 17-6.** Hemodynamic findings during exercise in a 55-year-old man with mitral regurgitation. Left ventricular (LV), pulmonary capillary wedge (PCW), and radial artery pressure tracings are shown before (A) and during (B) the sixth minute of supine bicycle exercise. PCW mean pressure and V wave increased substantially with exercise.

temic arterial (e.g., radial or femoral artery) mean pressure, and pulmonary capillary mean pressure simultaneously. Using a Honeywell Electronics-for-Medicine VR12 Recorder, we generally record at 100 or 200 gain for *all pressures*, so that all pressures may be visualized simultaneously (as shown in Fig. 17-6). Each minute, a brief recording of all three pressures on phasic at 25 to 50 mm/sec paper speed is accomplished, following which the pulmonary capillary and systemic arterial pressures are then returned to "mean," and the paper speed slowed to 5 to 10 mm/sec. The continuous observation and recording of pressures is extremely important, since it permits the accurate monitoring of any rise in filling pressure or fall in

arterial pressure during exercise and assures that catheters remain in correct position for measurements at peak exercise. After the patient has achieved a steady-state level of exercise for 4 minutes, simultaneous LV-systemic arterial, LV-PCW, and PCW-to-PA pullback pressures are recorded during minutes 4 to 6, after increasing the recorder speed to 50 mm/sec without attempting to rezero the transducers. The pulmonary capillary catheter is pulled back to the pulmonary artery and exercise cardiac output is measured by Fick or thermodilution technique, at which time arterial and pulmonary artery blood samples are drawn for measurement of oxygen saturation. After the blood samples are drawn, all pressures are redisplayed.

The right heart catheter is quickly pulled back directly to the right atrium, monitoring the displayed pressure waveform to permit measurement of mean and phasic right atrial pressure during exercise. The patient is then asked to stop cycling, and all transducers are again zeroed, without moving the transducers or the patient's position in the bicycle. The bicycle can then be removed and the return of any elevated filling pressures toward baseline can be monitored.

Cardiac output may be measured at rest and during the last 2 minutes of exercise utilizing the Fick principle, with collection of expired air as described in Chapter 8. As mentioned earlier, as an alternative to Douglas bag air collection, we have found it convenient and reliable to measure oxygen consumption at rest and during submaximal bicycle exercise using a servo-controlled instrument that measures time-averaged oxygen consumption ($\dot{V}O_2$) continuously, using a polarographic oxygen sensor (MRM oxygen consumption computer, Waters Instruments, Inc., Rochester, NY). This instrument, which has a response time of 10 seconds in detecting a step change in oxygen consumption, is ideal for making $\dot{V}O_2$ measurements during sustained effort. This device has advantages for dynamic exercise in the catheterization laboratory in that: (1) the clear plastic faceplate can be worn comfortably during exercise without the need for a mouthpiece or noseclip and adds no respiratory burden, and (2) it permits a continuous display of time-averaged $\dot{V}O_2$ during exercise so that both the level of exercise and establishment of a steady state can be monitored.[37] Alternatively, cardiac output can be assessed using an indicator-dilution technique (e.g., thermodilution, indocyanine green dye), and oxygen consumption can be estimated as the quotient of cardiac output and arteriovenous-oxygen difference.

We generally try to accomplish 6 minutes of dynamic exercise. Expired air is collected or MRM continuous $\dot{V}O_2$ measurements are recorded starting at the fourth minute into exercise, at which time a steady state has been established (Fig. 17-1). Obviously, the duration and intensity of the exercise must be tailored to fit the needs of the individual patient.

Precautions should be taken during exercise to insure patient safety. The electrocardiogram should be monitored constantly to avert serious arrhythmias, and exercise should be terminated if significant symptoms or greatly abnormal hemodynamic alterations occur. Little additional diagnostic information can be obtained by continuing the exercise to the point of producing acute pulmonary edema.

## ISOMETRIC EXERCISE

Lind and his colleagues reported more than 20 years ago that sustained isometric contraction of the forearm flexor muscles produces a cardiovascular reflex consisting of increases in heart rate, arterial blood pressure, and cardiac output.[38] The precise nature of this reflex is not completely understood, but it appears to require afferent neural impulses from the exercising extremity[39] and may be related to inhibition of vagal activity.[40] Although the cardiac output response may be blunted, the anticipated responses in heart rate and blood pressure are not blocked by administration of propranolol, indicating that more is involved than a simple increase in beta-adrenergic stimulation.[41] This lack of knowledge of specific mechanisms notwithstanding, the normal and abnormal hemodynamic responses to isometric exercise have been well-defined, making this a useful stress test in evaluating patients during cardiac catheterization.[42-45]

## Hemodynamic Response

The hemodynamic response to isometric handgrip exercise has been studied in a series of normal subjects and patients with heart disease.[42] Data obtained from 8 normal adult subjects are listed in Table 17-3. These data indicate that heart rate, systemic arterial pressure, and cardiac output increase significantly during isometric handgrip exercise. Systemic vascular resistance shows no change, indicating that the increase in systemic arterial pressure is due to the increased cardiac output rather than to a vasoconstrictor response. No significant or consistent change in stroke volume was observed, and there was no increase in left ventricular end-diastolic pressure. Contrast ventriculography studies in normal subjects have shown that handgrip exercise results in

**TABLE 17-3.** *Hemodynamic Observations During Isometric Handgrip in 8 Normal Subjects*

| Parameter | Control | Exercise |
|---|---|---|
| Heart rate (beats/min) | 79 ± 5 | 98 ± 8[*] |
| Aortic mean pressure (mmHg) | 94 ± 3 | 119 ± 5.5[*] |
| Stroke volume (ml/beat) | 66.5 ± 7 | 67 ± 8 |
| Stroke work (gm-meters) | 81 ± 8.8 | 104 ± 11[*] |
| Left ventricular end diastolic pressure (mmHg) | 6.8 ± 0.8 | 7.5 ± 1.2 |
| Systemic vascular resistance (dynes-sec-cm$^{-5}$) | 1606 ± 176 | 1645 ± 260 |
| Cardiac output (L/min) | 4.9 ± 0.4 | 6.4 ± 0.7 |

[*]Statistically significant change at p < .01 level. All values are expressed as mean ± standard error of the mean.

(Based on data from Grossman W et al: Changes in the inotropic state of the left ventricle during isometric exercise. Br Heart J 35:697, 1973.)

a decrease in left ventricular end-systolic and end-diastolic volumes and a slight increase in ejection fraction.[46] These hemodynamic and angiographic changes typify the expected normal response to isometric exercise.

## Left Ventricular Performance

Left ventricular performance is augmented during isometric exercise. This response may be due to both increased left ventricular myocardial contractility[42] and the Frank-Starling mechanism. Studies of myocardial mechanics performed during isometric exercise reveal increases in $\dot{V}_{max}$, the theoretic maximal velocity of contractile element shortening at zero load, and in left ventricular peak dP/dt.[42,47] Although these studies are subject to all of the criticisms surrounding the study of myocardial mechanics from intraventricular pressure recordings (as discussed in Chapter 20), they do constitute reasonable evidence for an increase in the inotropic state of the left ventricle in response to sustained isometric exercise. Further evidence for enhanced contractility may be derived by comparing left ventricular stroke work to changes in left ventricular filling pressure. Stroke work, a function of both pressure and stroke volume, is a useful parameter expressing the external work of the left ventricle. If increased stroke work

can be performed without a change in filling pressure, it is likely that an increase in inotropic state has occurred. Conversely, if increased stroke work is accomplished only at the expense of a significant increase in left ventricular filling pressure, it is reasonable to conclude that the Frank-Starling mechanism has been utilized to increase ventricular performance. In this context, left ventricular end-diastolic pressure is utilized as an approximation of end-diastolic left ventricular myocardial fiber tension.

Patients with heart disease and decreased left ventricular function or inotropic reserve commonly show an abnormal hemodynamic and contractile response to isometric exercise.[42] Although left ventricular peak dP/dt may increase in diseased hearts, changes are of less magnitude than in normal subjects. Left ventricular stroke work may increase, remain unchanged, or decrease in response to isometric exercise in pathologic states. This may by itself be evidence of compromised left ventricular function, but is more apparent when the change in stroke work is compared to the change in left ventricular end-diastolic pressure. Significant increases in left ventricular end-diastolic pressure are seen commonly in the abnormal response to isometric exercise[42] and indicate decreased inotropic reserve and dependence on the Frank-Starling mechanism in order to augment left ventricular performance.

In decompensated hearts, stroke work may not increase and may actually fall in spite of increased left ventricular filling pressures. This is an abnormal response, indicating poor left ventricular performance, and may be accompanied by a decrease in cardiac output and an increase in systemic vascular resistance. In patients with coronary artery disease, the rise in heart rate and blood pressure typically associated with handgrip exercise is accompanied by an abnormal increase in left ventricular end-diastolic volume and pressure, an increase in end-systolic volume, and the appearance or worsening of wall motion abnormalities.[11]

## Performing an Isometric Exercise Test

Isometric exercise is most commonly performed as sustained handgrip. The subject is first tested to evaluate his maximal voluntary contraction. A partially inflated sphygmomanometer cuff or a specially designed handgrip dynamometer* may be used. This testing may be done prior to cardiac catheterization and should be done well before the actual handgrip test. The patient must be coached and encouraged to grip as hard as possible at the time maximal voluntary contraction strength is determined. Baseline resting hemodynamic data should include heart rate, systemic arterial pressure (phasic and mean), left ventricular pressure, and cardiac output. Cardiac output is most easily determined for this form of exercise using the indicator dilution method (e.g., thermodilution, indocyanine green dye), or the Fick method with the continuous oxygen consumption measurement (MRM) technique.

Once baseline data are collected, the subject is asked to grip the dynamometer at a level of 30% to 50% of his previously determined maximal voluntary contraction. Some coaching is usually required to insure that the patient sustains the grip. It is important that the patient not do a Valsalva maneuver during handgrip exercise, and the respiratory pattern should be closely observed. Valsalva maneuver may be avoided simply by engag-

---

*Jamar Adjustable Dynamometer, Asimow Engineering Company, Los Angeles, CA.

ing the patient in conversation during the test. We have employed 50% maximal voluntary contraction for 3 minutes, and begin repeat measurements of pressures and cardiac output at 2 minutes and 30 seconds, so that measurements are completed at 3 minutes and the test may be terminated.

The electrocardiogram should be monitored continuously, for the appearance of arrhythmias with isometric exercise has been observed. Although the appearance of significant arrhythmia would be reason to halt the test, this has not been a problem in our experience.

## ISOPROTERENOL STRESS TEST

The infusion of the beta-agonist isoproterenol has been advocated as an alternative to dynamic or isometric exercise in the catheterization laboratory for evaluation of hemodynamic reserve during stress. The cardiovascular responses to isoproterenol infusion in normal subjects are similar to those of dynamic exercise and include an increase in heart rate and left ventricular systolic pressure, a fall in systemic vascular resistance, an increase in cardiac output, and an increase in left ventricular ejection fraction with a reduction of end-systolic and end-diastolic volumes.[48] The increase in cardiac output is largely met by an increase in heart rate with minimal change in stroke volume; however, if heart rate is held constant, the increase in cardiac output is accomplished by an augmentation of stroke volume.[9] Similar changes are generally seen even in patients with severely depressed myocardial function unless regional ischemia is provoked due to the presence of coronary artery disease. Thus, isoproterenol has the disadvantage of producing directionally similar changes in hemodynamics in both normal patients and patients with heart disease which may obscure the detection of impaired cardiovascular reserve. Furthermore, we have found that even low doses of isoproterenol infusion are frequently associated with distress due to sweating, a sensation of anxiety, and disturbing "palpitations" due to marked tachycardia in the absence of exertion. For these reasons, we generally prefer the stresses of dynamic or isometric exercise.

# REFERENCES

1. Weiner DA: Normal hemodynamic, ventilatory, and metabolic response to exercise. Arch Intern Med 143:2173, 1983.
2. Felig P, Wahren J: Fuel homeostasis in exercise. N Engl J Med 293:1078, 1975.
3. Wasserman K: Breathing during exercise. N Engl J Med 298:780, 1978.
4. Dexter L, et al: Effects of exercise on circulatory dynamics of normal individuals. J Appl Physiol 3:439, 1951.
5. Donald KW, Bishop JM, Cumming G, Wade OL: The effect of exercise on the cardiac output and circulatory dynamics of normal subjects. Clin Sci 14:37, 1955.
6. Sonnenblick EH, Braunwald E, Williams JF Jr, Glick G: Effects of exercise on myocardial force-velocity relations in intact unanesthetized man. Relative roles of changes in heart rate, sympathetic activity, and ventricular dimensions. J Clin Invest 44:2051, 1965.
7. Braunwald E, Goldblatt A, Harrison D, Mason D: Studies on cardiac dimensions in intact, unanesthetized man. Circ Res 13:448, 1963.
8. Gorlin R, et al: Effect of supine exercise on left ventricular volume and oxygen consumption in man. Circulation 32:361, 1965.
9. Ross, J Jr, Linhart JW, Braunwald E: Effects of changing heart rate in man by electrical stimulation of the right atrium: studies at rest, during exercise, and with isoproterenol. Circulation 32:549, 1965.
10. Thadani U, Parker JO: Hemodynamics at rest and during supine and sitting bicycle exercise in normal subjects. Am J Cardiol 41:52, 1978.
11. Slutsky R: Response of the left ventricle to stress: effects of exercise, atrial pacing, afterload stress and drugs. Am J Cardiol 47:357, 1981.
12. Crawford M, White D, Amon K: Echocardiographic evaluation of left ventricular size and performance during hand-grip and supine and upright bicycle exercise. Circulation 59:1188, 1979.
13. Tebbe V, et al: Changes in left ventricular diastolic function in coronary artery disease with and without angina pectoris assessed from exercise ventriculography. Clin Cardiol 3:19, 1980.
14. Slutsky R, et al: Peak systolic blood pressure/end-systolic volume in normal subjects and patients with coronary heart disease. Assessment at rest and during exercise. Am J Cardiol 46:813, 1980.
15. Bevegard S, Holmgren A, Jonsson B: The effect of body position on the circulation at rest and during exercise with special reference to the influence on stroke volume. Acta Physiol Scand 49:279, 1960.
16. Wilson M: Left ventricular diameter, posture and exercise. Circ Res 11:90, 1962.
17. Rerych R, et al: Cardiac function at rest and during exercise in normals and patients with coronary heart disease. Ann Surg 187:449, 1978.
18. Braunwald E, Ross J Jr: The ventricular end-diastolic pressure: Appraisal of its value in the recognition of ventricular failure in man. Am J Med 34:147, 1963.
19. Ross J Jr, et al: Left ventricular performance during muscular exercise in patients with and without cardiac dysfunction. Circulation 34:597, 1966.
20. Rodeheffer RJ, et al: Exercise cardiac output is maintained with advancing age in healthy human subjects: cardiac dilatation and increased stroke volume compensate for a diminished heart rate. Circulation 69:203, 1984.
21. Port S, Cobb FR, Coleman RE, Jones RH: Effect of age on the response of the left ventricular ejection fraction to exercise. N Engl J Med 303:1133, 1980.
22. Kuramoto K, et al: Comparison of hemodynamic effects of exercise and isoproterenol infusion in normal young and old men. Jpn Cir J 43:71, 1979.
23. Lakatta EG: Age-related alterations in the cardiovascular response to adrenergic mediated stress. Fed Proc 39:3173, 1980.
24. Reybrouck T, Amery A, Billiet L: Hemodynamic response to graded exercise after chronic beta-adrenergic blockade. J Appl Physiol 42:133, 1977.
25. Battler A, et al: Improvement of exercise-induced left ventricular dysfunction with oral propranolol in patients with coronary heart disease. Am J Cardiol 44:318, 1979.
26. Port S, Cobb F, Jones R: Effects of propranolol on left ventricular function in normal men. Circulation 61:398, 1980.
27. Crawford M, Lindenfield J, O'Rourke R: Effects of oral propranolol on left ventricular size and performance during exercise and acute pressure loading. Circulation 61:549, 1980.
28. Parker JO, Di Georgi S, West RO: A hemodynamic study of acute coronary insufficiency precipitated by exercise. Am J Cardiol 17:470, 1966.
29. McAllister BD, et al: Left ventricular performance during mild supine leg exercise in coronary artery disease. Circulation 37:922, 1968.
30. Grossman W, Barry WH: Diastolic pressure-volume relations in the diseased heart. Fed Proc 1980:148.
31. Thadani U, West RO, Mathew TM, Parker JO: Hemodynamics at rest and during supine and sitting bicycle exercise in patients with coronary artery disease. Am J Cardiol 39:776, 1977.
32. Carroll JD, Hess OM, Hirzel HO, Krayenbuehl HP: Dynamics of left ventricular filling at rest and during exercise. Circulation 68:59, 1983.
33. Epstein SE, et al: Characterization of the circula-

tory response to maximal upright exercise in normal subjects and patients with heart disease. Circulation 35:1049, 1963.

34. Franciosa JA, Leddy CL, Wilen M, Schwartz DE: Relation between hemodynamic and ventilatory responses in determining exercise capacity in severe congestive heart failure. Am J Cardiol 53:127, 1984.

35. Bache RJ, Wang Y, Jorgenson CR: Hemodynamic effects of exercise in isolated valvular aortic stenosis. Circulation 44:1003, 1971.

36. Richardson JW, Anderson FL, Tsargaris TJ: Rest and exercise hemodynamic studies in patients with isolated aortic stenosis. Cardiology 64:1, 1979.

37. Webb P, Troutman SJ Jr: An instrument for continuous measurement of oxygen consumption. J Appl Physiol 28:867, 1970.

38. Lind AR, et al: Circulatory effects of sustained voluntary muscle contraction. Clin Sci 27:229, 1964.

39. Donald KW, et al: Cardiovascular responses to sustained (static) contractions. Circ Res 20 (Suppl. 1):15, 1967.

40. Freyschuss U: Cardiovascular adjustments to somatomotor activities. Acta Physiol Scand (Suppl)342, 1970.

41. MacDonald HR, Sapru RP, Taylor SH, Donald KW: Effect of intravenous propranolol on the systemic circulatory response to sustained handgrip. Am J Cardiol 18:333, 1966.

42. Grossman W, et al: Changes in the inotropic state of the left ventricle during isometric exercise. Br Heart J 35:697, 1973.

43. Helfant RH, deVilla MA, Meister SG: Effect of sustained isometric handgrip exercise on left ventricular performance. Circulation 44:982, 1971.

44. Kivowitz C, et al: Effects of isometric exercise on cardiac performance: the grip test. Circulation 44:994, 1971.

45. Flessas AP, Ryan TJ: Cardiovascular responses to isometric exercise in patients with mitral stenosis. Comparison with normal subjects and patients with depressed ejection fraction: Arch Intern Med 142:1629, 1982.

46. Flessas A, et al: Effects of isometric exercise on the end-diastolic pressure, volumes and function of the left ventricle in man. Circulation 53:839, 1976.

47. Krayenbuehl HP, Rutishauser W, Schoenbeck M, Amende I: Evaluation of left ventricular function from isovolumic pressure measurements during isometric exercise. Am J Cardiol 29:323, 1972.

48. Krasnow N, et al: Isoproterenol and cardiovascular performance. Am J Med 37:514, 1964.

*chapter eighteen*

# Hemodynamic Stress Testing Using Pacing Tachycardia

RAYMOND G. MCKAY *and* WILLIAM GROSSMAN

A TRIAL pacing was first introduced in 1967 by Sowton and co-workers[1] as a stress test which could be used in the cardiac catheterization laboratory to evaluate patients with ischemic heart disease. Sowton noted that artificially increasing the heart rate by pacing the right atrium could usually induce angina in patients with symptomatic coronary artery disease. Moreover, he found that the degree of pacing stress needed to produce ischemia, defined in terms of the pacing rate and duration, was more or less reproducible in any given patient. Since Sowton's original description, numerous investigators have described characteristic pacing-induced electrocardiographic changes,[2-7] derangements of myocardial lactate metabolism,[3-4] hemodynamic abnormalities,[8-18] regional wall abnormalities,[19-20] and defects in thallium scintigraphy.[21-24] Although agreement on the overall usefulness of atrial pacing has not been uniform, it is clear that the technique can safely and reliably induce ischemia in most patients with coronary artery disease and that information obtained during the pacing-induced ischemic state can often be helpful in the diagnosis and treatment of the patient's underlying disease.

## HEMODYNAMIC EFFECTS OF PACING TACHYCARDIA

The principal form of stress that accompanies pacing tachycardia is an increase in myocardial oxygen consumption secondary to the increased heart rate and to an increase in myocardial contractility because of a Treppe effect.[25] Associated with this increase in myocardial oxygen consumption is a reflex coronary vasodilatation with an increase in myocardial blood flow.[26] Apart from these changes in oxygen demand and supply, pacing tachycardia appears to be associated with no major hemodynamic stress, at least in patients with normal coronary arteries. Artificially increasing the heart rate by pacing the right atrium is accompanied by a concomitant decrease in ventricular stroke volume, with little or no overall change in cardiac output. Moreover, there appears to be no significant change in ventricular afterload, venous return, or circulating catecholamines during pacing tachycardia. The physiology of pacing is thus distinctly different from that of dynamic or isometric exercise, where there is not only an increase in heart rate and in myocardial contractility, but also major changes in ventricular loading conditions and cardiac output in response to increased metabolic demands from the periphery.

Because of the differences in physiology between atrial pacing and exercise, each technique has relative advantages and disadvantages as a form of stress testing in the catheterization laboratory. Unlike pacing, exercise is associated with an increase in both heart rate and systolic blood pressure. As a result, exercise is usually capable of achieving a higher rate-pressure product (i.e., heart rate × peak systolic pressure) and represents a more severe form of stress with higher increases in myocardial oxygen consumption. On the other hand, pacing is not associated with exercise-induced changes in cardiac output or ventricular loading conditions, and the characterization of ventricular function is subsequently easier. In addition, atrial pacing is superior to exercise for evaluating myocardial metabolic function, since the rapid rise in arterial lactate levels that accompanies exercise may obscure abnormal patterns of myocardial lactate metabolism. Finally, unlike exercise, with the termination of pacing and the rapid diminution of myocardial oxygen requirement, myocardial ischemia almost always resolves rapidly (e.g., within 1 to 2 minutes) in the immediate post-pacing period. As a result, the physician has slightly more control over the amount of stress that the patient experiences with very little chance of prolonged ischemia occurring in the post-stress period.

Pacing has been used as a form of stress testing in patients with heart disease for over 15 years. Although the technique has been most useful in the assessment of patients with coronary artery disease, there have been isolated reports on the utility of the technique in patients with other forms of cardiac disease including valvular heart disease and cardiomyopathy. This chapter will focus primarily on the pathophysiology of pacing-induced ischemia and will only briefly touch on the potential use of the method in evaluating patients with other forms of cardiac dysfunction.

## METHOD FOR A PACING STRESS TEST

Atrial pacing protocols can usually be conducted in the cardiac catheterization laboratory without undue prolongation of the routine catheterization procedure and without significant added risk to the patient. In our laboratory, pacing is conducted following the routine diagnostic aspects of catheterization and usually extends the procedure by no more than 15 to 30 minutes, depending upon the details of the protocol. It is important that detailed planning of the protocol be made before the catheterization is begun to help incorporate the atrial pacing into the

routine catheterization as much as possible without unnecessary repetition of maneuvers and undue prolongation of arterial time. Thus, if pacing is to be conducted with monitoring of right-sided pressure and cardiac output, then two sites of venous access may need to be obtained at the beginning of the catheterization before systemic heparinization is achieved. Likewise, if pacing is to be conducted with simultaneous monitoring of left ventricular pressures, then coronary angiography should be performed prior to left ventriculography so that the left heart catheter can be left in place following the contrast ventriculogram, rather than in the reverse order so that the left ventricular catheter needs to be reinserted for the atrial pacing protocol.

The type of pacing catheter used for the pacing protocol can vary depending upon the type of information that is to be evaluated during the pacing procedure. In general, the pacing catheter can either be unipolar or bipolar. If pacing is to be conducted with simultaneous myocardial metabolic assessment, then a Gorlin pacing catheter that provides simultaneous pacing and coronary sinus lactate sampling is ideal for placement in the coronary sinus. Similarly, if assessment of myocardial oxygen consumption is to be made, then a coronary sinus pacing catheter with the capability of measuring coronary blood flow, such as the Baim catheter (Elecath, Rahway, NJ), may be used. If pacing is to be conducted with simultaneous measurement of left heart filling pressures and cardiac output, then both a pacing catheter and a second right heart catheter (typically, a thermodilution flow-directed catheter) may be inserted into the right heart.

The pacing catheter may be inserted either by venous cutdown or by percutaneous technique from the groin, the antecubital fossa, or the neck. Use of a coronary sinus pacing catheter usually requires a neck or arm approach for easier access into the coronary sinus.

Perhaps the most critical part of the atrial pacing technique is proper placement of the pacing lead, since accidental displacement of the pacing tip during pacing can disrupt the protocol. The pacing lead can be placed either at the superior vena cava-right atrial junction, the lateral right atrial wall, or in the coronary sinus. Placement of the pacing lead is most stable either at the superior vena cava-right atrial junction or in the coronary sinus, since displacement of the lead commonly occurs from the lateral atrial wall during spontaneous respiration. Stimulation on the phrenic nerve with subsequent diaphragmatic stimulation also occurs commonly with placement of the catheter against the lateral atrial wall. In our laboratory, to avoid problems with displacement of the pacing tip, a bipolar flared pacing catheter is used (Atri-pace I, Mansfield Scientific, Mansfield, MA). As shown in Figure 18-1, this catheter has two pacing leads that flare out in a V shape. At any given time at least one of the tips is in contact with the atrial wall and therefore disruption of the pacing due to respiration or the patient's motion is extremely unlikely.

Once the pacing catheter is positioned in the right atrium, it is connected to the pulse generator unit. This unit should be capable of a fixed rate mode, pacing at least to rates of 170 beats per minute, and a variable output from 0.5 to 10 milliamperes. Bipolar pacing catheters may be connected directly to the pacemaker unit or attached through extension wires with alligator clamps. Unipolar catheters should have their negative pole grounded to the skin using either a needle electrode or standard electrocardiographic plates.

Once the pacing catheter had been positioned properly and connected to the pulse generator, the ability of the pacemaker to stimulate the atrium and to control ventricular rate should be assessed. Initially, the output of the generator is set at 2 to 3 milliamperes, and the pacing rate is adjusted to 10 beats above the sinus rate. Pacing is then begun, and if there is ventricular capture, the pacing rate is increased by ten beats per minute every 5 seconds until a rate of 150 to 160 beats per minute is reached. Inadequate pacing may be secondary to an inadequate output of the pulse generator, improper lead positioning, or to the development of atrioventricular block. The output of the pulse generator may be increased, but in general stimulating energies in excess of 7 to 8 milliamperes frequently results in painful phrenic nerve stimulation. If excessively high energies are required for capture, the electrode lead should be repositioned. If atrioventricular block develops at higher stimulatory rates, 1 mg of intravenous atropine may be administered: this generally insures adequate atrioventricular conduction up to rates $\geq 140$ beats/minute.

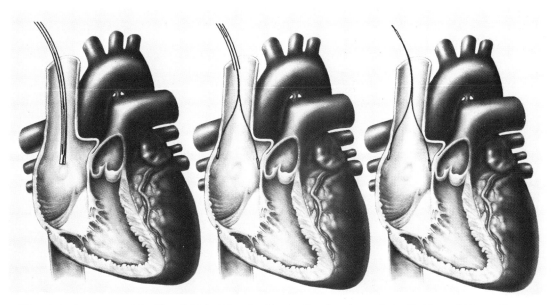

**Fig. 18-1.** Placement of the Mansfield Atri-Pace I, a bipolar flared pacing catheter that is useful for performing pacing stress tests. Stability of electrical capture is a strong point of this catheter.

Following proper lead positioning and an adequate trial of pacing to assess capture, the actual pacing protocol may be done. In our laboratory, a pacing stress test is usually begun approximately 20 beats per minute above the baseline rate, with increases in the pacing rate by 20 beats per minute every 2 minutes, until angina pectoris or characteristic hemodynamic alteration occurs or until 85% of maximum age-predicted heart rate is achieved. Placement of a thermodilution balloon-tip flow-directed catheter, a left heart catheter, and a radial arterial cannula prior to pacing allows for simultaneous assessment of right and left heart pressures, cardiac output measurement by thermodilution and/or Fick method, and determination of systemic and pulmonary vascular resistances. Assessment of left ventricular volumes may also be accomplished with standard angiographic, echocardiographic, or radionuclide techniques.

Following the induction of chest pain during pacing tachycardia, pacing may be continued at the same heart rate safely for up to 3 to 5 minutes, during which hemodynamic, metabolic, and electrocardiographic data may be obtained. Following the cessation of pacing, chest pain usually resolves quickly but may occasionally persist for up to 1 to 2 minutes following the return to sinus rhythm.

## PACING-INDUCED ANGINA

Initial reports on the use of atrial pacing suggested that pacing-induced angina was a sensitive marker for the presence of ischemic heart disease and could serve as a suitable ischemic endpoint of pacing protocols.[1] Specifically, the induction of angina was thought to mark a highly reproducible anginal threshold defined in terms of the pacing rate and duration. Subsequent investigators have found, however, that chest pain is neither a sensitive nor a specific indicator of the presence of coronary artery disease. Robson et al,[6] for example, demonstrated that chest pain could be elicited in 80% of patients with normal coronary arteries if they were paced at extremely high rates (in excess of 180 beats per minute). Moreover, Chandraratna[27] and others[7] have demonstrated the absence

of angina in patients with coronary artery disease who were stressed with pacing tachycardia at a significantly high rate. Similarly, in terms of defining anginal threshold according to the pacing rate and duration, as many as 20% of individuals have been shown to have considerable variation in these parameters.[28] In view of these results, it is clear that chest pain alone should not be used as a reliable marker for the presence of pacing-induced ischemia. Improved sensitivity and specificity of pacing-induced chest pain, however, are noted when additional evidence of ischemia such as pacing-induced electrocardiographic changes or myocardial metabolic abnormalities are noted.

## ELECTROCARDIOGRAPHIC CHANGES IN RESPONSE TO A PACING STRESS TEST

Like pacing-induced angina, the presence of ischemic ST segment depression during pacing tachycardia has not been previously regarded as a sensitive or specific marker for the presence of coronary artery disease. For example, in terms of sensitivity, Rios and Hurwitz compared pacing tachycardia and exercise in 50 patients and found diagnostic EKG changes with pacing in only 20% of patients in comparison to 83% of patients with exercise.[5] Similarly, in terms of specificity, Robson reported ST segment depression of 1.5 mm or more during pacing tachycardia in as many as 80% of patients with normal coronary arteries.[6] In addition to poor overall sensitivity and specificity, pacing tachycardia is associated with certain distortions of the electrocardiogram that sometimes make interpretation of ischemic ST segment changes difficult or impossible. Pacing is associated with prolongation of the PR interval in most patients and extreme prolongation of this interval can cause the pacemaker spike to fall within the ST segment of the preceding paced complex and thus obscure potential ST segment changes.

In spite of the previously reported poor utility of pacing-induced EKG changes, recent work from our laboratory has suggested an improved sensitivity and specificity of ischemic ST segment depression during pacing tachycardia *if certain technical guide-*

*lines of the pacing protocol are followed.*[7] Several earlier pacing trials that reported a low sensitivity of pacing EKG changes used only limited three-lead recording, and it is clear, at least with standard exercise testing, that sensitivity can be improved with full twelve-lead monitoring.[29,30] Other pacing trials reporting low sensitivity have used the induction of chest pain as an endpoint for the pacing stimulus; as previously mentioned, chest pain alone is not a reliable marker for pacing-induced ischemia. In terms of poor specificity, it is notable that pacing trials that have reported the presence of ST segment depression in patients with normal coronary arteries reported these changes at very high pacing rates, in excess of 180 beats per minute.

To re-evaluate the potential utility of pacing-induced EKG changes, pacing trials at our institution are conducted using the following guidelines. *First*, a twelve lead EKG is used for monitoring, and the EKG is regarded as positive for myocardial ischemia if at least 1 mm or more of horizontal or downsloping ST segment depression is produced. *Second*, pacing tachycardia is terminated when 85% of maximal age-predicted heart rate is achieved or when typical ischemic chest pain is accompanied by diagnostic EKG changes. *Finally*, if severe prolongation of the PR interval distorts the preceding ST segment changes, the EKG is considered positive for ischemia only if there is ST segment depression in the first 5 beats following the discontinuation of the pacing stimulus.

Using these guidelines, actual pacing protocols conducted at our institution have had an overall sensitivity and specificity of 94% and 83%, respectively, with regard to pacing-induced electrocardiographic changes. In addition, distortion of the ST segment by the pacing stimulus because of marked prolongation of the PR interval appears to occur infrequently when the peak pacing rate is no higher than 85% of the maximum age predicted heart rate. Moreover, in at least one subgroup of patients who were tested with both atrial pacing and standard treadmill exercise,[7] the concordance between pacing-induced and exercise-induced electrocardiographic changes was 90%. Examples of pacing-induced and exercise-induced electrocardiographic changes are shown for a patient with normal coronary arteries in Figure 18-2A and for a patient with coronary artery disease in Figure 18-2B.

## MYOCARDIAL METABOLIC CHANGES INDUCED BY A PACING STRESS TEST

Abnormal myocardial metabolism has been documented during pacing-induced ischemia by means of coronary sinus sampling and the subsequent measurement of coronary arterial and venous blood lactate. Since lactate production is a by-product of anaerobic glycolysis, its production by the heart and appearance within the coronary sinus is a sign of myocardial ischemia. Previous investigators have noted rapid increases in coronary sinus lactate during pacing tachycardia in patients with coronary artery disease, often before the appearance of angina.[3,4] On the cessation of pacing, the elevated coronary sinus lactates fall in an exponential manner, representing a washout of the accumulated myocardial lactate and diminished lactate production as normal oxygenation is restored. Monitoring of arterial lactate levels while coronary sinus lactate levels are rising usually shows little or no elevation, in marked contrast to arterial lactate levels during exercise. As a result, atrial pacing is superior to exercise for evaluating abnormal myocardial metabolic function, since rapidly rising arterial lactate levels during exercise may obscure abnormal patterns of myocardial lactate metabolism.

Monitoring of coronary sinus lactate during pacing protocols is most easily accomplished with a Gorlin pacing catheter. Placement of the Gorlin catheter in the coronary sinus can usually be confirmed by injection of a small amount of contrast medium. Care must be taken not to perforate either the coronary sinus or the great cardiac vein, as well as not to place the pacing tip of the catheter too distally, since placement of the distal catheter into the great cardiac vein may result in ventricular rather than atrial pacing.

Arterial and coronary venous blood lactate concentrations in response to a pacing stress test are illustrated in Figure 18-3. As can be seen, in the control state the concentration of coronary sinus blood lactate is lower than

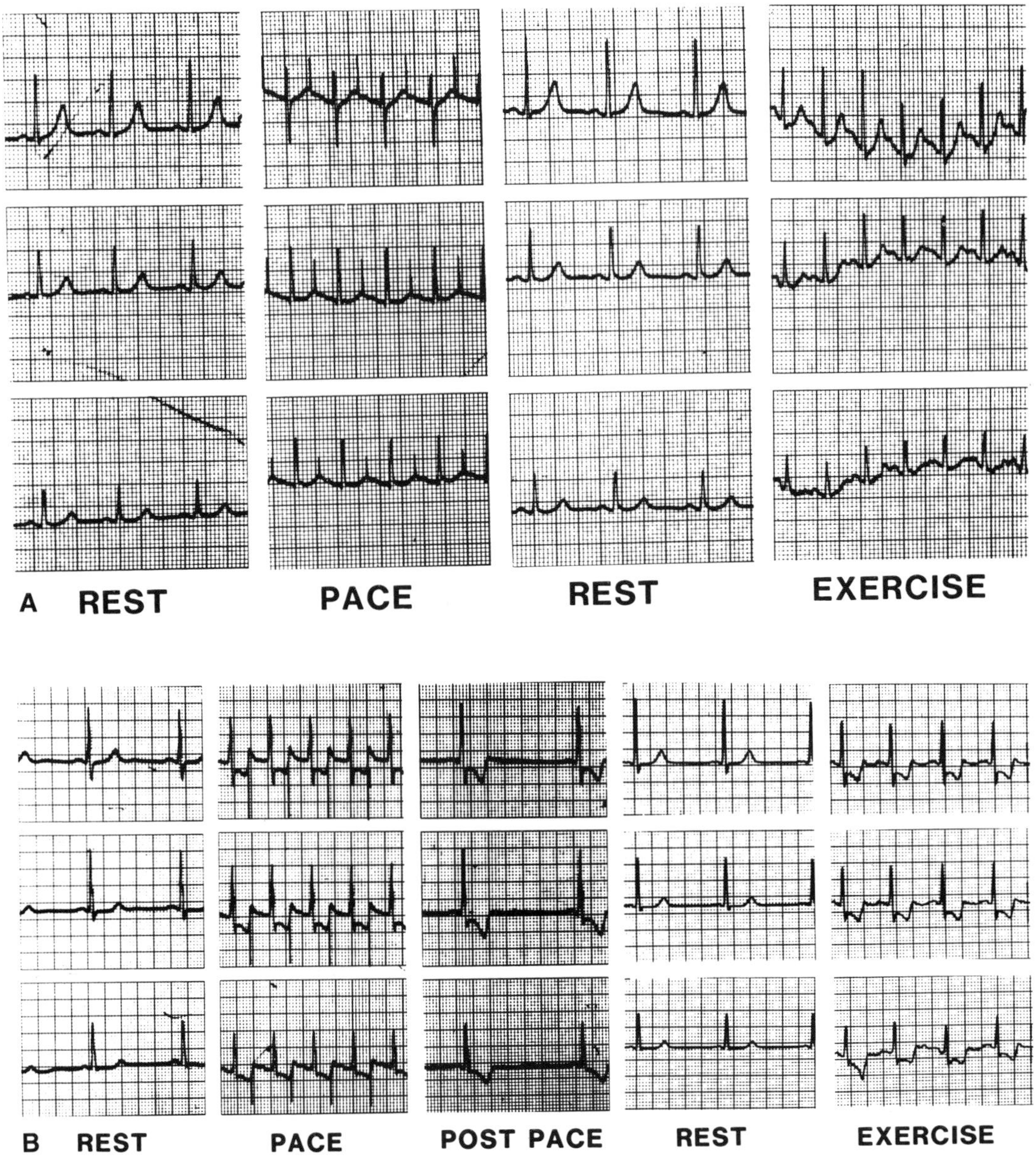

**Fig. 18-2.** (A) Electrocardiographic response to atrial pacing and exercise stress in a man with normal coronary arteries. From top to bottom, leads V4, V5, and V6 are monitored. (B) Comparison of electrocardiographic response to atrial pacing and exercise stress in a man with severe three-vessel coronary artery disease. Leads V4, V5, and V6 are monitored (top to bottom) as in A. ST depression occurs to the same degree with both types of stress. (Reprinted with permission from Heller GV, et al: The pacing stress test: a reexamination of the relation between coronary artery disease and pacing induced electrocardiographic changes. Am J Cardiol (54:50, 1984.)

lactate concentration in arterial blood, reflecting the fact that the heart normally consumes lactate as a fuel. During pacing tachycardia, coronary sinus blood lactate concentration rises progressively and exceeds arterial blood lactate concentration, reflecting a shift to anaerobic metabolism of the ischemic myocardium. The lactate falls rapidly after discontinuation of pacing, since the heart rate returns to control immediately.

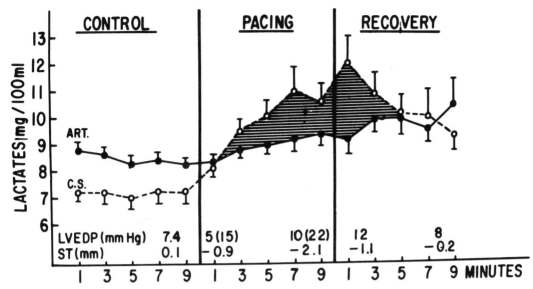

**Fig. 18-3.** Mean values for arterial (ART.) and coronary sinus (C.S.) blood lactate concentrate before (control), during and after pacing tachycardia in 17 patients with coronary artery disease. Left ventricular end-diastolic pressure (LVEDP) changes little during pacing tachycardia, but is elevated during brief periods of interruption of pacing (values in parentheses). ST segment depression developed progressively during pacing tachycardia and resolved in recovery. Lactate extraction shifted to lactate production during ischemia, and this persisted into recovery for a brief period. (Reproduced with permission from Parker JO, Chiong MA, West RO, Case RB: Sequential alterations in myocardial lactate metabolism, S-T segments, and left ventricular function during angina induced by atrial pacing. Circulation 40:113, 1969.)

## HEMODYNAMIC CHANGES DURING A PACING STRESS TEST

Previous investigators have described hemodynamic alterations associated with the pacing-induced ischemic state and have contrasted the hemodynamic changes seen in patients with normal coronary arteries with those observed in patients with significant coronary obstructive disease.[8-18]

Patients without ischemic heart disease who are stressed by atrial-paced tachycardia generally demonstrate no significant change in cardiac output, mean arterial pressure, arteriovenous oxygen difference, and systemic vascular resistance. Left ventricular end-diastolic pressure and pulmonary capillary wedge pressure generally fall during pacing tachycardia and then return toward prepacing baseline levels in the immediate post pacing period. Left ventricular end-diastolic and end-systolic volumes fall during pacing tachycardia with a decrease in stroke volume and no significant change in ejection fraction.

Patients with coronary artery disease who are paced to ischemia likewise manifest no significant change in cardiac output, mean arterial pressure, arteriovenous oxygen difference, or systemic vascular resistance. Some investigators have documented slight decreases in cardiac output with slight increases in mean arterial pressure, arterial venous oxygen difference and system resistance. These differences, however, probably are related to the intensity of pacing-induced ischemia, its duration before the measurement of hemodynamic variables, and the amount of myocardium that has become ischemic, with more extensive hemodynamic abnormalities occurring in the setting of more extensive myocardial ischemia. The most dramatic differences in pacing hemodynamics between patients with normal coronary arteries and those with coronary artery disease are seen in terms of left ventricular pressure-volume relationships during pacing tachycardia and in the immediate post-pacing period. Of note, left ventricular filling pressures do not show the progressive decrease seen in nonischemic patients, and elevations in pulmonary capillary wedge, mean pulmonary artery, and occasionally left ventricular end-diastolic pressure occur at maximum pacing. Most important, there is an abrupt rise in left ventricular end-diastolic pressure in the immediate post-pacing period. Similarly, ventricular end-diastolic and end-systolic volumes decrease less during pacing-induced tachycardia in patients with ischemic heart disease in comparison to normal subjects, and there is often a significant decrease in left-ventricular ejection fraction.

A recent study looking at pressure-volume relationships during pacing tachycardia conducted at our institution illustrates well the differences between nonischemic and ischemic hemodynamic responses to pacing.[31] In this study, 22 patients, including 11 patients with normal coronary arteries and 11 patients with significant coronary artery disease, underwent sequential atrial pacing with simultaneous monitoring of left ventricular pressure and ventricular volume measured from gated radionuclide ventriculography. Using synchronized left ventricular pressure tracings and radionuclide time-activity volume curves, three sequential pressure-volume diagrams were constructed for each patient corresponding to baseline, intermediate, and maximum pacing levels. All 11 pa-

tients with coronary artery disease demonstrated angina and significant ST segment depression at maximum pacing, but none of the 11 patients with normal coronary arteries showed any evidence of pacing-induced ischemia.

Figure 18-4 shows typical left ventricular pressure-volume curves for a patient with normal coronary arteries, stressed with pacing tachycardia. Notably, there is a progressive leftward shift for the loop with an increased heart rate and a progressive downward shift in the left ventricular diastolic pressure-volume limb of each pressure-volume curve. It is clear that changes in both systolic and diastolic function have occurred in these patients during pacing tachycardia. In terms of systolic function, the progressive leftward shift of the end-systolic portion of the loop presumably represents increased contractility secondary to a Treppe effect. Other investigators have likewise demonstrated a positive inotropic stimulus with increased heart rate, with increases in isovolumetric contraction indices (e.g., dP/dt) and ejection phase indices (e.g., circumferential fiber shortening) during pacing tachycardia.[25] With respect to diastolic function the progressive downward shift of the diastolic limbs in Figure 18-4 suggests that left ventricular distensibility has in-

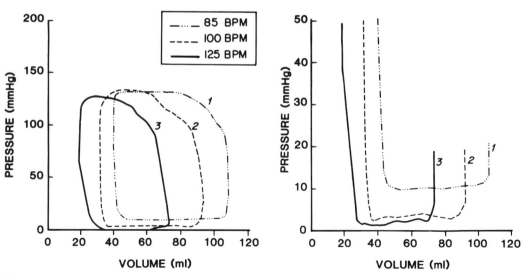

**Fig. 18-4.** Sequential left ventricular pressure-volume diagrams in a patient with normal coronary arteries in response to atrial pacing tachycardia at 3 increasing heart rates. See text for discussion. (Reproduced with permission from Aroesty JM, et al: Simultaneous assessment of left ventricular systolic and diastolic dysfunction during pacing-induced ischemia. Circulation 71:889, 1985.)

creased slightly during pacing tachycardia. Whether this downward shift is related to an increase in myocardial relaxation, an alteration in viscoelastic properties, or a change in factors extrinsic to the myocardium (e.g., right ventricle, pericardium) is not known. It is notable that some investigators have documented mild chronotropic increases in markers of diastolic relaxation such as peak negative dP/dt[32] and the time constant tau[33] in animals, and more recently the peak rate of posterior wall thinning[34] and left ventricular internal dimension change[35] in man.

In comparison to Figure 18-4, Figure 18-5 shows sequential left ventricular pressure-volume diagrams for a patient with coronary artery disease who was paced to ischemia. All patients in our study who developed chest pain and ischemic EKG changes demonstrated a similar pressure-volume pattern with an initial shift of the pressure-volume loop to the left at an intermediate heart rate, followed by a rightward shift at peak pacing when ischemia developed. In terms of systolic function, it is clear that pacing resulted in an initial Treppe effect with a leftward shift of the end systolic portion of the diagram at intermediate pacing, followed by systolic failure at peak pacing with an increase in ventricular volumes and a right-

ward shift in the end-systolic portion of the curve. Similarly, in terms of diastolic function, it is evident that the patient did not show a progressive downward shift of the diastolic limb of the left ventricular pressure-volume curve but actually experienced an upward shift at intermediate and peak pacing. In part the increase in LVEDP at peak pacing is related to systolic failure at peak pacing with an increase in ventricular volume. However, since the patient did not experience evidence of systolic failure at the intermediate pacing level, it is also clear that this patient has experienced a primary decrease in left ventricular diastolic distensibility so that pressure is higher at any given chamber volume throughout diastole.

Speculation has continued over the last two decades as to whether the increase in diastolic pressures during pacing-induced ischemia is related to a primary decrease in distensibility or is secondary to systolic failure with increases in ventricular volume. At present, it seems clear that both mechanisms play some role in the elevated diastolic pressures. Recent evidence suggests that changes in diastolic distensibility actually precede altered systolic function.[31]

The cause of the altered diastolic distensibility during pacing-induced ischemia has

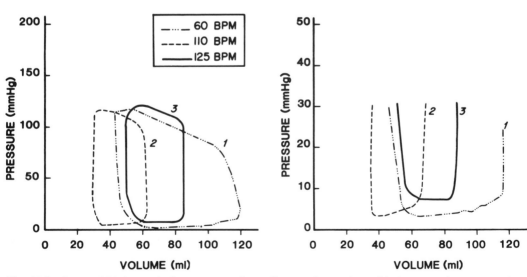

**Fig. 18-5.** Sequential left ventricular pressure-volume diagrams in a patient with three-vessel coronary artery disease who was paced at 3 increasing heart rates. The patient developed angina and ischemic S-T depression at peak pacing. See text for discussion. (Reproduced with permission from Aroesty, JM, et al.: Simultaneous assessment of left ventricular systolic and diastolic dysfunction during pacing-induced ischemia. Circulation 71:889, 1985).

been debated, and a number of different mechanisms[14–16, 36–37] have been proposed, including incomplete myocardial relaxation, altered diastolic tone, partial ischemic contracture of some myofibrils within the distribution of the stenotic or occluded coronary artery, altered right ventricular loading, and influence of the pericardium. At the present, it seems likely that relaxation of myocardial cells within the reversibly ischemic region is slowed and does not proceed to completion by end diastole.[37] This may be related to impaired diastolic calcium sequestration by sarcoplasmic reticulum, but data are insufficient to permit a firm conclusion.

The post-pacing rise in left ventricular end-diastolic pressure is perhaps the most concrete evidence of pacing-induced ischemia during atrial pacing protocols. In our laboratory this post-pacing rise is calculated on beats number 5 through 15 after discontinuation of pacing, with greater than a 5 mmHg increase in LVEDP in comparison to the prepacing baseline being considered abnormal. Figure 18-6 shows a typical post-pacing rise in LVEDP in a patient who experienced angina. Figures 18-7 and 18-8

summarize hemodynamic changes in patients with normal coronary arteries and those with ischemic heart disease in response to a pacing stress test.

## REGIONAL WALL MOTION ABNORMALITIES DURING A PACING STRESS TEST

Regional wall motion abnormalities during pacing-induced ischemia have been noted both with contrast ventriculography and gated radionuclide ventriculography. Using contrast ventriculography, Dwyer studied 8 patients with coronary artery disease who were paced to angina and found that three developed regional hypokinesis in one area, while the remaining five developed at least two separate areas of hypokinesis or akinesis.[19] In all cases, an associated coronary artery lesion could be identified in the vessel that supplied the area of the new regional wall motion abnormality. Similarly, Tzivoni et al using radionuclide ventriculography found that 9 out of 11 patients devel-

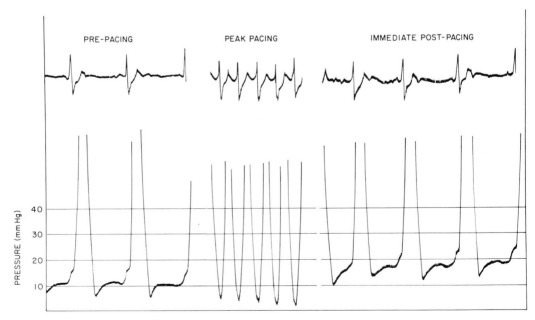

**Fig. 18-6.** Left ventricular end-diastolic pressure during atrial pacing tachycardia and in the immediate postpacing period. Left ventricular end-diastolic pressure increases substantially with resumption of sinus rhythm in this patient with coronary artery disease, who developed myocardial ischemia in response to pacing-induced tachycardia.

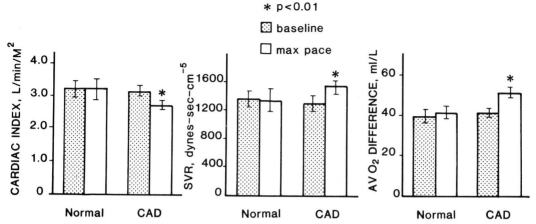

**Fig. 18-7.** Changes in cardiac index, systemic vascular resistance (SVR), and arteriovenous oxygen difference (AVO$_2$) in 5 patients with normal coronary arteries and 20 patients with coronary artery disease during pacing tachycardia. Patients with coronary disease showed a significant decrease in cardiac index and increase in SVR and AVO$_2$ difference during maximum pacing tachycardia. (Reprinted with permission from McKay RG, et al: The pacing stress test reexamined: Correlation of pacing-induced hemodynamic changes with the amount of myocardium at risk. J Am Coll Cardiol 3:1469, 1984.)

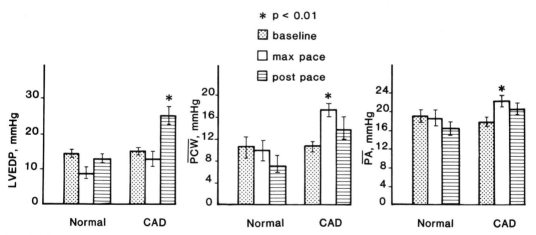

**Fig. 18-8.** Changes in left ventricular end-diastolic pressure (LVEDP), mean pulmonary capillary wedge pressure (PCW), and mean pulmonary artery pressure (PA) in 5 patients with normal coronary arteries and 20 patients with coronary artery disease during maximum pacing tachycardia and immediately after pacing. Patients with coronary disease showed significant elevation of PA and PCW at maximum pacing, and of LVEDP immediately after pacing. (Reprinted with permission from McKay RG, et al: The pacing stress test reexamined: Correlation of pacing-induced hemodynamic changes with the amount of myocardium at risk. J Am Coll Cardiol 3:1469, 1984.)

oped new regional wall motion abnormalities in response to pacing-induced ischemia.[20] However, the overall specificity and sensitivity of pacing-induced regional wall motion abnormalities have not been documented.

## THALLIUM SCINTIGRAPHY AND THE PACING STRESS TEST

A recent development that has improved the overall utility of atrial pacing as a stress test has been the incorporation of thallium scintigraphy into pacing protocols. In patients with normal coronary arteries, pacing tachycardia is associated with a homogeneous increase in myocardial oxygen consumption and a secondary increase in coronary blood flow. In patients with coronary artery disease, however, regional increases in myocardial blood flow may be limited by critical coronary stenoses. Since initial myocardial uptake of thallium-201 has been shown to reflect myocardial perfusion, myocardial ischemia induced by pacing tachycardia should theoretically be detectable by thallium scintigraphy. Although early reports on the simultaneous use of atrial pacing and thallium scintigraphy suggested serious limitations,[20,21] recent studies indicate that with appropriate methodology this approach is successful in detecting both reversible ischemia and infarcted myocardium.[22–24] For example, Weiss et al have reported an overall sensitivity of 100% of atrial pacing protocols utilizing thallium scintigraphy for detection of significant coronary stenoses.[22] Moreover, the authors noted that the technique could accurately demonstrate the site, extent, and severity of coronary artery disease.

To assess further the utility of combined atrial pacing and thallium scintigraphy, our laboratory has examined the correlation between pacing-induced and exercise-induced thallium defects in patients referred for evaluation of chest pain.[23] The overall sensitivity and specificity of thallium imaging after atrial pacing were excellent. Moreover, segment by segment comparison of the thallium scans after either pacing or exercise stress testing revealed a correlation of 83%.

Simultaneous use of thallium scintigraphy and atrial pacing tachycardia is accomplished in our laboratory by injection of 1.5 to 2.0 mCi of thallium-201 at peak pacing followed by continued pacing for at least an additional 5 minutes. In routine thallium-exercise testing, exercise is maintained for only 30 to 60 seconds after the injection of the radionuclide to allow the thallium to reach the myocardium. However, because of the rapid decrease in heart rate after the discontinuation of pacing and the subsequent rapid diminution of myocardial oxygen requirements, pacing is extended to 5 minutes. Following discontinuation of the pacing stimulus, while the patient is in the supine position, standard anterior, 40-degree left anterior oblique and 70-degree left anterior

oblique views are obtained immediately in the catheterization laboratory with a mobile scintillation camera. Repeat standard views are subsequently obtained 4 hours after the termination of the pacing protocol.

Figure 18-9 shows the arterial blood thallium activity curve obtained in patients during pacing tachycardia and the first 15 minutes after the discontinuation of pacing. The arterial activity is highest during the first minute after injection and decreases to approximately one tenth of the peak level within 5 minutes. The highest blood activity of thallium thus occurs well within the 5-minute pacing period following injection.

Figures 18-10, 18-11, and 18-12 show examples of pacing thallium scans in a patient with normal coronary arteries and in patients with coronary artery disease.

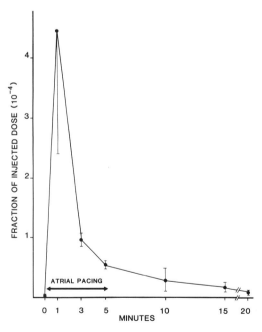

**Fig. 18-9.** Fraction of injected dose of thallium-201 in the arterial blood as a function of time after injection in 7 patients stressed with pacing tachycardia. Pacing was continued for the first 5 minutes of the sample collections. By 5 minutes, the arterial activity decreases to less than one tenth of the peak value. (Reprinted with permission from Heller GV, et al: The pacing stress test: thallium-201 myocardial imaging after atrial pacing. J Am Coll Cardiol 3:1197, 1984).

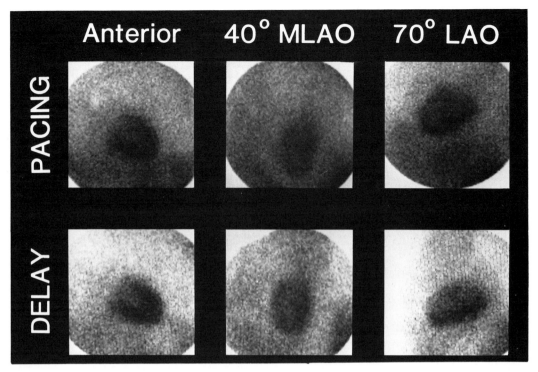

**Fig. 18-10.** Thallium scan during a pacing stress test in a patient with normal coronary arteries who was paced to a heart rate of 160 beats per minute. The patient did not develop chest pain or electrocardiographic changes. The thallium scintigram during pacing is identical with that at 4 hours later (Delay).

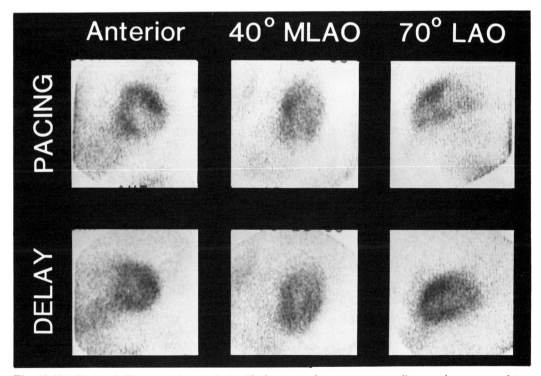

**Fig. 18-11.** Pacing thallium scan in a patient with three-vessel coronary artery disease who was paced to a heart rate of 150 beats per minute and who developed angina and electrocardiographic changes of ischemia. Scans show an inferoapical thallium defect which fills in 4 hours later (Delay).

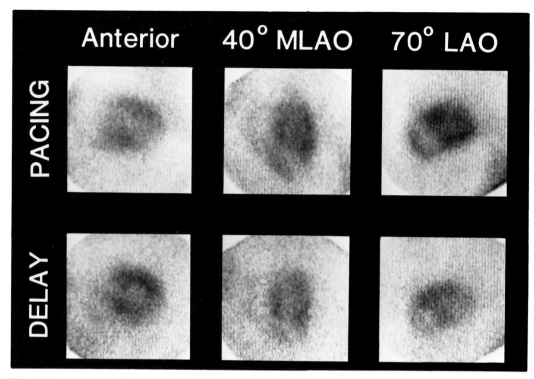

**Fig. 18-12.** Pacing thallium scan in a patient with a prior apical infarction who was paced to a heart rate of 150 beats per minute. The patient did not develop chest pain or electrocardiographic changes at maximum pacing. The scans show a fixed apical defect.

## CLINICAL USES OF ATRIAL PACING

The complete evaluation of a patient's cardiac function in the catheterization laboratory often requires an examination of the patient's performance under stressed conditions when electrocardiographic, metabolic, and hemodynamic abnormalities may manifest themselves fully. The role of stress testing is particularly important in the evaluation of patients with ischemic heart disease where, for example, it is often necessary to determine a patient's anginal threshold, the magnitude of hemodynamic impairment during ischemia, the efficacy of antianginal therapy, and a need for intervention therapy such as percutaneous coronary angioplasty or coronary bypass surgery. While standard dynamic and isometric exercise may serve as a form of stress for many patients, not all patients are able to exercise because of physical disabilities, old age, pulmonary disease, peripheral vascular disease, and possibly beta blockade. In each of these situations, atrial pacing may be used as a suitable form of stress.

## REFERENCES

1. Sowton GE, Balcon R, Cross D, Frick MH: Measurement of the angina threshold using atrial pacing. Cardiovasc Res 1:301, 1967.
2. Lau SH, et al: Controlled heart rate by atrial pacing in angina pectoris: a determinant of electrocardiographic S-T depressions. Circulation 38:711, 1968.
3. Parker JO, Chiong MA, West RO, Case RB: Sequential alterations in myocardial lactate metabolism, S-T segments, and left ventricular function during angina induced by atrial pacing. Circulation 40:113, 1969.
4. Helfant RH, et al: Differential hemodynamic, metabolic, and electrocardiographic effects in sub-

jects with and without angina pectoris during atrial pacing. Circulation 42:601, 1970.

5. Rios JC, Hurwitz LE: Electrocardiographic responses to atrial pacing and multistage treadmill exercise testing. Correlation with coronary anatomy. Am J Cardiol 34:986, 1976.

6. Robson RH, Pridie R, Fluck DC: Evaluation of rapid atrial pacing in diagnosis of coronary artery disease. Evaluation of atrial pacing test. Br Heart J 38:986, 1976.

7. Heller GV, et al: The pacing stress test: a reexamination of the relation between coronary artery disease and pacing induced electrocardiographic changes. Am J Cardiol 54:50, 1984.

8. Parker JO, Ledwich JR, West RO, Case RB: Reversible cardiac failure during angina pectoris. Circulation 34:745, 1969.

9. Linhart JW, Hildner FJ, Barold SS: Left heart hemodynamics during angina pectoris induced by atrial pacing. Circulation 40:483, 1969.

10. Khaja F, et al: Assessment of ventricular function in coronary artery disease by means of atrial pacing and exercise. Am J Cardiol 26:107, 1970.

11. Parker JO, Khaja F, Case RB: Analysis of left ventricular function by atrial pacing. Circulation 43:241, 1971.

12. McCans JL, Parker JO: Left ventricular pressure-volume relationships during myocardial ischemia in man. Circulation 48:775, 1973.

13. McLaurin LP, Rolett EL, Grossman W: Impaired left ventricular relaxation during pacing induced ischemia. Am J Cardiol 32:751, 1973.

14. Mann T, Brodie BR, Grossman W, McLaurin LP: Effect of angina on the left ventricular diastolic pressure-volume relationship. Circulation 55:761, 1977.

15. Barry WH, Brooker JZ, Alderman EL, Harrison DC: Changes in diastolic stiffness and tone of the left ventricle during angina pectoris. Circulation 49:225, 1974.

16. Mann T, Goldberg S, Mudge GH, Grossman W: Factors contributing to altered left ventricular diastolic properties during angina pectoris. Circulation 59:14, 1979.

17. Thadani U, et al: Clinical hemodynamic and metabolic responses during pacing in the supine and sitting postures in patients with angina pectoris. Am J Cardiol 44:249, 1979.

18. Slutsky R: Response of the left ventricle to stress: effects of exercise, atrial pacing, afterload stress and drugs. Am J Cardiol 47:357, 1981.

19. Dwyer EM: Left ventricular pressure-volume alterations and regional disorders of contraction during myocardial ischemia induced by atrial pacing. Circulation 42:1111, 1970.

20. Tzivoni D, et al: Diagnosis of coronary artery disease by multi-gated radionuclide angiography during right atrial pacing. Chest 80:562, 1981.

21. Vrobel TR, et al: Insensitivity of thallium 201 imaging in detecting pacing-induced myocardial ischemia (abstr.). Circulation 59 (suppl II):II, 1979.

22. Weiss AT, et al: Atrial pacing thallium scintigraphy in the evaluation of coronary artery disease. Isr J Med Sci 19:495, 1983.

23. Heller GV, et al: The pacing stress test: thallium-201 myocardial imaging after atrial pacing. J Am Coll Cardiol 3:1197, 1984.

24. McKay RG, et al: The pacing stress test reexamined: Correlation of pacing-induced hemodynamic changes with the amount of myocardium at risk. J Am Coll Cardiol 3:1469, 1984.

25. Ricci D, Orlick A, Alderman E: Role of tachycardia as an inotropic stimulus in man. J Clin Invest 63:695, 1979.

26. Holmberg S, Varnauskas E: Coronary circulation during pacing-induced tachycardia. Acta Med Scand 190:491, 1971.

27. Chandraratna PAN, et al: Spectrum of hemodynamic responses to atrial pacing in coronary artery disease. Br Heart J 35:1033, 1973.

28. Thadani U, et al: Are the clinical and hemodynamic events during pacing in patients with angina reproducible? Circulation 60:1036, 1979.

29. Chaitman BR, et al: Improved efficiency of treadmill exercise testing using multiple lead ECG system and basic hemodynamic exercise response. Circulation 57:71, 1978.

30. Chaitman BR, et al: The importance of clinical subsets in interpreting maximal treadmill exercise test results: the role of multiple lead ECG systems. Circulation 59:560, 1979.

31. Aroesty JM, et al: Simultaneous assessment of left ventricular systolic and diastolic dysfunction during pacing-induced ischemia. Circulation 71:889, 1985.

32. Karliner JS, et al: Pharmacological and hemodynamic influeneces on the rate of isovolumetric left ventricular relaxation in the conscious dog. J Clin Invest 60:511, 1977.

33. Weiss JL, Fredericksen JW, Weisfeldt ML: Hemodynamic determinants of the time-course of fall in canine left ventricular pressure. J Clin Invest 58:751, 1976.

34. Fifer MA, Borow KM, Colan S, Lorell BH: Left ventricular diastolic filling; contributions of heart rate, age, and extent of systolic shortening. Circulation 68 (III): III, 1983.

35. Bahler RC, Vrobel TR, Martin P: The relation of heart rate and shortening fraction to echocardiographic indexes of left ventricular relaxation in normal subjects. J Am Coll Card 2:926, 1983.

36. Grossman W, Barry WH: Diastolic pressure-volume relationship in the diseased heart. Fed Proc 39:148, 1980.

37. Sasayama et al: Changes in diastolic properties of the regional myocardium during pacing-induced ischemia in human subjects. J Am Coll Cardiol 5:599, 1985.

## chapter nineteen

# Measurement of Ventricular Volumes, Ejection Fraction, Mass, and Wall Stress

MICHAEL A. FIFER *and* WILLIAM GROSSMAN

ARDIAC angiography was introduced initially to provide qualitative information regarding anatomic abnormalities of the cardiovascular system. Subsequently, it became apparent that quantitative information derived from cineangiography could provide insight into *functional* abnormalities of the heart as well. Direct measurement of ventricular dimension, area, and wall thickness allows calculation of volume, ejection fraction, mass, and wall stress; assessment of volume-time, pressure-volume, and stress-volume relationships provides additional information regarding systolic and diastolic function of the ventricular chambers. The ventricular angiograms obtained by the techniques described in Chapter 14 can be used to derive quantitative descriptors of ventricular chamber size, mass, and wall stress.

## VOLUMES

### Technical Considerations

As discussed in detail in Chapter 14, ventriculograms are generally recorded on cine film at 30 to 60 frames/sec, and radiographic contrast agent is usually injected into the left

ventricle at rates of 8 to 15 ml/sec for a total volume of 40 to 50 ml. Alternatively, the left ventricle may be visualized from contrast injections into the pulmonary artery, the left atrium (by the transseptal technique), or, in cases of severe aortic insufficiency, the aortic root. Attention to catheter position and injection rate will minimize the occurrence of ventricular ectopy during contrast studies; this is important, since analysis of extrasystoles and post-extrasystolic beats cannot be used for proper assessment of basal ventricular function.

In the first step in calculating left ventricular chamber volume, the left ventricular outline or silhouette is traced. The ventricular silhouette should be traced at the *outermost margin of visible radiographic contrast* so as to include trabeculations and papillary muscles within the perimeter (Fig. 19-1). The aortic valve border is defined as a line connecting the inferior aspects of the sinuses of Valsalva.

To facilitate the calculation of left ventricular volume, the ventricle is usually approximated by an ellipsoid.[1,2] Alternatively, techniques based on Simpson's rule, which is independent of assumptions regarding ventricular shape, may be used;[3] these, however, are considerably more laborious unless com-

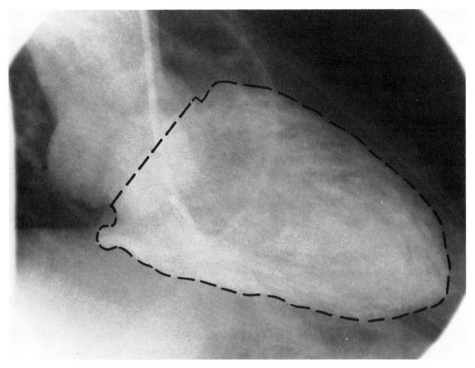

**Fig. 19-1.** Left ventriculogram in the 30° right anterior oblique projection. The ventricular outline has been traced, as indicated by the broken line.

puter techniques are used. Since the x-rays emanate from a point source, they are non-parallel; correction must therefore be made for magnification of the ventricular image onto the image intensifier. A further complicating factor is so-called pincushion distortion, i.e., greater magnification at the periphery than in the center of the image, resulting from spherical aberration of the electromagnetic lens system.[4] Finally, ventricular volumes calculated by most mathematical techniques overestimate true ventricular chamber volume, and regression equations must be used to correct for the overestimation.

## Biplane Methods

Biplane left ventriculography may be performed in the anteroposterior (AP) and lateral,[2] 30-degree right anterior oblique (RAO) and 60-degree left anterior oblique (LAO),[5] or angulated (e.g., 45-degree RAO and 60-degree LAO—25-degree cranial)[6] projec-

tions. Although a complex geometric shape, the left ventricle can be approximated with considerable accuracy by an ellipsoid[2] (Fig. 19-2). The volume of an ellipsoid is given by the equation:

$$V = \frac{4}{3}\,\pi\,\frac{L}{2}\,\frac{M}{2}\,\frac{N}{2} = \frac{\pi}{6}\,LMN \qquad (1)$$

where V is volume, L is the long axis, and M and N are the short axes of the ellipsoid. The long axis, L, is taken practically to be $L_{max}$, the longest chord that can be drawn within the ventricular silhouette in either projection. To determine M and N, each of the biplane projections of the left ventricle is approximated by an ellipse. M and N are the minor axes of these ellipses and have been drawn by hand by some investigators as perpendicular lines bisecting the long axes.[4] Alternatively, the *area-length method*, as introduced by Dodge and coworkers,[2] calculates M and N from the silhouette areas and long axis lengths in each projection, using the standard geometric formula for the area of an ellipse as a function of its major and

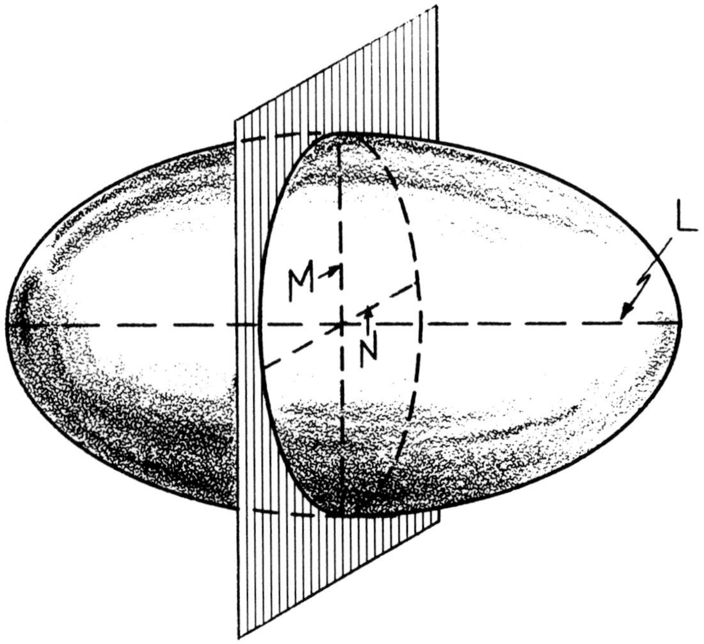

**Fig. 19-2.** Ellipsoid used as reference figure for the left ventricle. The long axis, L, and the short axes, M and N, are shown.

minor axes. Thus, for biplane oblique (RAO/LAO) left ventriculography the areas of the two ventricular silhouettes are given as:

$$A_{RAO} = \pi \frac{L_{RAO}}{2} \frac{M}{2} \quad \text{and} \quad A_{LAO} = \pi \frac{L_{LAO}}{2} \frac{N}{2}$$

$L_{RAO}$ and $L_{LAO}$ are the longest chords that can be drawn in the RAO and LAO silhouettes, respectively. The area of each traced silhouette (e.g., Fig. 19-1) is obtained by planimetry, and M and N are calculated by rearrangement as:

$$M = \frac{4A_{RAO}}{\pi L_{RAO}} \quad \text{and} \quad N = \frac{4A_{LAO}}{\pi L_{LAO}} \quad (2)$$

Combining equations 1 and 2:

$$V = \frac{\pi}{6} L_{max} \left( \frac{4A_{RAO}}{\pi L_{RAO}} \right) \left( \frac{4A_{LAO}}{\pi L_{LAO}} \right)$$
$$= \frac{8}{3\pi} \frac{A_{RAO} A_{LAO}}{L_{min}} \quad (3)$$

where $L_{min}$ is the shorter of $L_{RAO}$ and $L_{LAO}$. Since $L_{RAO}$ is nearly always greater than $L_{LAO}$, $L_{LAO}$ is usually substituted for $L_{min}$.

Equation 3 is derived for projections at right angles, or *orthogonal* projections, and is applicable to biplane oblique ventriculography in the 30-degree RAO and 60-degree LAO views, as just described, or for the older AP and lateral format. While it is not valid theoretically for nonorthogonal projections (e.g., RAO and angulated LAO), it has been demonstrated empirically to be useful in this situation as well.[6]

*Right* ventricular volumes have been calculated from biplane AP and lateral films using a modification of the Dodge area-length technique[7,8] or Simpson's rule.[8–10] Since right ventricular volumes are rarely calculated from cineangiographic studies today, the reader is referred elsewhere for methodologic details.[7–10]

## Magnification Correction: Calibration by Grid

When large cut film was used for angiocardiography, the degree of magnification of the ventricle on the film could be predicted if the x-ray-tube-to-ventricle and ventricle-to-film distances were known.[2] The techniques for calculation of ventricular volume and correction for magnification using large cut or roll film, rarely used today, were described in detail in the second edition of this textbook, and the interested reader is referred to that source for reference.

For cine techniques, the overall correction factor must account for a three-step process: magnification of the ventricle onto the surface of the image intensifier, minification of the image when recorded on 35 mm film, and remagnification of the image onto the screen of the cine projector. Correction for overall change in image size is best accomplished by filming a calibrated grid at the estimated level of the ventricle[11] and submitting the grid to the same three-step process.

The use of a calibrated grid is illustrated in Figure 19-3. In biplane studies, the level of the ventricle can be determined by placing lead markers on the face of each image intensifier and visually centering these markers using the ventricular catheter tip as reference. For single plane studies, the grid may be filmed at the level used as "zero" for pressure measurement (e.g., level of midchest) or at the actual level of the left ventricle as determined by the isocenter technique (described below). For calculation of the correction factor, the traced silhouette of the ventricle is placed over the projected image of the grid (which in Figure 19-3 consists of squares 1 cm$^2$ in area), and the squares that are closest to the image of the ventricle are planimetered (Fig. 19-3). The choice of squares near the projected image of the ventricle helps to correct for pincushion distortion at the edges of the cine frame. In the example shown in the figure, 30 squares were planimetered. If the projected (planimetered) area is $A_p$, and the actual area (number of squares) is $A_{true}$, then the linear correction factor (CF) is:

$$CF = \sqrt{A_{true}/A_p}$$

In the example in Figure 19-3, 30 squares were planimetered, so that $A_{true} = 30$ cm$^2$. In biplane studies, a correction factor must be calculated separately for each projection, yielding $CF_{RAO}$ and $CF_{LAO}$ in biplane oblique cineangiography. The linear correction factor is multiplied by the measured lengths, and the square of this correction factor is multiplied by planimetered areas to convert to true lengths and areas. Accordingly, the corrected volume of the ventricle is:

$$V = \frac{8}{3\pi} \frac{(CF_{RAO})^2 (CF_{LAO})^2}{CF_{LAO}} \frac{A_{RAO} A_{LAO}}{L_{LAO}}$$
$$= \frac{8 CF_{RAO}{}^2 CF_{LAO}}{3\pi} \frac{A_{RAO} A_{LAO}}{L_{LAO}} \qquad (4)$$

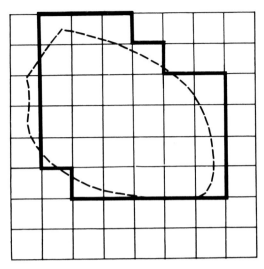

**Fig. 19-3.** Correction for magnification by use of a calibrated grid. The grid may be filmed at the level of the left ventricle (see text) after the catheterization is completed. For calculation, the grid (which consists of squares exactly 1 cm$^2$ in area) is traced from its projected image, and the squares that are closest in position to the image of the left ventricle on the left ventricular cineangiogram are planimetered. In this example, the left ventricular silhouette has been sketched in dotted lines for reference. As can be seen (bold outline), 30 squares were planimetered. See text for discussion and method of calculating correction factor.

## Magnification Correction without Grids

The introduction of certain newer biplane systems, (e.g., Phillips parallelogram system), in which the center of the ventricle is constrained by equipment design to be at the "isocenter" of the system, has allowed for magnification correction without the use of grids. This method is based on the assumption that the effects of pincushion distortion are minimal. As shown in Figure 19-4, when the ventricle is centered in both x-ray beams in such a system, its position in space is fixed (at "isocenter"). Furthermore, the horizontal tube-to-ventricle and ventricle-to-image intensifier distances are fixed and remain constant despite rotation and/or angulation of the beam. In one such system (Poly Diagnost C, N.V. Philips, Einthoven, The Netherlands), the vertical tube-to-ventricle distance is fixed, but movement of the vertical image

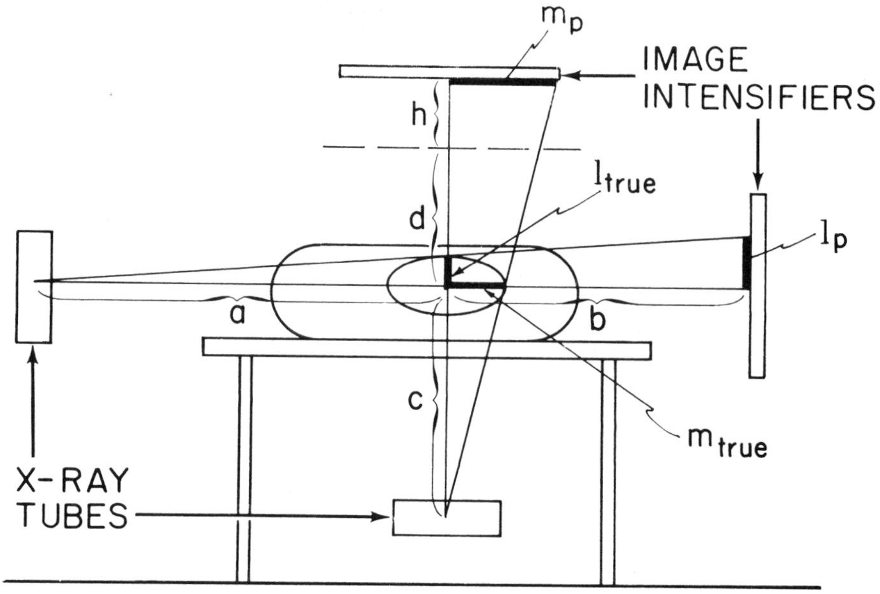

**Fig. 19-4.** Biplane isocenter system. When the patient is moved into a position that places the left ventricle at the isocenter, then the relationships between x-ray tubes, ventricle, and image intensifiers are fixed (as indicated by letters a to d), with the exception of h, the height of the vertical image intensifier above its lowest position. If h is known, the horizontal and vertical correction factors can then be calculated without the use of grids. See text for further explanation.

intensifier allows for variation in the ventricle-to-image intensifier distance.

As seen in Figure 19-4, for the horizontal image, the degree of magnification (projected length, $l_p$, relative to true length, $l_{true}$) of the ventricle onto the image intensifier is given by $(a + b)/a$, and will be the same for all patients (as will, of course, the minification of the image onto the film and the remagnification onto the projector screen). Thus, the horizontal or "lateral" CF can be determined once, and the same correction can be used for all patients (provided that no changes are made in the x-ray equipment or projector). For the vertical image, the degree of magnification is $(c + d + h)/c$; only h, the distance of the image intensifier above its lowest position, will vary from patient to patient. The vertical CF may be determined once for several values of h, and a chart may be constructed listing values of CF for each value of h. If h is measured during each patient study, then the vertical CF is known. Thus, if an isocenter biplane system is used and this approach is followed, it is unnecessary to film grids with each case.

## Regression Equations

Postmortem studies of hearts injected with contrast material have demonstrated that angiographic volumes calculated by equation 4 overestimate true left ventricular cavity volumes.[2,4,5,12] This overestimation is due in large part to the papillary muscles and trabeculae carneae, which do not contribute to blood volume but are nevertheless included within the traced left ventricular silhouette. Regression equations derived from these studies are used to adjust the calculated volumes. A list of the most commonly used regression equations is given in Table 19-1. For biplane studies in AP and lateral projections using large film techniques, the regression equation of Dodge and Sandler[13] (Table 19-1) is used. For children (in whom this regression equation may yield a negative volume), another formula has been suggested[14] (Table 19-1). For cine studies in the 60-degree RAO/30-degree LAO projections, Wynne et al. used postmortem casts, as shown in Figure 19-5, to derive the regression equation illustrated in Figure 19-6.[5]

**TABLE 19-1.** *Regression Equations to Correct for Overestimation in Calculation of Left Ventricular Volumes*

| Investigator | Angiographic Method | Age Group | Regression Equation |
|---|---|---|---|
| Wynne et al.[5] | Biplane cine RAO and LAO | Adults | $V_A = 0.989C_C - 8.1$ |
|  | Single plane cine RAO | Adults | $V_A = 0.938V_C - 5.7$ |
| Kennedy et al.[16] | Single plane cine RAO | Adults | $V_A = 0.81V_C + 1.9$ |
| Dodge et al.[2,13] | Biplane serial AP and lateral | Adults | $V_A = 0.928V_C - 3.8$ |
| Graham et al.[14] | Biplane cine AP and lateral | Children | $V_A = 0.733V_C$ |
| Sandler, Dodge[15] | Single plane serial AP | Adults | $V_A = 0.951V_C - 3.0$ |

$V_A$ = actual volume.
$V_C$ = calculated volume.

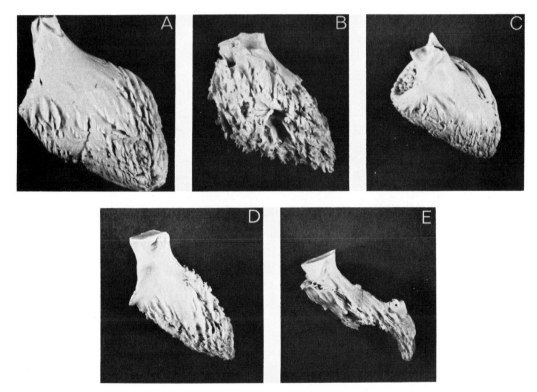

**Fig. 19-5.** Left ventricular casts made from fresh postmortem specimens of human hearts, using an encapsulant mixed with barium sulfate powder. The shape of the left ventricle only roughly approximates an ellipsoid of revolution; nevertheless, amazingly good correlation was obtained between true volume of these casts (measured by water displacement of the actual cast) and calculated volume using equations 1 and 2 (Fig. 19-6.) (From Wynne, J et al: Estimation of left ventricular volumes in man from biplane cineangiograms filmed in oblique projections. Am J Cardiol 41:726, 1978.)

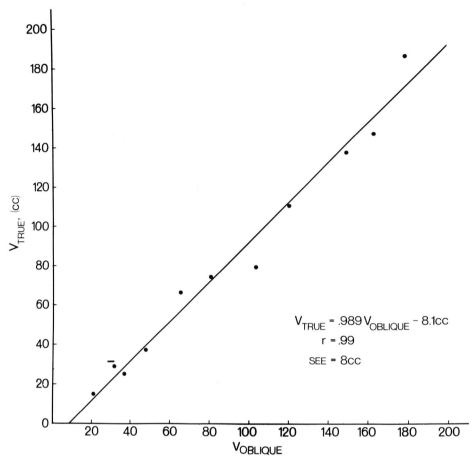

**Fig. 19-6.** Regression analysis for 11 human left ventricular casts of true volume ($V_{true}$) versus volume calculated from biplane oblique cine films of each cast ($V_{oblique}$), using equation 4. As can be seen, $V_{oblique}$ slightly overestimated $V_{true}$, although the correlation was excellent. (From Wynne, J et al: Estimation of left ventricular volumes in man from biplane cineangiograms filmed in oblique projections. Am J Cardiol 41:726, 1978.)

## Single Plane Methods

The area-length ellipsoid method for estimating left ventricular chamber volume has been modified for use when only single plane measurements obtained in the AP or RAO projection are available.[4,15,16] Inherent in single plane methods is the assumption that the left ventricular shape may be approximated by a prolate spheroid,[15] i.e., an ellipsoid in which the two minor axes are equal. Thus, it is assumed that the minor axis of the ventricle in the projection employed is equal to the minor axis in the orthogonal plane, which was not filmed. Recalling equation 1 for the general case of an ellipsoid:

$$V = \frac{\pi}{6} LMN$$

If only single plane (e.g., RAO) ventriculography is done, we assume that M = N, and that L in the plane presented is the true long axis of the ellipsoid. M is calculated from the single plane silhouette area (A) and L by the area-length method as M = 4A/πL. Thus, the single plane volume calculation becomes:

$$V = \frac{\pi}{6} LM^2 = \frac{\pi}{6} L \left( \frac{4A}{\pi L} \right)^2 = \frac{8A^2}{3\pi L} \quad (5)$$

With single plane techniques, it is difficult to locate precisely the center of the ventricle; thus, the correction factor is only approximate. Correction is usually accomplished by filming a calibrated grid at the estimated height of the center of the ventricle, as discussed previously. In our laboratories, the height of the grid is set at the midchest level when using equipment with which the isocenter cannot be determined. When using the parallelogram-C systems, which permit isocenter determination, a different technique is used. The parallelogram C-arm is rotated to 90° lateral position, and the x-ray table is raised or lowered by power control until the left ventricle (as judged by the left ventricular catheter tip) is centered on the fluoroscopic screen. The left ventricle is now "isocentered," and the table height is fixed in this position for left ventriculography. After ventriculography, the C-arm is returned to 0° and swung out to the side by rotating its pedestal base. Then, the grid is filmed at the level of the left ventricle above the floor (midface of the intensifier as determined during the isocenter procedure when the parallelogram C-arm had been rotated to a 90° lateral position). The grid height will always be the same when using the Phillips Polydiagnost C system, since in its 90° lateral position, the image intensifier face is always the same distance from the floor. The distance of the image intensifier face from the x-ray tube is variable, since the image intensifier slides up and down a track to permit adjustment of the distance between the patient's chest and the intensifier face. The intensifier tube position on its track during ventriculography should be recorded for each case, and held constant during filming of the grid. As discussed previously under biplane ventriculography, since the position of the image intensifier on its track is the only variable from case to case (grid height above the ground and x-ray generating tube position being fixed when using the Polydiagnost-C or similar systems), a series of correction factors could be calculated representing each image intensifier position, and grid filming would become unnecessary. This approach would neglect pincushion distortion, and introduce a small additional error into the volume calculation. Once a grid has been filmed, calculation of the correction factor is carried out using the same formula given under the discussion of biplane ventriculography.

Single plane techniques tend to overestimate volume significantly as compared to biplane methods, and this is reflected in the single plane regression equations (Table 19-1).

## EJECTION FRACTION AND REGURGITANT FRACTION

Visual inspection of the cine film generally allows for selection of those frames depicting maximum (end-diastolic) and minimum (end-systolic) ventricular volume. Ejection fraction (EF) is then calculated as:[17,18]

$$EF = (EDV - ESV)/EDV = SV/EDV \qquad (6)$$

where SV is the angiographic stroke volume.

In patients with aortic and/or mitral regurgitation, comparison of the angiographically determined stroke volume with the forward stroke volume determined by the Fick, indocyanine green dye, or (in the absence of concomitant tricuspid regurgitation) thermodilution technique yields the regurgitant stroke volume, that portion of the ejected volume that is regurgitated and thus does not contribute to the net cardiac output.[13] The regurgitant fraction (RF) is defined as:[17-19]

$$RF = \frac{SV_{angiographic} - SV_{forward}}{SV_{angiographic}} \qquad (7)$$

An assumption of this calculation is constancy of heart rate between determination of forward cardiac output and performance of left ventriculography. If the heart rate is substantially different at these times, a modified method for calculating RF must be used where the angiographic minute output ($SV_{angiographic} \cdot HR$) is substituted for angiographic stroke volume, and the forward minute output or cardiac output is substituted for the forward stroke volume. Because derivation of RF involves the difference between the two stroke volume measurements, both of which contain some degree of error, the error in RF itself may be quite significant; interpretation of this number should be influenced by qualitative assessment of the degree of regurgitation seen on the angiogram. In cases of combined aortic and mitral regurgitation, estimation of the relative contribution of the two lesions must be made from the cineangiograms.

## OTHER TECHNIQUES FOR MEASURING VENTRICULAR VOLUME AND EJECTION FRACTION: DIGITAL SUBTRACTION ANGIOGRAPHY AND THE IMPEDANCE CATHETER

Within the past several years, image enhancement by computerized digital subtraction techniques has been used to obtain left ventriculograms following peripheral intravenous administration of contrast material.[20-22] Peripheral injection of the contrast agent eliminates the problem of ventricular extrasystoles sometimes associated with direct injection of contrast material into the ventricular chamber. Alternatively, the image enhancement provided by the digital subtraction process permits direct left ventricular injections with small volumes of contrast agents,[22] possibly allowing multiple ventriculograms under varying conditions during a single catheterization procedure. Ventricular volume and ejection fraction may be calculated from digital subtraction ventriculograms using the area-length method,[21,22] as described for standard ventriculograms. Alternatively, ejection fraction may be determined by computer analysis of the attenuation of x-rays by the contrast agent within the ventricle;[23] this technique is independent of geometric assumptions regarding the shape of the ventricle.

Recently, a multielectrode catheter capable of measuring intracavitary electrical impedance has been introduced;[24] this catheter may prove to be useful for the measurement of ventricular volume and ejection fraction without the use of contrast agents. The catheter is shown in Figure 19-7 and consists of 12 platinum ring electrodes mounted at 1 cm intervals along the distal end of an 8 or 9F end-hole catheter. A $4\mu A$ current flows through the blood of the ventricular chamber between selected ring electrodes, and the voltage needed to drive this current reflects the instantaneous electrical impedance of the blood, which has shown to be a direct function of the blood volume. Validation studies[24] indicate that both LV and RV volumes can be measured by this technique. An illustration of the potential usefulness of this catheter in assessing LV pressure-volume relationship is shown in Figure 19-8.

## LEFT VENTRICULAR MASS

Measurement of left ventricular wall thickness, in addition to those parameters measured for volume determination, allows calculation of left ventricular wall volume and estimation of left ventricular mass (LVM). For these calculations, it is assumed that wall thickness is uniform throughout the ventricle. Wall thickness (h) is measured at end-diastole at the left ventricular free wall roughly two thirds of the distance from the aortic valve to the apex in the AP[25] or RAO[16] projection. Appropriate magnification correction is applied. The total volume of left ventricular chamber and wall, $V_{c+w}$, is approximated by that of the corresponding ellipsoid:

$$V_{c+w} = \frac{4}{3}\pi \left( \frac{L+2h}{2} \right)\left( \frac{M+2h}{2} \right)\left( \frac{N+2h}{2} \right)$$

$$= \frac{\pi}{6}(L+2h)\left( \frac{4A_{RAO}}{\pi L_{RAO}} + 2h \right) \cdot \left( \frac{4A_{LAO}}{\pi L_{LAO}} + 2h \right) \quad (8)$$

for biplane methods. As with h, appropriate correction for magnification must be applied to A and L so that $V_{c+w}$ represents the total volume of the left ventricular chamber and wall corrected for magnification. For single plane methods, it is assumed that $M = N$, yielding the single plane formula:

$$V_{c+w} = \frac{\pi}{6}(L+2h)\left( \frac{4A}{\pi L} + 2h \right)^2 \quad (9)$$

The volume of the chamber is calculated by the biplane or single plane technique. In order to exclude the volume of the papillary muscles and trabeculae from the chamber volume (and thus include their mass in LVM), the appropriate regression equation is applied, so that $V_c$ is the *regressed value* for chamber volume. Left ventricular mass, then, is calculated as:

$$LVM = 1.050V_w = 1.050(V_{c+w} - V_c) \quad (10)$$

where $V_w$ is wall volume, and 1.050 is the specific gravity of heart muscle. This method has been validated by postmortem examination of hearts;[25,26] however, it may not be accurate in the presence of marked right ventricular hypertrophy or pericardial effusion or thickening, where the accurate measurement of wall thickness from the RAO silhouette may be impossible. The left ventricular wall thickness may sometimes be seen quite well in the LAO projection in the region of the posterior wall, or it may be

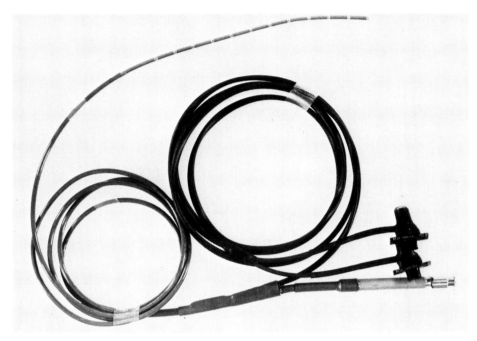

**Fig. 19-7.** Multielectrode impedance catheter for measurement of instantaneous chamber blood volume.[24] See text for description.

measured accurately by echocardiography. Values obtained by either of these methods may be used for the calculation of left ventricular mass.

## NORMAL VALUES

A number of investigators have reported normal values in adults and children for left ventricular volume, ejection fraction, wall thickness, and mass.[5,14,27–29] These are summarized in Table 19-2.

## WALL STRESS

While consideration of ventricular pressure and volume is useful for assessment of *ventricular* performance, direct evaluation of *myocardial* function requires attention to forces acting at the level of the individual myocardial fiber. In particular, correction must be made for differences in ventricular wall thickness and chamber radius (R), which modify the extent to which intraventricular pressure (P) is borne by the individ-

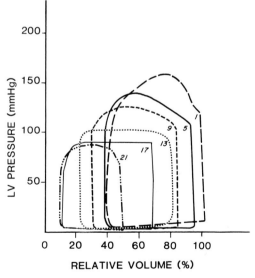

**Fig. 19-8.** Use of multielectrode impedance catheter, shown in Figure 19-7, to obtain LV pressure-volume loops every fourth beat during inhalation of amyl nitrite. (Reproduced with permission from McKay RG, et al: Instantaneous measurement of left and right ventricular stroke volume and pressure-volume relationships with an impedance catheter. Circulation 69:703, 1984.)

**TABLE 19-2.**  *Normal Average Values for Left Ventricular Parameters by Angiocardiography*

| Investigator | Angiographic Method | Number of Patients | Age Group | End-Diastolic Volume ($ml/m^2$) | End-Systolic Volume ($ml/m^2$) | Ejection Fraction | Wall Thickness (mm) | Mass (g) |
|---|---|---|---|---|---|---|---|---|
| Wynne et al.[5] | Biplane cine RAO-LAO | 17 | Adults | 72 ± 15 | 20 ± 8 | 0.72 ± 0.08 | — | — |
| Kennedy et al.[27] | Biplane serial AP and Lat | 16 | Adults | 70 ± 20 | 24 ± 10 | 0.67 ± 0.08 | 10.9 ± 2.0 | 167 ± 42 |
| Hood[28] | Biplane serial AP and Lat | 6 | Adults | 79 ± 11 | 28 ± 6 | 0.67 ± 0.07 | 8.5 ± 1.3 | 164 ± 35 |
| Hermann[29] | Biplane serial AP and Lat | 6 | Adults | 71 ± 20 | 30 ± 10 | 0.58 ± 0.05 | — | — |
| Graham[14] | Biplane cine AP and Lat | 19 | Children less than 2 yr | 42 ± 10 | — | 0.68 ± 0.05 | — | 96 ± 11* |
| Graham et al.[14] | Biplane cine AP and Lat | 37 | Children older than 2 yr | 73 ± 11 | — | 0.63 ± 0.05 | — | 86 ± 11* |

Mean ± SD
* $gm/m^2$

ual fiber; this is especially important in disease states characterized by ventricular hypertrophy or dilatation or both. Such a correction may be achieved by consideration of wall stress ($\sigma$).[30-33] Several formulae are commonly employed to calculate stress, all of which are related to the basic Laplace relation:

$$\sigma = \frac{PR}{2h} \qquad (11)$$

Assumptions regarding the shape of the ventricular chamber and the properties of the ventricular wall have led to a number of such formulae for wall stress components in the circumferential, meridional, and radial directions (Figure 19-9). Consideration of circumferential and meridional stress has been particularly useful for clinical applications. A representative formula for calculation of circumferential stress, $\sigma_c$, is:[31]

$$\sigma_c = \frac{Pb}{h}\left(1 - \frac{h}{2b}\right)\left(1 - \frac{hb}{2a^2}\right) \qquad (12)$$

where a and b are the major and minor semiaxes, respectively, at the midwall. Meridional stress, $\sigma_m$, may be calculated as:[32]

$$\sigma_m = \frac{PR}{2h(1 + h/2R)} \qquad (13)$$

where R is the internal chamber radius as bounded by the endocardial surface. For more detailed consideration of wall stress formulae, the reader is referred to reviews of the subject.[31,33]

Calculation of wall stress in disease states has provided information not apparent from consideration of pressure and volume data alone. For example, it has been demonstrated that peak stress does not necessarily occur at the same time in the cardiac cycle

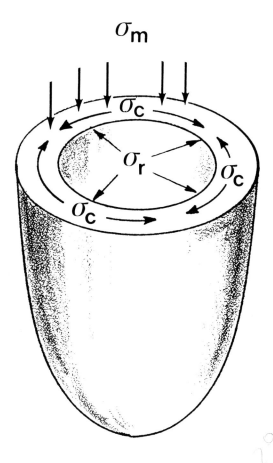

**Fig. 19-9.** Circumferential ($\sigma_c$), meridional ($\sigma_m$), and radial ($\sigma_r$) components of left ventricular wall stress for an ellipsoid model. The three components of wall stress are mutually perpendicular.

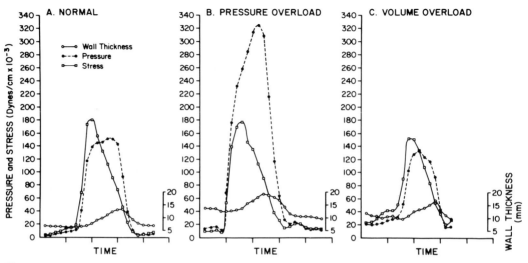

**Fig. 19-10.**   A comparison of changes in left ventricular pressure (solid dots), wall thickness (open dots), and meridional stress (open squares) throughout the cardiac cycle for representative normal, pressure-overloaded, and volume-overloaded ventricles. These parameters are plotted at 40-msec intervals. In all three types of ventricles, peak stress occurs earlier than peak pressure. In the pressure-overloaded ventricle (B), peak pressure is markedly elevated, but peak systolic stress and end-diastolic stress are normal. In the volume-overloaded ventricle (C), peak systolic stress is normal, but end-diastolic stress is elevated. (Reproduced with permission from Grossman W, Jones D, McLaurin LP: Wall stress and patterns of hypertrophy in the human left ventricle. J Clin Invest 56:56, 1974.)

as does peak pressure and that, in "compensated" pressure overload, the increase in ventricular pressure is offset by a proportional increase in wall thickness, such that wall stress remains normal (Fig. 19-10).[32]

## VOLUME-TIME AND PRESSURE-VOLUME CURVES

Left ventriculography performed with rapid filming rates has permitted construction of the ventricular volume-time curve[3,34] (Fig. 19-11). Calculation of the maximum slope of the early diastolic portion of the curve, i.e., the peak rate of early diastolic filling of the ventricle, has been suggested as an index of early diastolic function.[34]

Simultaneous measurement of ventricular pressure and volume allows construction of the pressure-volume diagram (Fig. 19-12).[35-38] The position and slope of the diastolic portion of the pressure-volume curve provide information regarding diastolic properties of the ventricle.[36,39] Construction of the systolic portion of the curve

is useful for analysis of the end-systolic pressure-volume relation, a measure of ventricular contractile function (see Chapter 20).

## REGIONAL LEFT VENTRICULAR WALL MOTION

The recognition that left ventricular regional dysynergy is a more sensitive marker of coronary artery disease than is depression of global function has led to attempts to quantify abnormalities of regional wall motion. Left ventriculography is performed in the RAO or RAO and LAO projections. The ventricle is divided into regions by one of two methods: (1) construction of lines perpendicular to the major axis that divide the major axis into equal segments (Fig. 19-13A);[40,41] or (2) construction of lines drawn from the midpoint of the major axis to the ventricular outline at intervals of a fixed number of degrees (Fig. 19-13B).[40,42] Extent of inward (or outward) movement of individual segments can then be measured, generally with the aid of computer techniques,

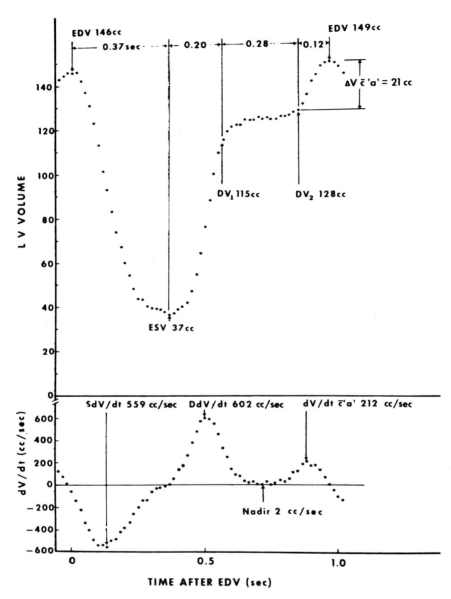

**Fig. 19-11.** Plots of left ventricular (LV) volume and the rate of change of volume (dV/dt) versus time calculated from a single-plane cineangiogram in a normal subject. The maximum value of dV/dt during diastole, i.e., the peak rate of diastolic filling (D dV/dt) of the ventricle, has been proposed as an index of early diastolic function. End-diastolic (EDV) and end-systolic (ESV) volumes are indicated. (Reproduced with permission from Hammermeister KE, Warbasse JR: The rate of change of left ventricular volume in man. Circulation 49:739, 1974.)

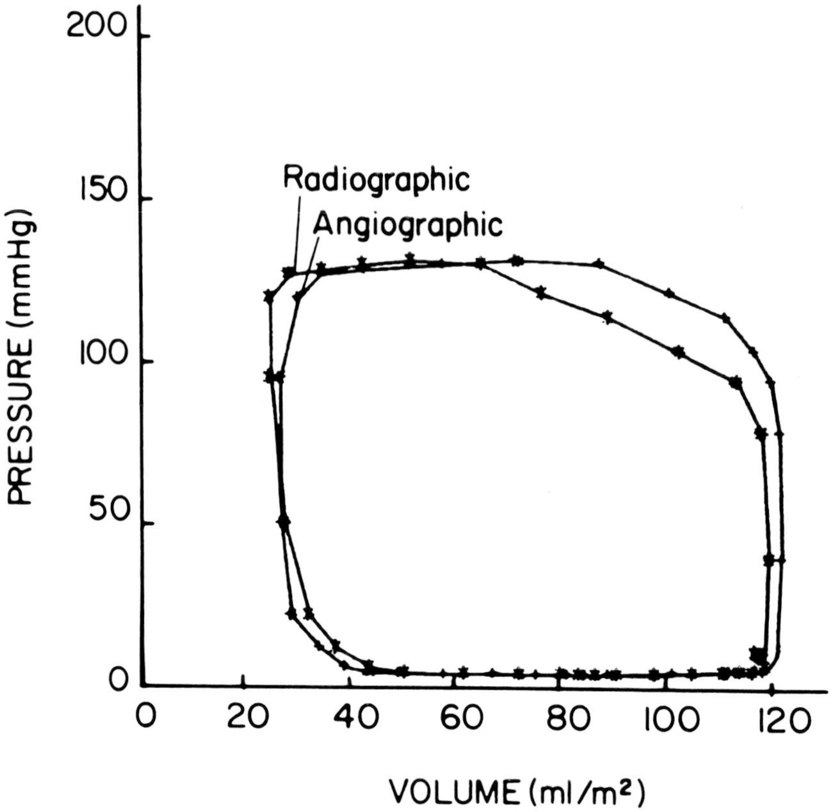

**Fig. 19-12.**  Pressure-volume diagram for the left ventricle. In this example, the diagram derived from single-plane cineangiography is compared to that constructed from radionuclide volume data. (Reproduced with permission from McKay RG, et al: Left ventricular pressure-volume diagrams and end-systolic pressure-volume relations in human beings. J Am Coll Cardiol 3:301, 1984.)

providing quantitative measures of hypokinesis, akinesis, and dyskinesis.

More recently, an automated method of processing the left ventricular cineangiogram has been reported by Sasayama and co-workers.[43-45] End-diastolic and end-systolic ventricular silhouettes are superimposed (Fig. 19-14), and 128 radial grids are drawn from the center of gravity of the end-diastolic silhouette to the endocardial margins. Measurement of the length of each radial grid between end-diastolic and end-systolic silhouettes serves as a measure of segmental systolic and diastolic function. Figure 19-14 illustrates this technique in a patient with coronary disease before (CON) and after (PCG) induction of angina pectoris by rapid atrial pacing. Simultaneously measured LV pressure (LVP) permits construction of segmental LV pressure-length loops for the normally perfused myocardial region (c and d), as well as for a region perfused by a stenotic coronary artery (a and b). Depressed wall motion develops during angina in region a/b, and compensatory hyperkinesis develops in region c/d.

Another approach has been proposed by Sheehan and colleagues at the University of Washington in Seattle. This approach, which has been applied by Mathey et al. to the study of myocardial salvage following thrombolytic therapy, measures wall motion along 100 chords constructed as perpendiculars to a center line drawn midway between the end diastolic and end systolic left ventricular contours.[46]

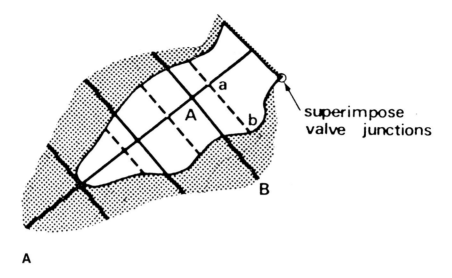

**A**

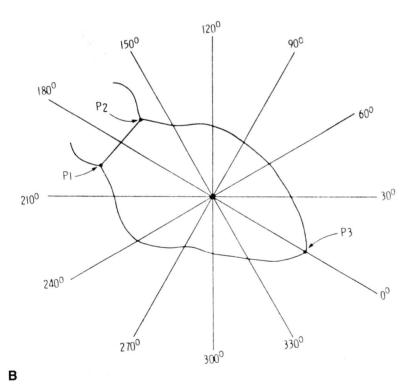

**B**

**Fig. 19-13.** Techniques for quantitative assessment of regional left ventricular wall motion. The ventricle, shown in a left lateral projection (A), may be divided into regions by constructing lines perpendicular to the major axis that divides the axis into equal segments. (Reproduced with permission from Sniderman AD, Marpole D, Fallen EL: Regional contraction patterns in the normal and ischemic left ventricle in man. Am J Cardiol 31:484, 1973.) Alternatively, lines may be drawn from the midpoint of the major axis to the ventricular outline at intervals of a fixed number of degrees (B). (Reproduced with permission from Cole JS, Holland PA, Glaeser DH: A semiautomated technique for the rapid evaluation of left ventricular regional wall motion. Cathet Cardiovasc Diagn 2:185, 1976.)

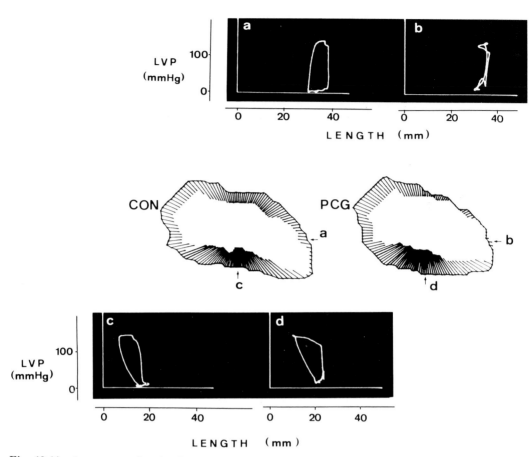

**Fig. 19-14.** Assessment of regional wall motion in the control state (CON) and after induction of angina pectoris by atrial pacing tachycardia (PCG). Left ventricular pressure (LVP)-length loops are plotted for a myocardial region distal to a stenotic coronary artery (a and b) and for a normally perfused region (c and d). (Reproduced with permission from Sasayama S, et al: Changes in diastolic properties of the regional myocardium during pacing-induced ischemia in man. J Am Coll Cardiol 5: 647, 1985.)

# REFERENCES

1. Arvidsson H: Angiocardiographic observations in mitral disease. Acta Radiol suppl 158, 1958.
2. Dodge HT, Sandler H, Ballew DW, Lord JD Jr.: The use of biplane angiocardiography for the measurement of left ventricular volume in man. Am Heart J 60:762, 1960.
3. Chapman CB, Baker O, Reynolds J, Bonte FJ: Use of biplane cinefluorography for measurement of ventricular volume. Circulation 18:1105, 1958.
4. Greene DG, Carlisle R, Grant C, Bunnell IL: Estimation of left ventricular volume by one-plane cineangiography. Circulation 35:61, 1967.
5. Wynne J, et al: Estimation of left ventricular volumes in man from biplane cineangiograms filmed in oblique projections. Am J Cardiol 41:726, 1978.
6. Rogers WJ, et al: Quantitative axial oblique contrast left ventriculography: validation of the method by demonstrating improved visualization of regional wall motion and mitral valve function with accurate volume determinations. Am Heart J 103:185, 1982.
7. Arcilla RA, Tsai P, Thilenius O, Ranninger K: Angiographic method for volume estimation of right and left ventricles. Chest 60:446, 1971.

8. Graham TP Jr., Jarmakani JM, Atwood GF, Canent RV Jr.: Right ventricular volume determinations in children. Normal values and observations with volume or pressure overload. Circulation 47:144, 1973.

9. Goerke RJ, Carlsson E: Calculation of right and left cardiac ventricular volumes. Method using standard computer equipment and biplane angiocardiograms. Invest Radiol 2:360, 1967.

10. Gentzler RD, Briselli MF, Gault JH: Angiographic estimation of right ventricular volume in man. Circulation 50:324, 1974.

11. Kasser IS, Kennedy JW: Measurement of left ventricular volumes in man by single-plane cineangiocardiography. Invest Radiol 4:83, 1969.

12. Rackley CE, Behar VS, Whalen RE, McIntosh HD: Biplane cineangiographic determination of left ventricular function: pressure-volume relationships. Am Heart J 74:766, 1967.

13. Sandler H, Dodge HT, Hay RE, Rackley CE: Quantitation of valvular insufficiency in man by angiocardiography. Am Heart J 65:501, 1963.

14. Graham TP Jr., Jarmakani JM, Canent RV Jr., Morrow MN: Left heart volume estimation in infancy and childhood. Reevaluation of methodology and normal values. Circulation 43:895, 1971.

15. Sandler H, Dodge HT: The use of single plane angiocardiograms for the calculation of left ventricular volume in man. Am Heart J 75:325, 1968.

16. Kennedy JW, Trenholme SE, Kasser IS: Left ventricular volume and mass from single-plane cineangiocardiogram. A comparison of anteroposterior and right anterior oblique methods. Am Heart J 80:343, 1970.

17. Arvidsson H, Karnell J: Quantitative assessment of mitral and aortic insufficiency by angiocardiography. Acta Radiol 2:105, 1964.

18. Miller GAH, Brown R, Swan HJC: Isolated Congenital mitral insufficiency with particular reference to left heart volumes. Circulation 29:356, 1964.

19. Jones JW, et al: Left ventricular volumes in valvular heart disease. Circulation 29:887, 1964.

20. Kruger RA, et al: Computerized fluoroscopy techniques for intravenous study of cardiac chamber dynamics. Invest Radiol 14:279, 1979.

21. Vas R, et al: Computer enhancement of direct and venous-injected left ventricular contrast angiography. Am Heart J 102:720, 1981.

22. Sasayama S, et al: Automated method for left ventricular volume measurement by cineventriculography with minimal doses of contrast medium. Am J Cardiol 48:746, 1981.

23. Tobis J, et al: Measurement of left ventricular ejection fraction by videodensitometric analysis of digital subtraction angiograms. Am J Cardiol 52:871, 1983.

24. McKay RG, et al: Instantaneous measurement of left and right ventricular stroke volume and pressure-volume relationships with an impedance catheter. Circulation 69:703, 1984.

25. Rackley CE, Dodge HT, Coble YD Jr, Hay RE: A method for determining left ventricular mass in man. Circulation 29:666, 1964.

26. Kennedy JW, Reichenbach DD, Baxley WA, Dodge HT: Left ventricular mass. A comparison of angiocardiographic measurements with autopsy weight. Am J Cardiol 19:221, 1967.

27. Kennedy JW, et al: Quantitative angiocardiography. I. The normal left ventricle in man. Circulation 34:272, 1966.

28. Hood WP Jr: Wall stress in the normal and hypertrophied human left ventricle. Am J Cardiol 22:550, 1968.

29. Hermann HJ, Bartle SH: Left ventricular volumes by angiocardiography: comparison of methods and simplification of techniques. Cardiovasc Res 4:404, 1968.

30. Sandler H, Dodge HT: Left ventricular tension and stress in man. Circ Res 13:91, 1963.

31. Mirsky I: Review of various theories for the evaluation of left ventricular wall stresses. *In* Mirsky I, Ghista DN, Sandler H (eds): Cardiac Mechanics. New York, John Wiley & Sons, Inc., 1974, p. 381.

32. Grossman W, Jones D, McLaurin LP: Wall stress and patterns of hypertrophy in the human left ventricle. J Clin Invest 56:56, 1974.

33. Yin FCP: Ventricular wall stress. Circ Res 49:829, 1981.

34. Hammermeister KE, Warbasse JR: The rate of change of left ventricular volume in man. II. Diastolic events in health and disease. Circulation 49:739, 1974.

35. Arviddson H: Angiocardiographic determination of left ventricular volume. Acta Radiol 56:321, 1961.

36. Dodge HT, Hay RE, Sandler H: Pressure-volume characteristics of diastolic left ventricle of man with heart disease. Am Heart J 64:503, 1962.

37. Bunnell IL, Grant C, Greene DG: Left ventricular function derived from the pressure-volume diagram. Am J Med 39:881, 1965.

38. McKay RG, et al: Left ventricular pressure-volume diagrams and end-systolic pressure-volume relations in human beings. J Am Coll Cardiol 3:301, 1984.

39. Grossman W, McLaurin LP: Diastolic properties of the left ventricle. Ann Intern Med 84:316, 1976.

40. Herman MV, Heinle RA, Klein MD, Gorlin R: Localized disorders in myocardial contraction. Asynergy and its role in congestive heart failure. N Engl J Med 277:222, 1967.

41. Sniderman AD, Marpole D, Fallen EL: Regional contraction patterns in the normal and ischemic left ventricle in man. Am J Cardiol 31:484, 1973.

42. Cole JS, Holland PA, Glaeser DH: A semiautomated technique for the rapid evaluation of left ventricular regional wall motion. Cathet Cardiovasc Diagn 2:185, 1976.
43. Sasayama, S, Nonogi H, Kawm C: Assessment of left ventricular function using an angiographic method. Jpn Circ J 46:1177, 1982.
44. Fujita M, et al: Automatic processing of cine ventriculograms for analysis of regional myocardial function. Circulation 63:1065, 1981.
45. Sasayama S, et al: Changes in diastolic properties of the regional myocardium during pacing-induced ischemia in human subjects. J Am Coll Cardiol 5:647, 1985.
46. Mathey DG, Sheehan FH, Schofer J, Dodge HT. Time from onset of symptoms to thrombolytic therapy: A major determinant of myocardial salvage in patients with acute transmural infarction. J Am Coll Cardiol 6:518, 1985.

*chapter twenty*

# Evaluation of Systolic and Diastolic Function of the Myocardium

WILLIAM GROSSMAN

━━━━━━━

A CRITICAL aspect of most cardiac catheterization procedures is the evaluation of myocardial function. At its simplest, this consists of a visual assessment of the left ventricular (LV) contractile pattern from the left ventriculogram, together with measurements of LV end-diastolic pressure. In laboratories such as ours, where most patients have right heart catheterization and cardiac output measurement as part of a standard cardiac catheterization procedure, additional information about LV function may be gleaned from the cardiac output, stroke volume, and pulmonary capillary wedge pressure, whereas right ventricular (RV) function is reflected in the values for right ventricular end-diastolic pressure (RVEDP) and right atrial pressure. Measurements of pressures and cardiac output give important information about overall cardiac function, but may shed little light on the question as to whether dysfunction is due to abnormal systolic or diastolic myocardial performance. This chapter will discuss some of the specific methods that can be used in the cardiac catheterization laboratory to examine myocardial performance in systole and diastole.

## SYSTOLIC FUNCTION
### Preload, Afterload, and Contractility

Systolic function of the myocardium is a reflection of the interaction of myocardial preload, afterload, and contractility. *Preload* is the load which stretches myofibrils during diastole and determines the end-diastolic sarcomere length. For the left ventricle, this load is often quantified as the LV end-diastolic pressure (EDP). This pressure, taken together with LV wall thickness (h) and radius (R) determines LV end-diastolic *wall stress* ($\sigma \sim$ PR/h) which is an estimate of the force stretching the myocardial fibers at end-diastole. The end-diastolic stress or "stretching force" is resisted by the intrinsic stiffness or elasticity of the myocardium, and the interaction of end-diastolic stretching force and myocardial stiffness determines the extent of end-diastolic sarcomere stretch. Thus, if the myocardium is diffusely fibrotic or infiltrated with amyloid, a very high end-diastolic stretching force may be required to produce even a normal end-diastolic sarcomere length. In such a case, LVEDP may be

301

very high (e.g., $> 25$ mmHg), and attempts to lower it by diuretic or venodilator therapy will lead to reduction in end-diastolic sarcomere stretch to subnormal values and a concomitant fall in cardiac output.

Changes in preload influence both the extent and velocity of myocardial shortening in experiments using isolated cardiac muscle preparations. Increased preload augments the extent and velocity of myocardial shortening at any given afterload. In the intact heart, the relationship is more complex, since increases in preload generally produce increases in LV chamber size and LV systolic pressure. Thus, *afterload* (the force resisting systolic shortening) is also increased, and this increase tends to blunt the increases in extent and velocity of myocardial shortening due to increased diastolic fiber stretch. This point will be discussed in more detail later in this chapter, under the section on ejection phase indexes of systolic function.

*Afterload*, the force resisting systolic shortening of the myofibrils, varies throughout systole as the ventricular systolic pressure rises and blood is ejected from the ventricular chamber. LV systolic stress approximates the force resisting myocardial fiber shortening within the wall of the ventricle. The theory and methods for calculation of wall stress are described in Chapter 19. End-systolic wall stress is considered by many to be the final afterload that determines the extent of myocardial fiber shortening, when preload and contractility are constant. Thus, an increase in end-systolic wall stress will result in a decrease in myocardial fiber shortening. For the intact ventricle, an increase in afterload (end-systolic wall stress) will result, therefore, in a fall in stroke volume and ejection fraction.

*Contractility* refers to that property of heart muscle that accounts for alterations in performance induced by chemical and hormonal changes, independent of preload and afterload. Contractility is generally used as a synonym for *inotropy:* both terms refer to the level of activation of cross bridge cycling during systole. Contractility changes are assessed in the experimental laboratory by measuring myocardial function (extent or speed of shortening, maximum force generation) while preload and afterload are held constant. In contrast to skeletal muscle, the strength of contraction of heart muscle can be increased readily by a variety of biochem-

ical and hormonal stimuli, some of which are listed in Table 20-1.

Increased myocardial contractility may be present in patients with hyperadrenergic states, thyrotoxicosis, and hypertrophic cardiomyopathy and in response to a variety of drugs. It is manifest by an increase in the speed and extent of myocardial contraction at constant afterload and preload.

The assessment of systolic function requires consideration of the simultaneous influence of afterload, preload, and contractility. Systolic function should *not* be regarded as synonymous with contractility. Major depression of systolic function may occur in the presence of normal contractility, as in conditions with so-called afterload excess discussed later in this chapter.

## Isovolumic Indices

One of the oldest and most widely used measures of myocardial contractility is the maximum rate of rise of LV systolic pressure, dP/dt. It was noted more than 50 years ago by Wiggers that in animal experiments the failing ventricle showed a reduction in the steepness of the upslope of the ventricular pressure pulse.[1-3] In 1962, Gleason and Braunwald first reported measurement of dP/dt in man.[4] They studied 40 patients with micromanometer catheters and found that maximum dP/dt in patients without hemodynamic abnormalities ranged from 841 to 1696 mmHg/sec in the left ventricle, and 223 to 296 mmHg/sec in the right ventricle. Interventions known to increase myocardial contractility, such as exercise and infusion of norepinephrine or isoproterenol, caused major increases in dP/dt. Increased heart rate produced by intravenous atropine also caused a rise in maximum dP/dt, and the authors attributed this to the "treppe" phenomenon described by Bowditch.[5] Acute increases in arterial pressure and afterload produced by infusion of the $\alpha$-adrenergic vasoconstricting agent methoxamine produced little change in dP/dt. These points are illustrated in Figures 20-1 and 20-2.

In normal subjects and in patients with no significant cardiac abnormality, maximum dP/dt increases significantly in response to isometric exercise,[6] dynamic exercise,[4] tachycardia by atrial pacing,[7,8] or by atropine,[4]

**TABLE 20-1.** *Hormones and Drugs That Influence Myocardial Contractility*

|  | Presumed Mechanism | Influence on Contractility |
|---|---|---|
| 1. Catecholamines with $\beta$ agonist activity | $\beta$ receptor stimulation $\rightarrow$ $\uparrow$ adenylate cyclase activity $\rightarrow$ $\uparrow$ cyclic AMP $\rightarrow$ $\uparrow Ca^{++}$ influx through sarcolemma $\rightarrow$ $\uparrow$ cytosolic $Ca^{++}$ | + |
| 2. Digitalis glycosides | Inhibition of $Na^+$-$K^+$ ATPase $\rightarrow$ $\uparrow$ intracellular $Na^+$ $\rightarrow$ $\uparrow Na^+/Ca^{++}$ exchange $\rightarrow$ $\uparrow$ cytosolic $Ca^{++}$ | + |
| 3. Calcium salts | $\uparrow$ Extracellular $Ca^{++}$ $\rightarrow$ $\uparrow Ca^{++}$ influx via slow channels and $Na^+/Ca^{++}$ exchange $\rightarrow$ $\uparrow$ cytosolic $Ca^{++}$ | + |
| 4. Caffeine | Multiple actions:<br>(1) local release of catecholamines<br>(2) inhibition of sarcoplasmic reticular $Ca^{++}$ uptake<br>(3) inhibition of phosphodiesterase $\rightarrow$ $\uparrow$ cyclic AMP<br>(4) $\uparrow$ sensitivity of contractile proteins to $Ca^{++}$ | + |
| 5. Milrinone, amrinone, other bipyridines | Phosphodiesterase inhibition $\rightarrow$ $\uparrow$ cyclic AMP $\rightarrow$ $\uparrow$ cytosolic $Ca^{++}$ | + |
| 6. Thyroid hormone | Increases myosin ATPase activity by altering production of certain myosin isozymes | + |
| 7. Calcium blocking agents (verapamil, nifedipine, D600, diltiazem) | Block $Ca^{++}$ entry via slow channels | − |
| 8. Barbiturates, Ethanol | Depress contractility by unknown mechanism | − |

$\beta$-agonists,[4] and digitalis glycosides.[9] Relatively few studies have been done in humans assessing the changes in dP/dt induced by alterations in afterload and preload, but those studies that have been done indicate that maximum positive dP/dt tends to increase slightly (6 to 8%) with moderate increases in LV preload[10] and shows little change with methoxamine-induced increases[4] or nitroprusside-induced decreases[11] in mean arterial pressure of 25 to 30 mmHg. Extensive studies in animals have examined the influence of changes in afterload, preload, and contractility on maximum dP/dt.[10,12–15] These studies generally show that maximum dP/dt rises with increases in

afterload and preload, but the changes were quite small (<10%) in the physiologic range.

As discussed in Chapter 9, accurate measurement of dP/dt requires a pressure measurement system with excellent frequency-response characteristics. Micromanometer catheters are generally required to achieve this frequency-response range.[16] Differentiation of the ventricular pressure signal can be achieved by (1) analog techniques on-line (Figs. 20-1 and 20-2), using an RC differentiating circuit;[4,10] (2) computer digitization of the analog LV pressure tracing and subsequent differentiation of a polynomial best fit to the averaged LV isovolumic pressure;[17] or (3) computer digitization of the analog LV

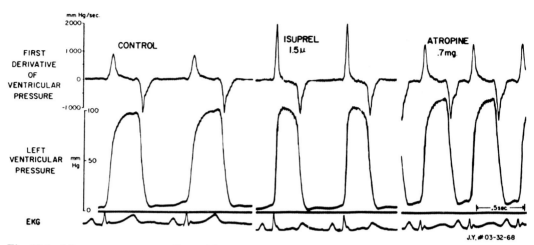

**Fig. 20-1.** Micromanometer recordings of left ventricular pressure and its first derivative, dP/dt, in a patient with normal left ventricular function. Isoproterenol markedly increases contractility with large increments in positive dP/dt. Atropine produces tachycardia, which results in a treppe effect and a rise in +dP/dt above control. (Reproduced, with permission, from Gleason WL, Braunwald E: Studies on the first derivative of the ventricular pressure pulse in man. J Clin Invest 41:80, 1962.)

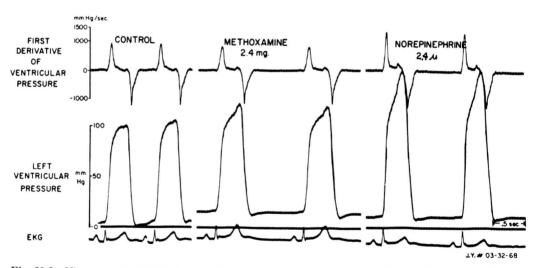

**Fig. 20-2.** Micromanometer recordings of left ventricular (LV) pressure and dP/dt, as in Figure 20-1. Methoxamine raises arterial and LV systolic pressure, but does not increase +dP/dt. In contrast, the combined α and β adrenergic effects of norepinephrine increase with LV systolic pressure and +dP/dt. (Reproduced, with permission, from Gleason WL and Braunwald E: Studies on the first derivative of the ventricular pressure pulse in man. J Clin Invest 41:80, 1962.)

pressure tracing with subsequent Fourier analysis and differentiation.[18]

In addition to dP/dt, several other isovolumic indices have been introduced in an attempt to obtain a pure contractility index, completely independent of alterations in preload and afterload.[10,19–26] Of these indices,

the maximum value of [(dP/dt)/P], where P is LV pressure, has been utilized by several groups over the past 15 years. On theoretical grounds, the quantity (dP/dt)/P has been related to the velocity of contractile element shortening, $V_{CE}$; the mathematical basis for this relation is given by several authors[20,21,23,27] and is not given here in detail. A fundamental problem with the utilization of (dP/dt)/P as a measure of contractile element velocity is that the mathematics upon which this concept is based are highly model-dependent and require knowledge of the compliance of series and parallel elastic elements. From a *practical* standpoint, although (dP/dt)/P does directly reflect changes in contractility (e.g., it increases with isoproterenol or calcium infusion), it is very sensitive to alterations in preload.[10] Thus, (dP/dt)/P falls during dextran infusion in animals and in response to increased venous return (passive straight leg raising) in man.[10] This preload sensitivity can be abolished if the P used in calculating (dP/dt)/P is "developed" LV pressure (total LV intraventricular pressure minus LVEDP), which corrects for shifts in preload.

The maximum value of (dP/dt)/P is sometimes called $V_{PM}$; as mentioned, it reflects changes in contractility directly, but is related inversely to changes in preload. Nevertheless, if an intervention produces an increase in $V_{PM}$ at a time when LVEDP is unchanged or rising, an increase in contractility has almost certainly occurred.

Other isovolumic indices include (peak dP/dt)/IIT (where IIT = integrated isovolumic tension), (dP/dt)/CPIP (where CPIP = common developed isovolumic pressure), $V_{max}$ (the extrapolated value of (dP/dt)/P versus P, when P = 0); (dP/dt)/$P_D$ when developed LV pressure, $P_D$ = 5, 10, or 40 mmHg; and the fractional rate of change of power (which involves the second derivative of LV pressure). The reader is referred elsewhere for more information on these less commonly used isovolumic indices.[19,22,23,25,27]

While changes in dP/dt reflect acute changes in inotropy in a given individual, the usefulness of dP/dt is reduced when attempting to compare one individual with another, especially when there has been chronic LV pressure or volume overload. Thus, peak dP/dt is generally increased in patients with chronic aortic stenosis even though contractility is normal in most of these patients. To account for chronic changes in LV geometry and mass that occur with chronic LV overload some investigators have examined the rate of rise of systolic wall stress.[17] The peak value of d$\sigma$/dt may be employed as a contractility index, as may the spectrum plot which relates d$\sigma$/dt to instantaneous $\sigma$ (Fig. 20-3).

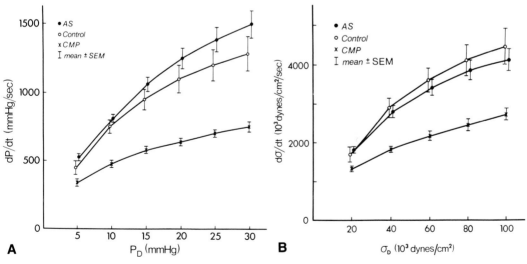

**Fig. 20-3.** Left ventricular (LV) isovolumic indexes of contractility. (A) Rate of pressure development (dP/dt) as a function of LV developed pressure ($P_D$). Mean values in control subjects (open circles), patients with aortic stenosis (AS, closed circles), and those with dilated cardiomyopathy (CMP, crosses) are shown. Brackets represent standard errors of the mean (SEM). (B) Rate of wall stress development (d$\sigma$/dt) as a function of LV developed stress ($\sigma_D$) for the same groups. There are no significant differences for patients with AS compared to controls, although patients with CMP clearly show depressed values for dP/dt and d$\sigma$/dt at all levels of $P_D$ and $\sigma_D$. (Reproduced, with permission, from Fifer MA et al: Myocardial contractile function in aortic stenosis as determined from the rate of stress development during isovolumic systole. Am J Cardiol 44:1318, 1979.)

## Pressure-Volume Analysis

Since the time of Otto Frank and Ernest Starling, pressure-volume diagrams have been used to analyze ventricular function. The normally contracting left ventricle ejects blood under pressure, and the relationship of its pressure generation and ejection can be expressed in a plot of LV pressure against volume (Fig. 20-4). As can be seen in Figure 20-4, end-diastole is represented by point A, isovolumic contraction by line AB, aortic valve opening by point B, ejection by line BC, end ejection and aortic valve closure by point C, isovolumic relaxation by line CD, mitral valve opening by point D, and LV diastolic filling by line DA.

***Stroke Work.*** The area ABCD enclosed within the PV diagram in Figure 20-4 is the external LV stroke work (SW), represented mathematically as ∫PdV. Although the calculation of LVSW is most accurate when derived by integrating the area within complete PV diagrams, a practical approximation can be obtained as:

$$LVSW = (\overline{LVSP} - \overline{LVDP})SV(0.0136) \qquad (1)$$

where $\overline{LVSP}$ and $\overline{LVDP}$ are the mean LV systolic and diastolic pressures in mmHg, SV is

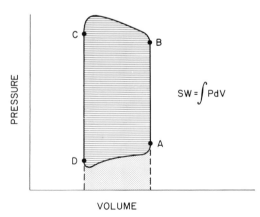

**Fig. 20-4.** Diagram of ventricular pressure (P) plotted against simultaneous ventricular volume (V) for a single cardiac contraction. For the left ventricle, point A represents end-diastole, segment AB is isovolumic contraction, point B is aortic valve opening, segment BC is LV ejection, point C is aortic valve closure and represents end-ejection, segment CD is isovolumic relaxation, point D is mitral valve opening, and segment DA is LV filling. LV stroke work (SW) is the cross-hatched area, while the stippled area is diastolic work done on the left ventricle by right ventricle and left atrium. See text for details.

the LV total stroke volume in ml, and 0.0136 is a constant for converting mmHg · ml into gm-m. LVSP and LVDP may be obtained from planimetry as shown in Figure 20-5. When the total LV stroke volume is the same as the forward stroke volume, SV may be calculated as cardiac output ÷ heart rate. In patients where LV total stroke volume differs from forward stroke volume (e.g., mitral or aortic regurgitation, ventricular septal defect), the PV diagram may differ substantially in configuration from that shown in Figure 20-4, and LVSW cannot be calculated from equation 1. Instead, planimetric integration of the entire PV plot will be required.

If LV pressure tracings are not available, in the absence of major regurgitation SW can be approximated using aortic and pulmonary capillary wedge pressures as:

$$LVSW = (\overline{AoSP} - \overline{PCW})SV(0.0136) \qquad (2)$$

where $\overline{AoSP}$ and $\overline{PCW}$ are the aortic systolic mean pressure (planimetered from the aortic pressure tracing, Fig. 20-5) and the mean pulmonary capillary wedge pressure. Since the mean systemic arterial pressure closely approximates $\overline{AoSP}$, a further approximation may be made by substituting mean arterial pressure ($\overline{Ao}$) for $\overline{AoSP}$.

LVSW is a reasonably good measure of LV systolic function in the absence of volume or pressure overload conditions, both of which may substantially increase calculated LVSW. The normal LVSW in adults is approximately 90 ± 30 gm · m (mean ± S.D.); in patients with dilated cardiomyopathy or heart failure from extensive prior myocardial infarction, LVSW is often less than 40 gm-m. Values less than 25 gm-m indicate severe LV systolic failure and when LVSW is less than 20 gm-m the prognosis is grave.

LVSW is a measure of total LV chamber function and can be considered to reflect myocardial contractility only when the ventricle is reasonably homogeneous in its composition, as in most patients with dilated cardiomyopathy. For patients with coronary artery disease and extensive myocardial infarction, LVSW may be depressed even though there remain well perfused areas of the myocardium with normal contractility.

***Ejection Phase Indices.*** LV systolic function can be assessed using only the volume data from the PV diagram. Thus, one of the most widely used indices of LV systolic

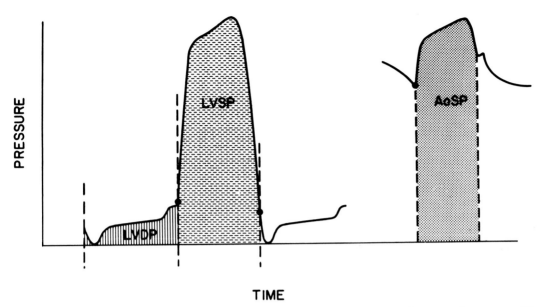

**TIME**

**Fig. 20-5.** Left ventricular (LV) and aortic (Ao) pressure tracings, illustrating areas planimetered to measure LV mean systolic pressure (LVSP), mean diastolic pressure (LVDP), and aortic mean systolic pressure (AoSP). LVSP is the area contained under the LV pressure curve, bounded by perpendicular lines defining end-diastole and mitral valve opening; LVDP is the diastolic area similarly defined. AoSP is the area contained under the Ao pressure curve, bounded by perpendicular lines defining aortic valve opening and closure.

performance is the *ejection fraction* (EF), which is defined as:

$$EF = (LVEDV - LVESV)/LVEDV \quad (3)$$

where LVEDV and ESV are the LV end-diastolic and end-systolic volumes, respectively. In the cardiac catheterization laboratory, LVEF is most often derived from the LV angiogram, as discussed in Chapter 19. If the EF is divided by the ejection time (ET), measured from the aortic pressure tracing, the quotient is called *mean normalized systolic ejection rate* (*MNSER*).

$$MNSER = \frac{(LVEDV - LVESV)}{(LVEDV)(ET)} \quad (4)$$

Finally, another ejection phase index of LV systolic function is velocity of circumferential fiber shortening, $V_{CF}$.[28,29] This is calculated as the rate of shortening of a theoretical LV myocardial fiber in a circumferential plane at the midpoint of the long axis of the ventricle. For convenience, mean $V_{CF}$ is used most often, rather than instantaneous or peak $V_{CF}$. Mean $V_{CF}$ is obtained as end-diastolic endocardial circumferential fiber length ($\pi D_{ED}$) minus end-systolic endocardial circumferential fiber length ($\pi D_{ES}$), di-

vided by ET and normalized for end-diastolic circumferential fiber length:

$$V_{CF} = (\pi D_{ED} - \pi D_{ES}/\pi D_{ED}(ET)$$
$$= (D_{ED} - D_{ES})/D_{ED}(ET) \quad (5)$$

$D_{ED}$ and $D_{ES}$ are end-diastolic and end-systolic minor axis dimensions. Although $V_{CF}$ can be calculated from angiographic data using the area-length method ($D = 4A/\pi L$), it is most commonly calculated from values for D measured by echocardiography. Normal values for isovolumic and ejection phase indices are given in Table 20-2.

Ejection phase indices are obtained easily from LV angiography and can also be derived reliably from a variety of noninvasive techniques such as radionuclide ventriculography and echocardiography. The most widely used ejection phase index, the *ejection fraction*, is generally depressed when myocardial contractility is diminished. However, the ejection indices are heavily dependent on preload and afterload and cannot be regarded as reliable indices of contractility in conditions associated with altered loading conditions. Thus, increases in preload cause the EF (and other ejection indices) to rise: consequently, left ventricular EF may be in-

**TABLE 20-2.**  *Evaluation of Left Ventricular Systolic Performance: Normal Values for Some Isovolumic and Ejection Phase Indices*

| Contractility Indices | | Normal Values (mean ± S.D.) | References |
|---|---|---|---|
| *Isovolumic Indices:* | | | |
| Maximum dP/dt | | 1610 ± 290 mmHg/sec | 7 |
| | | 1670 ± 320 mmHg/sec | 26 |
| | | 1661 ± 323 mmHg/sec | 19 |
| Maximum (dP/dt)/P) | | 44 ± 8.4 sec$^{-1}$ | 19 |
| $V_{PM}$ or peak $\left[\dfrac{dP/dt}{28P}\right]$ | | 1.47 ± 0.19 ML/sec | 26 |
| dP/dt/DP at DP = 40 mmHg | | 37.6 ± 12.2 sec$^{-1}$ | 19 |
| *Ejection Phase Indices:* | | | |
| LVSW | | 81 ± 23 gm-m | 6 |
| LVSWI | | 53 ± 22 gm-m/M$^2$ | 30 & 31, combined |
| | | 41 ± 12 gm-m/M$^2$ | 32 |
| EF | angio: | 0.72 ± 0.08 | 33 |
| MNSER | angio: | 3.32 ± 0.84 EDV/sec | 19 |
| | echo: | 2.29 ± 0.30 EDV/sec | 34 |
| Mean $V_{CF}$ | angio: | 1.83 ± 0.56 ED circ/sec | 19 |
| | | 1.50 ± 0.27 ED circ/sec | 29 |
| | echo: | 1.09 ± 0.12 ED circ/sec | 34 |

dP/dt = rate of rise of left ventricular (LV) pressure; DP = developed LV pressure; ML = muscle lengths; MNSER = mean normalized systolic ejection rate; ED = end-diastolic; V = volume; circ = circumference; EF = ejection fraction.

creased in patients with mitral or aortic regurgitation, severe anemia, or other causes of increased diastolic LV inflow and may mask underlying deterioration of myocardial contractility. Conversely, increases in afterload cause the EF to fall: consequently, left ventricular EF may be low in patients with severe aortic stenosis or other causes of increased resistance to systolic ejection and may falsely suggest underlying depression of myocardial contractility.

In actual practice, acute elevation of LV preload causes some increase in LV chamber size and aortic pressure, and these increases in afterload (systolic $\sigma$ resisting shortening) tend to decrease the EF and other ejection indices, offsetting the rise in EF which a pure rise in preload would produce. Thus, Rankin and co-workers produced changes in venous return by total body tilt in normal subjects:[34] despite substantial changes in LV end-diastolic dimension and volume, there were no significant changes in EF, MNSER or $V_{CF}$. Similarly, acute elevation of afterload by raising aortic pressure causes an increase in LVEDP, and the resultant rise in preload (end-diastolic fiber stretch) tends to increase the EF and other ejection indices, offsetting the fall in EF produced by a pure rise in afterload. These physiologic adjustments explain why the ejection indices are much more useful clinically than might be expected on the basis of studies in the isolated heart or muscle preparation.

An LV ejection fraction of less than 0.40 indicates depressed LV systolic pump function, and if there is no abnormal loading to account for it, an LVEF ≤ 0.40 can be taken to signify depressed myocardial contractility. An LVEF of <0.20 corresponds to severe depression of LV systolic performance and is normally associated with a poor prognosis. Interpretation of EF and other ejection indices is improved by consideration of the ventricular preload and afterload, and the latter are defined most precisely by end-diastolic and end-systolic wall stresses, respectively.

### End-Systolic Pressure-Volume, and σ-Length Relations.

Over the past 10 to 15 years, several groups have shown that the LV end-systolic pressure-volume, pressure-diameter and σ-length relationships accurately reflect myocardial contractility, independent of changes in ventricular loading.[35-39] The fundamental principle of end-systolic pressure-volume analysis is that at end-systole there is a single line relating LV chamber pressure to volume, unique for the level of contractility and independent of loading conditions. The LV end-systolic PV line can be generated by producing a series of PV loops (such as the one in Figure 20-4), over a range of loading conditions (Fig. 20-6). The line connecting the upper left hand corners of the individual PV diagrams is the end-systolic PV line. This line is characterized by a slope and by an x-axis intercept, called $V_o$ (the extrapolated end-systolic volume when end-systolic pressure is zero). Current evidence indicates that an increase in contractility shifts the end-systolic PV line to the left

with a steeper slope, and a depression in contractility is associated with a displacement of the line downward and to the right, with a reduced slope. While there is some uncertainty as to the meaning of $V_o$, it is agreed generally that an increase in slope of the end systolic PV line is a sensitive indicator of an increase in contractility. Unfortunately, the technique of end-systolic analysis may not be as useful in comparing one subject with another as in comparing values in one subject to those measured in the same subject after an intervention. The end-systolic PV lines for groups of patients with normal, intermediate, and depressed LV contractility are shown in Figure 20-7.

To measure the end-systolic PV line one can use aortic dicrotic notch pressure as end-systolic LV pressure and minimum LV chamber volume as end-systolic volume. LV volume can be measured by angiography, using either direct LV injection or right-sided injection with image enhancement by digital subtraction angiography. Alternatively, LV volume can be measured by radionuclide techniques, ultrasonic techniques, or a specially designed impedance catheter.[40]

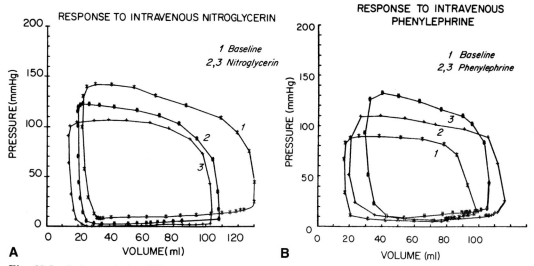

**Fig. 20-6.** Left ventricular (LV) pressure-volume plots constructed using radionuclide ventriculography to measure LV volume simultaneous with measurement of LV pressure during cardiac catheterization. (A) Three sequential plots measured during baseline and at two sequential doses of intravenous nitroglycerin to lower LV pressure. (B) Similar plots in a patient whose baseline LV systolic pressure was low: in this case phenylephrine was used in increasing doses to produce three levels of systolic loading. The upper left hand (end-systolic) corners of the three pressure-volume plots in each panel define a straight line, the LV end-systolic pressure-volume line. See text for discussion. (Reproduced, with permission, from McKay RG et al: Left ventricular pressure-volume diagrams and end-systolic pressure-volume relations in human beings. J Am Coll Cardiol 3:301, 1984.)

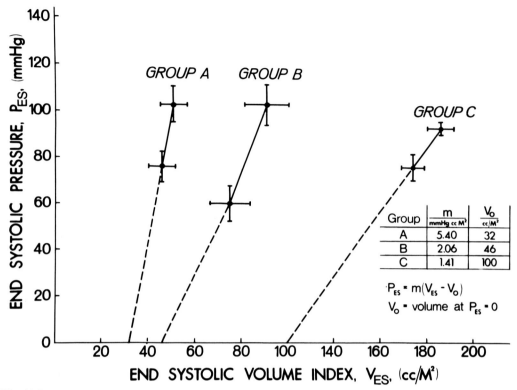

**Fig. 20-7.** Left ventricular end-systolic pressure ($P_{ES}$) plotted against end-systolic volume index ($V_{ES}$) at two levels of loading for each of 3 patient groups: Group A, patients with normal LV contractile function; Group B, patients with moderate depression of LV contractile performance; Group C, patients with marked depression of LV contractility. Depressed contractility shifts the $P_{ES} - V_{ES}$ relation to the right, with a reduced slope (m) and intercept ($V_O$) of the relation for each group. (Reproduced, with permission, from Grossman W, et al: Contractile state of the left ventricle in man as evaluated from end-systolic pressure-volume relations. Circulation 45:845, 1977.)

***Stress-shortening Relations.*** Another approach to the assessment of LV systolic performance and myocardial contractility involves measuring the extent of cardiac muscle shortening and relating this shortening to the systolic wall stress ($\sigma$) resisting shortening.

If a ventricle is presented with progressively increasing resistance to ejection, $\sigma$ rises while extent of myocardial shortening declines. Thus, a plot of systolic $\sigma$ (horizontal axis) against myocardial shortening expressed as EF, $V_{CF}$, or %$\Delta$D (vertical axis) yields a tight inverse relationship (Fig. 20-8). Data from studies of individual patients may then be compared with these normal values. In Figure 20-8, if the point relating end-systolic $\sigma$ ($\sigma_{ES}$) and %$\Delta$D for a given patient lies within the confidence lines of the normal population, myocardial contractility is likely to be normal; however, if the $\sigma_{ES}$-%$\Delta$D point lies below the normal range, contractility is depressed even though %$\Delta$D may be normal. Figure 20-9 shows that the LV end-systolic wall stress–%$\Delta$D relationship is shifted upward by an increase in contractility resulting from a dobutamine infusion. One caution concerning the $\sigma_{ES}$-%$\Delta$D relationship is that it is preload sensitive. That is, increases in preload will increase %$\Delta$D for any level of $\sigma_{ES}$. There is some evidence that when $V_{CF}$ is substituted for %$\Delta$D, the preload dependence of the stress-shortening relationship is attenuated or abolished.

Plots of systolic wall stress against LV ejection fraction have been analyzed for patients with a variety of conditions, including LV pressure overload (Fig. 20-10). In these plots, comprised of multiple individual data points (each point relating LV wall $\sigma$ and EF

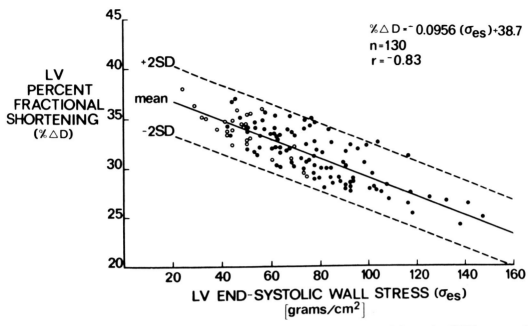

**Fig. 20-8.** Relationship between LV end systolic wall stress ($\sigma_{ES}$) and % fractional shortening (%$\Delta$D) measured by echo for 130 control points measured at rest (open circles) or during methoxamine infusion (closed circles). The inverse relationship defines normal LV myocardial contractility. (Reproduced, with permission, from Borow KM, et al: Left ventricular end-systolic stress-shortening and stress-length relations in humans. Am J Cardiol 50:1301, 1982.)

for an individual patient) an inverse systolic $\sigma$-EF relationship is apparent for patients with chronic LV pressure-overload. This suggests that the depressed LVEF in some of these individuals is due to excessive systolic $\sigma$; that is, the load resisting systolic shortening is abnormally high and is responsible for a reduced extent of shortening. This combination of high $\sigma$ and low EF is sometimes referred to as "afterload mismatch"[41–43] and implies that hypertrophy has been inadequate to return systolic wall stress to its relatively low normal level. Patients in whom LVEF is diminished out of proportion to any increase in systolic wall stress can be assumed to have depressed myocardial contractility (Fig. 20-11).

The advantage of $\sigma$-shortening analysis over PV diagram analysis is that wall $\sigma$ takes into consideration changes in LV geometry and muscle mass that occur in response to chronic alterations in loading. Thus, a systolic pressure of 250 to 300 mmHg imposed acutely on a normal left ventricular chamber would result in considerable reduction in LVEF, perhaps down to the 20 to 30% range.

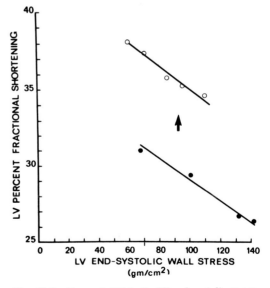

**Fig. 20-9.** Upward shift in the LV end-systolic stress-shortening relation resulting from dobutamine infusion. See text. (Reproduced, with permission, from Borow KM, et al: Left ventricular end-systolic stress-shortening and stress-length relations in humans. Am J Cardiol 50:1301, 1982.)

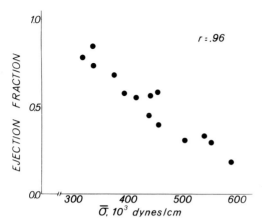

**Fig. 20-10.** Left ventricular (LV) ejection fraction plotted against mean systolic circumferential wall stress, $\bar{\sigma}$, for 14 patients with pure aortic stenosis (normal coronary arteries, no other valve disease) and varying degrees of LV decompensation. The inverse relationship is consistent with afterload excess as a principal cause of the decreased ejection fraction. (Reproduced, with permission, from Gunther S, Grossman W: Determinants of ventricular function in pressure-overload hypertrophy in man. Circulation 59:679, 1979.)

This change occurs since in the absence of any increase in LV wall thickness or decrease in chamber radius, systolic $\sigma$ would more than double in response to such an acute pressure-overload, and this would lead to a major reduction in LVEF. However, if the increase in systolic pressure to 250 to 300 mmHg occurs gradually and is matched by the development of sufficient hypertro-

phy in the appropriate pattern, systolic wall $\sigma$ will remain normal and therefore fiber shortening and LVEF will not decrease. Thus, in the presence of significant hypertrophy and/or altered LV geometry, $\sigma$-shortening analysis may have considerable value.

## DIASTOLIC FUNCTION

### Left Ventricular Diastolic Distensibility: Pressure-Volume Relationship

As pointed out by Henderson in 1923: "In the heart, diastolic relaxation is a vital factor and not merely the passive stretching of a rubber bag. Being vital, it is variable."[44] Analysis of diastolic function today requires appreciation of the fact that diastolic compliance is variable and may change substantially in a given patient from one minute to the next. Diastolic function is summated physiologically in the relation between LV pressure and volume during diastole (Fig. 20-4, segment DA). Traditionally, an upward shift in this diastolic PV relation is regarded as indicating increased LV diastolic chamber *stiffness* and a downward shift indicates decreased stiffness or increased LV diastolic chamber *compliance*. In the terminology of physics and engineering, stiffness, and its opposite, compliance, relate a change in pressure ($\Delta P$) to a change in volume ($\Delta V$); therefore, some investigators have

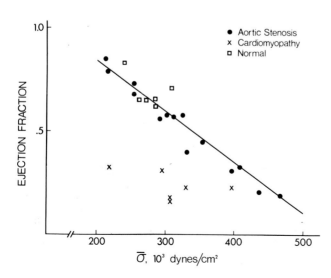

**Fig. 20-11.** Plot of LV ejection fraction against systolic $\bar{\sigma}$, similar to Figure 20-10, but including patients with aortic stenosis (solid dots), dilated cardiomyopathy (crosses), and normal ventricular function (open squares). The regression line was constructed from the patients with normal LV function and those with aortic stenosis. See text for discussion. (Reprinted, with permission, from Gunther S., Grossman W: Determination of ventricular function in pressure overload hypertrophy in man. Circulation 59:679, 1979.)

restricted these terms to refer to the *slope* of the diastolic PV relation. In this regard, as seen in segment DA of Figure 20-4, LV diastolic stiffness ($\Delta P/\Delta V$) is low early in diastole and rises steadily throughout diastolic filling.

Figure 20-12 shows theoretical LV diastolic PV plots for patients with normal, stiff, and compliant ventricular chambers. Several major problems arise when stiffness and compliance are defined strictly in terms of the slope of the diastolic PV diagram. First, in some clinical conditions the LV diastolic PV plot may shift upward in a parallel fashion (e.g., during angina pectoris), without a noticeable change in slope. These patients have increased LV filling pressure often with normal chamber volumes, and from a hydrodynamic point of view the LV chamber must be regarded as presenting increased resistance to diastolic filling. To say that LV diastolic stiffness and compliance are normal in such individuals because the upward shift has been a parallel one, without slope change, seems inappropriate. In some cases, patients may have a downward shift in the LV diastolic PV plot (e.g., following nitroprusside infusion in patients with heart failure) with an increase in the steepness of the plot; again, to say that such patients exhibit increased LV diastolic stiffness seems inappropriate, since they are requiring a lower filling pressure to achieve the same diastolic chamber dimension and fiber stretch. Thus, the LV diastolic PV plot can show changes of two types: *displacement* or movement of the entire relationship upward, downward, or laterally, and *configuration change*, including change in curvature. In our studies, we have referred to upward or downward displacement changes as being associated with a change in *ventricular distensibility*. Thus, if the LV diastolic PV plot shifts upward, as is common during attacks of angina pectoris, we would say that the LV chamber has become *less distensible;* a higher diastolic pressure is required to fill or distend the chamber to its prior volume. Similarly, a downward shift in the diastolic PV plot, as occurs commonly during nitroprusside infusion in patients with heart failure, would be said to indicate an increase in LV diastolic distensibility. The changes in curvature and/or configuration that may accompany these displacement changes are difficult to quantify and to interpret.[45]

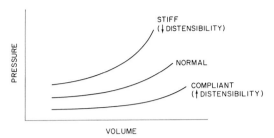

**Fig. 20-12.** Diagrammatic representation of ventricular diastolic pressure-volume relations for normal, stiff, and compliant ventricles. See text for discussion.

A variety of formulae have been developed for analyzing the curvature of the LV diastolic PV plot.[45–50] These generally assume that the curvature is exponential, an assumption which is often but not always reasonable. Diastolic PV and P-segment length (SL) plots constructed from a series of *end*-diastolic points have been utilized in animal experiments to assess LV diastolic compliance,[49,51] and this technique is having its first application to clinical studies. When a series of end-diastolic PV or P-SL points are plotted, the relation is more strictly exponential, and application of mathematical models and analysis is more easily justified by the good agreement of measured data and mathematical predictions.

Factors that influence the position of the LV diastolic PV plot (that is, factors that influence LV diastolic *distensibility*) are listed in Table 20-3. Factors extrinsic to the LV chamber may influence the diastolic PV plot in striking fashion. Constrictive pericarditis and pericardial tamponade are associated with a striking upward shift in the diastolic PV relation. In dogs with experimental tamponade, it has been shown that this upward shift is a *parallel* shift, without substantial change in curvature. When distended, the right ventricle can decrease LV diastolic distensibility by exerting an extrinsic pressure on the LV chamber in diastole, through the shared interventricular septum, which may actually bulge into the LV chamber. Acute RV infarction causes dilatation of the RV chamber which in the presence of an intact, previously unstressed pericardium may lead to extrinsic compression of the LV in diastole with a hemodynamic pattern resembling cardiac tamponade.[52] The effect of increased RV loading on LV diastolic distensibility is an

**TABLE 20-3.** *Factors That Influence LV Diastolic Chamber Distensibility*

I. Factors extrinsic to the LV chamber
 A. Pericardial restraint
 B. Right ventricular loading
 C. Coronary vascular turgor (erectile effect)
 D. Extrinsic compression by tumor, pleural pressure, etc.

II. Factors intrinsic to LV chamber
 A. Passive elasticity of LV wall (stiffness or compliance when myocytes are completely relaxed)
  1. Thickness of LV wall
  2. Composition of LV wall (muscle, fibrosis, amyloid, hemosiderin) including both endocardium and myocardium
  3. Temperature, osmolality
 B. Active elasticity of LV wall due to residual cross-bridge activation (cycling and/or latch state) through part or all of diastole:
  1. Slow relaxation affecting early diastole only
  2. Incomplete relaxation affecting early, mid- and end-diastolic distensibility
  3. Diastolic tone, contracture, or rigor
 C. Elastic recoil (diastolic suction)
 D. Viscoelasticity (stress relaxation, creep)

example of ventricular interaction, which is more prominent in the presence of an intact and relatively snug pericardium. In fact, in animal experiments it is difficult to demonstrate diastolic ventricular interaction once the pericardium has been opened widely.[53]

Coronary vascular turgor can influence LV diastolic chamber stiffness.[54] The LV wall has a rich blood supply, and engorgement of the capillaries and venules with blood makes the wall relatively stiff: for obvious reasons, this has been referred to as the erectile effect. While the erectile effect is probably not of much importance when coronary blood flow and pressure (the two components determining the degree of turgor) are in the physiologic range, a marked fall in coronary flow and pressure (as occurs distal to a coronary occlusion when collateral flow is poor

or absent) is associated with a decrease in stiffness of the affected myocardium and an increase in LV diastolic distensibility.

Extrinsic compression of the heart by tumor may cause decreased LV diastolic distensibility and may mimic cardiac tamponade. An example of this is presented in Chapter 27.

When an upward shift in the diastolic PV relation is present and the extrinsic factors listed in Table 20-3 cannot clearly explain the altered distensibility, a change in one of the intrinsic determinants of LV distensibility is likely to be present. Altered passive elasticity due to amyloidosis or diffuse fibrosis may cause a restrictive cardiomyopathic pattern, with high LV diastolic pressure relative to volume in the presence of reasonably well-preserved systolic function. Clinically, heart failure may be present. Endomyocardial biopsy of RV or LV may be needed to establish the diagnosis (see Chapter 31).

Abnormal diastolic relaxation can cause the diastolic PV relation to shift upward strikingly. During angina pectoris, a 10 to 15 mmHg rise in average LV diastolic pressure may occur with little or no change in diastolic volume; if this persists for a sufficient duration ($\geq 10$ to 20 minutes), pulmonary edema may result. Such episodes of "flash pulmonary edema" in patients with essentially normal LV systolic function and normal LV chamber size are generally indicative of a large mass of ischemic myocardium[55] and suggest three-vessel or left main coronary obstruction. The decreased LV distensibility during ischemia may be prevented in many patients by a $Ca^{++}$ channel blocking agent.[56] The mechanism of impaired myocardial relaxation during the ischemia of angina pectoris is not understood completely, but may be associated with diastolic $Ca^{++}$ overload of the ischemic myocytes, in part due to ischemic dysfunction of the sarcoplasmic reticulum.[57] During the ischemia of acute coronary occlusion, an upward shift of the diastolic PV relation may occur if sufficient collateral blood flow is present to permit continued systolic contraction of the ischemic segment. However, if ischemia is sufficiently severe to cause complete akinesis of the affected myocardium, altered distensibility does not occur: "incomplete" relaxation can occur only in myocytes where there has been systolic cross-bridge activation. Also, the marked decrease in coronary vascular turgor distal to a coronary occlusion with poor or absent collaterals, together with local accumulation of $H^+$, contributes to an increase in regional distensibility, so that the net effect on the ventricular diastolic PV relation may be one of no change.

Impaired relaxation with decreased LV diastolic distensibility is also seen in patients with hypertrophic cardiomyopathy, and during angina pectoris in patients with aortic stenosis and normal coronary arteries.

## Indices of LV Diastolic Relaxation Rate

There has been much attention in recent years to measures of LV diastolic relaxation during the isovolumic relaxation period and during early diastolic filling. A listing of some of these indices and their normal values is given in Table 20-4. The time course of LV pressure decline following aortic valve closure is altered in conditions known to be as-sociated with abnormalities of myocardial relaxation.[50]

***Isovolumic Pressure Decay.*** One of the simplest ways of quantifying the time course of LV pressure decline is to measure the maximum rate of pressure fall, peak $-dP/dt$. Although peak $-dP/dt$ is altered by conditions that change myocardial relaxation, it is also altered by changes in loading conditions. For example, peak LV $-dP/dt$ increases (that is, rises in absolute value) when aortic pressure rises. Thus, an increase in LV $-dP/dt$ from $-1500$ mmHg/sec to $-1800$ mmHg/sec could be due to an increase in the rate of myocardial relaxation, a rise in aortic pressure, or both. However, an increase in peak $-dP/dt$ at a time when aortic pressure is unchanged or declining signifies an improvement of LV relaxation. LV peak $-dP/dt$ is decreased during the myocardial ischemia of either angina pectoris or infarction, and is increased in response to beta adrenergic stimulation and the new bipyridine inotrope milrinone.[58] It is not increased by digitalis glycosides.

**TABLE 20-4.** *Evaluation of Left Ventricular Diastolic Performance: Normal Values for Some Indices of Relaxation and Filling*

|  | Normal Values | Reference |
|---|---|---|
| Peak $-dP/dt$ | $2660 \pm 700$ mmHg/sec | 7 |
|  | $2922 \pm 750$ mmHg/sec | 67 |
|  | $1864 \pm 390$ mmHg/sec | 68 |
|  | $1825 \pm 261$ mmHg/sec | 69 |
| T (logarithmic method, equation 7) | $38 \pm 7$ msec | 67 |
|  | $33 \pm 8$ msec | 68 |
|  | $31 \pm 3$ msec | 69 |
| T (derivative method, equations 8 and 9) | $55 \pm 12$ msec | 69 |
| $P_B$ (derivative method, equations 8 and 9) | $-25 \pm 9$ mmHg | 69 |
| PFR | $3.3 \pm 0.6$ EDV/sec | 63 |
| Time to PFR | $136 \pm 23$ msec | 63 |
| Peak $-dh/dt$ (posterior wall) | $8.4 \pm 3.0$ cm/sec | 64 |
|  | $8.2 \pm 3.7$ cm/sec | 66 |

Peak $-dP/dt$ = maximum rate of LV isovolumic pressure decline; T = time constant of LV isovolumic relaxation, calculated assuming both zero pressure intercept (equation 7) and variable pressure ($P_B$) intercept (equations 8 and 9); PFR = LV peak filling rate, from radionuclide ventriculography, normalized to end-diastolic volumes (EDV)/sec; Peak $-dh/dt$ = maximum rate of posterior wall thinning, measured by echo.

### *Time Constant of Relaxation.*

Because of the load dependency of peak $-dP/dt$, and the fact that it uses information from only 1 point on the LV pressure-time plot, newer indices have been introduced that analyze the time course of LV isovolumic pressure fall more completely. In 1976, Weiss et al. introduced the time constant T (or tau) of LV isovolumic pressure decline.[59] They pointed out that LV isovolumic pressure decline could be fit by the equation:

$$P = e^{At+B} \qquad (6)$$

where P is LV isovolumic pressure, t is time after peak negative $dP/dt$, and A and B are constants. This can also be expressed as:

$$\ln P = At + B \qquad (7)$$

A plot of ln LV pressure versus time allows calculation of the slope A, a negative number whose units are $sec^{-1}$. The time constant tau or T of isovolumic pressure fall is then defined as $-1/A$, expressed in milliseconds, and is the time that it takes P to decline $1/e$ of its value. Studies by the Johns Hopkins group have suggested that myocardial relaxation is normally complete by approximately 3.5 T after the onset of isovolumic relaxation. The normal value for T as calculated using a plot of LnP-versus-t is 25 to 40 msec in man. Thus, by 140 msec after the dicrotic notch, LV diastolic PV relations should be determined primarily by passive elastic properties of the myocardium. Since the normal LV diastolic filling period is >400 msec, it is unlikely, according to this concept, that late and end diastolic PV relations are still influenced by the relaxation process. There is now considerable evidence, however, that even in the normal myocardium cross-bridge cycling persists to some extent throughout diastole. This resting myocardial activity or tone makes it difficult to know what significance to apply to the concept that relaxation is complete at 3.5 T. Nevertheless, it is important to emphasize that the relaxation process does progress with time through diastole, so that slowing of the process (prolongation of T) or shortening of the diastolic filling period (e.g., tachycardia) will result in a greater resistance to early and even late diastolic filling.

An approach to the measurement of T that has become more widely accepted in recent years uses a more general equation to describe LV isovolumic pressure decline:[60]

$$P = P_o e^{-t/T} + P_B \qquad (8)$$

In this formulation, if diastole were infinite in duration ($t = \infty$), P decays to a residual pressure $P_B$. In the initial formulation by Weiss et al,[59] P always declines toward zero in long diastoles. The more general formula allows for 2 variables; tau or T (which equals $-1/A$) and $P_B$. Work by Carroll and co-workers,[61] as well as other groups,[58] have shown that both $P_B$ and T can vary with physiologic maneuvers (e.g., exercise, ischemia). The biologic meaning of $P_B$ is uncertain, although there has been speculation that it may reflect the level of diastolic myocardial tone. A problem with both $P_B$ and T is that there is experimental evidence that the speed of this relaxation process itself is altered by myofiber stretch that occurs after mitral valve opening.

When T is to be derived from the formulae that assume a variable pressure intercept ($P_B$), the calculation is often accomplished by taking the first derivative:[60]

$$P = P_o e^{-t/T} + P_B$$
$$dP/dt = -\frac{1}{T}(P - P_B) \qquad (9)$$

Here, a plot of $dP/dt$ vs $(P - P_B)$ has the slope $-1/T$.

T may be prolonged from slow myocardial relaxation, but asynchrony of the relaxation process within the ventricular chamber may also result in a prolongation of T. In addition, T is probably not completely independent of loading conditions, although the influence of altered loading is relatively small.

### *Peak Filling Rate.*

After mitral valve opening, ventricular filling usually proceeds briskly with an initial rapid filling phase, a middle slow filling phase, and a terminal increase in filling rate associated with atrial systole. The rapid filling phase may be characterized by a maximum or peak filling rate (PFR) and by time to PFR. PFR is usually determined by plotting LV volume against time, fitting the initial portion of this plot after mitral valve opening to a third (or higher) order polynomial, and solving for the first derivative of this polynomial. LV volume for this calculation may be obtained from the LV cineangiogram, or from radionuclide techniques. As one might expect, PFR is preload dependent: interventions that raise left atrial pressure increase PFR; interventions that reduce pulmonary venous return and left atrial pressure cause PFR to decrease. However, an increase in PFR that occurs when LV filling pressure (pulmonary capillary wedge pressure, left atrial pressure, or LV diastolic pressure) is unchanged or falling can reasonably be taken as an indication that LV relaxation has improved. Thus, PFR has been shown to decrease during angina pectoris when LV filling pressure is increasing; since the rise in LV filling pressure by itself would cause an increase in PFR, the fall in PFR which is actually observed most likely indicates slowed relaxation of the myocardium, consistent with the other findings in this condition (fall in peak negative dP/dt, prolongation of T) suggesting impaired relaxation of the ischemic myocardium. PFR is reduced in patients with coronary stenoses, even in the absence of overt ischemia, and improves following coronary angioplasty.[62] PFR is also reduced in patients with hypertrophic cardiomyopathy and improves following administration of a calcium blocking agent.[63] PFR is usually normalized for end-diastolic volume (EDV) and expressed as EDV/sec. Thus, cardiac dilatation by itself will tend to depress PFR, exaggerating its preload-dependence.

***Rate of Wall Thinning.*** Another index of diastolic function, which is similar in some ways to PFR, is the peak rate of diastolic LV wall thinning. This can be measured echocardiographically by plotting posterior or septal wall thickness against time, fitting the data to a polynomial and taking the first derivative.[64-66] The posterior wall thickness, h, and its first derivative, dh/dt, reflect regional diastolic function of the posterior wall myocardium. An advantage of peak negative dh/dt as opposed to PFR is that peak negative dh/dt assesses regional myocardial function while PFR describes behavior for the whole ventricle and will be insensitive when equal and opposite changes in diastolic function are occurring in different parts of the LV chamber. Peak negative dh/dt decreases during angina, even though LV filling pressure rises.[66]

A variety of other indices of diastolic myocardial relaxation have been proposed. Most are imperfect, as are the ones discussed above. However, important information about diastolic relaxation and distensibility can usually be gleaned from examination of the parameters discussed in this chapter, taken in the context of the clinical setting and other hemodynamic findings in an individual patient.

# REFERENCES

1. Wiggers CJ: Studies on the cardiodynamic actions of drugs. I. The application of the optical methods of pressure registration in the study of cardiac stimulants and depressants. J Pharmacol Exp Ther 30:217, 1927.
2. Wiggers CJ: Studies on the cardiodynamic actions of drugs. II. The mechanism of cardiac stimulation by epinephrin. J Pharmacol Exp Ther 30:233, 1927.
3. Wiggers CJ, Stimson B: Studies on the cardiodynamic actions of drugs. III. The mechanism of cardiac stimulation by digitalis and g-strophanthin. J Pharmacol Exp Ther 30:251, 1927.
4. Gleason WL, Braunwald E: Studies on the first derivative of the ventricular pressure pulse in man. J Clin Invest 41:80–91, 1962.
5. Bowditch HP: Uber die Eigenthumlichkeiten der Reizarbeit, welche die Muskelfasern des Herzens zeigen. Ber Verh der kongiglich sachsischen ges Wissenschaften zu Leipzig 23: 652, 1871.
6. Grossman W, et al: Changes in inotropic state of the left ventricle during isometric exercise. Br Heart J 35:697, 1973.

7. McLaurin LP, Rolett EL, Grossman W: Impaired left ventricular relaxation during pacing induced ischemia. Am J Cardiol 32:751, 1973.
8. Graber JD, Conti CR, Lappe DL, Ross RS: Effect of pacing-induced tachycardia and myocardial ischemia on ventricular pressure-velocity relationships in man. Circulation 46:74, 1972.
9. Mason DT, Braunwald E: Studies on digitalis. IX. Effects of ouabain on the nonfailing human heart. J Clin Invest 42:1105, 1963.
10. Grossman W, et al: Alterations in preload and myocardial mechanics. Circ Res 31:83, 1972.
11. Brodie BR, Grossman W, Mann T, McLaurin LP: Effects of sodium nitroprusside on left ventricular diastolic pressure-volume relations. J Clin Invest 59:59, 1977.
12. Wallace AG, Skinner NS, Mitchell JH: Hemodynamic determinants of the maximal rate of rise of left ventricular pressure. Am J Physiol 205:30, 1963.
13. Zimpfer M, Vatner SF: Effects of acute increases in left ventricular preload on indices of myocardial function in conscious, unrestrained and in-

tact, tranquilized baboons. J Clin Invest 67:430, 1981.

14. Broughton A, Korner PI: Steady-state effects of preload and afterload on isovolumic indices of contractility in autonomically blocked dogs. Cardiovasc Res 14:245, 1980.

15. Barnes GE, Horwitz LD, Bishop VS: Reliability of the maximum derivatives of left ventricular pressure and internal diameter as indices of the inotropic state of the depressed myocardium. Cardiovasc Res 13:652, 1979.

16. Gersh BJ, Hahn CEW, Prys-Roberts C: Physical criteria for measurement of left ventricular pressure and its first derivative. Cardiovasc Res 5:32, 1971.

17. Fifer MA, et al: Myocardial contractile function in aortic stenosis as determined from the rate of stress development during isovolumic systole. Am J Cardiol 44:1318, 1979.

18. Arentzen CE, et al: Force-frequency characteristics of the left ventricle in the conscious dog. Circ Res 42:64, 1978.

19. Peterson KL, et al: Comparison of isovolumic and ejection phase indices of myocardial performance in man. Circulation 49:1088, 1974.

20. Grossman W, et al: New technique for determining instantaneous myocardial force-velocity relations in the intact heart. Circ Res 28:290, 1971.

21. Mirsky I, Pasternac A, Ellison RC: General index for the assessment of cardiac function. Am J Cardiol 30:483, 1972.

22. Falsetti HL, Mates RE, Green DG, Bunnel IL: $V_{max}$ as an index of contractile state in man. Circulation 43:467, 1971.

23. Mason DT: Usefulness and limitations of the rate of rise of intraventricular pressure (dp/dt) in the evaluation of myocardial contractility in man. Am J Cardiol 23:516, 1969.

24. Mehmel H, Krayenbuehl HP, Rutishauser W: Peak measured velocity of shortening in the canine left ventricle. J Appl Physiol 29:637, 1970.

25. Stein PD, McBride GG, Sabbah HN: The fractional rate of change of ventricular power during isovolumic contraction. Derivation of haemodynamic terms and studies in dogs. Cardiovasc Res 9:456, 1975.

26. Krayenbuehl HP, et al: High-fidelity left ventricular pressure measurements for the assessment of cardiac contractility in man. Am J Cardiol 31:415, 1973.

27. Sonnenblick EH, Parmley WW, Urshel CW: The contractile state of the heart as expressed by force-velocity relations. Am J Cardiol 23:488, 1969.

28. Paraskos JA, et al: A non-invasive technique for the determination of velocity of circumferential fiber shortening in man. Circ Res 29:610, 1971.

29. Karliner JS, et al: Mean velocity of fiber shortening. A simplified measure of left ventricular myocardial contractility. Circulation 44:323, 1971.

30. Ross J Jr, et al: Left ventricular performance during muscular exercise in patients with and without cardiac dysfunction. Circulation 34:597, 1966.

31. Ross J Jr, Braunwald E: The study of left ventricular function in man by increasing resistance to ventricular ejection with angiotensin. Circulation 29:739, 1964.

32. McLaurin LP, et al: A new technique for the study of left ventricular pressure-volume relations in man. Circulation 48:56, 1973.

33. Wynne J, et al: Estimation of left ventricular volumes in man from biplane cineangiograms filmed in oblique projections. Am J Cardiol 41:726, 1978.

34. Rankin LS, Moos S, Grossman W: Alterations in preload and ejection phase indices of left ventricular performance. Circulation 51:910, 1975.

35. Suga H, Sagawa K, Shoukas AA: Load independence of the instantaneous pressure-volume ratio of the canine left ventricle and effects of epinephrine and heart rate on the ratio. Circ Res 32:314, 1973.

36. Weber KT, Janicki JS, Reeves RC, Hefner LL: Factors influencing left ventricular shortening in isolated canine heart. Am J Physiol 230:419, 1976.

37. Grossman W, et al: Contractile state of the left ventricle in man as evaluated from end-systolic pressure-volume relations. Circulation 45:845, 1977.

38. Mehmel HC, et al: The linearity of the end-systolic pressure-volume relationship in man and its sensitivity for assessment of left ventricular function. Circulation 63:1216, 1981.

39. Borow KM, Green LH, Grossman W, Braunwald E: Left ventricular end-systolic stress shortening and stress-length relations in human. Normal values and sensitivity to inotropic state. Am J Cardiol 50:1301, 1982.

40. McKay RG, et al: Instantaneous measurement of left and right ventricular stroke volume and pressure-volume relationships with an impedance catheter. Circulation 69:703, 1984.

41. Ross J Jr: Afterload mismatch and preload reserve: a conceptual framework for the analysis of ventricular function. Progr Cardiovasc Dis 18:255, 1976.

42. Gunther S, Grossman W: Determinants of ventricular function in pressure-overload hypertrophy in man. Circulation 59:679, 1979.

43. Grossman W: Cardiac hypertrophy: Useful adaptation or pathologic process? Am J Med 69:576, 1980.

44. Henderson Y: Volume changes of the heart. Physiol Rev 3:165, 1923.

45. Glantz SA: Computing indices of diastolic stiffness has been counterproductive. Fed Proc 39:162, 1980.

46. Gaasch WH, et al: Left ventricular stress and compliance in man. With special reference to normalized ventricular function curves. Circulation 45:746, 1972.

47. Mirsky I: Assessment of diastolic function: suggested methods and future considerations. Circulation 69:836, 1984.

48. Mirsky I, Pasipoularides A: Elastic properties of normal and hypertrophied cardiac muscle. Fed Proc 39:156, 1980.

49. Rankin JS, et al: Viscoelastic properties of the diastolic left ventricle in the conscious dog. Circ Res 41:37, 1977.

50. Grossman W, McLaurin LP: Diastolic properties of the left ventricle. Ann Intern Med 84:316, 1976.

51. Momomura SI, Bradley AB, Grossman W: Left ventricular diastolic pressure-segment length relations and end-diastolic distensibility in dogs with coronary stenoses: an angina physiology model. Circ Res 55:203, 1984.

52. Lorell BH, et al: Right ventricular infarction. Clinical diagnosis and differentiation from cardiac tamponade and constriction. Am J Cardiol 43:465, 1979.

53. Glantz SA, et al: The pericardium substantially affects the left ventricular diastolic pressure-volume relationship in the dog. Circ Res 42:433, 1978.

54. Vogel WM, et al: Acute alterations in left ventricular diastolic chamber stiffness. Role of the "Erectile" effect of coronary arterial pressure and flow in normal and damaged hearts. Circ Res 51:465, 1982.

55. McKay RG, et al: The pacing thallium test reexamined: correlation of pacing-induced hemodynamic changes with the amount of myocardium at risk. J Am Coll Cardiol 3:1469, 1984.

56. Lorell BH, Turi Z, Grossman W: Modification of left ventricular response to pacing tachycardia by nifedipine in patients with coronary artery disease. Am J Med 71:667, 1981.

57. Paulus WJ, Serizawa T, Grossman W: Altered left ventricular diastolic properties during pacing-induced ischemia in dogs with coronary stenosis. Potentiation by caffeine. Circ Res 50:218, 1982.

58. Monrad ES, et al: Improvement in indices of diastolic performance in patients with congestive heart failure treated with milrinone. Circulation 70:1030, 1984.

59. Weiss JL, Frederiksen JW, Weisfeldt ML: Hemodynamic determinants of the time-course of fall in canine left ventricular pressure. J Clin Invest 58:751, 1976.

60. Raff GL, Glantz SA: Volume loading slows left ventricular isovolumic relaxation rate. Circ Res 48:813, 1981.

61. Carroll JD, Hess OM, Hirzel HO, Krayenbuehl HP: Exercise-induced ischemia: The influence of altered relaxation on early diastolic pressures. Circulation 67:521, 1983.

62. Bonow RO, et al: Improved left ventricular diastolic filling in patients with coronary artery disease after percutaneous transluminal coronary angioplasty. Circulation 66:1159, 1982.

63. Bonow RO, et al: Effects of verapamil on left ventricular systolic function and diastolic filling in patients with hypertrophic cardiomyopathy. Circulation 64:787, 1981.

64. Mason SJ, et al: Exercise echocardiography: Detection of wall motion abnormalities during ischemia. Circulation 59:50, 1979.

65. St. John Sutton MG, Tajik AJ, Smith HC, Ritman EL: Angina in idiopathic hypertrophic subaortic stenosis. Circulation 61:561, 1980.

66. Bourdillon PD, et al: Increased regional myocardial stiffness of the left ventricle during pacing-induced angina in man. Circulation 67:316, 1983.

67. Pouleur H, et al: Force-velocity-length relations in hypertrophic cardiomyopathy: Evidence of normal or depressed myocardial contractility. Am J Cardiol 52:813, 1983.

68. Hirota Y: A clinical study of left ventricular relaxation. Circulation 62:756, 1980.

69. Thompson DS, et al: Analysis of left ventricular pressure during isovolumic relaxation in coronary artery disease. Circulation 65:690, 1982.

*chapter twenty one*

# Evaluation of Myocardial Blood Flow and Metabolism

ARLENE B. BRADLEY *and* DONALD S. BAIM

O VER the past three decades several techniques have been developed for the measurement of myocardial blood flow in conscious man. Although such measurements are not usually of clinical value in individual patients, they have resulted in significant advances in our knowledge of the regulation of the coronary circulation.

## REGULATION OF CORONARY BLOOD FLOW

Myocardial perfusion is controlled by a variety of metabolic and neuronal factors, which influence driving pressure and coronary resistance. Quantitatively, coronary arterial flow may be expressed as the ratio between transmyocardial perfusion pressure and coronary vascular resistance. Total coronary vascular resistance (CVR) is, in turn, the sum of three physiologically distinct components, $R_1$, $R_2$, and $R_3$.[1] $R_1$ is the resistance of the epicardial coronary conductance vessels. In the absence of fixed stenoses or spasm, $R_1$ contributes only a small percentage to total coronary resistance. The autoregulatory resistance, $R_2$, is the major component of coronary resistance and results primarily from arteriolar smooth muscle tone. The compressive resistance, $R_3$, results from the compression of coronary vessels by intramyocardial pressure during systole, accounting for the

observation that myocardial blood flow occurs primarily during diastole.

The mean coronary vascular resistance over the cardiac cycle can be calculated from the mean coronary artery flow and the coronary perfusion pressure, i.e., CVR = driving pressure/flow. In patients with normal ventricular filling pressures, the coronary driving pressure may be approximated by the mean aortic pressure (MAP) alone. When ventricular filling pressures are elevated, however, use of the mean aortic pressure tends to overestimate perfusion pressure, and one of two corrections may be in order: The first corrects for elevations in right atrial pressure (RAP), since the coronary sinus drains into the right atrium, i.e., perfusion pressure = MAP − RAP.[1] Recent studies have shown, however, that even use of right atrial pressure tends to overestimate perfusion pressure when left ventricular end diastolic pressure (LVEDP) or pulmonary capillary wedge pressure (PCWP) is increased. Elevations in LVEDP raise intramyocardial diastolic pressure and thereby elevate the zero-flow pressure ($P_{zf}$) (Fig. 21-1).[2] According to the vascular "waterfall" model of coronary blood flow, the difference between intramyocardial pressure and right atrial pressure has no effect on flow (just as the height of a waterfall does not influence the flow of water over its brink).[3] When there are substantial elevations of left ventricular filling pressure, therefore, myocardial driving pressure may be more appropriately described by the second equation, i.e., perfusion pressure = MAP − PCWP.

The heart is an obligatorily aerobic organ, relying almost exclusively on oxidative metabolism to supply its energy needs. Although the myocardium may increase oxygen extraction slightly during severe stress,[4] myocardial oxygen extraction is already nearly maximal at rest (coronary venous oxygen saturation being typically only 25 to 35%). Thus, changes in myocardial oxygen demand must be met by proportional alterations in myocardial blood flow. Furthermore, coronary autoregulation must permit adequate myocardial perfusion despite alterations in perfusion pressure. When coronary perfusion pressure declines, coronary arteriolar resistance promptly falls in order to maintain flow. This autoregulatory capacity of the coronary vasculature requires the availability of coronary vascular reserve— the potential to increase coronary blood flow by a reduction in the arteriolar resistance $R_2$. The vasodilatory reserve capacity of the nor-

mal coronary circulation allows coronary flow to increase four- to sixfold under maximal stress.[5-7]

Coronary vasomotion due to physiologic or pharmacologic stimuli may affect either the epicardial coronary arteries or the arteriolar vasculature.[8,9] These effects must be distinguished, since vasodilation of a stenotic or spastic large vessel may improve myocardial perfusion, but excessive vasodilation of the arterioles beyond a severe stenosis may redistribute blood flow away from the endocardium and cause ischemia via coronary steal.[10] Observations of coronary vasomotion should also differentiate between "primary" and "secondary" vasoconstriction or vasodilation: "Primary" vasomotion signifies alteration of myocardial perfusion in the absence of any significant change in myocardial oxygen demand. In contrast, "secondary" vasomotion refers to changes in coronary blood flow which occur in response to alterations in myocardial oxygen consumption (Fig. 21-2).[11]

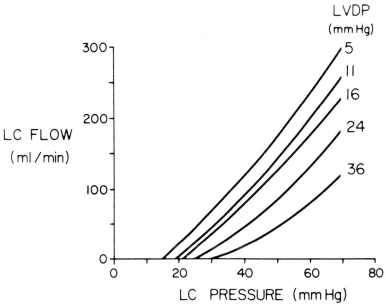

**Fig. 21-1.** Capacitance-free left circumflex coronary artery (LC) pressure-flow relationships at increasing levels of preload. As left ventricular diastolic pressure (LVDP) increases from 5 to 36 mmHg, the zero-flow pressure ($P_{zf}$) at which LC arterial flow ceases rises from 15 to 30 mmHg. For constant coronary arterial inflow pressures, this rise in zero-flow pressure would imply a marked reduction in coronary perfusion pressure = MAP − $P_{zf}$. (From Aversano T, et al: Preload-induced alterations in capacitance-free diastolic pressure-flow relationships. Am J Physiol 246:H410, 1984, with permission.)

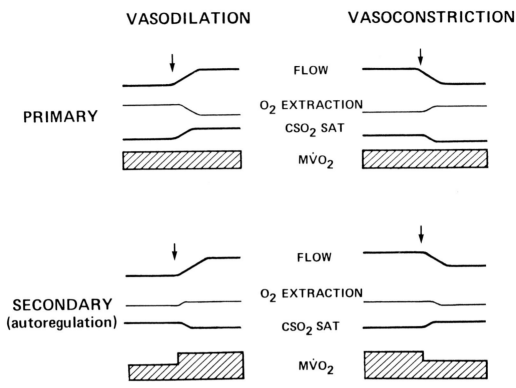

**Fig. 21-2.**   Primary and secondary coronary vasomotion as determined by the simultaneous measurement of coronary blood flow (FLOW) and coronary venous oxygen saturation (CSO$_2$SAT). Primary vasodilation causes a rise in flow at constant myocardial oxygen consumption (M$\dot{V}$O$_2$), resulting in lowered transmyocardial oxygen extraction and a rise in coronary sinus oxygen saturation. In contrast, in *secondary* coronary vasodilation an increase in myocardial oxygen consumption obligates a secondary rise in coronary blood flow with either constant or reduced coronary sinus oxygen saturation. (From Baim DS, Rothman MT, and Harrison DC: Simultaneous measurement of coronary venous blood flow and oxygen saturation during transient alterations in myocardial oxygen supply and demand. Am J Cardiol 49:743, 1982, with permission.)

## MYOCARDIAL METABOLISM

The energy requirements of the heart are primarily a function of the mechanical activity of the myocardium, and depend in particular on (1) the tension developed and sustained during ventricular contraction, (2) the rate of force development, and (3) the frequency of force generation per unit time.[4] In contrast, basal metabolism of the noncontractile heart consumes only 15 to 20% of total myocardial oxygen consumption, and electrical activity requires less than 1%.[12] Chemical energy is stored in the high-energy phosphate bonds of ATP for immediate use or is conserved as creatine phosphate. Under physiologic aerobic conditions, the myocardium oxidizes a variety of substrates for the generation of high-energy phosphates. These are, in order of decreasing utilization, free fatty acids (65%), glucose (15%), lactate and pyruvate (12%), and amino acids (5%).[13–14]

Under aerobic conditions, glycolysis plays only a minor role in myocardial metabolism. Thus, lactate is not normally produced by the heart. Rather, 10 to 30% of arterial lactate is extracted during a myocardial passage, is converted to pyruvate, and is oxidized via the Krebs cycle.[15]

Myocardial ischemia and anoxia result in diminished oxidative phosphorylation. High-energy phosphate stores are depleted, leading to an accumulation of ADP, AMP, and purine nucleosides. These ATP breakdown products enhance glycogenolysis and glycolysis for the anaerobic production of ATP. This process results in the generation of pyruvate. Under anoxic conditions the pyruvate-lactate equilibrium shifts toward lactate formation, resulting in net transmyocardial lactate production rather than extraction.[16]

The introduction of coronary sinus catheterization has facilitated the study of myocardial metabolism in man. Myocardial ischemia is probably the most prevalent disorder affecting cardiac metabolism. Coronary sinus sampling studies have demonstrated an increase in oxygen extraction,[17] glucose uptake,[18] potassium,[19] and purine nucleoside release[20] during ischemia, as well as a decrease in free fatty acid[21] and lactate extraction.[22] Accurate assessment of whole blood lactate levels requires special handling and buffering at the time of sampling to avoid errors due to ongoing metabolism.[23] Although early work appeared to show a good correlation between angina and lactate production,[24] there have been difficulties in monitoring regional manifestations of ischemia via nonselective coronary sinus catheterization. More disturbing is the observation by Apstein et al. that under conditions of "steady-state" ischemia and optimal coronary sinus sampling,[25] changes in the coronary sinus lactate level did not reliably measure sequential changes in the degree or amount of ischemia.

The recent introduction of positron emission tomography promises to contribute significantly to the study of regional myocardial metabolism under a variety of conditions.

## METHODS

The methods available for the evaluation of coronary flow include (1) measuring epicardial coronary blood flow velocity, (2) assessing myocardial tissue perfusion and metabolism, and (3) monitoring coronary venous outflow. Major attention will be devoted to those modalities that can be currently employed in the cardiac catheterization laboratory.

## Epicardial Blood Flow Velocity

***Electromagnetic Flowmeters.*** The electromagnetic flowmeter is based on Faraday's law of induction, which states that a conductor, e.g., blood, moving in a magnetic field will produce an electric field that is perpendicular to both the magnetic field and the direction of the conductor's movement. Furthermore, the magnitude of the electric field is proportional to the velocity of the conductor.[26] Electromagnetic flowmeter probes have been affixed to cardiac catheters to assess aortic blood flow velocity.[27] To date, however, these flow probes can be used for the measurement of coronary blood flow only when placed directly around an epicardial coronary artery. This allows intraoperative monitoring of aortocoronary bypass graft flows but does not permit measurement of coronary blood flow in conscious man.

***Doppler Velocity Probes.*** The Doppler flowmeter functions on the principle of the Doppler shift. Sound waves reflected from moving particles (e.g., red blood cells) undergo a shift in sound frequency that is linearly proportional to the velocity of the particles. Single piezoelectric crystals are used to transmit and receive pulsed high frequency sound waves. The magnitude of the Doppler shift is electronically determined to allow the measurement of instantaneous phasic blood flow velocity.[28,29] A human velocity probe mounted on a silicone suction cup has been recently developed for use at the time of open heart surgery to allow measurement of native epicardial coronary artery or coronary bypass graft blood flow velocity.[30]

The Doppler flowmeter has also been adapted for use in conscious humans by affixing piezoelectric crystals to the tips of coronary catheters. When positioned at the ostium of either the right or the left coronary artery, these catheter-mounted flowmeters can measure total right or left coronary phasic flow velocity. Furthermore, some of the Doppler catheter systems allow simultaneous coronary arterial pressure measurement or the infusion of vasoactive agents and radiographic contrast materials.[31,32]

The catheter-mounted pulsed ultrasonic flow probe affords a high frequency response and a stable zero flow reference point. Furthermore, coronary flow velocity following physiologic or pharmacologic stimuli can be measured repeatedly.[32] The ultrasonic flow probe measures flow velocity only, which may underestimate actual volume flow if coronary cross-sectional area changes during interventions,[33] and does not allow assessment of regional or transmural myocardial perfusion.

*Videodensitometry.* This technique allows the measurement of epicardial coronary flow during coronary angiography of conscious patients. Biplanar filming permits assessment of the epicardial coronary cross-sectional area. Blood flow velocity is obtained by monitoring the change of radiographic contrast density as a function of time at two points along a given coronary artery. Coronary blood flow is then determined as the product of cross-sectional area and flow velocity (Fig. 21-3). Although the frequency response of this technique is insufficient to detect the phasic aspects of coronary blood flow, the flow response to repeated interventions can be followed.[34,35]

A major drawback of videodensitometry is the expensive technology required for compensation of density variations that occur secondary to cardiac and respiratory cycles. Furthermore, the vasodilatory properties of currently available radiographic contrast

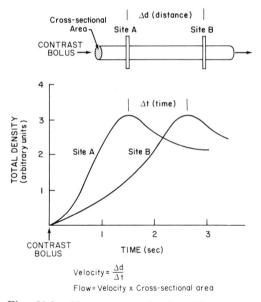

Fig. 21-3. Measurement of epicardial coronary blood flow by videodensitometry. Following intracoronary injection of a bolus of radiographic contrast agent, contrast density is measured as a function of time at two sites (A and B) along a coronary artery. The sites monitored should ideally be in the same plane along a relatively straight portion of the artery with no interposing branches and have similar cross-sectional areas. Blood flow velocity is derived from the transit time ($\Delta t$), and volume flow is then calculated as the product of velocity and cross-sectional area.

agents may distort actual blood flow measurement values.[36] In analogy to the previously described modalities for measuring epicardial coronary flow, videodensitometry does not differentiate between regional and transmural perfusion inhomogeneities.

## Myocardial Tissue Perfusion and Metabolism

*Microspheres.* Since the first reported use of radioactive microspheres for evaluating transmural myocardial blood flow in laboratory animals in 1969,[37] microsphere studies have become the standard technique for the quantitation of total coronary blood flow and the assessment of regional and transmural myocardial perfusion. This method is based on the assumption that microsphere distribution and entrapment will mimic red blood cell flow and thus be proportional to myocardial perfusion. Animal studies typically employ 9 to 15 $\mu$ plastic microspheres that incorporate gamma-emitting radioactive labels. Up to nine labels can be employed, allowing serial measurements during several interventions. The major disadvantage of the quantitative microsphere method is that it requires scintillation well-counting of myocardial tissue and is thus inapplicable for clinical studies of human myocardial perfusion.[38]

In contrast, qualitative microsphere studies have been performed in conscious humans. Human studies generally utilize biodegradable particles such as albumin- and dextran microspheres, or macroaggregates of albumin, labeled with Tc-99m or In-113m. These labeled microparticles are injected directly into the coronary circulation at the time of coronary angiography, and myocardial perfusion is assessed by precordial scintigraphy. The resulting scintigram reflects distribution of the regional blood flow within the area subtended by the injected artery. This technique yields only a qualitative assessment of flow distribution. Only two interventions can be observed, and myocardial perfusion imaging does not permit the assessment of transmural blood flow. Lastly, the spatial resolution obtained with the intracoronary microsphere technique is similar to that obtained during myocardial perfusion scintigraphy with intravenous Tl-201.[39,40] Recently, positron-emitting biodegradable C-11 albumin microspheres have been developed. If administered and mixed in the left ventricular chamber, a timed arterial withdrawal of these microspheres, coupled with emission-tomographic evaluation of myocardial tracer distribution, should allow regional and transmural quantitation of human myocardial perfusion in the future.[41]

***Potassium Congeners.*** Myocardial perfusion scintigraphy has been performed in humans primarily with the potassium analogs Ce-129, Rb-81, and Tl-201. After intravenous injection, their initial myocardial distribution is determined by the product of regional coronary blood flow and the tissue extraction fraction.[39,42] Tl-201, which is extracted by the myocardium via the sodium-potassium ATPase system, has been the most useful indicator of regional myocardial perfusion, particularly when combined with exercise stress testing.[43] Better spatial resolution of the precordial scintigram can be obtained by injecting a tracer such as Tl-201 or Rb-82 directly into the coronary circulation during coronary angiography.[44] Rb-82 is particularly useful in this regard in view of its short (75 second) half-life, allowing sequential scintigrams to be obtained. Thus, patients can be studied at rest and following a hyperemic stimulus such as atrial pacing.[45] Intracoronary Tl-201 or Rb-82 do not permit quantitative assessment of coronary blood flow, and transmural distribution of blood flow cannot be evaluated.

***Videodensitometry.*** Recently, videodensitometry has also been adapted to allow qualitative assessment of regional myocardial blood flow reserve.

Myocardial contrast appearance time (MCAT) is defined as the time from the onset of contrast injection to its maximal incremental appearance within a region of myocardium.[46,47] Radiographic contrast injection is standardized by intraarterial injection of a fixed amount of contrast at a given rate using an ECG-gated power injector. Image processing involves digitization and gated interval differencing of consecutive end-diastolic arteriogram frames. The MCAT is determined by histographic analysis of the resulting functional images.

The relationship between regional coronary flow and MCAT is based on the following two equations:

regional myocardial blood flow
  = regional distributional volume/MCAT

$$\frac{\text{regional blood flow at A}}{\text{regional blood flow at B}} = \frac{\text{MCAT}_A}{\text{MCAT}_B}$$

for a comparison of regional blood flows in basal state (A) and after an intervention (B). The second equation is based on the assumption that the distributional volume of myocardial perfusion does not change within a given region.[46,48]

Although this method allows qualitative assessment of changes in myocardial perfusion, it does not provide adequate assessment of regional or transmural myocardial perfusion inhomogeneities. Furthermore, the vasodilatory properties of available radiographic contrast agents may affect flow measurements.[36] A major disadvantage of this method is the expensive equipment required for image processing.

***Clearance Methods.*** The clearance techniques used for the measurement of myocardial perfusion permit quantitative assessment of blood flow per gram of myocardial tissue in conscious humans,[49] and allow quantitation of regional perfusion inhomogeneities. The clearance method derives from the Fick principle for both tracer uptake (saturation) and washout (desaturation):

myocardial tracer *saturation*
  = coronary blood flow × mean (arterial
    − coronary venous) tracer concentration.

myocardial *desaturation*
      = coronary blood flow
      × mean (coronary venous
      − arterial) tracer difference.

Thus, coronary blood flow measurements require monitoring of systemic arterial and coronary venous tracer levels during myocardial saturation or desaturation (Fig. 21-4).[1,50]

Individual procedures vary with respect to the indicators employed, the method of administration, and the method of analysis of the indicator. Ideally, indicators should be physiologically inert, should diffuse rapidly across the capillary endothelium to allow myocardial tissue saturation and desaturation, be detectable by coronary sinus sampling or precordial scintigraphy, and have minimal recirculation. The tracers used can be divided into two categories: substances

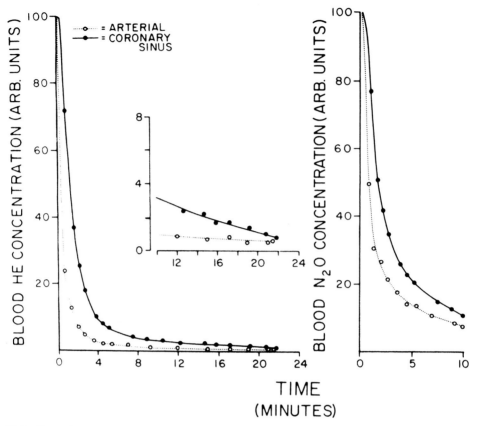

**Fig. 21-4.** Systemic arterial (open circles) and coronary sinus (closed circles) desaturation curves for helium (HE) and nitrous oxide (N₂O). Myocardial blood flow per 100 g N₂O (F/W) = 100 times the difference in coronary venous helium concentrations at two points in time ($\Delta C_v$) divided by the area between the venous and arterial desaturation curves in that period of time $_0\int^t (C_v - C_a)$. (From Klocke FJ, et al: Average coronary blood flow per unit weight of left ventricle in patients with and without coronary artery disease. Circulation 50:547, 1974, with permission.)

that diffuse like water (H₂O-15 and I-131-antipyrine), and inert gases (He, Ar, Kr-85, Xe-133, as well as H₂, N₂, and N₂O).[50]

Xe-133 is currently the tracer most frequently used. The inert gas is dissolved in saline solution and injected directly into the coronary circulation at the time of coronary angiography. The gamma radiation emitted by the radioisotope within the heart is recorded subsequently by a multicrystal scintillation camera, allowing visualization of isotope washout. The initial Xe-133 washout from each region of myocardium is a computer-derived monoexponential equation, and the slope or clearance constant of the initial washout curve is determined. Myocar-

dial blood flow (F) in ml/100 g · min is then derived by the Kety formula:

$$F = k \cdot l/r$$

where k is the myocardial Xe-133 clearance constant, l is the blood:myocardium partition coefficient for Xe-133, and r is the specific gravity of the myocardial tissue. Regional myocardial blood flow distribution can be correlated with the angiographically delineated coronary anatomy (Fig. 21-5).[51–53]

The inert gas washout method cannot measure transmural distribution of myocardial perfusion. Additional technical limitations of this technique are that the blood-tissue coefficient for xenon is difficult to

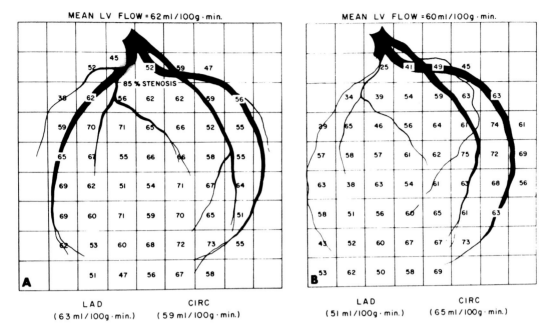

**Fig. 21-5.** Xe-133 precordial scintigram in the LAO projection following selective injection of the tracer into the left coronary artery. (A) Despite the presence of an 85% stenosis of the proximal left anterior descending coronary artery, regional myocardial perfusion rates were similar throughout the left ventricle. (B) Three months following an anterior myocardial infarction, this same patient has a 100% proximal LAD occlusion. Regional myocardial flow rates distal to the occlusion are lower compared to the remainder of the ventricle. (From Cannon PJ, Weiss MB, Sciacca RR: Myocardial blood flow in coronary artery disease: Studies at rest and during stress with inert gas washout techniques. Prog Cardiovasc Dis 20:95, 1977, with permission.)

determine accurately. Furthermore, xenon is eight to ten times more soluble in fat than in cardiac muscle. This differential solubility may affect the initial xenon washout curves, resulting in an underestimation of flow. Similarly, repeated flow measurements with 133-Xe will result in xenon accumulation in fat tissue, rendering multiple sequential flow measurements unreliable.

***Positron Emission Tomography.*** Although positron emission tomography (PET) is a noninvasive, expensive, and not widely available mode for the evaluation of myocardial perfusion, it will be briefly discussed here inasmuch as it offers quantitative information on regional and transmural coronary blood flow supply in conscious humans. More importantly, PET may in the future contribute importantly to our understanding of myocardial metabolism in various human disease states.

The unstable isotopes C-11, O-15, N-13, and F-18 that are used in the study of myo-cardial perfusion emit positrons upon radio-active decay. Subsequent positron-electron annihilation gives off paired 511 kev annihilation photons in opposite directions which are detected simultaneously by two scintillation detectors positioned 180 degrees apart (coincidence detection). Typically, one or more circular rings of these detectors surround the patient. This circular positron camera allows data collection from all angles simultaneously, allowing the electronic reconstruction of tomographic myocardial slices with a spatial resolution ranging from 4 to 20 millimeters.[54]

Myocardial perfusion studies employing PET have employed $H_2O$-15, Rb-82, and N-13-ammonia as radiotracers. The short (75 second) half-life of Rb-82 makes it a particularly useful tracer for sequential studies of myocardial perfusion following serial interventions. In contrast, metabolically specific substrates such as C-11-palmitate, C-11-glucose, and F-18-deoxyglucose have been used as radiotracers in the investigation of oxygen utilization and metabolic pathways.[55,56]

At present, PET is still primarily a research tool. Its major disadvantage is the substantial capital investment required for the installment of a positron camera. Furthermore, an on-site cyclotron is required for generation of the very short-lived positron radionuclides.

## Coronary Venous Flow

***Coronary Sinus Thermodilution and Oximetry.*** Measurement of coronary venous flow is one of the most sensitive and practical techniques to quantitate stable as well as rapidly changing levels of regional myocardial blood flow.

In contrast to the predominantly diastolic flow in the coronary arteries, coronary venous flow occurs primarily in systole (Fig. 21-6). Studies of the coronary venous anatomy in the dog, as well as postmortem studies in humans, have shown that coronary sinus flow is derived predominantly from left ventricular free wall venous drainage and

consitutes 80 to 85% of left coronary inflow. Approximately two thirds of left anterior descending coronary artery flow drains into the great cardiac vein, which is the continuation of the anterior interventricular vein as it reaches the atrioventricular groove (Fig. 21-7). The great cardiac vein becomes the coronary sinus per se at the site of the valve of Vieussens and the oblique vein of Marshall, a left atrial venous remnant of the embryonic left-sided superior vena cava. The remaining portion of left anterior descending arterial drainage enters the coronary sinus in combination with blood from the circumflex territory via the left marginal vein and circumflex venous branches. Significantly, only a very small percentage of left circumflex venous flow reaches the great cardiac vein. Thus great cardiac vein flow represents primarily left anterior descending venous drainage. In contrast, coronary sinus flow represents an admixture of both left anterior descending and left circumflex coronary artery outflow.[57,58]

Measurement of coronary venous flow is based on the thermodilution principle with the assumption that the heat lost from the measurement system between the site of in-

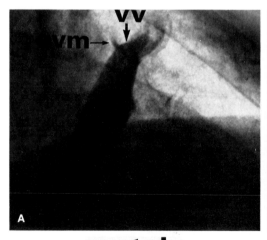
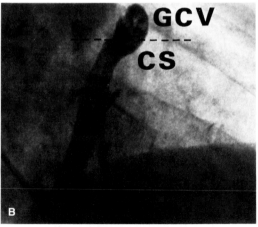

## systole                    diastole

**Fig. 21-6.** Coronary venogram in the RAO projection. The catheter tip is at the junction of the coronary sinus (CS) with the great cardiac vein (GCV). (A) During ventricular systole, outflow of unopacified venous blood from the great cardiac vein silhouettes the valve of Vieussens (VV) at the CS–GCV junction. The oblique vein of Marshall (OVM), the remnant of the embryonic left-sided superior vena cava, lies adjacent to the valve of Vieussens and is filled by contrast agent. (B) During ventricular diastole, contrast refluxes beyond the valve of Vieussens to fill the great cardiac vein. Furthermore, several small marginal veins are seen to fill in retrograde fashion. (From Bradley AB, Baim DS: Measurement of coronary blood flow in man: Methods and implication for clinical practice. Cardiovasc Clinics 14 (3):67, 1984, with permission.)

# RAO

# LAO

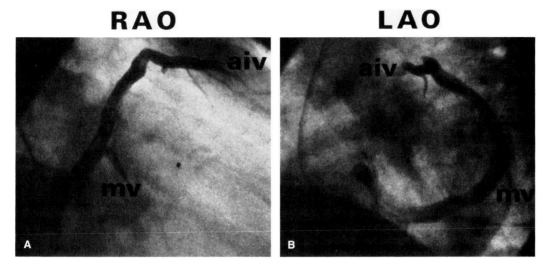

**Fig. 21-7.** Coronary venous anatomy in the RAO and LAO projection. The catheter tip is in the great cardiac vein. Contrast injection reveals the origin of the anterior interventricular vein (aiv) and a single marginal vein (mv). (From Bradley AB, Baim DS: Measurement of coronary blood flow in man: Methods and implications for clincial practice. Cardiovasc Clinics 14 (3):67, 1984, with permission.)

jection and the sensing thermistor is negligible. Thus the heat lost by the bood equals the heat gained by the indicator. A thermally insulated 7F catheter injects fluid at room temperature upstream in the coronary sinus for 30 to 60 seconds at a rate of 35 to 55 ml per minute to ensure turbulent mixing with coronary venous blood. While most investigators have used a large (200 cc) Harvard pump to deliver the injectate, we have also found the Medrad Mark IV angiographic injector, which is available in most catheterization laboratories, to be an excellent substitute. Coronary venous flow is then computed according to the formula first introduced by Ganz and recently modified by Baim (Fig. 21-8):[11,59]

$$Q = F \times C \times (T_M - T_I)/(T_B - T_M)$$

where Q is coronary venous flow; F is the rate of injection of thermodilution indicator; $T_M$, $T_I$, and $T_B$ are temperatures of the mixture; injectate, and blood respectively; C is the ratio of the specific heats of blood and injectate and is equal to 1.08 for 5% dextrose injection and 1.19 for normal saline injection.

Modifications in the initial catheter design have enhanced the clinical utility of coronary venous flow measurements. The presence of two sampling thermistors allows for the simultaneous selective measurement of left anterior descending coronary artery flow as well as more proximal coronary sinus flow, via a catheter whose tip is positioned in the great cardiac vein. Incorporation of pacing electrodes in the thermodilution catheter has facilitated the study of human myocardial blood flow changes in response to pacing-induced alterations in myocardial oxygen demand.[60] A further adaptation of the thermodilution catheter is the flow-oximetry catheter, in which optical fibers permit continuous reflectance measurements of great cardiac vein oxygen saturation (Fig. 21-9). Thus, regional left anterior descending coronary blood flow and myocardial oxygen extraction (A $O_2$ − CS $O_2$) can be continuously and simultaneously monitored. Regional myocardial oxygen consumption (MVO$_2$) can be determined for the territory subtended by the left anterior descending artery:[61]

$$M\dot{V}O_2 = Q \times (A\,O_2 - CS\,O_2)$$

This allows changes in coronary flow (Q) to be differentiated into "primary" or myocardial oxygen demand-independent vasomotion and "secondary" or autoregulatory vasomotion[11] and permits correlation of these flow changes with alterations in myocardial metabolism.

Coronary sinus thermodilution is a simple, inexpensive, and safe technique for studies

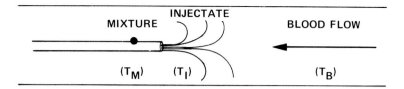

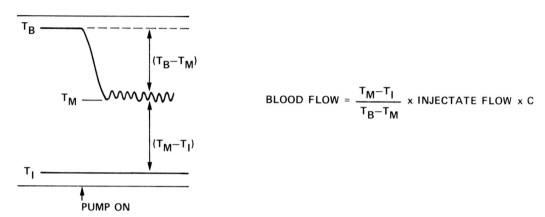

$$\text{BLOOD FLOW} = \frac{T_M - T_I}{T_B - T_M} \times \text{INJECTATE FLOW} \times C$$

**Fig. 21-8.** Schematic diagram of the thermodilution technique. The thermal indicator (INJECTATE) at temperature $T_I$ is infused at a fixed rate, typically 50 ml per minute. The ensuing turbulence causes mixing of the injectate with coronary venous blood at temperature $T_B$, resulting in a mixture at temperature $T_M$. The temperatures monitored by the catheter-tip ($T_B$ and $T_M$) and injectate ($T_I$) thermistors are recorded continuously on a uniform temperature scale. Since the heat lost by the blood is gained by the injectate, coronary venous flow can be calculated using the respective measured temperatures, the rate of indicator injection, and a constant derived from the specific heats of blood and injectate. (From Bradley AB, Baim DS: Measurement of coronary blood flow in man: Methods and implications for clinical practice. Cardiovasc Clinics 14 (3):67, 1984, with permission.)

of regional and global myocardial flow and metabolism in conscious humans. The measurements obtained correlate well with electromagnetic flow measurements.[62] Multiple and frequent serial measurements can be taken with a frequency response that is sufficiently rapid to detect transient changes in flow and oxygen extraction. The technique does not permit evaluation of transmural inhomogeneities in myocardial perfusion.

The coronary sinus catheter, either Wilton-Webster (Altadena, CA) or Baim catheter (Electro-catheter, Rahway, NJ) for measurement of blood flow, or Gorlin catheter (USCI, Billerica, MA) for blood sampling and pacing only, can be placed successfully in approximately 90% of patients using a combination of fluoroscopy, contrast injection, and pressure monitoring. The "classic" approach to the sinus has been via the left arm. From the left arm, a catheter with a single curve easily enters the ostium of the coronary sinus

which is located slightly above and behind the tricuspid annulus. Although the coronary sinus can also be cannulated from the right arm or even the femoral venous approach (using the reverse-loop technique), the preferred approach in our laboratory involves percutaneous placement via the right internal jugular vein. This approach allows excellent catheter control by virtue of its proximity to the coronary sinus and the absence of intervening vascular curvatures to compromise torque transmission.

While direct entry is possible by advancement of the catheter tip with a posteromedial orientation, our approach is to point the catheter toward the right atrial border, rotate the catheter counterclockwise, and advance it slightly to enter the right ventricle. Following slight additional counterclockwise rotation, the catheter is then slowly withdrawn until an atrial pressure trace is restored. Upon gentle readvancement of the catheter,

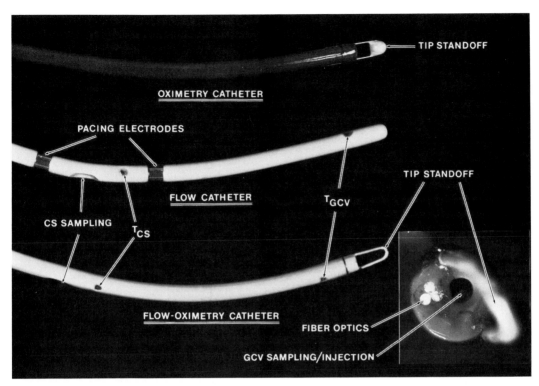

**Fig. 21-9.** Coronary venous oximetry, thermodilution flow, and combined flow-oximetry catheters (top to bottom). The flow and flow-oximetry catheters have the following features in common: two lumens for indicator injection or sampling at the great cardiac vein (see insert) and coronary sinus sites and two great cardiac vein ($T_{GCV}$) and coronary sinus ($T_{CS}$) thermistors for regional flow determinations. The flow catheter in addition has two pacing electrodes. Both the oximetry and flow-oximetry catheters have fiberoptic bundles for continuous measurement of great cardiac vein oxygen saturation. (From Baim DS, Rothman MT, Harrison DC: Simultaneous measurement of coronary venous flow and oxygen saturation during transient alterations in myocardial oxygen supply and demand. Am J Cardiol 49:743, 1982, with permission.)

it will either reenter the right ventricle (whereupon the same maneuver is repeated with additional counterclockwise rotation), or it will cannulate the coronary sinus.

Successful coronary sinus entry will be confirmed by the maintenance of a right atrial pressure trace as the catheter is smoothly advanced across the heart border. In doing so, the catheter can usually be easily positioned at the origin of the anterior interventricular vein, where its position relative to venous tributaries can be assessed by gentle injection of contrast agent (Figs. 21-7 and 21-10). When slight resistance during catheter advancement is encountered, this usually signifies catheter impingement upon a venous branch or the valve of Vieussens, which lies at the junction of the coronary sinus and the great cardiac vein. If slight withdrawal of the catheter and gentle con-

trast injection confirms an intravascular position, a soft-tipped 0.018-inch guide wire (ACS) can be advanced gently through the endhole of the coronary sinus catheter. The wire will usually bypass the anatomic obstacles, allowing advancement of the catheter over the wire. It should be understood that the coronary sinus is a thin-walled venous structure which can be perforated if excessive force is applied, although this complication is rare in experienced hands.

Accurate and reproducible coronary venous flow measurements require stable positioning of the catheter in order to avoid variations in temperature reading due to fluctuating flow contributions from venous tributaries near the thermistors. The coronary sinus thermistor needs to be positioned at some distance (2 to 3 cm) from the sinus ostium to avoid contamination of the true

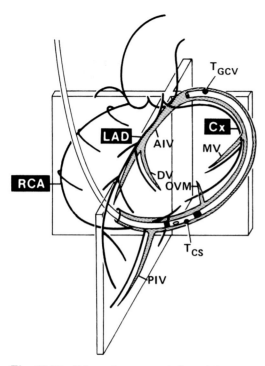

**Fig. 21-10.** Schematic representation of the coronary venous system in relation to the coronary artery anatomy: diagonal vein (DV), anterior interventricular vein (AIV), marginal vein (MV), oblique vein of Marshall (OVM), posterior interventricular vein (PIV), and the right, left anterior descending, and circumflex coronary arteries (RCA, LAD, Cx, respectively). (From Baim DS, Rothman MT, Harrison DC: Simultaneous measurement of coronary venous flow and oxygen saturation during transient alterations in myocardial oxygen supply and demand. Am J Cardiol 49:743, 1982, with permission.)

coronary sinus temperature profile by right atrial blood reflux. In our experience, the most satisfactory position for the tip of the coronary sinus catheter is near the point where the anterior interventricular vein meets the great cardiac vein. This position provides selective measurement of LAD-territory outflow and is well beyond the entry point of lateral wall venous drainage.

In the future, coronary sinus catheterization may assume not only a diagnostic but also therapeutic function. Recent studies in animal models have suggested that intermittent balloon-catheter coronary sinus occlusions during ischemia can salvage jeopardized myocardium. In the animal laboratory, this process apparently occurs without any

change in antegrade or collateral-dependent blood flow;[63] it may rather be the result of retrograde venous blood flow. Venous blood perfusion of the ischemic region may effect some, albeit minimal, oxygen delivery, supply metabolic substrates, and wash out harmful products of ischemia.[64] Alternatively, *synchronous diastolic coronary venous retroperfusion* with arterial blood in animals has been shown to protect against myocardial ischemia and limit infarct size.[65] Studies involving coronary sinus occlusion and retroperfusion are currently being extended to clinical situations.

## MEASUREMENT OF MYOCARDIAL PERFUSION IN CLINICAL SITUATIONS

### Coronary Artery Disease

Because of the large vasodilatory reserve of the coronary arterioles, resting myocardial flow may remain normal in the face of decreased coronary perfusion pressure when the epicardial coronary arteries are stenosed. Thus, studies in animal models have demonstrated that normal resting coronary flow is preserved until epicardial coronary stenoses reduce internal diameter by more than 80 to 90%.[66] However, coronary *reserve* is eroded by stenoses as moderate as 50 to 60% (Fig. 21-11). Therefore, to assess the hemodynamic severity of a coronary stenosis, measurements are needed not only of resting coronary flow but also of coronary reserve capacity by maximally dilating the coronary arteriolar bed.

Using Xe-133 clearance methods, Cannon and his co-workers found normal resting myocardial flow in patients with single vessel coronary disease.[53] Similar findings were reported by Fuchs et al.,[67] using the thermodilution technique. Resting great cardiac vein flows of patients with isolated left anterior descending artery stenoses were found to match those of normal controls. With graded pacing tachycardia, great cardiac vein flow showed a steady increase in the controls as well as in the patients with left anterior descending coronary stenoses until the final pacing increment. At that point, whereas the control group continued to increase flow, patients with stenoses had no further rise in

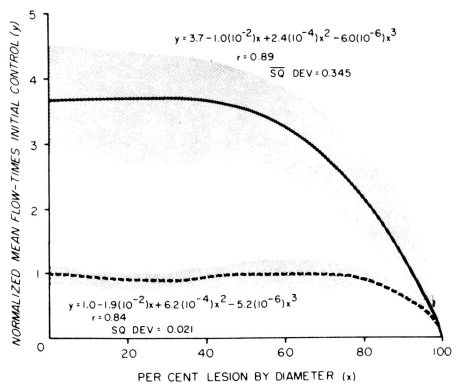

**Fig. 21-11.** Resting coronary blood flow and coronary vascular reserve as a function of precentage of diameter stenosis. Resting coronary flow is preserved in the face of increasing coronary stenoses and declines only as the epicardial coronary diameter is obstructed by more than 85%. In contrast, coronary vascular reserve begins to fall with lesions greater than 40% and is virtually absent for stenoses greater than 90%. (From Gould KL, Kelley KO: Physiological significance of coronary flow velocity and changing stenosis during coronary vasodilation in awake dogs. Circ Res 50:695, 1982, with permission.)

great cardiac vein flow and developed angina and electrocardiographic changes suggesting that their coronary reserve capacity had been exhausted.[67]

In contrast to the findings in single vessel disease, Cannon and Klocke, using Xe-133 and He clearance methods, respectively, found a systematic reduction in left ventricular perfusion per unit weight in patients with double and triple vessel coronary artery lesions even at rest.[53,68] These findings contrast with the thermodilution measurements of Yoshida and Ganz who found that coronary blood flow in patients with multivessel coronary disease was normal at rest.[60]

These conflicting observations might be reconciled by the finding of increased left ventricular mass in patients with coronary artery disease.[69,70] Chen and co-workers have provided evidence that this increased wall thickness and mass is associated with decreased wall stress and thus lower myocardial oxygen demand. The result would be a reduction of resting myocardial flow per unit weight which would not be detectable by thermodilution measurements.[71]

Inasmuch as patients with coronary artery disease need to expend their coronary vascular reserve in order to preserve normal resting flow, they appear to be more sensitive to a variety of vasoconstrictor stimuli.[72–74]

## Coronary Artery Spasm

Myocardial blood flow during spontaneous or pharmacologically induced coronary artery spasm has been evaluated using primarily coronary sinus thermodilution or oximetry techniques. These studies have demonstrated that episodes of silent or symptomatic ischemia at rest are not preceded by a change in the hemodynamic determinants of myocardial oxygen consumption. Rather, fiberoptic reflectance measurements of coronary sinus oxygen saturation have shown a primary reduction in coronary sinus oxygen saturation before any of the conventional signs of myocardial ischemia such as diminished systolic function, electrocardiographic changes, and angina ensued.[75,76] Similar observations have been made with thermodilution measurements.[77] These have also documented an overshoot of coronary flow coincident with a fall in coronary arteriovenous oxygen extraction upon spontaneous resolution of spasm, consistent with a reactive hyperemic response to spasm-induced ischemia.[78]

## Chest Pain Syndromes

Up to 30% of patients referred for diagnostic cardiac catheterization experience angina-like symptoms despite the finding of normal coronary arteries and the absence of inducible focal epicardial coronary spasm.[79,80] Using the argon clearance method, Opherk et al.[81] identified a group of such patients who had normal resting myocardial blood flows; however, the coronary vasodilatory capacity of these patients, as assessed by their response to intravenous dipyridamole, was inadequate. Schwartz and co-workers[82] studied coronary flow responses to intravenous ergonovine in a group of these patients. Despite a rise in the determinants of oxygen demand in response to ergonovine, a subgroup of these patients showed no change in coronary sinus flow, and in half of the patients coronary sinus flow actually fell. Furthermore, Cannon et al.[83] found a diminished vasodilatory reserve capacity in these patients in response to pacing tachycardia. This diminished reserve capacity was accentuated by cold pressor testing and intravenous ergonovine administration.[83]

## Myocardial Hypertrophy

Patients with hypertrophied ventricles frequently exhibit signs of myocardial ischemia

such as exertional angina and S-T segment depressions on their resting or exercise electrocardiograms. This may occur in the absence of atherosclerotic coronary artery stenoses. Using Xe-133 clearance techniques, Weiss et al.[84] found decreased left ventricular perfusion per unit weight in patients with hypertrophic cardiomyopathy when compared to control patients. Total resting coronary blood flow was estimated by multiplying measured flow by estimated myocardial mass and was found to be increased relative to controls.[84] The decreased perfusion per unit weight was considered to be a reflection of diminished myocardial wall stress in the hypertrophied ventricles and thus did not provide an explanation for the patients' ischemic symptoms. Since angina might also be the result of impaired coronary vascular reserve resulting from inadequate hyperplasia of the coronary vascular bed, numerous recent studies of myocardial perfusion in hypertrophied ventricles have also provided an assessment of reserve capacity. Using thermodilution techniques, Pichard and associates confirmed that patients with severe left ventricular hypertrophy secondary to aortic stenosis or aortic regurgitation have increased resting coronary flow; however, coronary reserve as measured by contrast-induced hyperemia was significantly diminished.[85,86]

## Dilated Cardiomyopathy

Weiss and co-workers found decreased resting myocardial perfusion per unit weight in patients with congestive (dilated) cardiomyopathy using Xe-133 clearance techniques.[84] Thermodilution techniques have been employed to assess the effect of inotropic agents on myocardial oxygen consumption and myocardial perfusion in patients with congestive heart failure. A rise in left ventricular contractility would be expected to obligate a "secondary" rise in coronary blood flow. This has been described following dobutamine administration to patients with congestive heart failure.[87] In contrast, Benotti and associates found that even though amrinone acutely increased cardiac index and left ventricular stroke work, coronary blood flow and oxygen consumption actually decreased, suggesting that the oxygen cost of increased myocardial contractility was more than offset by a fall in left ventricular wall stress.[88] Recent studies of milrinone in congestive heart failure have shown a similar reduction in myocardial oxygen demand, associated with a "primary" rise in coronary blood flow inasmuch as coronary sinus fiberoptic oximetry revealed a simultaneous fall in transmyocardial oxygen extraction. This "primary" dilation of the myocardial vasculature may have been either the result of the vasodilatory properties of milrinone or of withdrawal of alpha-constrictor tone upon improvement in hemodynamic parameters.[89]

# Percutaneous Transluminal Coronary Angioplasty

Whereas electromagnetic and Doppler flow probes have been used routinely in coronary artery bypass surgery to assess adequacy of bypass graft flow, measurements of coronary flow have thus far been employed during coronary angioplasty only as investigative tools. Great cardiac vein and coronary sinus thermodilution techniques have permitted the observation of postocclusion reactive hyperemia in conscious humans during the procedure. Numerous investigators have demonstrated that as the luminal stenosis severity is reduced during repeated balloon inflations, coronary reserve capacity is restored progressively as manifested by a rise in the magnitude of reactive hyperemia.[90–92] An analogous functional assessment of improvement in coronary vasodilatory reserve was provided by Williams and co-workers.[93,94] These investigators found that after successful angioplasty, pacing tachycardia achieved higher myocardial oxygen consumption, higher peak coronary blood flow, normalization of lactate extraction, absence of angina, and restoration of basal coronary alpha-adrenergic tone.[93,94]

# SUMMARY

The techniques currently available for the measurement of coronary blood flow in conscious humans are relatively limited when compared to the modalities available in the animal laboratory. They have, however, played a pivotal role in elucidating the physiology and pathophysiology of the human coronary circulation. At present, clearance techniques as well as coronary sinus thermodilution measurements, appear to be the most practical approaches to measuring coronary flow in the cardiac catheterization laboratory. In the future, quantitative evaluation of myocardial perfusion will continue to be important in a number of clinical situations, such as those listed in Table 21-1.

**TABLE 21-1.** *Clinical Applications of Coronary Blood Flow and Metabolic Studies*

1. Assessment of the hemodynamic severity of coronary stenoses
2. Study of coronary collateral function
3. Evaluation of anginal chest pain syndromes and small vessel disease
4. Determination of coronary reserve capacity in a variety of primary myocardial diseases
5. Monitoring of blood flow in patients undergoing therapeutic angiographic procedures such as coronary angioplasty and thrombolysis
6. Investigation of the metabolic and coronary hemodynamic effects of vasoactive and inotropic agents.

# REFERENCES

1. Klocke FJ: Coronary blood flow in man. Prog Cardiovasc Dis 19:117, 1976.
2. Aversano T, Klocke FJ, Mates RE, Canty JM: Preload-induced alterations in capacitance-free diastolic pressure-flow relationships. Am J Physiol 246:H410, 1984.
3. Permutt S, Riley RL: Hemodynamics of collapsible vessels with tone: the vascular waterfall. J Appl Physiol 18:924, 1963.
4. Weber KT, Janicki JS: The metabolic demand and oxygen supply of the heart: Physiologic and clinical considerations. Am J Cardiol 44:722, 1979.
5. Rubio R, Berne RM: Regulation of coronary blood flow. Prog Cardiovasc Dis 18:105, 1975.

6. Bache RJ, Dymek DJ: Local and regional regulation of coronary vascular tone. Prog Cardiovasc Dis 24:191, 1981.

7. Klocke FJ: Measurement of coronary blood flow and degree of stenosis: Current clinical implications and continuing uncertainties. J Am Coll Cardiol 1:31, 1983.

8. Macho P, Vatner SF: Effects of nitroglycerin and nitroprusside on large and small coronary vessels in conscious dogs. Circulation 64:1101, 1981.

9. Vatner SF, Hintze TH: Effects of a calcium-channel antagonist on large and small coronary arteries in conscious dogs. Circulation 66:579, 1982.

10. Cohen MV: Coronary steal in awake dogs: a real phenomenon. Cardiovasc Res 16:339, 1982.

11. Baim DS, Rothman MT, Harrison DC: Simultaneous measurement of coronary venous blood flow and oxygen saturation during transient alterations in myocardial oxygen supply and demand. Am J Cardiol 49:743, 1982.

12. Scheuer J, Penpargkul S: Myocardial metabolism. *In* Willerson S, Sanders C (ed): Clinical Cardiology. New York, Stratton, 1977.

13. Bing RJ: The metabolism of the heart. Harvey Lect 50:27, 1954.

14. Opie LH: Metabolism of the heart in health and disease, Part I. Am Heart J 76:685, 1968. Part II 77:100, 1969. Part III 77:383, 1969.

15. Krasnow N, et al: Myocardial lactate and metabolism. J Clin Invest 41:2075, 1962.

16. Brachfeld N: Characterization of the ischaemic process by regional metabolism. Am J Cardiol 37:467, 1976.

17. Messer JV, et al: Pattern of human myocardial oxygen extraction during rest and exercise. J Clin Invest 41:725, 1962.

18. Most AS, Gorlin R, Soeldner JS: Glucose extraction by the human myocardium during pacing stress. Circulation 45:92, 1972.

19. Case RB, Nasser MG, Crampton RS: Biochemical aspects of early myocardial ischaemia. Am J Cardiol 24:766, 1969.

20. Fox AC, et al: Release of nucleosides from canine and human hearts as an index of prior ischemia. Am J Cardiol 43:52, 1979.

21. Scheuer J: Myocardial metabolism in cardiac hypoxia. Am J Cardiol 19:385, 1967.

22. Cohen LS, et al: Coronary heart disease: Clinical, cinearteriographic, and metabolic correlations. Am J Cardiol 17:153, 1966.

23. Livesley B, Atkinson L: Accurate quantitative estimation of lactate in whole blood. Clin Chemistry 20:1578, 1974.

24. Helfant RH, et al: Coronary heart disease. Differential hemodynamic, metabolic, and electrocardiographic effects in subjects with and without angina pectoris during atrial pacing. Circulation 42:601, 1970.

25. Apstein CS, Gravino F, Hood WB: Limitations of lactate production as an index of myocardial ischemia. Circulation 60:877, 1979.

26. Khouri EM, Gregg DE: Miniature electromagnetic flowmeter applicable to coronary arteries. J Appl Physiol 18:224, 1963.

27. Klinke WP, et al: Use of catheter-tip velocity-pressure transducer to evaluate left ventricular function in man: Effects of intravenous propranolol. Circulation 61:946, 1980.

28. Hartley CJ, Cole JS: An ultrasonic pulsed Doppler system for measuring blood flow in small vessels. J Appl Physiol 37:626, 1974.

29. Franklin D, et al: A system for radiotelemetry of blood pressure, blood flow and ventricular dimensions from animals: A summary report. Proceedings of the International Telemetry Conference, Washington, DC, 1971.

30. Wright CB, et al: Intraoperative evaluation of the functional significance of coronary obstructions. *In* Rapaport E (ed): Cardiology Update, New York, Elsevier Biomedical, 1983.

31. Cole JS, Hartley CJ: The pulsed Doppler coronary artery catheter. Preliminary report of a new technique for measuring rapid changes in coronary artery flow velocity in man. Circulation 56:18, 1977.

32. Wilson RF, et al: Transluminal subselective measurement of coronary artery blood flow velocity and vasodilator reserve in man. Circulation 72:82, 1985.

33. Gould KL, Kelley KO: Physiological significance of coronary flow velocity and changing stenosis geometry during coronary vasodilation in awake dogs. Circ Res 50:695, 1982.

34. Rutishauser W et al: Evaluation of roentgen cinedensitometry for flow measurements in models and in intact circulation. Circulation 36:951, 1967.

35. Smith HC, Strum RE, Wood EH: Videodensitometric system for measurement of vessel blood flow, particularly in the coronary arteries, in man. Am J Cardiol 32:144, 1973.

36. Gould KL, Lipscomb K, Calvert C: Compensatory changes in the distal coronary vascular bed during progressive coronary constriction. Circulation 51:1085, 1975.

37. Domenech RJ, et al: Total and regional coronary blood flow measured by radioactive microspheres in conscious and anesthetized dogs. Circ Res 25:581, 1969.

38. Heymann MA, et al: Blood flow measurements with radionuclide-labeled particles. Prog Cardiovasc Dis 20:55, 1977.

39. Adelstein SJ, Maseri A: Radioindicators for the study of the heart: Principles and applications. Prog Cardiovasc Dis 20:3, 1977.

40. Ritchie JL, et al: Myocardial imaging with indium-

113m and technetium-99m-macroaggregated albumin: New procedure for identification of stress-induced regional ischemia. Am J Cardiol 35:380, 1975.

41. Wilson RA, et al: Validation of quantitation of regional myocardial blood flow in vivo with [11]C-labeled human albumin microspheres and positron emission tomography. Circulation 70:717, 1984.

42. Zaret BL: Myocardial imaging with radioactive potassium and its analogs. Prog Cardiovasc Dis 20:81, 1977.

43. Bailey IK, et al: Thallium-201 myocardial perfusion imaging at rest and during exercise. Comparative sensitivity to electrocardiography in coronary artery disease. Circulation 55:79, 1976.

44. Markis JE, et al: Myocardial salvage after intracoronary thrombolysis with streptokinase in acute myocardial infarction. N Engl J Med 305:777, 1981.

45. Selwyn AP, et al: Relation between regional myocardial uptake of rubidium-82 and perfusion: Absolute reduction of cation uptake in ischemia. Am J Cardiol 50:112, 1982.

46. Vogel R, et al: Application of digital techniques to selective coronary arteriography: Use of myocardial contrast appearance time to measure coronary flow reserve. Am Heart J 107:153, 1984.

47. LeGrand V, et al: Reversibility of coronary collaterals and alteration in regional coronary flow reserve after successful angioplasty. Am J Cardiol 54:453, 1984.

48. O'Neill WW, et al: Criteria for successful coronary angioplasty as assessed by alterations in coronary vasodilatory reserve. J Am Coll Cardiol 3:1382, 1984.

49. Bing RJ, et al: The measurement of coronary blood flow, oxygen consumption, and efficiency of the left ventricle in man. Am Heart J 38:1, 1949.

50. Bassingthwaighte JP: Physiology and theory of tracer washout techniques for the estimation of myocardial blood flow: Flow estimation from tracer washout. Prog Cardiovasc Dis 20:165, 1977.

51. Cannon PJ, Dell RB, Dwyer EM: Regional myocardial perfusion rates in patients with coronary artery disease. J Clin Invest 51:978, 1972.

52. Cannon PJ, et al: Measurement of regional myocardial blood flow in man: Description and critique of the method using Xenon-133 and a scintillation camera. Am J Cardiol 36:783, 1975.

53. Cannon PJ, Weiss MB, Sciacca RR: Myocardial blood flow in coronary artery disease: Studies at rest and during stress with inert gas washout techniques. Prog Cardiovasc Dis 20:95, 1977.

54. Holman L: Nuclear cardiology. *In* Braunwald E (ed): Heart Disease. A textbook of Cardiovascular Medicine. Philadelphia, W.B. Saunders, 1984.

55. Berger HJ, Zaret BL: Nuclear Cardiology. N Engl J Med 305:799, 1981.

56. Brownell GL et al: Positron tomography and nuclear magnetic resonance imaging. Science 215:619, 1982.

57. Roberts DL, Nakazawa HK, Klocke FJ: Origin of great cardiac vein and coronary sinus drainage within the left ventricle. Am J Physiol 230:486, 1976.

58. Nakazawa HK, Roberts DL, Klocke FJ: Quantitation of anterior descending vs. circumflex venous drainae in the canine great cardiac vein and coronary sinus. Am J Physiol 234:H163, 1978.

59. Ganz W, et al: Measurement of coronary sinus blood flow by continuous thermodilution in man. Circulation 44:181, 1971.

60. Yoshida S, et al: Coronary hemodynamics during successive elevation of heart rate by pacing in subjects with angina pectoris. Circulation 44:1062, 1971.

61. Baim DS, Rothman MT, Harrison DC: Improved catheter for regional coronary sinus flow and metabolic studies. Am J Cardiol 46:997, 1980.

62. Pepine CJ, et al: In vivo validation of a thermodilution method to determine regional left ventricular blood flow in patients with coronary disease. Circulation 58:795, 1978.

63. Gross L, Blum L: Effect of coronary artery occlusion on dog's heart with total coronary sinus ligation. Proc Soc Exp Biol Med 32:1578, 1935.

64. Ciuffo AA, et al: Intermittent obstruction of the coronary sinus following coronary ligation in dogs reduces ischemic necrosis and increases myocardial perfusion. *In* Mohl W, Wolner E, Glogar D (ed): The Coronary Sinus, New York, Springer, 1984.

65. Drury JK, et al: Synchronized coronary venous retroperfusion: A safe and effective treatment of acute myocardial ischemia. *In* Mohl W, Wolner E, Glogar D (ed): The Coronary Sinus. New York, Springer, 1984.

66. Gould KL, Lipscomb K: Effects of coronary stenoses on coronary flow reserve and resistance. Am J Cardiol 34:48, 1974.

67. Fuchs RM, et al: Coronary flow limitation during development of ischemia. Effect of atrial pacing in patients with left anterior descending coronary artery disease. Am J Cardiol 48:1029, 1981.

68. Klocke FJ, et al: Average coronary blood flow per unit weight of left ventricle in patients with and without coronary artery disease. Circulation 50:547, 1974.

69. Titus JL, et al: Sudden unexpected deaths as the initial manifestation of ischemic heart disease. Clinical and pathologic observations. Am J Cardiol 26:662, 1970.

70. Scott RF, Briggs TS: Pathological findings in prehospital deaths due to coronary atherosclerosis. Am J Cardiol 29:782, 1972.

71. Chen PH, et al: Left ventricular myocardial blood

flow in multivessel coronary artery disease. Circulation 66:537, 1982.

72. Mudge GH, et al: Reflex increase in coronary vascular resistance in patients with ischemic heart disease. N Engl J Med 295:1333, 1976.

73. Mudge GH, et al: Comparison of metabolic and vasoconstrictor stimuli on coronary vascular resistance in man. Circulation 59:544, 1979.

74. Friedman PL, et al: Coronary vasoconstrictor effect of indomethacin in patients with coronary-artery disease. N Engl J Med 305:1171, 1981.

75. Chierchia S, et al: Sequence of events in angina at rest: Primary reduction in coronary flow. Circulation 61:759, 1980.

76. Chierchia S, et al: Impairment of myocardial perfusion and function during painless myocardial ischemia. J Am Coll Cardiol 1:924, 1983.

77. Feldman RL, Conti CR, Pepine CJ: Regional coronary venous flow responses to transient coronary artery occlusion in human beings. J Am Coll Cardiol 2:1, 1983.

78. Ricci DR, et al: Reduction of coronary blood flow during coronary artery spasm occurring spontaneously and after provocation by ergonovine maleate. Circulation 57:392, 1978.

79. Ockene IS, et al: Unexplained chest pain in patients with normal coronary arteriograms. N Engl J Med 303:1249, 1980.

80. Kemp HG, et al: The anginal syndrome associated with normal coronary arteriograms: report of a six year experience. Am J Med 54:735, 1973.

81. Opherk D, et al: Reduced coronary dilatory capacity and ultrastructural changes of the myocardium in patients with angina pectoris but normal coronary arteriograms. Circulation 63:817, 1981.

82. Schwartz AB, et al: Variability in coronary hemodynamics in response to ergonovine in patients with normal coronary arteries and atypical chest pain. J Am Coll Cardiol 1:797, 1983.

83. Cannon RO, et al: Angina caused by reduced vasodilator reserve of the small coronary arteries. J Am Coll Cardiol 1:1359, 1983.

84. Weiss MB, et al: Myocardial blood flow in congestive and hypertrophic cardiomyopathy: Relationship to peak wall stress and mean velocity of circumferential fiber shortening. Circulation 54:484, 1976.

85. Pichard AD, et al: Coronary flow studies in patients with left ventricular hypertrophy of the hypertensive type. Evidence for an impaired coronary vascular reserve. Am J Cardiol 47:547, 1981.

86. Pichard AD, et al: Coronary vascular reserve in left ventricular hypertrophy secondary to chronic aortic regurgitation. Am J Cardiol 51:315, 1983.

87. Bendersky R, et al: Dobutamine in chronic ischemic heart failure: alterations in left ventricular function and coronary hemodynamics. Am J Cardiol 48:554, 1981.

88. Benotti JR, et al: Effects of amrinone on myocardial energy metabolism and hemodynamics in patients with severe congestive heart failure due to coronary artery disease. Circulation 62:28, 1980.

89. Monrad ES, et al: Effects of milrinone on coronary hemodynamics and myocardial energetics in patients with congestive heart failure. Circulation 71:972, 1985.

90. Hartzler GO, et al: Coronary blood-flow responses during successful percutaneous transluminal coronary angioplasty. Mayo Clin Proc 55:45, 1980.

91. Rothman MT, et al: Coronary hemodynamics during percutaneous transluminal coronary angioplasty. Am J Cardiol 49:1615, 1982.

92. Serruys PW, et al: Left ventricular performance, regional blood flow, wall motion, and lactate metabolism during transluminal angioplasty. Circulation 70:25, 1984.

93. Williams DO, et al: Restoration of normal coronary hemodynamics and myocardial metabolism after percutaneous transluminal coronary angioplasty. Circulation 62:653, 1980.

94. Williams DO, et al: Coronary circulatory dynamics before and after successful coronary angioplasty. J Am Coll Cardiol 1:1268, 1983.

# chapter twenty two

# Intracardiac Electrophysiology

### JOHN P. DIMARCO

T HE DEVELOPMENT of catheter techniques for intracardiac recording and stimulation has greatly enhanced our knowledge of the mechanisms responsible for cardiac arrhythmias in man. Since the first description of the clinical use of His bundle recordings in 1969,[1] cardiac electrophysiologists have described methods for assessing sinus node function, atrioventricular (AV) conduction, and the mechanisms of atrial and ventricular tachyarrhythmias.[2,3] Although many questions remain unanswered, stimulation techniques have also been used in serial fashion to predict the future clinical efficacy of pharmacologic and nonpharmacologic modes of antiarrhythmic therapy. This chapter will attempt to provide a general introduction to the techniques of clinical electrophysiology.

## EQUIPMENT

Like all other catheterization procedures, intracardiac electrophysiologic studies must be performed in an environment that ensures patient safety and comfort during the procedure. The room should be large enough for a patient litter, fluoroscopy unit, instrument table, stimulator and recording equipment. An emergency cart that carries a monitor-defibrillator, supplies to allow manually assisted ventilation, and emergency drug stocks should be accessible for immediate use. Wall outlets for oxygen and suction should be conveniently located. Although portable fluoroscopy equipment is adequate

for many procedures, multiplane fluoroscopy is required if left or right ventricular catheter mapping is to be performed. All electrical devices should be adequately grounded with individual leakage currents of less than 10 microamps and connected to circuits that have immediate backup in case of power failure.

Intracardiac electrograms are displayed on a multichannel oscilloscope-recorder. An instrument for these studies should permit simultaneous display of three or four surface ECG leads and a minimum of five intracardiac channels. Amplifiers for the intracardiac channels are usually filtered below 30 and above 500 or 1000 Hz for standard procedures and should be free of significant line noise at a sensitivity of at least 0.05 mV/cm, preferably at 0.02 mV/cm. Some types of recording (i.e., sinus node electrograms) require different filter settings, and one or more specialized amplifiers may be required. Although bipolar recordings are used for most purposes, unipolar recordings may occasionally be of interest. The technique for obtaining unipolar recordings will vary with different recording systems. Each channel should have a standard calibration signal. Electrical signals are either recorded directly onto recording paper or are stored on FM magnetic tape for subsequent retrieval and analysis. The printer should be capable of producing high quality tracings at paper speeds up to 200 mm/sec. Intracardiac stimulation may be performed using one of several commercial devices. The stimulator should be capable of delivering a minimum of 3 extrastimuli after either an externally-sensed event or after a drive train of delivered stimuli. The impulses delivered should be of a constant current. Most laboratories use a stimulus width of 1 to 2 msec and a current intensity set at 2 to 5 times diastolic threshold. The ability to deliver longer pulse widths (up to 10 msec) or higher currents may be useful if special techniques such as transesophageal pacing are to be performed.

## CATHETERIZATION TECHNIQUES

Diagnostic electrophysiologic procedures usually require insertion of between two and five multipolar, 6 or 7 French electrode catheters into the heart (Fig. 22-1). The catheters themselves are made of woven Dacron and have three to six platinum ring electrodes positioned near the distal tip. We commonly use quadripolar catheters with an interelectrode spacing of 0.5 or 1.0 cm with the distal ring at the tip of the catheter. This permits bipolar stimulation and recording from each catheter. Other electrode configurations may be useful for selected purposes. Each electrode is then connected to a switch box which directs signals from the recording

poles to the oscilloscope-recorder and transmits impulses from the stimulator.

The patient is brought to the laboratory in a fasting state. If possible, prior antiarrhythmic therapy will have been discontinued and the drugs allowed to wash out for 5 half-lives. Oral or intravenous benzodiazepines may be used to allay anxiety when necessary. Both groins are sterilely prepared and draped, and the skin overlying the femoral vessels is anesthetized with 0.5 or 1% lidocaine. Excessive amounts of lidocaine should be avoided, since significant amounts may be absorbed systemically, thus potentially affecting the results obtained.[4] The femoral artery is palpated about 1 to 2 cm below the iliac crease, using the anatomic guideline described in Chapter 5. A small skin incision is made with a scalpel blade, and the subcutaneous tissue is dilated with a hemostat. A guide wire is then inserted into the common femoral vein using the Seldinger technique (see Chapter 5). An appropriately sized introducing sheath is then passed over the guide wire, and the electrode catheter is passed through the sheath to the inferior vena cava. A second catheter may be inserted using the same procedure on the opposite groin. When three or more electrode catheters are re-

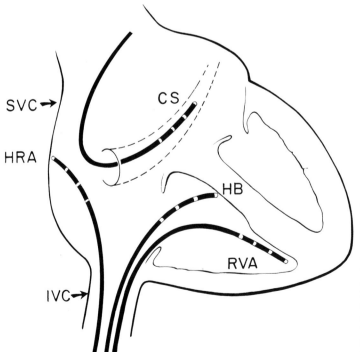

**Fig. 22-1.** Diagram of standard catheter positions for electrophysiologic studies. Quadripolar catheters to the high right atrium (HRA), the right ventricular apex (RVA), and the bundle of His (HB) are usually inserted via the femoral veins and inferior vena cava (IVC). Left atrial recording and stimulation are usually performed with a catheter in the coronary sinus (CS). (SVC, superior vena cava.)

quired for the study, second sheaths usually may be inserted into the right and/or left femoral vein for the third and fourth catheters. A puncture is made about 1 cm proximal to the prior insertion site, and a second sheath is inserted over a guide wire. If a catheter has already been advanced through the first sheath, the possibility of puncturing the thin walls of the initial sheath during the second puncture will be minimized.

Once the catheters have been inserted, they are advanced to the heart under fluoroscopic guidance (Fig. 22-1). The catheters usually employed in these studies are somewhat more rigid than are the catheters used for most other catheterization procedures, and care must be taken to avoid vessel perforation. One catheter is usually positioned high in the right atrium at its junction with the superior vena cava (Fig. 22-1). This places the catheter just adjacent to the sinus node. A second catheter is positioned in the right ventricular apex (Fig. 22-1). The distal and proximal poles of these catheters are used for right atrial and right ventricular stimulation and recording, respectively.

The bundle of His lies in the high membranous septum, and a local electrogram containing the His bundle potential may be recorded with the catheter tip positioned just across the tricuspid valve. In practice, the catheter should be advanced into the right ventricular cavity and connected to the oscilloscope for monitoring. The catheter is then slowly withdrawn until the characteristic bi- or triphasic His bundle potential is recognized before the onset of ventricular depolarization (Fig. 22-2). Small movements of the catheter or by the patient may cause the His bundle potential signal to be lost or even cause the catheter to flip back into the atrium, and it is occasionally necessary to reposition this catheter one or more times during the procedure. His bundle recording may also be performed using a superior approach by making a figure six-shaped loop with the catheter across the tricuspid valve, but this technique is considerably more difficult and yields a less stable recording than the transfemoral approach. In rare cases, His bundle recording may be performed using a catheter positioned either just above or just below the noncoronary cusp of the aortic valve.

Most electrophysiologic studies for assessment of AV conduction, sinus node function, or ventricular tachycardia do not require left atrial recording. However, analysis of atrial activation patterns and responses to left atrial stimulation may be critical for the evaluation of supraventricular arrhythmias or preexcitation patterns. Left atrial activity is most commonly recorded using a catheter placed in the coronary sinus. Although coronary sinus catheterization via a femoral approach is possible, it is technically easier to perform from either a subclavian or an internal jugular site. In some patients a medial left antecubital vein will also allow suitable access. Occasionally, a catheter may be placed in the left atrium through a patent foramen ovale from a transfemoral approach. This may provide more convenient left atrial access in some patients.

## BASELINE INTERVALS

As illustrated in Figure 22-2, a number of standard measurements may be made from the initial recordings obtained. The PA interval is measured from the onset of the P wave on the ECG to the first rapid atrial deflection on the His bundle electrogram. We have not found measurement of the PA interval to be a clinically valuable exercise. It has not been possible to directly record AV nodal activation with a catheter. Therefore, AV nodal conduction time has been approximated as the interval from onset of septal atrial activation to the onset of the His bundle potential (AH interval). His Purkinje conduction time is measured as the interval from the onset of the His bundle potential to the first point of ventricular activity on either the surface ECG leads or on the ventricular electrogram (HV interval). The normal ranges for these intervals in our laboratory are given in Table 22-1.

## Sinus Node Function

Sinus node dysfunction may be diagnosed when marked sinus bradycardia and tachycardia are recorded during routine ambulatory electrocardiography. However, these findings may appear only intermittently or may not be associated with symptoms. In patients with intermittent symptoms and inconclusive findings during ambulatory moni-

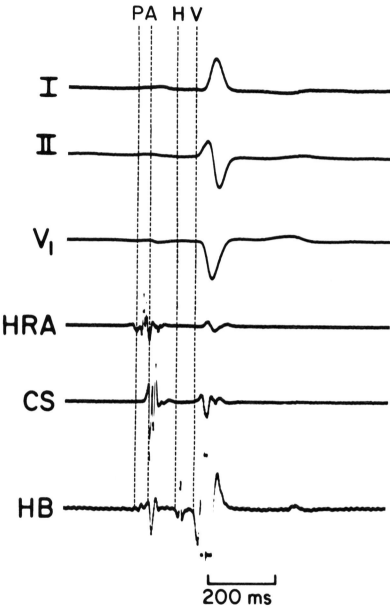

**Fig. 22-2.** Normal conduction intervals. Three surface electrocardiographic leads (I, II, and $V_1$) are displayed simultaneously. In addition, a high right atrial (HRA) electrogram, a coronary sinus (CS) electrogram, and a His bundle (HB) electrogram are also displayed. The PA interval is measured from the onset of the P wave on the surface ECG to the first rapid atrial deflection on the His bundle electrogram. AV nodal conduction time is approximated as the interval from onset of septal atrial activation to the onset of the His potential (AH interval). His Purkinje conduction time is measured as the HV interval, where V is the first point of ventricular activity on either the surface ECG or ventricular electrogram.

toring, firm conclusions about the need for implantation of a permanent pacemaker are difficult. For this reason, a number of tests of sinus node function have been used clinically. Those most commonly used are an as-

sessment of the response of the sinus node to overdrive stimulation (sinus node recovery time) and the direct or indirect measurement of sinoatrial conduction times.[5]

***Sinus Node Recovery Time.*** If cardiac

**TABLE 22-1.** *Normal Electrophysiologic Parameters*

Intervals

| | |
|---|---|
| PA | 25–50 msec |
| AH | 60–140 msec |
| HV | 30–55 msec |
| His Duration | 10–25 msec |

Effective Refractory Periods

| | |
|---|---|
| Atrium | 200–270 msec |
| AV node | 280–450 msec |
| Ventricle | 200–270 msec |

Corrected Sinus
Node Recovery Time ..... <525 msec
Sinoatrial Conduction
Time (Total) ............ 100–210 msec

tissue with intrinsic automaticity is repetitively depolarized by impulses conducted from another source, its intrinsic automaticity will be suppressed transiently after the external drive is discontinued. This phenomenon has been termed overdrive suppression, and the response of the sinus node to overdrive stimulation has been used as a measure of sinus node automaticity.[6]

In practice, a pacing catheter is positioned in the high right atrium and, beginning at a cycle length just below the intrinsic sinus cycle length, 30 to 60 second trains of pacing are delivered. The delay between the last stimulus to the onset of atrial activity originating near the high right atrial catheter is termed the *sinus node recovery time* (SNRT) (Fig. 22-3).

For the SNRT to accurately reflect the effects of overdrive suppression on the sinus node, each stimulus must conduct into the sinus node and depolarize it. In addition, the magnitude of overdrive suppression may vary with different rates of pacing in an individual subject. Maximum sensitivity is therefore achieved if pacing at each cycle length is repeated twice and if cycle lengths ranging from just below the patient's sinus cycle length to 300 msec are tested. The sinus node recovery time is dependent upon the intrinsic sinus cycle length, and most authors report a corrected sinus node recovery time (CSNRT) calculated by subtracting the basic sinus cycle length (SCL) from the recovery time (CSNRT = SNRT − SCL). The upper limit of normal for a measured CSNRT in our laboratory is 525 msec. As mentioned above, this test assumes that the last atrial stimulus has penetrated the sinus node and depolarized it. This may not always be true. In such cases, unexplained pauses after the first intrinsic beat may occur. When such secondary pauses are greater than 525 msec above the intrinsic sinus cycle length, they should be considered to be markers of abnormal sinus node recovery.

***Sinoatrial Conduction.*** In some patients, sinus node automaticity is normal, but conduction of the impulse to the atrium is blocked or delayed. Both direct and indirect

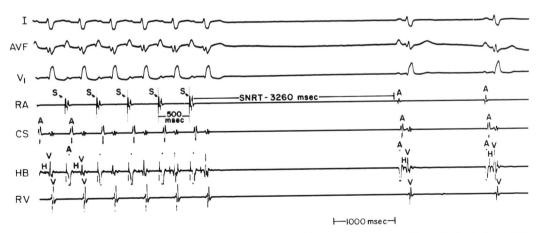

**Fig. 22-3.** Abnormal sinus node recovery time in a patient with recurrent syncope. The end of a train of right atrial stimuli at a cycle length of 500 msec is shown. A 3260 msec pause follows the termination of pacing. The intrinsic sinus cycle length was 1140 msec giving a markedly abnormal corrected SNRT of 2120 msec. (RA, right atrium; CS, coronary sinus; HB, His bundle; RV, right ventricle; S, stimulus artifact; SNRT, sinus node recovery time.)

methods for assessing sinoatrial conduction have been described.

Two indirect methods for measuring sinoatrial conduction times have been used. The Strauss method measures the delay in atrial recovery after a single atrial premature depolarization introduced during sinus rhythm.[7] Single atrial premature stimuli ($A_2$) are delivered during stable sinus rhythm ($A_1$-$A_1$) beginning with the initial coupling interval just below the sinus cycle length ($A_1$-$A_1$). Four zones of response may be identified as the extrastimulus is made progressively more premature. In zone 1, the premature beat ($A_2$) depolarizes the atrium, but the sinus node itself has already depolarized. Thus the impulse exiting from the sinus node collides with the stimulated impulse, and the interval from the premature beat to the next sinus beat ($A_2$-$A_3$) is fully compensatory, i.e., $(A_1$-$A_2) + (A_2$-$A_3) = 2\ (A_1$-$A_1)$. If the extra stimulus is moved earlier, the impulse will penetrate the sinus node and reset it. The $A_2$-$A_3$ return cycle therefore is composed of three periods, the time for penetration into the node, the reset interval, and the time for conduction out of the node. The reset interval should be the same as the basic cycle length, ($A_1$-$A_1$). Therefore, $(A_2$-$A_3) - (A_1$-$A_1)$ = conduction time (in) + conduction time (out). In practice either total sinoatrial conduction times [$SACT_{TOTAL} = (A_2$-$A_3) - (A_1$-$A_1)$] or, if one assumes equal antegrade and retrograde conduction, unidirectional sinoatrial conduction times

$$SACT_{A\ or\ R} = \frac{(A_2\text{-}A_3) - (A_1\text{-}A_1)}{2}$$

are reported. As the $A_1$-$A_2$ interval is further shortened, $A_2$-$A_3$ shortens to less than $A_1$-$A_1$. This shortening is done by either interpolation (zone 3) or reentry (zone 4). The most reliable and reproducible values for sinoatrial conduction time are obtained with $A_1$-$A_2$ intervals in the latter half of zone 2.

A second method for estimating sinoatrial conduction has been proposed by Narula et al.[8] The atrium is paced at a rate slightly above the intrinsic sinus rate for eight consecutive beats, and the interval from the last paced beat to the next sinus beat is measured. The basic cycle length is then subtracted from this interval, and the mean of several such determinations is used as an estimate of $SACT_{TOTAL}$.

Recently a direct method for estimating sinoatrial conduction has been developed.[9] An electrode catheter is placed at the junction of the superior vena cava and the high right atrium adjacent to the expected location of the sinus node. With appropriate gain (0.05 mV/cm) and filtering (0.1 to 50 Hz), a low amplitude deflection can be seen to precede both the P wave and the local atrial electrogram. This deflection is thought to represent the sinus node electrogram, and the time from its first deflection to the onset of atrial activation has been used as a direct measure of sinoatrial conduction. Values obtained with this method are in general agreement with those obtained by the indirect methods described. The upper limit of normal for a directly or indirectly measured total SACT in our laboratory is 210 msec.

The clinical value of electrophysiologic testing in patients with suspected sinus node dysfunction has been disappointing. Although an abnormal SNRT is a relatively specific marker for patients with significant sinus node dysfunction, it is frequently normal in patients with a clear history of symptomatic sinus bradyarrhythmias. Measurement of sinoatrial conduction times has also not proven valuable as a test to screen patients for suspected sinus node dysfunction. At present, ambulatory monitoring remains the most reliable guide to therapy in patients with disorders of sinus node function, and the tests outlined are used chiefly to confirm or clarify other clinical findings.

## AV Conduction

The specialized AV conduction system consists of the AV node, the common bundle of His, the bundle branches, and the distal Purkinje fiber network. In most cases, the mechanism responsible for a prolongation in AV conduction can be deduced from standard electrocardiographic criteria. Analysis of AV conduction intervals as outlined previously may also be of value. In certain situations, however, it may be useful to assess the responses of the AV conduction system to both incremental atrial stimulation and to atrial extrastimuli.

Atrial pacing is usually performed from the right atrium, but coronary sinus pacing may also be used. Pacing is started at a cycle length just below the sinus cycle length, and the cycle length is decreased by 50 msec every 30 to 60 seconds. The onset of AV nodal Wenckebach and the point at which 2:1 AV nodal block develops should be noted. In adults, the development of AV nodal Wenckebach at a cycle length of greater than 500 msec or less than 300 msec is considered abnormal. It must be remembered that drugs, age, and autonomic tone all have profound effects on AV nodal conduction, and these factors must be considered in interpreting the data.

During incremental atrial pacing, the HV interval usually remains constant. The development of block within or below the bundle of His during atrial pacing, particularly at a pacing cycle length of >400 msec, is an abnormal finding.[10] Rate-related bundle branch block may also be observed during incremental atrial pacing, and its demonstration may be of value for the interpretation of wide complex beats or tachycardias of uncertain origin.

The clinical value of His bundle recording remains controversial, since moderate prolongation of the HV interval is commonly found. In asymptomatic patients with bundle branch block, HV intervals of under 80 to 100 msec have not been associated with a high rate of progression to complete heart block.[11] However, as illustrated in Figure 22-4, His bundle recording is frequently help-ful for explaining atypical electrocardiographic patterns of AV block.

The effective, relative, and functional refractory periods of the AV conduction system may be measured using the atrial extrastimulus method. A stimulation train of eight atrial beats ($A_1$) at a constant cycle length is followed by a single premature stimulus ($A_2$). The drive train is repeated after a 2 to 6-second pause, and the extrastimulus is introduced at progressive decrements of 10 to 20 msec. The effective refractory period (ERP) of the AV node is defined as the longest $A_1$-$A_2$ interval that captures the atrium but fails to conduct to the bundle of His. The relative refractory period is the atrial premature interval that results in a measurable increase in the AH interval over that measured during the drive train. The functional refractory period is the shortest interval between His bundle depolarizations ($H_1$-$H_2$) that results from any $A_1$-$A_2$.

The response of the AV node to premature stimuli usually yields a relatively smooth curve when $A_2$-$H_2$ intervals are plotted against $A_1$-$A_2$ intervals. In some patients, however, the curve may be discontinuous (Fig. 22-5), and longitudinal dissociation of conduction due to dual pathways in the AV node has been postulated as the underlying mechanism.[12] This phenomenon can be demonstrated in many patients with paroxysmal supraventricular tachycardia (SVT) due to

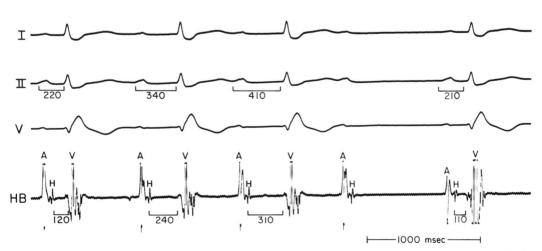

**Fig. 22-4.** Infra-Hisian Wenckebach block. The tracings were obtained in a 31-year-old man with Wenckebach Type, second-degree AV block on his ECG and a history of syncope. Intracardiac recordings documented that the site of conduction delay was below the bundle of His (HB) despite the Wenckebach periodicity. Note that all the conduction delay occurs within the HV interval.

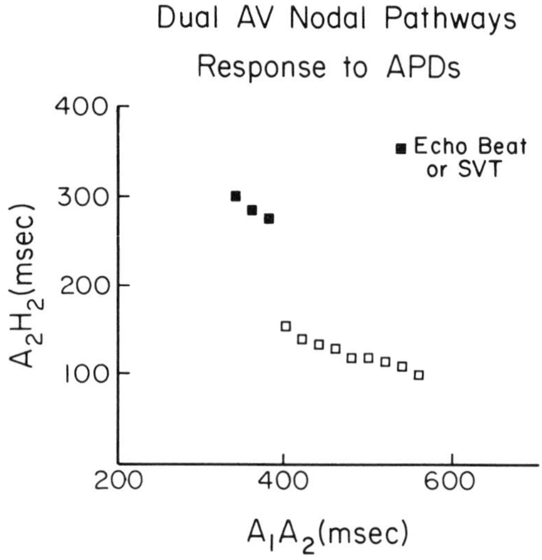

## Dual AV Nodal Pathways
## Response to APDs

**Fig. 22-5.** AV conduction in a patient with dual AV nodal pathways. The $A_2H_2$ intervals are plotted against the $A_1A_2$ intervals. The sudden increase in $A_2H_2$ signifies a shift in conduction to the slow pathway as the refractory period of the faster pathway is reached.

AV nodal reentry but can also be observed in some patients without a history of SVT.

## PROGRAMMED CARDIAC STIMULATION

Many chronic cardiac tachyarrhythmias are due to the reentry of impulses over fixed circuits within the heart. Reentry depends upon dissociation of conduction and refractory properties of contiguous tissue enabling unidirectional block to occur in one limb of the circuit and slow conduction in the opposite limb. If conduction in the initially blocked circuit recovers after an appropriate interval, it will conduct an impulse that has completed the circuit in retrograde fashion. If the tissue proximal to the region of initial block has recovered excitability, a reentrant beat will be initiated. Premature stimulation, by decreasing the time allowed for tissues to recover, is able to induce reentrant arrhythmias by enhancing the inhomogeneity of conduction and refractory properties of adjacent tissues.

A number of factors will influence the results of programmed cardiac stimulation

**TABLE 22-2.** *Factors Affecting Results of Programmed Stimulation*

Site of stimulation
Intensity and duration of stimuli
Number of extrastimuli
Cycle lengths of drive trains
Rate and duration of burst pacing
Definition of a positive response
Use of provocative stimuli
Population studied

(Table 22-2). These factors may all interact in a fashion that has not been totally characterized. As a result, it is often difficult to compare results obtained in different laboratories that employ different stimulation protocols. At the present time there is no general agreement on the techniques that afford the highest sensitivity without sacrificing specificity. The stimulation protocol we currently use is outlined below.

***Atrial Stimulation.*** Single ($S_2$) and double ($S_2$-$S_3$) atrial extrastimuli are introduced during sinus rhythm and after eight beats of atrial pacing at cycle lengths of 600 and 400 msec. A pause of 2 to 6 seconds is allowed to occur between successive drive trains. The initial $S_1$-$S_2$ interval is set to put $S_2$ in late diastole, and the interval is decreased in 10 or 20 msec decrements until $S_2$ no longer captures. This defines the atrial effective refractory period (ERP) for that cycle length. The $S_1$-$S_2$ interval is then set at 50 msec above the atrial ERP, and the $S_2$-$S_3$ interval is set equal to that $S_1$-$S_2$ interval. $S_2$-$S_3$ is then decreased in 10 msec decrements until $S_3$ is refractory. $S_1$-$S_2$ is then shortened by 10 msec until $S_3$ captures. The sequence is repeated until $S_2$ no longer captures. In patients with supraventricular arrhythmias, atrial premature stimulation is repeated from the left atrium using the same protocol. Finally, bursts of atrial pacing at rates up to 300 beats per minute may be used to assess the point at which AV conduction delay occurs and the effects of conduction delay on arrhythmia initiation. When indicated, bursts of rapid atrial pacing at rates up to 800 per minute may be used to induce atrial flutter or atrial fibrillation.

***Ventricular Stimulation.*** Single, double, and triple ventricular extrastimuli are delivered to the right ventricular apex during both sinus rhythm and ventricular pacing at cycle lengths of 600 and 400 msec. The coupling intervals are varied in a similar manner to the sequence described above. Recently, we have modified our protocol to include a series of double extrastimuli after an abrupt cycle length change from 400 to 600 msec following the seventh beat of the drive train.[13] We have also eliminated nonsynchronous bursts of rapid ventricular pacing, although many laboratories continue to use this mode of stimulation. If no arrhythmia is initiated with right ventricular apical stimulation, stimulation is repeated from a second right ventricular site, usually the outflow tract. Rarely, isoproterenol infusion or left ventricular stimulation may be required to reproduce a patient's clinical arrhythmia.

## Supraventricular Arrhythmias

Programmed atrial and ventricular stimulation is frequently useful in patients with a history of supraventricular arrhythmias. These studies can be used to define the mechanism responsible for the arrhythmia, to localize any extranodal pathways that might be involved, to assess risk for more serious arrhythmias in patients with Wolff-Parkinson-White syndrome, to measure the effects of drug therapy, and to provide a guide for attempts to interrupt a pathway required for arrhythmia propagation either surgically or with catheter techniques.[12,14–16]

## Paroxysmal Supraventricular Tachycardia

Four electrophysiologic mechanisms account for the majority of cases of supraventricular tachycardia (SVT) that occur clinically.[14] Patients with each type will manifest characteristic patterns of responses to atrial and ventricular stimulation (Table 22-3). Evaluation should determine the mode(s) of stimulation required to initiate and terminate the tachycardia, the requirements of atria or ventricles for tachycardia initiation and continuation, the atrial activation sequence during SVT, and the effects of atrial and ventricular stimulation during tachycardia. In addition, it is often helpful to evaluate the effects of drugs or physical maneuvers on the tachycardia.

Reentry within the AV node is the most common cause for recurrent SVT. The tachycardia circuit involves antegrade conduction over a "slow" antegrade AV nodal pathway and retrograde conduction over a "fast" pathway. With atrial premature stimulation, dual AV nodal pathways can often be demonstrated (Fig. 22-5). Initiation of AV nodal re-entrant SVT usually occurs after either atrial or ventricular premature beats that produce a critical AV nodal conduction delay or during atrial pacing that results in Wenckebach block. As the antegrade refractory period of the fast pathway is reached, the AH interval abruptly prolongs because the slow pathway is then used for antegrade conduction. If SVT is initiated, retrograde septal atrial activation will often occur simultaneously with ventricular activation. The septal atrial deflection on the His bundle electrogram will often be obscured by ventricular activity, but left and right atrial activation will indicate a normal retrograde activation pattern. Since the reentry circuit is located within the AV node, AV dissociation may occur and may be demonstrated with premature stimulation during tachycardia.

The second most common form of recurrent SVT involves antegrade conduction over the AV node and retrograde conduction over an extranodal pathway. This arrhythmia mechanism may be documented in patients with manifest preexcitation (Wolff-Parkinson-White syndrome) and in patients whose accessory pathways conduct only in the retrograde fashion (concealed bypass tracts). Initiation occurs when an atrial extrastimulus encounters antegrade block in the accessory pathway and causes prolonged AV conduction through the normal pathway. An example is shown in Figure 22-6. Initiation may also occur when a ventricular extrastimulus blocks retrogradely in the His-Purkinje system and conducts over the accessory pathway only. Atrial activation during SVT will depend upon the location of the accessory pathway, and a precise location may be determined if atrial activity is recorded from multiple sites (Fig. 22-7). If eccentric activation is not seen and the first retrograde activity is recorded at the AV junction, it is necessary to confirm the pres-

**TABLE 22-3.** *Characteristics of Common Forms of Supraventricular Tachycardia*

| Arrhythmia | Mode of Initiation | Requirement for Atria/Ventricle | P Wave Morphology and Position | Atrial Activation Sequence | Notes |
|---|---|---|---|---|---|
| AV nodal reentry | APD, VPD AP | Neither | Retrograde, obscured by QRS | Caudocephalad, AVJ earliest | Dual pathways common |
| AV reentry in patients with WPW or CBT | APD, VPD AP, VP | Both | Variable, after QRS | Depends on AP location | Smooth AV nodal conduction ipsilateral BBB increases CL |
| Intraatrial reentry | APD, AP | Atria | Variable, PR related to rate | Depends on location | AV block common |
| Sinoatrial reentry | APD | Atria | Normal, PR related to rate | Identical to sinus | AV block may occur |

Abbreviations: AP = atrial pacing; APD = atrial premature depolarizations; AV = atrioventricular; AVJ = atrioventricular junction; CBT = concealed bypass tract; SVT = supraventricular tachycardia; VP = ventricular pacing; VPD = ventricular premature depolarizations; WPW = Wolff-Parkinson-White syndrome.

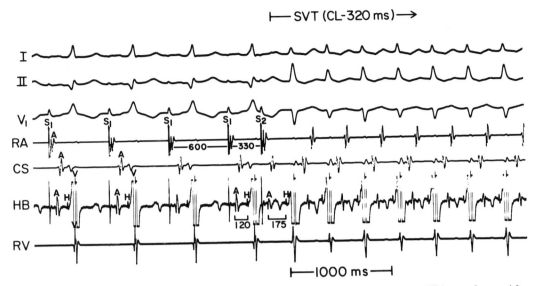

**Fig. 22-6.** Initiation of AV reciprocating tachycardia in a patient with Wolff-Parkinson-White syndrome. After eight atrially paced beats at a cycle length of 600 msec, a single atrial premature stimulus (S$_2$) is introduced. Antegrade block is produced in the accessory pathway, and AV conduction is via the normal pathway. The impulse then can engage the left-sided pathway in the retrograde conduction, and the reentrant circuit is completed. (SVT, supraventricular tachycardia; CL, cycle length; RA, right atrium; CS, coronary sinus; HB, His bundle; RV, right ventricle.)

ence of a septal bypass tract by preexciting the atrium during SVT with a premature ventricular stimulus instituted at the time of antegrade His bundle activation. Since ventricular activation is required before the accessory pathway can be entered, atrial activity will follow ventricular activity, and the development of bundle branch block ipsilateral to the pathway will increase the tachycardia cycle length. Contralateral bundle branch block will not affect cycle length. Both atria and ventricle are required for the arrhythmia circuit and AV dissociation should not occur.

Sinus node reentry and intraatrial reentry are the two other common forms of SVT. Both are independent of AV nodal conduction delay and may continue despite AV block. Other pertinent features of these arrhythmias are listed in Table 22-3.

Paroxysmal supraventricular tachycardia may also be caused by increased automaticity in an ectopic atrial focus, by reentry over multiple accessory pathways, and by atypical patterns in patients with preexcitation. Discussion of the characteristics of these arrhythmias is beyond the scope of this chapter.

## Atrial Flutter and Fibrillation

Intracardiac recordings and programmed stimulation are of less value in other atrial arrhythmias. Atrial flutter may be diagnosed by recording discrete atrial depolarizations with a constant cycle length ranging between 240 and 180 msec. Bursts of rapid atrial pacing, usually at rates between 320 and 420 beats per minute, will terminate flutter in about two thirds of patients if atrial capture can be achieved.[17] It is frequently difficult to confirm atrial capture at these rapid pacing rates using only a surface ECG, and we have preferred to monitor a local electrogram from the recording poles of the catheter during each attempt at termination. We have also noted that it is often necessary to try pacing from several different sites within the atrium before successful termination of the arrhythmia can be achieved. Atrial fibrillation and some cases of atrial flutter cannot be terminated with burst pacing, and the value of serial drug testing by repeated attempts to initiate arrhythmia in these patients has not been proven. For these reasons, electrophysiologic studies in patients with paroxysmal atrial flutter or fibrillation

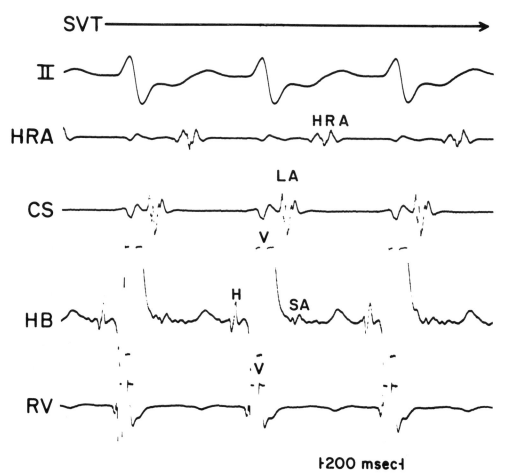

**Fig. 22-7.** Atrial activation sequence in supraventricular tachycardia (SVT) due to a concealed bypass tract. The tracings are high speed recordings made during SVT. Note that the first retrograde atrial activity recorded after ventricular depolarization is from the left atrium (LA) as recorded on the coronary sinus (CS) catheter. High right atrial (HRA) and septal right atrial (SA) activation is recorded later. (CS, coronary sinus; HB, His bundle; RV, right ventricle.)

as their only rhythm disturbance are only occasionally useful.

## Accessory Pathways

In patients with preexcitation, it is necessary to measure the effective refractory period of the accessory pathway for both antegrade and retrograde conduction and to localize the pathway. The effective refractory period of the pathway may be defined as the shortest coupling interval after which an extrastimulus cannot be conducted over the pathway. During atrial decremental extra-stimulation in patients with preexcitation, the QRS will become more and more bizarre as the contribution of conduction over the accessory pathway to ventricular activation becomes more pronounced. Once the effective refractory period of the pathway is reached, either no AV conduction will occur or, if the ERP of the pathway is relatively long, the PR length and the QRS will normalize as conduction is shifted to the normal AV conduction system. It is also advisable to attempt to initiate atrial fibrillation in these patients, since the shortest PR interval measured during atrial fibrillation approximates the antegrade ERP of the accessory pathway and correlates with the risk of future occurrence of a life-threatening arrhythmia.[18]

The location of the accessory pathway can be determined best by atrial activation mapping during either SVT or ventricular stimulation. The earliest site of atrial activation found correlates with the location of the accessory pathway. Atrial stimulation from this site should also result in the shortest possible stimulus-to-ventricle activation time and usually shows the greatest degree of preexcitation at any given pacing cycle length.

## Ventricular Arrhythmias

The successful use of electrophysiologic studies in patients with supraventricular arrhythmias led several groups of investigators to employ a similar approach in patients with recurrent ventricular tachycardia and ventricular fibrillation.[19–21] However, many questions about the optimal methods for evaluating such patients remain unanswered, and the role of such studies in these patients has not been completely defined.

The ventricular stimulation protocol used in our laboratory has been outlined. Like any other stimulation protocol, it attempts to reach a compromise between sensitivity and specificity. Sensitivity is increased if more extrastimuli are used,[22–24] if several sites are stimulated,[25,26] if stimulus intensity is increased, and if either nonsustained, polymorphic runs of ventricular tachycardia or ventricular fibrillation are accepted as positive responses.[27,28] However, any attempts to increase sensitivity through the use of more aggressive stimulation protocols have resulted in decreased specificity, i.e., when the stimulation protocol is used in patients without a history of prior arrhythmia, "positive" responses are obtained. In addition, an aggressive stimulation protocol may make suppression of the arrhythmia at subsequent drug testing difficult or impossible, thereby limiting the value of electrophysiologic testing for evaluating therapy.[29]

The definition of a positive response is also difficult, since there is not a clearly defined separation in response to a reasonably sensitive stimulation protocol between populations with and without prior arrhythmias. All investigators would agree that sustained, monomorphic ventricular tachycardia that is morphologically identical to a clinically documented arrhythmia is a positive response. Unfortunately, a 12 lead ECG during tachycardia with the patient off antiarrhythmic drug therapy is available in only a small number of patients and such a correlation cannot always be made. It has been our practice to define the reproducible initiation of >30 nonstimulated ventricular beats in response to 1, 2, or 3 extrastimuli as a positive response. Patients who have more than 10 nonstimulated beats in response to 1 or 2 extrastimuli will almost always manifest sustained arrhythmias if triple extrastimuli are used. However, in all patients with a history of sustained ventricular tachycardia, it is important to try to reproduce the clinically documented arrhythmia. Therefore, we recommend that the stimulation protocol always be carried out either to its conclusion or to initiation of a sustained arrhythmia. When these definitions are used, a ventricular arrhythmia can be reproducibly initiated with our protocol in over 90% of patients with coronary artery disease and a history of ventricular tachycardia and in about 60 to 75% of patients with ventricular fibrillation. Lower percentages of successful initiation are observed in other forms of heart disease.

***Initial Study.*** Antiarrhythmic therapy should be discontinued, and the patient should be observed in a monitored setting until serum concentrations are undetectable. Sinus node function and AV conduction should be assessed routinely, and several recording catheters should be used to exclude SVT with aberrancy as the mechanism for any arrhythmia. Programmed ventricular stimulation is then performed according to the protocol outlined. If a sustained ventricular arrhythmia is initiated, the patient's ability to tolerate the arrhythmia should be evaluated immediately. Some laboratories routinely record intraarterial pressure during these studies, but we have not found this necessary except during catheter mapping procedures. If the arrhythmia is poorly tolerated, attempts should be made to terminate it with bursts of rapid ventricular pacing beginning at a cycle length just below that of the tachycardia (Fig. 22-8). In well-tolerated tachycardias, single or double extrastimuli may produce termination with less risk of acceleration. If syncope or severe chest pain develops or if the tachycardia either cannot be terminated with drugs or pacing or accel-

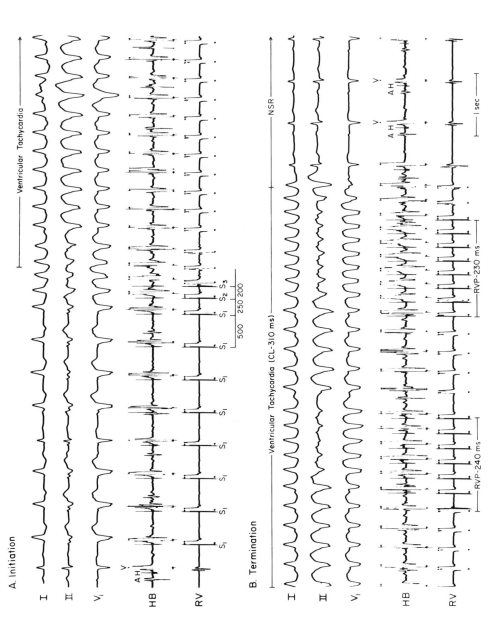

**Fig. 22-8.** Electrophysiologic study in a patient with recurrent ventricular tachycardia. (A) Sustained ventricular tachycardia is initiated by double extrastimuli ($S_2 S_3$) after eight paced beats at a cycle length of 500 msec. (B) Two bursts of rapid ventricular pacing (RVP) are delivered. The first fails to terminate the arrhythmia, but the second at a shorter cycle length is effective and sinus rhythm is restored. Note that the His bundle (HB) electrogram shows an absent His potential and AV dissociation during tachycardia.

erates when pacing is attempted, direct current countershock should be used. We have found it helpful to monitor response to countershock by watching the intraventricular electrogram as opposed to a surface ECG lead, since its signal will not be distorted by muscle activity due to the countershock or to seizure activity.

Electrophysiologic studies may be employed in serial fashion to evaluate the effects of antiarrhythmic drugs or surgical procedures. If several studies are performed within a short period, an indwelling pacing wire may be left in position, but the catheter should be changed if more than 48 hours have elapsed since the initial insertion or if there has been any increase in pacing threshold. During a drug trial, programmed ventricular stimulation using the original protocol is repeated. Although some laboratories advocate stimulation at multiple sites during each drug trial, it has been our practice to use only the site from which ventricular tachycardia was initiated at the original study. Suppression of the ability to induce an arrhythmia has correlated well with subsequent protection from recurrent arrhythmias in our experience[30] and in that of others.[19–21, 31–33]

***Nonpharmacologic Therapy.*** The concept that sustained ventricular tachycardia (VT) is due to reentry in a small area of the ventricle has led to a number of innovative nonpharmacologic approaches to its control. If patients are able to tolerate their arrhythmia, an electrode catheter can be inserted retrogradely into the left ventricle, and bipolar recordings can be made from multiple sites. In this manner, activation sequence maps of the ventricle during tachycardia can be generated and the site of earliest activity can be identified. In patients with coronary artery disease, these areas have usually been found within the border zones of ventricular aneurysms or scars resulting from prior myocardial infarction. Surgical excision, cryoablation, and, more recently, catheter ablation at these areas have been reported to prevent further episodes of ventricular tachycardia.[34–36] In each situation, the efficacy of the intervention may be assessed with repeat programmed ventricular stimulation. Further refinement of these techniques may improve the prognosis for many patients who cannot be optimally managed with drug therapy alone.

Another approach that is under study is the use of implantable devices to terminate arrhythmias. Initially, attempts were made to prevent the occurrence of arrhythmia by chronic pacing at rates above the intrinsic sinus rate. This approach proved to be unsuccessful in most cases. However, since most chronically recurring ventricular tachycardias are due to reentry and can be terminated with pacing, there has been considerable interest in the development of permanent pacemakers with antitachycardia capabilities.[37] These devices may be patient-activated with a magnet or an external transmitter or may be programmed to function automatically if a certain ventricular rate is detected. Some new devices can adjust the pacing stimulus that they deliver if the tachycardia is not terminated with the programmed setting. Unfortunately, acceleration of arrhythmia may occur unpredictably during attempts to terminate an arrhythmia with pacing, and this factor has limited the application of chronically implanted antitachycardia pacemakers. Occasional patients with atrial arrhythmias may, however, be managed successfully with such units. The planned introduction of an implantable device that has the capacity for both antitachycardia pacing and defibrillation if ventricular fibrillation is precipitated will be a major advance in the management of selected patients with recurrent, life-threatening arrhythmias.

## COMPLICATIONS OF ELECTROPHYSIOLOGIC STUDIES

One of the purposes of an electrophysiologic study is to reproduce a patient's clinical arrhythmia. In many cases, these arrhythmias cause hemodynamic deterioration which, if not promptly terminated, might result in death. For this reason, it is critically important to evaluate carefully every patient prior to study for factors that might complicate any attempt at resuscitation. We try to screen out patients with unstable ischemia, uncompensated heart failure, severe, uncorrected valvular lesions, metabolic abnormalities, or drug toxicity in whom provocation of an arrhythmia might lead to irreversible collapse. By taking these precautions we have been able to perform studies safely even in patients with advanced heart disease.

If these precautions are taken, the complications of the electrophysiologic studies should be similar to those of any other catheterization procedure. The most common complications reported in one series were deep venous thrombosis and pulmonary embolism.[38] These complications were presumably related to femoral vein catheterization and occurred primarily in elderly patients with congestive heart failure. Some laboratories use full heparinization during every study, but we have found that routine use of subcutaneous heparin (5000 U q 12 h)

has minimized this complication. We do recommend, however, full heparinization during the procedure in patients otherwise at high risk for thrombotic complications and for all studies involving left-sided catheterization. We have observed only 2 cases of deep venous thrombosis in our last 400 patients.

Other potential complications include infection related to indwelling catheters, cardiac or blood vessel perforation, and cerebral or systemic emboli with left atrial or ventricular catheterization. The incidence of these complications should be extremely low if careful catheter techniques are employed.

# REFERENCES

1. Scherlag BJ, et al: Catheter technique for recording His bundle activity in man. Circulation 39:13, 1969.
2. Fisher JD: The role of electrophysiologic testing in the diagnosis and treatment of patients with known and suspected bradycardias and tachycardias. Prog Cardiovasc Dis 24:25, 1981.
3. Michelson EL, Dreifus LS: Present status of clinical electrophysiologic studies: Introduction— What studies are necessary. PACE 7:421, 1984.
4. Nattel S, Rinkenberger RL, Lehrman LL, Zipes DP: Therapeutic blood lidocaine concentration after local anesthesia for cardiac electrophysiologic studies. N Engl J Med 301:418, 1979.
5. Strauss HC, et al: Current diagnostic and therapeutic maneuvers in patients with sinus node disease. *In* Rappaport E (ed.): Cardiology Update— 1983. New York, Elsevier, 1983, pp 193–218.
6. Mandell W, Hayakawa H, Danzig R, Marcus HS: Evaluation of sinoatrial function in man by overdrive suppression. Circulation 44:59, 1971.
7. Strauss HC, Saroff AL, Bigger JT, Jr, Giardina EGV: Premature atrial stimulation as a key to the understanding of sinoatrial conduction in man. Circulation 47:86, 1973.
8. Narula OS, et al: A new method for measurement of sinoatrial conduction time. Circulation 58:706, 1978.
9. Reiffel JA, et al: The human sinus node electrogram. A transvenous catheter technique and a comparison of directly measured and indirectly estimated sinoatrial conduction time in adults. Circulation 62:1324, 1980.
10. Dhingra RC, et al: Significance of block distal to the His bundle induced by atrial pacing in patients with chronic bifacicular block. Circulation 60:1455, 1979.
11. McAnulty JH, et al: Natural history of "high-risk" bundle branch block. N Engl J Med 307:137, 1982.
12. Denes P, et al: Demonstration of dual A-V nodal pathways in patients with paroxysmal supraventricular tachycardia. Circulation 48:549, 1973.
13. Denker S, et al: Facilitation of ventricular tachycardia induction with abrupt changes in ventricular cycle length. Am J Cardiol 53:508, 1984.
14. Josephson ME, Kastor JA: Supraventricular tachycardia: mechanisms and management. Ann Intern Med 87:346, 1977.
15. Gallagher JJ, et al: Wolff-Parkinson-White syndrome. The problem, evaluation and surgical correction. Circulation 51:767, 1975.
16. Gallagher JJ, et al: Catheter technique for closed-chest ablation of the atrioventricular conduction system. N Engl J Med 306:194, 1982.
17. Wells JL Jr, MacLean WAH, James TN, Waldo AL: Characterization of atrial flutter. Studies in man after open heart surgery using fixed atrial electrodes. Circulation 60:665, 1979.
18. Klein GJ, et al: Ventricular fibrillation in the Wolff-Parkinson-White syndrome. N Engl J Med 301:1080, 1979.
19. Horowitz LN, et al: Recurrent sustained ventricular tachycardia. 3. Role of the electrophysiologic study in selection of antiarrhythmia therapy. Circulation 58:987, 1978.
20. Mason JW, Winkle RA: Accuracy of the ventricular tachycardia-induction study for predicting long-term efficacy and inefficacy of antiarrhythmic drugs. N Engl J Med 303:1073, 1980.
21. Ruskin JN, DiMarco JP, Garan H: Out-of-hospital cardiac arrest. Electrophysiologic observations and selection of long-term antiarrhythmic therapy. N Engl J Med 303:607, 1980.
22. Josephson ME, Horowitz LN, Spielman SR,

Greenspan AM: Electrophysiologic and hemodynamic studies in patients resuscitated from cardiac arrest. Am J Cardiol 46:948, 1980.

23. Mann DE, et al: Induction of clinical ventricular tachycardia using programmed stimulation: value of third and fourth extrastimuli. Am J Cardiol 52:501, 1983.

24. Brugada P, Abdollah H, Heddle B, Wellens HJJ: Results of a ventricular stimulation protocol using a maximum of 4 premature stimuli in patients without documented or suspected ventricular arrhythmias. Am J Cardiol 52:1214, 1983.

25. Buxton AE, et al: Role of triple extrastimuli during electrophysiologic study of patients with documented sustained ventricular tachyarrhythmias. Circulation 69:532, 1984.

26. Doherty JU, et al: Programmed ventricular stimulation at a second right ventricular site: an analysis of 100 patients with special reference to sensitivity, specificity and characteristics of patients with induced ventricular tachycardia. Am J Cardiol 52:1184, 1983.

27. Morady F, Hess D, Scheinman MM: Electrophysiologic drug testing in patients with malignant ventricular arrhythmias: importance of stimulation at more than one ventricular site. Am J Cardiol 50:1055, 1982.

28. Swerdlow CD, Winkel RA, Mason JW: Prognostic significance of the number of induced ventricular complexes during assessment of therapy for ventricular arrhythmias. Circulation 68:400, 1983.

29. Brugada P, Green M, Abdollah H, Wellens HJJ: Significance of ventricular arrhythmias initiated by programmed ventricular stimulation: the importance of the type of arrhythmia induced and the number of premature stimuli required. Circulation 69:87, 1984.

30. Swerdlow CD, et al: Decreased incidence of antiarrhythmic drug efficacy at electrophysiologic study associated with the use of a third extrastimulus. Am Heart J 104:1004, 1982.

31. DiMarco J, et al: Non-arrhythmic events limit the predictive accuracy of electrophysiologic studies in patients with ventricular tachyarrhythmias. Circulation 70:SII, 1984 (abstr).

32. Swerdlow CD, Winkle RA, Mason JW: Determinants of survival in patients with ventricular tachyarrhythmias. N Engl J Med 208:1346, 1983.

33. Platia E, Reid PR: Comparison of programmed electrical stimulation and ambulatory electrocardiographic (Holter) monitoring in the management of ventricular tachycardia and ventricular fibrillation. J Am Coll Cardiol 4:493, 1984.

34. Miller JM, Kienzle MG, Harken AH, Josephson ME: Subendocardial resection for ventricular tachycardia: predictors of surgical success. Circulation 70:624, 1984.

35. Winston SA, et al: Catheter ablation of ventricular tachycardia. Circulation 70:SII, 1984 (abstr).

36. Hartzler GO: Electrode catheter ablation of refractory focal ventricular tachycardia. J Am Coll Cardiol 2:1107, 1983.

37. Fisher JD, Kim SG, Waspe LE, Matos JA: Mechanisms for the success and failure of pacing for termination of ventricular tachycardia: clinical and hypothetical considerations. PACE 6:1095, 1983.

38. DiMarco JP, Garan H, Ruskin JN: Complications in patients undergoing electrophysiologic procedures. Ann Intern Med 97:490, 1982.

# PART VI
*Profiles of Hemodynamic and Angiographic Abnormalities in Specific Disorders*

*chapter twenty three*

# Profiles in Valvular Heart Disease

WILLIAM GROSSMAN

T HE CARDIAC valves have as their function the maintenance of unidirectional flow, thus ensuring that the energy released during myocardial contraction is efficiently transformed into the circulation of blood around the body. When the valves become diseased, compensatory mechanisms are brought into play in order to maintain the circulation commensurate with the metabolic needs of the body. These mechanisms, chief amongst which are dilatation and hypertrophy, are not without clinical costs, and it is these costs that are responsible for the major manifestations of valvular heart disease.

Valvular disease results in either incompetence of the valve with regard to its function of maintaining unidirectional flow (i.e., valvular insufficiency and regurgitation), or obstruction to the forward and natural course of the circulation (i.e., stenosis). Although mixed stenosis and insufficiency, both of moderate degree, frequently coexist in a particular valve, severe stenosis and severe insufficiency cannot both be present in the same valve. Thus, the $0.5\,cm^2$ valvular orifice of a patient with severe calcific aortic stenosis may barely allow 50 to 60 ml to be ejected from the left ventricle during systole, and this only at a left ventricular systolic pressure of 200 to 300 mmHg. The tiny fixed orifice cannot be expected to permit more than mild regurgitation in the subsequent diastole, where the driving force is an aortic diastolic pressure of 80 mmHg.

Valvular heart disease may be considered to impose two different types of stress on the cardiac chamber proximal to the lesion. These are either pressure overload (increased afterload), or volume overload (increased preload). The former is generally the result of a valvular stenosis, and the latter of valvular insufficiency. Both pressure and volume overload serve as stimuli for the heart to call upon compensatory mechanisms. As mentioned, chief amongst these mechanisms are hypertrophy (which allows the generation of greater systolic force and at the same time tends to normalize wall stress by increasing wall thickness), and dilatation (which enables increased strength and extent of shortening by the Frank-Starling mechanism). These mechanisms preserve the circulation at the cost of increased myocardial oxygen needs and elevated ventricular filling pressures, leading to clinical evidence of ischemia and congestive heart failure.

In this chapter, we shall discuss the hemodynamic and angiographic findings in pa-

Note: some material in this chapter has been retained from the first and second editions, to which Dr. Lewis Dexter had contributed.

tients with valvular heart disease. We have found it useful to apply the general physiologic principles discussed above in the interpretation of catheterization data obtained in patients with disordered valve function. This approach will generally enable the physician to unravel even the most complicated of problems.

## MITRAL STENOSIS

The orifice area of the normal mitral valve is about 4.5 cm$^2$. As a result of chronic rheumatic heart disease, the orifice becomes progressively smaller. This leads to two circulatory changes.[1] The first is the development of a pressure gradient across the valve, the left ventricular mean diastolic pressure remaining at its normal level of about 5 mmHg and the left atrial mean pressure rising progressively, reaching about 25 mmHg when the orifice of the mitral valve is reduced to approximately 1.0 cm$^2$. The second circulatory change is a reduction of blood flow across the valve—i.e., cardiac output. The normal resting output of 3.0 L/min/m$^2$ usually falls to about 2.5 L/min/m$^2$ when the valve size is 1.0 cm$^2$. A rise of left atrial pressure necessitates a similar rise of pressure in pulmonary veins and pulmonary capillaries, and pulmonary edema occurs when the pulmonary capillary pressure exceeds the oncotic pressure of normal plasma, which is about 25 mmHg.

Pulmonary vascular complications practically never occur in mitral stenosis until the mitral valve area approaches 1.0 cm$^2$, i.e., when the resting left atrial pressure approaches 25 mmHg. After this point, reactive changes in the pulmonary arteriolar bed frequently develop and pose a progressive obstruction to blood flow through the lungs.

As pulmonary vascular obstruction becomes increasingly severe, the pulmonary arterial pressure rises and occasionally may exceed the systemic pressure. In the extreme, the pulmonary vascular resistance can rise to 25 or 30 times normal. Despite substantial hypertrophy, the right ventricle cannot cope with the enormous pressure load imposed upon it, dilates and fails.

***The "Second Stenosis."*** Thus, in mitral stenosis, two "stenoses" eventuate—first at the mitral valve and second in the arterioles of the lung. The hemodynamic findings in patients with tight mitral stenoses with and without major pulmonary vascular disease are illustrated in Figure 23-1. As can be seen, the *second stenosis* (Fig. 23-1, bottom panel) has resulted in a 70-mmHg mean pressure gradient across the lungs, giving a pulmonary vascular resistance of 1866 dynes-sec-cm$^{-5}$. Work-up of the patient with mitral stenosis should include an assessment of both these obstructions.

## Catheterization Protocol

The usual indication for cardiac catheterization in patients with mitral stenosis is that the patient is being considered a candidate for corrective surgery by the clinician. Catheterization should be a combined right and left heart procedure, in which the following measurements and calculations are made:

1. Simultaneous left ventricular diastolic pressure, left atrial (or pulmonary capillary wedge) diastolic pressure, heart rate, diastolic filling period and cardiac output. From these, the size of the orifice of the mitral valve may be calculated (see Chapter 11 for details of the orifice area calculation).

2. If the transmitral pressure difference is less than 5 mmHg, the error of calculation of the mitral valve orifice area is appreciable. The circulatory measurements should be repeated under circumstances of stress (exercise, tachycardia induced by isoproterenol or pacing) in order to increase the pressure difference across the mitral valve.

3. Simultaneously, or in close order, pulmonary arterial mean pressure, left atrial (or pulmonary capillary wedge) mean pressure, and cardiac output for the calculation of pulmonary vascular resistance.

4. Right ventricular systolic and diastolic pressures for assessment of right ventricular function.

5. If *other lesions* are suspected (e.g., mitral regurgitation, aortic valve disease, left atrial myxoma), they too must be evaluated. In this regard, it should be pointed out that certain lesions tend to occur in combination with mitral stenosis. In my experience, many (if not most) patients with severe mitral stenosis have had some degree of aortic regurgitation. Also, al-

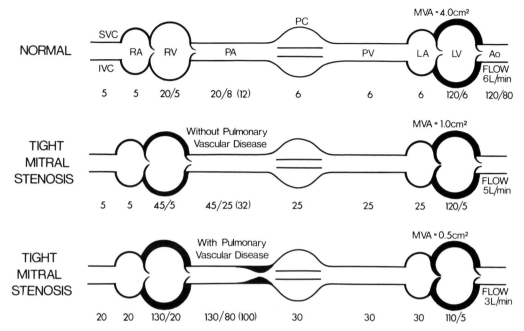

**Fig. 23-1.** Diagrammatic representation of circulation in patients with normal hemodynamics (upper panel), tight mitral stenosis (middle panel), and tight mitral stenosis with pulmonary vascular disease and the development of a *second stenosis* at the pulmonary arteriolar level (bottom panel). See text for discussion.

though it is rare, tricuspid stenosis should always be looked for in the patient with severe mitral stenosis, since it is only seen in association with this condition.

The following case studies illustrate the different clinical and hemodynamic syndromes seen in patients with mitral stenosis. The first is a typical example of a very symptomatic patient with "tight" mitral stenosis, normal pulmonary vascular resistance, and a normal-sized heart (stage II, Fig. 23-2). The second is an example of a relatively asymptomatic patient with more severe mitral stenosis, a five- to tenfold increase of pulmonary vascular resistance, and an enlarged heart due principally to enlargement of the right ventricle (stage III, Fig. 23-2). The third represents terminal mitral stenosis with an extreme degree of pulmonary vascular resistance, pulmonary hypertension and right ventricular failure (stage IV, Fig. 23-2).

## Case 1

### *Tight Mitral Stenosis with Normal Pulmonary Vascular Resistance.* A. R.,

a 35-year-old woman, had chorea as a child and was thereafter asymptomatic until two years prior to admission, when she noted the onset of exertional dyspnea. This progressed to the point of her having to stop after climbing one flight of stairs slowly. She had had

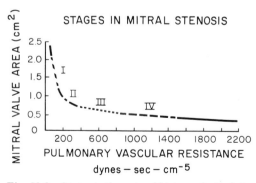

**Fig. 23-2.** Stages in the natural history of mitral stenosis. As the mitral orifice progressively narrows, pulmonary vascular resistance increases. This increase is slow at first, but when the mitral valve area becomes "critical" (less than 1 cm$^2$) the increase is rapid, reflecting the development of a second stenosis at the level of the precapillary pulmonary arterioles. Clinical correlations are discussed in the text.

one recent episode of coughing up a table-spoon of pure red blood. Her most trouble-some symptom had been paroxysmal atrial fibrillation over a period of several months. She had had orthopnea and one episode of paroxysmal nocturnal dyspnea.

On physical examination, she was in no apparent distress. Blood pressure was 130/70 and pulse rate was 80. The rhythm was nor-mal sinus. There was no venous distension, lungs were normal, the PMI was in the fifth interspace in the midclavicular line. $S_1$ was accentuated. At the apex, there was a grade 1 pansystolic murmur, an opening snap, and a grade 2 diastolic rumble with presystolic accentuation. The liver edge was at the cos-tal margin, and there was no edema.

The ECG was within normal limits.

The roentgenogram showed a normal-sized heart, an enlarged left atrium, a mild degree of pulmonary vascular redistribution, no calcification in the region of the mitral valve, and was otherwise normal.

Cardiac catheterization revealed the fol-lowing:

| | |
|---|---|
| Body surface area, $m^2$ | 1.78 |
| $O_2$ consumption, ml/min | 180 |
| A-V $O_2$ difference, ml/L | 40 |
| Cardiac output, L/min | 4.5 |
| Heart rate/min | 76, NSR |
| Stroke volume ml/beat | 72 |
| Pressures, mmHg: | |
| Brachial artery | 130/70, $\overline{90}$ |
| Left ventricle | 130/8 |
| Diastolic mean | 6 |
| Diastolic filling period, sec/beat | 0.42 |
| Pulmonary capillary wedge, mean | 24 |
| Diastolic mean | 20 |
| Pulmonary artery | 40/22, $\overline{28}$ |
| Right ventricle | 40/6 |
| Right atrium, mean | 4 |
| Pulmonary vascular resistance, dynes-sec-cm$^{-5}$ | 71 |
| Calculated mitral valve area, $cm^2$ | 1.0 |

Cineangiography of the left ventricle re-vealed no mitral regurgitation.

*Interpretation.* This patient was symp-tomatic because of her increased left atrial pressure and atrial arrhythmia. She had not yet developed the "second stenosis" at the precapillary pulmonary arteriolar level, dis-cussed previously. Thus, her pulmonary ar-tery pressure elevation was purely a conse-quence of the increased left atrial and pulmonary venous pressures, and the pulmo-nary vascular resistance was normal (<120 dynes-sec-cm$^{-5}$). In the spectrum of patients with mitral stenosis, she would fall into stage II of Figure 23-2.

## Case 2

***Severe Mitral Stenosis, Moderately Elevated Pulmonary Vascular Resis-tance, Few Symptoms, Fatigue Syn-drome.*** E. C. was a 42-year-old woman without any history of acute rheumatic fever. She was asymptomatic until she was 19 years old, when during the last month of her first pregnancy, she developed pulmonary congestion. She responded well to therapy and remained asymptomatic thereafter, even during three subsequent pregnancies. How-ever, during her fifth pregnancy, age 37, dyspnea, orthopnea, paroxysmal nocturnal dyspnea, and one episode of hemoptysis of pure red blood occurred at the seventh month, necessitating hospitalization through term. Thereafter she improved but became progressively tired with loss of energy and drive. She became less thorough in her housework and in her attention to the children's clothes and lost her previous meticulousness. If she pushed herself, she would become somewhat short of breath on a flight of stairs, but it was fatigue more than breathlessness that bothered her.

She was well-nourished and had a malar flush. Her blood pressure was 115/70; her pulse, 90 and irregularly irregular. Respira-tions were 15. There was no pulmonary or peripheral congestion. The neck veins were just visible at the clavicles with the patient sitting upright. The PMI was in the fifth inter-space just outside the midclavicular line. The impulse was normal. A prominent paraster-nal heave was present. $S_1$ was accentuated. No apical systolic murmur was present. There was an opening snap and a grade 2 apical diastolic rumble.

The ECG showed right ventricular hyper-trophy and atrial fibrillation.

X-ray examination showed the heart to be moderately enlarged, due to enlargement of the left atrium and right ventricle. The pul-monary arteries were prominent, and there was a moderate degree of pulmonary vascular redistribution.

The findings at cardiac catheterization were as follows:

| | |
|---|---|
| Body surface area, m$^2$ | 1.41 |
| O$_2$ consumption, ml/min | 188 |
| A-V O$_2$ difference, ml/L | 51 |
| Cardiac output, L/min | 3.7 |
| Heart rate/min | 85, AF |
| Stroke volume, ml/beat | 44 |
| Pressures, mmHg | |
|   Brachial artery | 120/62, $\overline{84}$ |
|   Left ventricle | 120/7 |
|     Diastolic mean | 5 |
|     Diastolic filling period, | |
|       sec/beat | 0.38 |
|   Pulmonary capillary | |
|     wedge, mean | 27 |
|     Diastolic mean | 23 |
|   Pulmonary artery | 82/32, $\overline{51}$ |
|   Right ventricle | 82/10 |
|   Right atrium, mean | 8 |
| Pulmonary vascular | |
|   resistance, | |
|     dynes-sec-cm$^{-5}$ | 520 |
| Calculated mitral valve | |
|   area, cm$^2$ | 0.7 |

***Interpretation.*** This patient's symptoms were initially due to elevated left atrial pressure when, during her fifth pregnancy, she developed hemoptysis, orthopnea, and paroxysmal nocturnal dyspnea. Subsequently, however, her major symptom was fatigue, associated with a reduced cardiac output and an increased arteriovenous O$_2$ difference. The orthopnea and paroxysmal dyspnea had receded somewhat despite the fact that her pulmonary capillary pressure was at the pulmonary edema level. This is a common, although poorly understood, phenomenon in patients with mitral stenosis when pulmonary vascular disease begins to occur. Thus, this patient was beginning to develop the "second stenosis" discussed previously, and this is apparent from the elevated pulmonary vascular resistance (520 dynes-sec-cm$^{-5}$). In the spectrum of patients with mitral stenosis, she would be representative of stage III of Figure 23-2.

## Case 3

***Terminal Mitral Stenosis With Severe Pulmonary Hypertension.*** C. A., a 47-year-old woman, had had acute rheumatic fever at eight years of age and a murmur ever since. She did well thereafter until five years ago, when she noticed exertional dyspnea and paroxysmal nocturnal dyspnea. Four years ago, these symptoms worsened. Orthopnea and ankle edema appeared. Her symptoms then improved for nearly two years, only to return about two months prior to admission. Since then, despite a good cardiac regimen, she had had to lead a bed-chair-bathroom existence.

On examination, she was cachectic, dyspneic, and orthopneic. Acrocyanosis was evident. Blood pressure was 96/72; pulse rate, 90 and irregularly irregular; respirations, 32. Neck veins were distended to the angle of the jaw, "V" waves were prominent, and there were bibasilar rales. The PMI was in the anterior axillary line. The apex impulse was normal, but a parasternal heave was present. S$_1$ was loud. Systole was silent. An opening snap was present, and there was a barely audible mitral diastolic murmur with appreciable presystolic accentuation. The pulmonary component of S$_2$ was loud and palpable. The liver was two fingerbreadths below the costal margin and was tender. There was considerable pitting edema to the knees.

The ECG showed atrial fibrillation, right axis deviation, and right ventricular hypertrophy.

Roentgenograms showed a large heart with prominent left atrium, right ventricle, pulmonary arteries, pulmonary vasculature, and Kerley B lines.

Cardiac catheterization revealed the following:

| | |
|---|---|
| Body surface area, m$^2$ | 1.4 |
| O$_2$ consumption, ml/min | 201 |
| A-V O$_2$ difference, ml/L | 110 |
| Cardiac output, L/min | 1.8 |
| Pulse rate | 92, AF |
| Stroke volume, ml/beat | 17 |
| Pressures: mmHg | |
|   Brachial artery | 108/70 |
|   Left ventricle | 108/12 |
|     Diastolic mean | 10 |
|     Diastolic filling period, | |
|       sec/beat | 0.36 |
|   Pulmonary capillary | |
|     wedge, mean | 33 |
|     Diastolic mean | 31 |
|   Pulmonary artery | 125/65; $\overline{75}$ |

|  |  |
|---|---|
| Right ventricle | 125/20 |
| Right atrium, mean | 19 |
| Pulmonary vascular resistance, dynes-sec-cm$^{-5}$ | 1838 |
| Calculated mitral valve area, cm$^2$ | 0.3 |

*Interpretation.* This patient had symptoms of left atrial hypertension five years prior to her catheterization, suggesting that she was in stage II (see Fig. 23-2) of mitral stenosis at that time. At the time of presentation to us, she had evidence of advanced right heart failure and pulmonary hypertension. This woman has "two stenoses," and both are severe: the mitral orifice area is less than one tenth normal at 0.3 cm$^2$, and the pulmonary arteriolar (vascular) resistance is approximately 18 times normal at 1838 dynes-sec-cm$^{-5}$! She is in late stage IV of mitral stenosis, as diagrammed in Figure 23-2.

## MITRAL REGURGITATION

The normal mitral valve is extraordinarily competent. Mitral incompetence, failure of the valve to prevent regurgitation of blood from the left ventricle to the left atrium during ventricular systole, may be due to functional or anatomic inadequacy of any one of the components of the mitral valve apparatus, which consists of two valve leaflets, two papillary muscles with their chordae tendineae, and the valve ring or annulus.[2]

Mitral regurgitation may occur when there is destruction or deformation of the valve leaflets as a result of rheumatic fever or bacterial endocarditis. Mitral regurgitation begins during "isometric" ventricular contraction and continues throughout systole, thus giving rise to a holosystolic murmur. A fibromyxomatous process in the mitral valve annulus and chordae tendineae may give rise to the "floppy valve syndrome." There may or may not be other evidence of Marfan's syndrome in these patients. The papillary muscles are usually normal but there is a marked redundancy of the valve leaflets and chordae with resulting prolapse into the left atrium during systole and accompanying regurgitation.

The papillary muscles are particularly vulnerable to ischemia from coronary artery disease as well as to damage from viral myo-

carditis. The posterior papillary muscle derives its blood supply from the right coronary and left circumflex arteries. Ischemic dysfunction of this muscle may occur in association with either an inferior or posterolateral myocardial infarction. Less frequently, ischemic involvement of the anterior papillary muscle in an anterior or anterolateral infarction produces mitral regurgitation. Papillary-chordal integrity is maintained to a point when the left ventricle dilates. The common occurrence of a mitral regurgitant murmur in patients with large left ventricles, however, may reflect a simple anatomic loss of this integrity, an involvement of the papillary muscle with the same disease that causes the left ventricle to dilate, or an abnormality of contraction of the mitral annulus.

Mitral regurgitation from whatever cause implies a *double outlet to the left ventricle:* during systole, blood exits through both aortic and mitral valves. Total left ventricular output rises, that going into the aorta may fall, and that regurgitating through the mitral valve depends largely upon the size of the regurgitant orifice, left atrial compliance, the systolic mean pressure difference between left ventricle and left atrium, and the duration of systole. Although hypertension aggravates and lowering of blood pressure lessens mitral regurgitation, the most important factor is probably the size of the regurgitant orifice.

In patients with mitral regurgitation, cardiac catheterization is important to provide a complete hemodynamic and angiographic assessment of the severity of the valvular lesion.

## Hemodynamic Assessment[3-8]

First, it is important to assess the hemodynamic consequences of the mitral regurgitation by measuring cardiac output and right and left heart pressures.

*Interpretation of V Waves in the Pulmonary Wedge Tracing.* With *acute* mitral regurgitation (e.g., ruptured chordae tendineae), giant V waves will be seen in the left atrial or pulmonary artery pressure tracing (Fig. 23-3). In this regard, our Fellows and Residents frequently ask, "How large must a V wave be in order to be diagnostic of severe mitral regurgitation?" In my experience, V

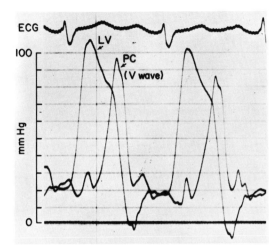

**Fig. 23-3.** Left ventricular (LV) and pulmonary capillary wedge (PC) pressure tracings taken in a patient with ruptured chordae tendineae and acute mitral insufficiency. The giant V wave results from regurgitation of blood into a relatively small and noncompliant left atrium. Electrocardiogram (ECG) illustrates the timing of the PC V wave, whose peak follows ventricular repolarization, as manifested by the T wave of the ECG.

waves up to twice the mean left atrial pressure can be seen in the absence of any mitral regurgitation. The patient with left ventricular failure from any cause may have a distended, noncompliant left atrium and the *normal V wave* (which is due to left atrial filling from the pulmonary veins during left ventricular systole) will be prominent in this circumstance.[7] When pulmonary blood flow is increased, the normal V wave increases in prominence correspondingly: this is particularly striking in acute ventricular septal defect complicating myocardial infarction, in which enormous V waves ($\geq$50 mmHg) can be seen in the absence of any mitral regurgitation.

V waves *greater than twice the mean* left atrial (or pulmonary wedge) pressure are suggestive of severe mitral regurgitation, and when the height of *the V wave is three times the mean wedge* or left atrial pressure, a diagnosis of severe mitral regurgitation is virtually certain (Fig. 23-3). I hasten to point out, however, that the absence of a prominent V wave by no means rules out severe mitral regurgitation. Slowly developing chronic mitral regurgitation commonly leads to marked left atrial enlargement, and the dilated left atrium can accept an enormous

regurgitant volume per beat *without any increase in mean pressure or height of the V wave.*[9] Also, the level of afterload, as determined by systemic vascular resistance, may greatly affect the height of the regurgitant or V wave in patients with mitral regurgitation.[4] As seen in Figure 23-4, a patient with severe mitral regurgitation had a V wave of 48 mmHg at a time when LV systolic pressure was approximately 140 mmHg. With sodium nitroprusside (right hand panel, Fig. 23-4), the LV systolic pressure came down to 120 mmHg and the V wave was essentially abolished.[10,11] Although this patient's regurgitant fraction was reduced with sodium nitroprusside (from 80% to 64%), it still remained in the range of severe mitral regurgitation (see below).

***Exercise Hemodynamics.*** Another important hemodynamic parameter in the assessment of mitral regurgitation is the forward cardiac output. Low cardiac output is common in advanced mitral regurgitation and may account for much of the clinical picture. If resting cardiac output is near normal, and if the patient's primary symptoms are related to exertion (i.e., easy fatigability and dyspnea on exertion), dynamic exercise during cardiac catheterization may be revealing. If the symptoms are cardiac in origin, the patient will usually fail to increase cardiac output appropriately with exercise; i.e., the increase in cardiac output will be $\leq$80% predicted (see formula for prediction of cardiac output increase with exercise in Chapter 17). In addition, pulmonary wedge or left atrial mean pressure will rise with exercise, commonly reaching levels $\geq$35 mmHg by 4 to 5 minutes of supine bicycle exercise, even if the control value was nearly normal. A case demonstrating this point is illustrated in Figure 17-6, Chapter 17.

## Angiographic Assessment

The second objective of cardiac catheterization in patients with mitral regurgitation is the angiographic assessment of the severity of the regurgitation by left ventriculography. The assessment may be qualitative, by noting the degree of opacification of the left atrium due to regurgitation back through the incompetent valve, using a scale of 1+ (mild), 2+ (moderate), 3+ (moderately severe), and 4+

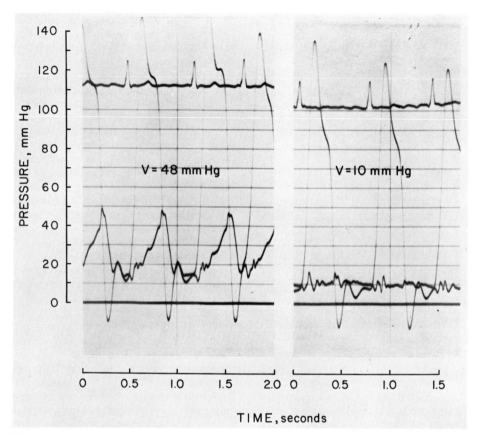

**Fig. 23-4.** Left ventricular and pulmonary capillary wedge pressures before (left) and during (right) an infusion of sodium nitroprusside in a patient with severe mitral regurgitation. This illustrates the sensitivity of the V wave height to LV afterload in patients with mitral regurgitation. See text for discussion. (From Harshaw CW et al: Reduced systemic vascular resistance as therapy for severe mitral regurgitation of valvular origin. Ann Intern Med 83:312, 1975.)

(severe) regurgitation. These grades are essentially subjective, but certain criteria can be used to enhance consistency of their usage. Regurgitation that is 1+ essentially clears with each beat and never opacifies the entire left atrium. When regurgitation is 2+ (moderate), it does not clear with one beat and generally does opacify the entire left atrium (albeit faintly) after several beats; however, opacification of the left atrium does not equal that of the left ventricle. In 3+ regurgitation (moderately severe), the left atrium is completely opacified and achieves equal opacification with the left ventricle. In 4+ regurgitation (severe), opacification of the entire left atrium occurs within one beat, the opacification becomes progressively

more dense with each beat, and contrast can be seen refluxing into the pulmonary veins during left ventricular systole.

***Regurgitant Fraction.*** The angiographic assessment of severity of mitral regurgitation may also be made more quantitative by calculation of the *regurgitant fraction.* This entails measurement of total left ventricular stroke volume (TSV) from the left ventriculogram and the amount that goes forward by way of the aorta to the body (the forward stroke volume, FSV) by Fick or indicator-dilution technique. The TSV is calculated as the difference between end-diastolic and end-systolic left ventricular volumes (EDV − ESV = TSV), as described in Chapter 19. Regurgitant stroke volume (RSV, regurgitant volume/beat) is then given, as RSV = TSV − FSV. Regurgitant fraction (RF) is then calculated as RF = RSV/TSV.

The accuracy of these calculations depends upon many factors. Since FSV is calculated by dividing cardiac output by heart rate at the time of the Fick (or other) cardiac output determination, it is an average stroke volume. The particular beat chosen from the left ventriculogram for volume determination must therefore be an "average" or representative beat; alternatively, volumes from multiple beats must be calculated and averaged. Thus, in patients with atrial fibrillation or extrasystoles during ventriculography, the regurgitant stroke volume and regurgitant fraction may be highly inaccurate, and we do not calculate them in such patients. It should also be obvious that the accuracy of the regurgitant fraction depends upon a similar physiologic state prevailing between the cardiac output and angiographic phases of the catheterization procedure. An increase in arterial blood pressure may substantially increase the mitral regurgitation and decrease forward output. Therefore, if blood pressure or other hemodynamic variables change significantly between the time of cardiac output determination and left ventriculography, it is pointless to calculate regurgitant fraction. Finally, regurgitant fraction quantifies at best the *total* amount of regurgitation. Thus, if a patient has both mitral and aortic regurgitation, the regurgitant fraction gives an assessment of the regurgitation due to *both* lesions combined.

A study from the University of Texas at Dallas analyzed the interrelationship of qualitative and quantitative angiographic grading in 230 patients with either aortic or mitral regurgitation.[12] These authors showed a stepwise correlation between actual regurgitant volume (L/min/M$^2$) and 1+ to 4+ regurgitation graded visually, using the definitions given in this chapter. For the 147 patients with mitral regurgitation, 1+ regurgitation was associated with a mean regurgitant flow of 0.61 L/min/M$^2$, 2+ regurgitation with 1.14 L/min/M$^2$, 3+ regurgitation with 2.14 L/min/M$^2$, and 4+ regurgitation with 4.60 L/min/M$^2$ and the regurgitant fractions showed similar correlation (L. David Hillis, M.D., personal communication). However, there was considerable scatter in the data so that much overlap of actual flow values existed.

Within the context of these caveats and qualifications, we regard the regurgitant fraction to be a useful parameter in the quantitative assessment of mitral regurgitation. In general, RF <20% is mild, 20% to 40% is moderate, 40% to 60% is moderately severe, and >60% is severe mitral regurgitation.

The third objective of cardiac catheterization in patients with mitral regurgitation is the assessment of left ventricular function by measuring the left ventricular diastolic pressure and more importantly by measuring the left ventricular ejection fraction and end-systolic volume. As others have emphasized, the nearer the preoperative ejection fraction is to normal, the greater is the degree of postoperative restoration to full activity. Specific parameters of left ventricular function are discussed in Chapters 19 and 20.

## Catheterization Protocol

1. Right heart catheterization for evaluation of right atrial pressure (to detect possible tricuspid valve disease or right ventricular failure), pulmonary artery pressure (degree of pulmonary hypertension), and wedge pressure (V wave height). In severe, acute mitral regurgitation, a V wave may actually be seen in the pulmonary artery as a second or late systolic hump in the pressure wave form.[8]

2. Left heart catheterization for measurement of LVEDP and assessment of gradients (if any) across mitral or aortic valves. A characteristic of severe mitral regurgitation is that the LVEDP is usually much lower than the LA or PCW mean pressure. In contrast, in LV failure due to cardiomyopathy or coronary artery disease, LVEDP is usually close to or equals the PCW mean pressure, while in aortic regurgitation or LV aneurysm, LVEDP is usually much higher than PCW mean pressure.

3. Cardiac output by Fick or indicator-dilution technique. This measures the fraction of blood going out via the aorta to the body, and by itself yields no information about regurgitant flow. The response of forward cardiac output to dynamic exercise may provide useful information, however, because patients with severe mitral regurgitation are generally incapable of increasing forward output commensurate with the

needs of the body, as estimated by the increased oxygen consumption (see Chapter 17).

4. Cineangiography of the left ventricle is the definitive method for evaluating mitral regurgitation. By this method, it is possible to measure the total left ventricular volumes and regurgitant fraction, as discussed previously.

5. Pharmacologic intervention. An infusion of sodium nitroprusside (Fig. 23-4) often has a dramatic and salutary effect on the hemodynamic abnormalities in mitral regurgitation and may have both therapeutic and diagnostic value. Although TSV may not change, RSV decreases and FSV increases, leading to increased cardiac output.

## Case 4

G. A. was a 59-year-old woman with no history of rheumatic fever in childhood. She was healthy and active until six months prior to admission, when she noticed both dyspnea and lower chest discomfort on mild exertion but no other symptoms of heart failure. There was no past history of bacterial endocarditis.

On physical examination, she had normal body habitus. Blood pressure was 130/70; pulse, 80 and regular. The jugular veins were not distended, the carotid pulsations were normal and the lungs were clear. The apical impulse was diffuse; $S_1$ was diminished. There was a grade 3 apical pansystolic murmur transmitted to the axilla. No opening snap, $S_3$, or diastolic murmurs were heard. There were no aortic murmurs.

The ECG showed normal sinus rhythm, complete right bundle branch block, and left axis deviation.

Roentgenograms showed enlargement of the left ventricle and left atrium. No valvular calcification was seen.

Cardiac catheterization, left ventricular angiography, and coronary angiography were performed with the following findings:

| | |
|---|---|
| Body surface area, m$^2$ | 1.95 |
| O$_2$ consumption, ml/min | 200 |
| A-V O$_2$ difference, ml/L | 52 |
| Cardiac output, L/min | |
|     Total left ventricular | |
|         output (angiographic) | 10.4 |
|     Forward flow (Fick) | 3.9 |
|     Regurgitant flow | 6.5 |
| Heart rate/min | 67 |
| Stroke volume, ml/beat | |
|     End-diastolic LV volume, | |
|         ml (angiography) | 197 |
|     End-systolic LV volume, | |
|         ml (angiography) | 42 |
|     Total LV stroke volume, | |
|         ml (angiography) | 155 |
|     Forward stroke volume, | |
|         ml (Fick) | 58 |
|     Regurgitant stroke | |
|         volume, ml | 97 |
|     Ejection fraction | |
|         (155 ÷ 197) | 0.79 |
|     Regurgitant fraction | |
|         (97 ÷ 155) | 0.63 |
| Pressures: mmHg | |
|     Brachial artery | 140/84, $\overline{105}$ |
|     Left ventricle | 140/14 |
|         Systolic mean | 112 |
|         Systolic ejection | |
|             period, sec/beat | 0.28 |
|     Pulmonary capillary | |
|         wedge, mean | 12 |
|         V wave | 24 |
|     Pulmonary artery | 30/14, $\overline{19}$ |
|     Right ventricle | 30/6 |
|     Right atrium, mean | 4 |
| Pulmonary vascular | |
|     resistance, | |
|         dynes-sec-cm$^{-5}$ | 143 |

Left ventricular cineangiography showed an excellent and uniform contraction of the left ventricle and a large regurgitant jet into the left atrium, which was completely filled within one beat. The mitral valve did not prolapse into the left atrium.

Coronary arteriograms with selective injections into both left and right coronary arteries revealed normal vasculature, no irregularities or narrowings and normal run-off.

***Interpretation.*** Mitral regurgitation was identified and quantified. There were no other valvular lesions. Although the left ventricular diastolic pressure and end-diastolic volume were above normal, the left ventricle contracted uniformly and vigorously as judged by cineangiography. The ejection fraction of 0.79 and the end-systolic volume were normal. The slight elevation of pulmonary vascular resistance was mainly related to the low pulmonary blood flow (forward cardiac output) of 3.9 L/min (cardiac index = 2.0 L/min/M$^2$). The cause of the mitral regurgitation was not determined.

## AORTIC STENOSIS

Aortic stenosis may be valvular, subvalvular, or supravalvular. Valvular aortic stenosis is most often of the acquired calcific type, which develops on the substrate of a congenitally deformed (e.g., bicuspid) aortic valve. Valvular aortic stenosis may also be present from birth or may develop as a consequence of rheumatic fever. Subaortic stenosis is of various types. Supravalvular stenosis is rare. All produce a significant systolic pressure difference between the left ventricle and the aorta.[13-16] In subaortic stenosis, the gradient is between the main portion of the left ventricle and its outflow tract, although in "tunnel" subaortic stenosis there may be no discrete subvalvular chamber. In supravalvular stenosis, the gradient is between the proximal and distal aorta just beyond the aortic valve. It is important surgically to identify the site and nature of the obstruction in each instance. This is determined by both hemodynamics and angiography. In addition, left ventricular function and the presence or absence of aortic and mitral regurgitation should be evaluated. The left ventricle becomes progressively hypertrophied in aortic stenosis. The cardiac output is well maintained until the left ventricle dilates and fails; it then becomes progressively reduced. The following discussion will focus on valvular aortic stenosis in the adult.

The cardinal indications for cardiac catheterization in anticipation of surgery for all three types of aortic stenosis are left ventricular failure, angina pectoris, or syncope. Some believe that coronary angiography should be performed in all of these patients who are over 50. Others reserve coronary angiography for those who have angina.

## Hemodynamic Assessment

In the hemodynamic assessment of valvular aortic stenosis, primary importance should be placed on obtaining simultaneous measurement of pressure and flow across the aortic valve. As discussed in Chapter 11,

this permits calculation of the aortic orifice or valve area (AVA). In the average adult with symptomatic aortic stenosis, AVA will be reduced to ≤0.7 cm$^2$. Occasionally a valve of 0.8 to 0.9 cm$^2$ will result in a symptomatic presentation, especially when there is concomitant coronary artery disease or hypertension, or when the absolute value of cardiac output is high (e.g., a large patient, anemia, fever, or thyrotoxicosis). When AVA is ≤0.5 cm$^2$, severe aortic stenosis is present and cardiac reserve is minimal or absent.

Most patients with aortic stenosis, particularly those with the clinical presentation of angina and/or syncope, will have a normal cardiac output/index, normal right heart and PCW mean pressures, and normal LV ejection fraction. The LVEDP will usually be increased, reflecting a stiff LV chamber, and there will be a prominent A wave in PCW, LA, and LV pressure tracings (Fig. 23-5). In more advanced cases, LV ejection fraction and cardiac output are depressed, and right heart and PCW mean pressures are elevated. Severe pulmonary hypertension with right heart failure, ascites, and edema may come to dominate the picture. In these patients, the low output state may lead to a reduction

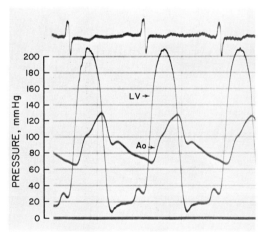

**Fig. 23-5.** Left ventricular (LV) and aortic (Ao) pressure tracings in an elderly man with severe calcific aortic stenosis. The large A wave in the LV tracing is consistent with decreased compliance of the massively hypertrophied ventricle. The LV pressure was measured with a micromanometer catheter, and aortic pressure was measured with a fluid-filled catheter system attached via tubing to a P23Db transducer. This accounts in part for the delay in onset of Ao upstroke relative to LV pressure rise.

in the intensity of the characteristic systolic murmur, obscuring the diagnosis.

An interesting hemodynamic finding, described by Carabello, and co-workers,[17] is a rise in arterial blood pressure during left heart catheter pull-back in patients with severe aortic stenosis (Fig. 23-6). Pressure tracings from 42 patients with aortic stenosis who underwent continuous arterial pressure recording during left heart catheter pull-back (withdrawal from LV to central aorta of a catheter that had been placed in the LV by retrograde technique) were examined. Increases in peripheral arterial pressure of ≥5 mmHg were noted during withdrawal of the retrograde catheter from left ventricle to central aorta in 15 of the 42 patients. Fifteen of 20 patients (75%) with AVA ≤ 0.6 cm² demonstrated this phenomenon, but none of 22 patients with AVA ≥ 0.7 cm² showed such an increase. It was concluded that a rise in peak arterial pressure during LV catheter withdrawal is an ancillary hemodynamic finding of critical aortic stenosis (Fig. 23-6). Although the mechanism of this phenomenon is uncertain, partial obstruction of an already narrowed aortic orifice by the retrograde catheter and relief of this obstruction with catheter withdrawal may be operative.

## Angiographic Assessment

In patients with aortic stenosis, left ventriculography can yield important information, and we believe that it should generally be part of the catheterization procedure. It must be emphasized, however, that patients with LV failure and high PCW pressures due to aortic stenosis may not tolerate the radiographic contrast load of left ventriculography. Adequate preventriculography preparation (e.g., IV furosemide, morphine, or oxygen), as outlined in Chapter 14, is mandatory in such patients, and ventriculography should not be done in such patients without careful consideration of risk vs benefit. The value to be obtained from left ventriculography includes assessment of the mitral valve (is there significant mitral regurgitation?), detection of regional wall motion abnormalities or LV aneurysm indicative of major coronary disease, and overall assessment of LV function. In addition, wall thickness and LV mass may be measured from the ventriculogram.

Aortography is generally not required in the patient with aortic stenosis, unless the gradient is small and the aortic pulse pressure is wide. Selective coronary arteriogra-

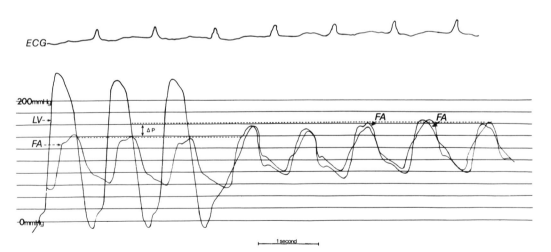

**Fig. 23-6.** Left ventricular (LV) and femoral artery (FA) pressure tracings in a patient with severe aortic stenosis (aortic valve area, 0.4 cm²). During pull-back of the retrograde catheter from LV to ascending aorta, the peak systolic femoral artery pressure can be seen to increase (ΔP) by approximately 20 mmHg. This sign is seen only in patients with aortic valve areas <0.6 cm². The mechanism of this phenomenon is believed to be partial obstruction of an already narrowed aortic orifice by the retrograde catheter and relief of this obstruction with catheter withdrawal. (From Carabello BA et al: Changes in arterial pressure during left heart pull-back in patients with aortic stenosis. Am J Cardiol 44:424, 1979.)

phy should be done in most patients with acquired calcific aortic stenosis, especially if chest pain is present.

## Catheterization Protocol

1. Right heart catheterization for measurement of right heart pressures and cardiac output.

2. Left heart catheterization for measurement of pressure gradient across aortic valve, LVEDP, and assessment of presence or absence of a transmitral gradient (concomitant mitral stenosis). Retrograde crossing of a tight aortic valve may be difficult. From the *brachial approach,* I have been successful in crossing a tight aortic valve most often using a Sones catheter. The Cordis polyurethane Sones catheter has high torque control and tapers to a 5.5 French tip, which can often be negotiated across a stenotic aortic valve without the aid of a guide wire. When a guide wire is required, a 0.35-inch diameter straight wire passes easily through the Sones catheter and can help in crossing the aortic valve.

With a *femoral approach,* the use of a pigtail catheter together with a straight guide wire protruded a short distance beyond the catheter tip is my standard first approach to retrograde catheterization of the left ventricle in the patient with aortic stenosis: this method is illustrated on page 69 (Fig. 5-8). On occasion, a right or left Judkins coronary catheter used together with a straight guide wire is successful in crossing a tight aortic valve in a patient with aortic stenosis. We recently had one patient in whom all these approaches failed, but a left L-2 Amplatz catheter with straight guide wire was successfully introduced in retrograde catheterization of the left ventricle in a patient with calcific aortic stenosis and a very eccentric aortic valve orifice.

If these approaches are not successful (or are not desirable in a particular patient), a transseptal approach may be utilized. In some laboratories, the transseptal approach is the primary technique for patients with aortic stenosis.

3. Angiography following the guidelines just discussed.

Angiography[18] also demonstrates the stenotic orifice of the valve during systole as outlined by a jet of contrast material injected into the aorta. The valve cusps may appear irregular, their mobility may be reduced, and the number of cusps may frequently be identified. In congenital aortic stenosis, the valve often forms a funnel during systole. The ascending aorta is dilated (poststenotic dilatation), but the subvalvular area is widely patent. A subaortic membrane, with a small central orifice, or a subvalvular muscular ring may be seen. The characteristic changes of idiopathic hypertrophic subaortic stenosis may be observed. In supravalvular stenosis, the narrowing of the proximal aorta can be seen.

Aortography also can be helpful in evaluation of the patient with aortic stenosis. In "pure" aortic stenosis (no concomitant aortic regurgitation), aortography often demonstrates a negative jet of radiolucent blood exiting focally from the left ventricle. In congenital aortic stenosis, there may be upward doming of the aortic valve leaflets which together with the central negative jet gives the so-called Prussian helmet sign (Fig. 23-7). In the patient with aortic stenosis when some aortic regurgitation is also present, aortography permits a rough quantitation of the se-

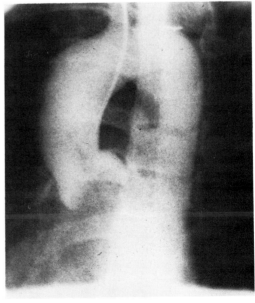

**Fig. 23-7.** Aortogram in a young man with congenital aortic stenosis; 45-degree LAO cine projection. Catheter positioned clear of the aortic valve. Systolic frame shows doming of the valve cusps with negative jet of blood (the Prussian helmet sign). Note also the poststenotic dilatation of the ascending aorta.

verity of the regurgitation. If new catheter technqiues (e.g., laser, balloon angioplasty) become successful in the nonoperative treatment of pure aortic stenosis, determination of the extent of associated aortic regurgitation may become important in clinical decision making. Hemodynamic assessment can often detect the presence of mixed significant aortic stenosis and regurgitation, as illustrated by the patient whose pressure tracings are shown in Figure 23-8. This 78-year-old man had the unusual combination of hemodynamically significant aortic stenosis (70 mmHg gradient) *and* significant aortic regurgitation (3+, regurgitant fraction 48%).

## Case 5

*Aortic Stenosis Without Appreciable Cardiomegaly.* L.C. was a 48-year-old married woman with a history of rheumatic fever in childhood. Six months prior to admission, she noted increasing exertional dyspnea and decreased exercise tolerance. She had had dizziness, but no syncope or angina.

Physical examination was normal except for the heart. There was a somewhat forceful apex impulse in the midclavicular line in the fifth interspace. Rhythm was regular. $S_1$ and $S_2$ were normal. The only murmur was a grade 2 ejection type systolic murmur, maximal along the left sternal border transmitted to apex and into the carotids. No thrill was detected. The carotid pulsations were plateau in quality.

The ECG revealed left ventricular hypertrophy and strain.

Roentgenography showed a heart of normal overall size. There was a little rounding in the region of the left ventricle. The other cardiac chambers appeared normal, as did the lungs. At fluoroscopy there was calcification in the region of the aortic valve.

The findings at cardiac catheterization were as follows:

| | |
|---|---|
| Body surface area, $m^2$ | 1.87 |
| $O_2$ consumption, ml/min | 225 |
| A-V $O_2$ difference, ml/L | 40 |
| Cardiac output, L/min | 5.6 |
| Heart rate/min | 70 |
| Stroke volume, ml/beat | 80 |

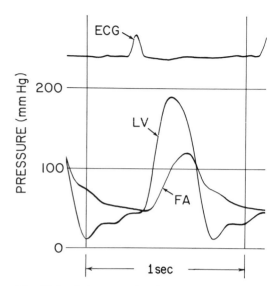

**Fig. 23-8.** Left ventricular (LV) and femoral artery (FA) pressure tracings in a 78-year-old man with increasing dyspnea on exertion and one episode of pulmonary edema. In this case, femoral artery and central aortic pressures were nearly superimposable. There is a 70 mmHg peak-to-peak systolic gradient, but there is also unusually rapid aortic diastolic runoff with equilibration (diastasis) of end-diastolic LV and FA pressures. This latter finding suggested significant aortic regurgitation, which was confirmed by aortography.

| Pressures, mm Hg | |
|---|---|
| Brachial artery | 100/66 |
| Systolic mean | 84 |
| Left ventricle | 176/16 |
| Systolic mean | 140 |
| Diastolic mean | 10 |
| Systolic ejection period, sec/beat | 0.35 |
| Pulmonary capillary wedge, mean | 10 |
| Pulmonary artery | 25/11, $\overline{15}$ |
| Right ventricle | 25/5 |
| Right atrium, mean | 5 |
| Pulmonary vascular resistance, dynes-sec-cm$^{-5}$ | 72 |
| Calculated aortic valve area, cm$^2$ | 0.7 |
| Ejection fraction | 0.69 |

Cineangiography showed a vigorously contracting normal-sized left ventricle and a calcified aortic valve with three cusps. The cusps were almost immobile. A jet was seen passing through the valve which almost immediately became obscured by the radio-pacity of the aorta. There was a rather discrete poststenotic dilation of the ascending aorta just above the aortic valve.

**Interpretation.** The severely stenotic calcified valve in this woman was probably rheumatic in origin. The left ventricle contracted well, as indicated by an ejection fraction of 0.69 and a normal cardiac output. The elevated end-diastolic pressure at rest was compatible with a decreased compliance from hypertrophy.

## Case 6

*Aortic Stenosis With Appreciable Cardiomegaly.* A. H., a 77-year-old man, was well until three years before admission, when exertional dyspnea, orthopnea, fatigue, and peripheral edema appeared. Despite therapy, these symptoms increased progressively to the point of invalidism. He had mild angina, and had had two syncopal episodes.

On physical examination, the blood pressure was 110/80; the pulse, 78 and regular; respirations, 24. The carotids were of small volume with slow upstroke and downstroke. Neck veins were moderately distended. There were bibasilar rales to the angles of the scapulae. The PMI was in the sixth interspace 2 cm within the anterior axillary line, diffuse and forceful. There was no parasternal heave. A grade 2/6 aortic systolic ejection murmur was heard all along the left sternal border and over both carotid arteries. The liver was two fingerbreadths below the costal margin. There was slight pitting edema of both lower legs. The ECG showed left ventricular hypertrophy and strain pattern.

Roentgenography showed enlargement of the left ventricle, calcification in the region of the aortic valve, moderate redistribution of vascular markings to the upper lobes of the lung, and small amount of pleural fluid on the right.

Cardiac catheterization yielded the following results:

| | |
|---|---|
| Body surface area, m$^2$ | 1.76 |
| O$_2$ consumption, ml/min | 218 |
| A-V O$_2$ difference, ml/L | 81 |
| Cardiac output, L/min | 2.7 |
| Heart rate/min | 90 |
| Stroke volume, ml/beat | 30 |

| | |
|---|---|
| Pressures, mmHg | |
| Brachial artery | 135/78 |
| Systolic mean | 100 |
| Left ventricle | 184/35 |
| Systolic mean | 140 |
| Diastolic mean | 28 |
| Systolic ejection period, sec/beat | 0.27 |
| Pulmonary capillary wedge, mean | 29 |
| Pulmonary artery | 75/40, $\overline{52}$ |
| Right ventricle | 75/12 |
| Right atrium, mean | 10 |
| Pulmonary vascular resistance, dynes-sec-cm$^{-5}$ | 683 |
| Calculated aortic valve area, cm$^2$ | 0.4 |
| Ejection fraction | 0.30 |

Left ventriculography was performed only after pretreatment with intravenous furosemide, and showed a large dilated left ventricle with uniformly poor contractions in systole. There was no mitral or aortic regurgitation. The aortic valve had two cusps that appeared ragged and were heavily calcified. There was considerable dilation of the ascending aorta. Left ventriculography was tolerated well, and coronary angiography (two injections of the left coronary artery and one injection of the right coronary artery) revealed the absence of significant coronary artery obstruction.

**Interpretation.** There was severe calcific aortic stenosis as indicated by a calculated valve area of 0.4 cm$^2$. Severe left ventricular failure was present, as indicated by left ventricular dilatation, high left ventricular mean and end-diastolic pressures, uniformly poor contraction by cineangiography, an ejection fraction of only 0.30, and a very low cardiac output. The aortic obstruction was severe, and the left ventricle was so decompensated that it generated a peak systolic pressure of only 184 mmHg (instead of 250 to 300 mmHg, as would be expected with a normal cardiac output), and the transaortic mean pressure difference was only 40 mmHg.

The pulmonary capillary wedge pressure of 29 mmHg explained the rales heard at both lung bases as well as the patient's shortness of breath. The pulmonary hypertension was due in part to the elevated left ventricular diastolic pressure (passive rise), and in part to reactive pulmonary hypertension as revealed by the finding of a pulmonary vascular resistance of 683—more than five times normal.

The pressure load on the right ventricle resulted in its decompensation, as indicated by a mild elevation of the right ventricular diastolic and right atrial pressures. The clinical counterpart was slight distension of neck veins, enlarged liver and edema.

## AORTIC REGURGITATION

The dynamic effects of aortic regurgitation are due to regurgitation of blood from aorta to left ventricle in diastole. The magnitude of the regurgitation depends on the size of the regurgitant orifice, the pressure difference between aorta and left ventricle in diastole, and the duration of diastole. The size of the regurgitant aperture may be as large as $1.0 \text{ cm}^2$, but regurgitation is generally severe when it is more than $0.5 \text{ cm}^2$. The total left ventricular stroke volume increases and equals that which supplies the body (forward flow), plus that which is regurgitated. The amount of blood regurgitated may be as much as 60% or more of the systolic discharge and usually occurs mainly in early diastole.

### Hemodynamic Assessment

The large stroke volume entering the aorta with systole produces an elevated systolic pressure, whereas the regurgitation produces a lowered aortic diastolic pressure (Fig. 23-9). Left ventricular work load increases progressively with the magnitude of regurgitation. This is due not only to the raised stroke volume and to the rise of systolic pressure, but also to the high intramyocardial tension that must be developed by the dilated ventricle in order to produce a given pressure (LaPlace's law). Dilatation and hypertrophy of the left ventricle are invariable consequences of aortic regurgitation. The heart may become the largest encountered in cardiac pathology—the so-called cor bovinum. Up to a point, the forward output is well maintained. The addition of blood regurgitated to the normal inflow from the left atrium increases the diastolic

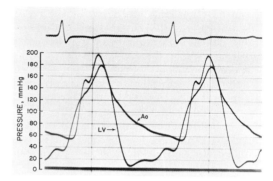

**Fig. 23-9.** Left ventricular (LV) and aortic (Ao) pressure tracings in a patient with severe aortic insufficiency secondary to rheumatic heart disease. In this condition, the aortic and left ventricular pressures may equalize in late diastole, a phenomenon occasionally termed "diastasis."

volume of the left ventricle, leading to a more forceful contraction (Starling's law). With time the fraction of end-diastolic volume ejected per beat (ejection fraction) becomes diminished, reflecting impaired myocardial function. Furthermore, the left ventricle may operate with an excessive end-systolic volume—another index of left ventricular dysfunction.

***Premature Mitral Valve Closure.*** The reflux of blood into the left ventricle in diastole encounters that streaming through the mitral valve from the left atrium. The mitral valve may close prematurely because the regurgitating blood may raise the left ventricular diastolic pressure to exceed that in the left atrium. This is particularly common in acute aortic regurgitation, in which sudden onset of severe regurgitation into a normal-sized left ventricle leads to striking elevations in LV diastolic pressure (Fig. 23-10). In the case illustrated in Figure 23-10, LVEDP approaches 50 mmHg, and LV diastolic pressure exceeds left atrial (or wedge) pressure for nearly half of diastole. This reversal of pressures is associated with premature mitral valve closure, which may be seen on the left ventriculogram.

Another example of premature closure of the mitral valve in association with severe aortic regurgitation is shown in Figure 23-11. These tracings were recorded during cardiac catheterization of a 71-year-old man who had previously had aortic valve replacement for aortic stenosis. After doing extremely well for more than 5 years, he suddenly devel-

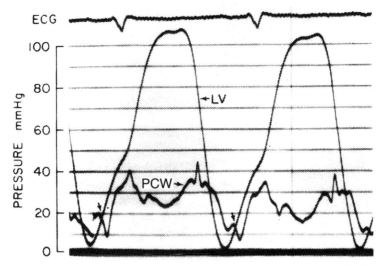

**Fig. 23-10.** Left ventricular (LV) and pulmonary capillary wedge (PCW) pressures in a patient with acute aortic regurgitation due to infective endocarditis. Note the unusual wave form of the LV pressure with its striking late diastolic rise, loss of clear A wave, and high elevation of LVEDP (approximately 45 to 50 mmHg). LV diastolic pressure rises in late diastole to exceed left atrial and pulmonary wedge pressures (arrow), forcing premature closure of the mitral valve. (From Mann T et al: Assessing the hemodynamic severity of acute aortic regurgitation due to infective endocarditis. N Engl J Med 293:108, 1975.)

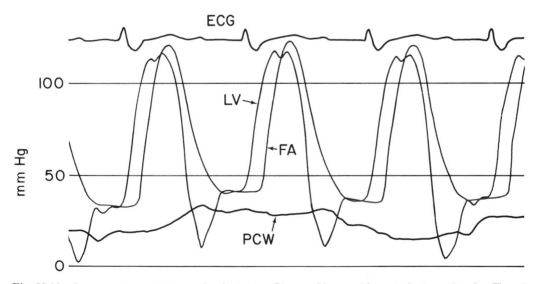

**Fig. 23-11.** Severe aortic regurgitation developing in a 71-year-old man with a prosthetic aortic valve. There is diastasis between left ventricle (LV) and aorta. Also, LV diastolic pressure exceeds pulmonary capillary wedge (PCW) pressure early in diastole. Femoral artery = FA. See text for details.

oped marked shortness of breath and a new murmur of aortic regurgitation. Pressure recordings show that left ventricular diastolic pressure exceeds left atrial (pulmonary capillary wedge pressure) by the end of the first ⅓ of the diastolic filling period. Also, complete diastasis of aortic and left ventricular pressures occurs by mid-diastole, at which point aortic regurgitation ceases, since there is no longer any gradient driving the regurgitant flow. As expected, this patient's diastolic murmur was blowing in quality, decrescendo, and ended by mid-diastole.

***Acute vs Chronic Aortic Regurgitation.*** The typical hemodynamic findings in acute vs chronic aortic regurgitation have been reported by Mann et al,[19] and are presented in Table 23-1. As can be seen, widened pulse pressure is characteristic only of chronic aortic regurgitation, reflecting both the enormous stroke volume associated with this condition, and the tachycardia commonly seen in patients with acute aortic regurgitation. This may give rise to a situation where there exists a high *end*-diastolic pressure in the noncompliant left ventricle in the presence of little if any elevation of the mean pressure in the left atrium. With time and with the severity of the leak, the *mean* dia-stolic pressure of the ventricle rises, and when this happens, the clinical counterpart is left ventricular failure.

Another hemodynamic finding in aortic regurgitation is the amplification of peak systolic pressure in peripheral arteries (especially the femoral and popliteal), so that peak systolic femoral artery pressure may exceed central aortic pressure by 20 to 50 mmHg. This is essentially an exaggeration of a normal phenomenon (see Chapter 9), but emphasizes the importance of central aortic pressure measurement in aortic regurgitation.

## Angiographic Assessment

Aortic cineangiography yields a graphic demonstration of the severity and dynamics of the regurgitation. Qualitative assessment is subjective, as for mitral regurgitation. We use a scale of 1+ to 4+ employing the following definitions to aid discrimination of these four degrees of regurgitation. In 1+ regurgitation (mild), a small amount of contrast material enters the left ventricle in diastole; it is essentially cleared with each beat and never fills the ventricular chamber. More

**TABLE 23-1.** *Comparison of Hemodynamic and Angiographic Findings in Acute and Chronic Aortic Regurgitation*

|  | Acute AR | Chronic AR | P Value |
|---|---|---|---|
| Age (years) | 33 ± 14 | 40 ± 15 | NS |
| Regurgitant fraction | 0.6 ± 0.1 | 0.7 ± 0.1 | NS |
| LVEDP (mmHg) | 41 ± 12 | 36 ± 13 | NS |
| Ejection fraction | 0.6 ± 0.1 | 0.6 ± 0.1 | NS |
| Heart rate (beats/min) | 108 ± 15 | 71 ± 14 | <0.01 |
| LV volumes (ml/m²) |  |  |  |
| EDV | 146 ± 28 | 264 ± 64 | <0.01 |
| ESV | 57 ± 23 | 101 ± 42 | <0.02 |
| TSV | 89 ± 22 | 163 ± 57 | <0.01 |
| Aortic pressure (mmHg): |  |  |  |
| Systolic | 110 ± 14 | 155 ± 26 | <0.01 |
| Diastolic | 56 ± 11 | 50 ± 6 | NS |
| Mean | 78 ± 12 | 90 ± 8 | <0.02 |
| Pulse pressure (mmHg) | 55 ± 7 | 105 ± 22 | <0.01 |
| Systemic Vascular Resistance |  |  |  |
| (dynes-sec-cm⁻⁵) | 1326 ± 372 | 1341 ± 461 | NS |

Mean ± SD; EDV, ESV and TSV are LV end-diastolic, end-systolic and total stroke volumes; AR, aortic regurgitation; LVEDP, left ventricular end-diastolic pressure. (Modified from Mann et al: Assessing the hemodynamic severity of acute aortic regurgitation due to infective endocarditis. N Engl J Med 293:108, 1975.)

contrast material enters with each diastole in 2+ (moderate) regurgitation, and faint opacification of the entire chamber occurs. With moderately severe (3+) regurgitation, the LV chamber is well opacified, and equal in density with the ascending aorta. Severe (4+) aortic regurgitation is characterized by complete, dense opacification of the LV chamber on the first beat, and there is the appearance that the left ventricle is more densely opacified than the ascending aorta.

Quantitative assessment of aortic regurgitation involves calculation of the regurgitant fraction (RF), as described in Chapter 19. The same scale of interpretation holds, with RF <20% corresponding to mild regurgitation; 20% to 40%, moderate; 40% to 60%, moderately severe; and >60%, severe aortic regurgitation.

Part of the angiographic assessment of aortic regurgitation involves assessment of the aortic valve leaflets (mobility, calcification, number of cusps), the ascending aorta (extent and type of dilatation), and possible associated abnormalities (e.g., coronary lesions, sinus of Valsalva aneurysm, dissecting aneurysm of the aorta, and ventricular septal defect). All these aspects are best evaluated in the LAO view.

## Catheterization Protocol

1. Right heart catheterization for measurement of right heart pressures and cardiac output.

2. Left heart catheterization for measurement of central aortic pulse pressure, LVEDP, detection of transvalvular gradients (if any), of diastasis between LV and aorta, if this is present (Fig. 23-11), and of relative height of LVEDP compared to PCW or LA mean pressure.

3. Angiography, including left ventriculography, aortography, and possibly coronary angiography (if indicated clinically).

4. If resting hemodynamics are normal, consider stress intervention, such as dynamic exercise.

## TRICUSPID REGURGITATION

Tricuspid regurgitation can be functional or organic. Functional tricuspid regurgita-

tion is thought to be due to right ventricular dilatation and failure as a result of excessive right ventricular afterload. Most commonly this is due to pulmonary hypertension from mitral stenosis, left ventricular failure, cor pulmonale, or pulmonary embolism.

"Organic" tricuspid regurgitation implies disease of the tricuspid valve or its supporting apparatus, and is most commonly seen with rheumatic heart disease, bacterial endocarditis, or right ventricular infarction.

## Hemodynamic Assessment

In tricuspid regurgitation, either organic or functional, the primary hemodynamic finding is a large systolic wave in the right atrial pressure tracing. Tracings of jugular venous pulsations have distinguished A, C, and V waves in the normal subject; in the patient with moderate tricuspid regurgitation there is a fourth pulsation, the S wave. This systolic wave precedes and blends with the normal ventricular filling (V) wave, and in severe tricuspid regurgitation, the S and V waves form a single regurgitant systolic wave (Fig. 23-12). As can be seen in Figure 23-12, the right atrial pressure tracing in severe tricuspid regurgitation resembles the right ventricular pressure tracing. In the most extreme cases, the pressure tracings are virtually superimposable, which is to be expected, since the right atrium and ventricle are physiologically a common chamber in such cases.

The hemodynamic distinction between organic and functional tricuspid regurgitation is difficult. Generally, if the right ventricular systolic pressure exceeds 60 mmHg, the tricuspid regurgitation is functional, with right ventricular systolic pressures of ≤40 mmHg, there is an organic component. This distinction is of practical importance in terms of surgical correction, since functional tricuspid regurgitation will improve substantially solely with correction of the right ventricular hypertension (e.g., following corrective surgery for mitral stenosis), whereas the patient with major organic tricuspid regurgitation may not survive cardiac surgery unless the operation includes tricuspid valve replacement or tricuspid annuloplasty.

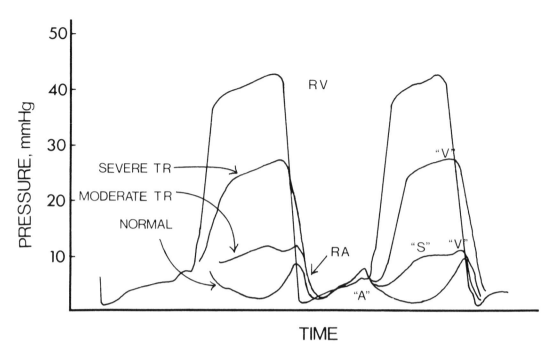

**Fig. 23-12.** Right ventricular (RV) and right atrial (RA) pressure tracings in patients with normal RA pressure, moderate tricuspid regurgitation (moderate TR), and severe TR. The A and V waves are depicted as nearly equal in the normal RA pressure tracing. The regurgitant S wave can barely be distinguished from the V wave in moderate TR and blends in completely with the V wave in severe TR. Note that in severe TR, the RA pressure resembles the RV wave form.

## Angiographic Assessment

The angiographic demonstration of tricuspid regurgitation is generally accomplished by right ventricular cineangiography in the RAO projection, as discussed in Chapter 14. Some artificial tricuspid regurgitation is seen due to the presence of the catheter across the tricuspid valve, but this is usually minor. It is important to choose a catheter type, position, and injection rate that will avoid extrasystoles, since a run of ventricular tachycardia will make it impossible to evaluate the degree of tricuspid regurgitation; these considerations are discussed in Chapter 14. We like the Grollman, pigtail or Eppendorf catheters situated in mid-RV or RV outflow tract, with injection rates of 12 to 18 ml/sec depending on RV size and irritability. A scale of 1+ to 4+ is used to grade the severity of tricuspid regurgitation, using criteria of definition similar to those described for mitral regurgitation. In some circumstances, a right atrial cineangiogram in RAO projection can be used for assessment of tricuspid regurgi-

tation; in this instance, a negative jet (unopacified blood) from RV to RA shows the regurgitation. A catheter technique for assessing tricuspid regurgitation using a specially shaped no. 7 NIH catheter has recently been described with excellent results in a series of 60 patients.[20]

Cardiac catheterization protocol depends upon the associated conditions.

## TRICUSPID STENOSIS

Previously, this rare condition was seen only in patients with rheumatic heart disease and mitral stenosis. Today, however, stenosis of a prosthetic tricuspid valve (placed originally as treatment for tricuspid regurgitation) accounts for the majority of the cases seen in most major medical centers. The clinical diagnosis may be difficult, especially if the patient is in atrial fibrillation. Diagnosis is aided by the characteristic finding of an increased jugular venous pressure with blunting or absence of the Y descent. One patient seen by the author had severe stenosis of the mitral, aortic, and tricuspid valves. This was a 43-year-old woman with a history of repeated bouts of rheumatic fever in childhood, whose major complaint was fatigue and "blackouts."

## Hemodynamic Assessment

The sine qua non of tricuspid stenosis is a pandiastolic gradient across the tricuspid valve. The gradient is usually small (4 to 8 mmHg) and may be missed unless a careful assessment is made. Two catheters (or a single catheter with double lumen) and simultaneous measurement of RA and RV pressures should be employed if there is any doubt about the presence of this condition. However, a careful RV to RA pull-back using a standard catheter will serve to confirm or eliminate this diagnosis with reliability in most cases. The tricuspid valve area is calculated using the formula given in Chapter 11. Tricuspid stenosis is usually of clinical and hemodynamic significance when the tricuspid valve area is $<1.3 \, \text{cm}^2$.

## Angiographic Assessment

The valve is usually calcified and shows decreased mobility. There may be associated right atrial dilatation and some tricuspid regurgitation.

Cardiac catheterization protocol depends on associated lesions.

## PULMONIC STENOSIS AND REGURGITATION

Pulmonic stenosis is essentially a congenital condition and is discussed in Chapter 28. Pulmonic regurgitation is usually functional and a consequence of severe pulmonary hypertension. When the pulmonary artery pressure exceeds 100 mmHg systolic, there is usually some pulmonic regurgitation. This may lead to widening of the pulmonary artery pulse pressure and an increase in RVEDP. Angiographic assessment of pulmonic regurgitation is difficult, since the angiographic catheter lying across the pulmonic valve may cause artifactual regurgita-

tion. Cineangiography in RAO or LAO projection with contrast injection at 20 to 25 ml/sec into the main pulmonary artery will demonstrate the pulmonic valve and allow some assessment of regurgitation.

Cardiac catheterization protocol depends on associated conditions.

## RELATIVE STENOSIS OF PROSTHETIC VALVES

An unusual case of *relative* tricuspid stenosis, mitral stenosis and aortic stenosis in a 60-year-old man is shown in Figure 23-13 and illustrates an important point concerning function of prosthetic cardiac valves. This man had mitral valve replacement with a Harken disc valve in 1969 for rheumatic mitral regurgitation. He then did well until 1980 when he presented with left and right heart failure and was found at cardiac catheterization to have severe aortic and tricuspid regurgitation, but normal function of the mitral prosthetic valve. Aortic valve replacement (Starr-Edwards prosthesis) and tricuspid valve replacement (porcine prosthesis) led to improvement, but over the following years he required large amounts of diuretic therapy to remain free of edema and pulmonary congestion. Echocardiographic assessment of his prosthetic valves demonstrated apparently normal function, and left ventricular contraction was vigorous.

Because of persistent left and right heart failure, cardiac catheterization was undertaken in 1985. The porcine tricuspid valve was crossed antegrade with a Swan-Ganz catheter, and the Starr-Edwards aortic prosthesis was crossed retrograde with a Sones catheter to obtain the pressure measurements shown in Figure 23-13. As can be seen, significant pressure gradients were present across tricuspid, mitral, and aortic prostheses. However, a surprising finding was an elevated cardiac output, measured both by Fick and thermodilution methods. Oxygen consumption index was 148 ml/min/$M^2$ and arteriovenous oxygen difference was 29 ml $O_2$/L giving a Fick cardiac index of 5 L/min/$M^2$ and a cardiac output of 10 L/min. Using the Gorlin formula (Chapter 11), calculated aortic valve area was $1.3 \, \text{cm}^2$, mitral valve was $1.6 \, \text{cm}^2$ and tricuspid valve area was $2.4 \, \text{cm}^2$: these values were all consistent with

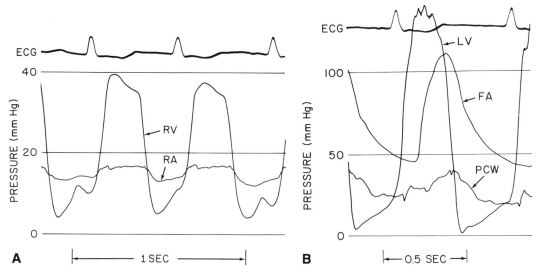

**Fig. 23-13.** Pressure tracings in a 60-year-old man with high cardiac output and significant pressure gradients across normally functioning tricuspid, mitral, and aortic valve prostheses. (A) From the right ventricle (RV) and right atrium (RA). (B) From the left ventricle (LV), femoral artery (FA), and pulmonary capillary wedge position (PCW).

the known effective orifice areas of the particular prosthetic valves implanted, and did not signify prosthetic valve dysfunction or stenosis. Thus, a *high cardiac output state* caused substantial pressure gradients to occur across the patient's three prosthetic valves, resulting in the clinical picture of biventricular failure. Thyroid function tests were normal and a search for other causes of high output state (e.g., arteriovenous fistula, Paget's disease) was unrevealing. This patient responded nicely to thiamine supplementation, beta blockade, and diuretic therapy with spironolactone and furosemide: evidence of high output state receded and a vigorous diuresis ensued.

## Catheter Passage Across Prosthetic Valves

As illustrated in the case just described, it has become routine to cross prosthetic valves with catheters in an attempt to assess their function or the function of other valves. Published reports have documented the safety of this procedure in a large number of patients[21,22] with a variety of prosthetic valves. Based on my own experience and

anecdotal experience reported to me by many others, I offer the following guidelines.

First, porcine valves may be crossed retrograde or antegrade safely with a variety of catheters. For retrograde crossing of a *porcine prosthetic valve* in the aortic position, a pigtail catheter is generally my first approach. The pigtail catheter tip is rested on top of the valve's leaflets as they protrude into the aorta high above the sewing ring and is gently advanced until it prolapses into the left ventricular chamber. Antegrade crossing of a *porcine tricuspid prosthesis* is accomplished easily using a balloon-flotation catheter, as described in the preceding section. Retrograde crossing of a *ball valve* (e.g., Starr-Edwards) prosthesis in the aortic position may be accomplished easily using a 7F or 8F Sones catheter with or without guidewire assistance. The pigtail catheter also may be advanced into the left ventricle over a guide wire across a ball valve prosthesis, but the wire should be reinserted for catheter withdrawal, to avoid hooking the pigtail on the metal cage. Although some operators have crossed *low profile disc-valve prostheses* (e.g., Bjork-Shiley valve) retrograde without complications,[21] I have heard of instances where catheter entrapment occurred with retrograde crossing of such valves. Also, Dr. Viking Bjork has specifically stated that the Bjork-Shiley valve must not be crossed retrograde, based on his own large experience. When restudy has been required in his patients, a transseptal approach has been used. Accordingly, it is my practice never to attempt to cross a Bjork-Shiley valve (or any low profile disc valve prosthesis) retrograde.

# REFERENCES

1. Lewis BM, et al: Clinical and physiological correlations in patients with mitral stenosis. Am Heart J 43:2, 1952.
2. Selzer A: Nonrheumatic mitral regurgitation. Mod Concepts Cardiovasc Dis 48:25, 1979.
3. Braunwald E: Mitral regurgitation. Physiologic, clinical and surgical considerations. N Engl J Med 281:425, 1969.
4. Braunwald E, Welch GH Jr, Morrow AG: The effects of acutely increased systemic resistance on the left atrial pressure pulse: a method for the clinical detection of mitral insufficiency. J Clin Invest 37:35, 1958.
5. Brody W, Criley JM: Intermittent severe mitral regurgitation. Hemodynamic studies in a patient with recurrent acute left-sided heart failure. N Engl J Med 183:673, 1970.
6. Baxley WA, Kennedy JW, Feild B, Dodge HT: Hemodynamics in ruptured chordae tendineae and chronic rheumatic mitral regurgitation. Circulation 48:1288, 1973.
7. Pichard AD, et al: Large V waves in the pulmonary wedge pressure tracing in the absence of mitral regurgitation. Am J Cardiol 50:1044, 1982.
8. Grose R, Strain J, Cohen MV: Pulmonary arterial V waves in mitral regurgitation: Clinical and experimental observations. Circulation 69:214, 1984.
9. Fuchs RM, Heuser RP, Yin FCP, Brinker JA: Limitations of pulmonary wedge V waves in diagnosing mitral regurgitation. Am J Cardiol 49:849, 1982.
10. Harshaw CW, Munro AB, McLaurin LP, Grossman W: Reduced systemic vascular resistance as therapy for severe mitral regurgitation of valvular origin. Ann Intern Med 83:312, 1975.
11. Grossman W, et al: Lowered aortic impedance as therapy for severe mitral regurgitation. JAMA 230:1011, 1974.
12. Croft et al: Limitations of qualitative angiographic grading in aortic or mitral regurgitation. Am J Cardiol 53:1593, 1984.
13. Gorlin R, et al: Dynamics of the circulation in aortic vavular disease. Am J Med 18:855, 1955.
14. Samet P, Bernstein WH, Litwak RS: The effect of exercise upon the mean systolic left ventricular-brachial artery gradient in aortic stenosis.
15. Kroetz FW, et al: The effect of atrial contraction on left ventricular performance in valvular aortic stenosis. Circulation 35: 852, 1967.
16. Hancock EW: Differentiation of valvar and subvalvar aortic stenosis. Circulation 20:709, 1959.
17. Carabello BA, Barry WH, Grossman W: Changes in arterial pressure during left heart pullback in patients with aortic stenosis: a sign of severe aortic stenosis. Am J Cardiol 44:424, 1979.
18. Baron MG: Angiographic diagnosis of valvular stenosis. Circulation 44:143, 1971.
19. Mann T, McLaurin LP, Grossman W, Craige E: Assessing the hemodynamic severity of acute aortic regurgitation due to infective endocarditis, N Engl J Med 293:108, 1975.
20. Lingamneni R, et al: Tricuspid regurgitation: clinical and angiographic assessment. Cath Cardiovasc Diag 5:7, 1979.
21. Karsh et al: Retrograde left ventricular catheterization in patients with an aortic valve prosthesis. Am J Cardiol 41:893, 1978.
22. Kosinski EJ, Cohn PF, Grossman W, Cohn LH: Severe stenosis occurring in antibiotic sterilised homograft valves. Br Heart J 40:194, 1978.

# chapter twenty four

# Profiles in Coronary Artery Disease

RICHARD C. PASTERNAK

CORONARY angiography, left ventriculography, and hemodynamic measurements are integral to the evaluation of many patients with suspected or known coronary artery disease. In addition to the diagnostic value of these studies, they are useful for prognostic purposes and for planning therapeutic interventions such as coronary artery bypass surgery. More recently, coronary angiography has been performed in association with newer forms of therapy, such as percutaneous transluminal coronary angioplasty (PTCA) and thrombolysis, thus expanding cardiac catheterization beyond its role as a diagnostic procedure into the realm of therapeutics. The evaluation of ventricular function by angiography and the measurement of hemodynamics allow for the assessment of possible mechanical compromise induced by coronary artery disease. Additionally, the effect of pharmacologic or mechanical therapies can be determined accurately, and therapeutic regimens may be adjusted based on the results of these studies.

***Coronary angiography*** itself remains the most definitive way to make the diagnosis of coronary artery disease. While often the diagnosis of coronary artery disease can be made from the history or by noninvasive techniques, angiography may be necessary for diagnostic purposes in patients with recurrent chest pain and atypical features of coronary disease. Important prognostic information can be obtained by defining the coronary anatomy. Although the most simple prognostic system is based on the number of coronary vessels diseased, more complex systems have been proposed.[1] However, none are so widely used as the "one-, two-, or three-vessel disease" categorization.[2] A more accurate determination of prognosis may be made by combining information about ventricular function and various other clinical factors with coronary pathoanatomy.[3] Definition of the coronary anatomy is an absolute necessity prior to coronary artery bypass surgery, and it is an integral part of percutaneous transluminal coronary angioplasty. Additionally, in selected patients, the diagnosis of coronary artery spasm can be made by provocative testing with ergonovine.

***Left ventriculography*** is useful for defining prognosis in patients with coronary artery disease. For prediction of survival, analysis of left ventricular function, as determined from a left ventricular cineangiogram, is probably more useful than the definition of the number of diseased coronary vessels.[4] The determination of baseline left ventricular function also affects the choice of therapeutic approaches—both mechanical and pharmacologic ones. Ventriculography is useful for the detection of complications of coronary artery disease such as mitral regurgitation or ventricular aneurysm. Finally, left ventriculography may be important in defining the relationship between coronary pathoanatomy and electrocardiographic evidence of myocardial infarction. For example, a total coronary artery occlusion may occur in the absence of any myocardial damage leaving a patient with normal left ventricular function (and a normal electrocardiogram) as long as the portion of heart muscle initially supplied by the occluded artery is adequately supplied by collaterals. Conversely, only minimal narrowing of a coronary artery may be present following an acute myocardial infarction if recanalization of a coronary artery thrombus or relaxation of prolonged coronary spasm has occurred. In such patients, extensive myocardial dysfunction may be demonstrated by left ventriculography, and the electrocardiogram may show Q waves indicative of transmural infarction, in spite of the absence of a critical coronary artery stenosis.

*Hemodynamic measurements* may aid in the evaluation of abnormalities caused by coronary artery disease. Assessment of the presence and degree of systolic and diastolic dysfunction may be important in devising a medical program that involves choosing from a wide variety of drugs with quite different pharmacologic actions. As has already been discussed in detail (Chapter 18), pacing may be combined with hemodynamic studies, lactate measurements, and even thallium scintigraphy in the evaluation of certain patients with coronary disease. Such studies are particularly useful when noninvasive testing has failed to lead to clear diagnostic conclusions or the effect of a particular therapy needs to be assessed relatively rapidly.

To illustrate these points, several cases across the spectrum of coronary artery disease will be described. The cases are representative profiles of patients referred to the Cardiac Catheterization Laboratory for evaluation or management. Before the discussion of cases, a brief review of catheterization procedures for patients with ischemic heart disease is presented.

## CATHETERIZATION PROTOCOL

For patients with suspected or known coronary artery disease the catheterization procedure itself is generally standardized regardless of the exact indications for the study. In many laboratories combined right and left heart procedures are performed on most patients. Right heart catheterization is undertaken both to assess the hemodynamics and to provide access to the central circulation for diagnostic and therapeutic pharmacologic maneuvers. We generally perform right-sided catheterization using a balloon-tipped flow-guided catheter which is inserted via a brachial vein or through a sheath in the femoral vein. If the measurements of right heart hemodynamics and saturations are deemed unnecessary, then access to the central circulation should still be provided through a well-secured, large bore venous cannula. Left heart catheterization is performed by either the brachial or femoral techniques as outlined in previous chapters. Patients undergoing complete cardiac catheterization usually have the study undertaken in the following sequence:

1. The right heart catheter is inserted and right atrial, right ventricular, and pulmonary arterial pressures are measured. Superior vena cava, right atrial, and pulmonary arterial saturations are determined. The balloon of the flow-directed catheter is then inflated, and pulmonary capillary wedge pressure is measured. The mean wedge pressure is recorded, as well as the height of the A wave and V wave, and the balloon is then deflated.

2. Left heart catheterization is then performed, and measurements of central aortic, left ventricular systolic, and end diastolic pressures are made.

3. Cardiac output is determined by either the Fick method (during measurement or estimation of oxygen consumption) or by the thermodilution technique (see Chapter 8).

4. Contrast left ventriculography is undertaken with careful attention to segmental wall motion, inclusion of the entire ventricular silhouette for calculation of ejection fraction, and attention to the left atrium for detection of the presence of mitral regurgitation (see Chapter 14).

5. Selective cineangiography of the coronary arteries is then undertaken. Angiograms are filmed in multiple projections. When ste-

noses are noted, views providing a minimum of vessel overlap are performed to optimally outline lesions (see Chapter 13).

6. Further interventions such as atrial pacing or ergonovine testing are performed in some patients, following the routine diagnostic procedures.

Although the above procedures are usually followed in sequence for routine diagnostic cases, modification of this sequence or the procedures is appropriate in certain circumstances, particularly when the patient is critically ill. In the latter instance, the procedure is often tailored to allow obtaining the most *important* information first. For example, in a patient with refractory unstable angina in whom left main coronary artery stenosis is suspected, angiography of the left coronary artery system may be performed prior to left ventriculography or right coronary artery cineangiography. In occasional patients, left ventriculography is omitted, such as when severe renal disease exists (meriting a minimum use of contrast agent) or when severe ventricular dysfunction is present and the risk of further hemodynamic compromise is greater than the need to obtain angiographic information. In the latter case information from a two-dimensional echocardiogram or radionuclide ventriculogram can often be substituted for left ventricular cineangiography.

## CASE STUDIES

## Atypical Chest Pain—Normal Coronary Arteries

Registry data from the Society of Cardiac Angiography indicate that the frequency of finding normal coronary arteries at cardiac catheterization is about 20% with an additional 8% of patients having minimal disease.[5] However, these rates vary considerably in different laboratories. This variability undoubtedly reflects differing referral practices, and the extent to which noninvasive testing is utilized prior to cardiac catheterization. While assessment of the relative risk/benefit ratio is always necessary when one considers the use of an invasive test, there are situations when cardiac catheterization is appropriate for patients with atypical symptoms and a low risk of coronary artery disease, even after careful noninvasive screening.

Patients with recurrent chest pain not typical for classic angina pectoris may occasionally present a difficult problem even for the most experienced clinician. Studies of patients found to have normal coronary arteries at cardiac catheterization, many of whom have atypical chest pain, have failed to provide a unifying pathophysiologic explanation for this problematic syndrome.[6] Individual causes or relationships that have been identified include: mitral valve prolapse, costochondritis, esophageal spasm, epicardial coronary artery spasm, abnormally reduced coronary reserve, cardiomyopathy (of various types), and occult atherosclerotic coronary disease (i.e., undetectable by conventional angiography).[6-10] An extremely good prognosis has been noted in patients with either classic angina or atypical chest pain who are found to have angiographically normal or near normal coronary arteries.[6] Thus, the performance of coronary angiography to place such a patient in this favorable prognostic group may become necessary for either clinical or professional (such as for airline pilots) reasons. The following case demonstrates some of these issues and findings in one such patient.

*Case 1.* A 42-year-old woman with a family history of coronary artery disease has had chest pain for three years. She experienced similar chest pain 20 years earlier, but was then symptom free until chest pain recurred intermittently over the course of the last three years. Her pain occurs both at rest and with exertion, and at times it is relieved by nitroglycerin. She has never experienced syncope, does not complain of dyspnea on exertion, but has noted that palpitations occur during periods when the chest pain is more frequent. On three separate occasions she has been hospitalized following prolonged episodes of chest pain. On each admission a myocardial infarction was ruled out. Physical examination is entirely normal with the exception of an early systolic click. Resting ECG shows T wave inversions in the inferior leads. Exercise stress testing reveals fluctuating T wave changes with hyperventilation, but no significant ST segment deviation is seen with maximal exercise. A two-dimension echocardiogram demonstrates moderate prolapse of both the anterior and posterior mitral valve leaflets. A Doppler echocardiogram does not show mitral regurgitation.

At cardiac catheterization hemodynamic measurements and cardiac output are normal. Left ventriculography reveals normal motion of all walls with a calculated ejection fraction of 0.62. Prolapse of the posterior mitral leaflet is demonstrated on the ventriculogram (Fig. 24-1). No mitral regurgitation is seen. Coronary arteriograms are normal. Ergonovine testing fails to produce chest pain, ECG changes, or angiographic evidence of coronary artery spasm. Impression: Mitral valve prolapse and normal coronary arteries.

***Illustrative Points.*** The appropriate approach to most patients with mitral valve prolapse is one of reassurance and beta-blocker therapy to control both the symptoms of palpitations (which may be due to either supraventricular tachyarrhythmias or ventricular arrhythmias) and chest pain.

It is occasionally necessary to undertake cardiac catheterization to rule out coronary artery disease, even in patients with a low probability of that diagnosis. This case demonstrates the potential difficulty faced in managing some patients with chest pain. If the chest pain is in part characteristic of myocardial ischemia, if noninvasive testing is equivocal, and particularly if certain risk factors are present, the physician may be confronted with the potential for recurrent hospital admissions to rule out myocardial infarction. Although cardiac catheterization is probably not appropriate after the first such admission, invasive testing may become necessary before the decision can be made *not* to hospitalize such a patient each time chest pain occurs. In this case, the demonstration of normal coronary arteries allows the clinician to safely and confidently provide the necessary reassurance when confronted with an anxious and uncomfortable patient complaining of chest pain.

The diagnosis of mitral valve prolapse is usually made easily, without left ventriculography. In this case both the physical examination, which demonstrated a systolic click, and the echocardiogram were consistent with mitral valve prolapse. While the echocardiogram is probably the most sensitive diagnostic technique for demonstrating this abnormality, occasionally evidence of mitral valve prolapse may be found only by physical examination or left ventricular cineangiography. Mitral leaflet prolapse, such as demonstrated in this case, is most commonly due to myxomatous degeneration of the mitral valve apparatus.[11] However, papillary muscle dysfunction due to either myocardial ischemia or infarction is another frequent cause of mitral valve prolapse.[12] These papil-

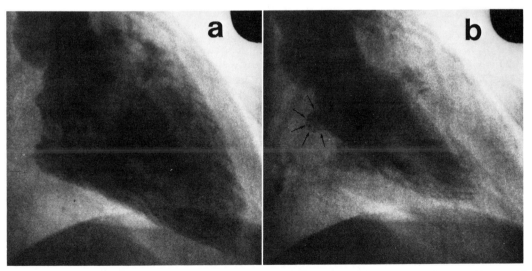

**Fig. 24-1.** Diastolic (a) and systolic (b) frames of a right anterior oblique left ventriculogram in a 42-year-old woman with chest pain (Case 1). Left ventricular contraction pattern is normal. Note prolapse (leftward bulging) of the posterior leaflet of the mitral valve (arrows, b) during systole.

lary muscle abnormalities are usually caused by coronary artery disease and most often occur in the context of more widespread evidence of myocardial dysfunction.

Whether or not mitral valve prolapse is present, patients with chest pain and normal coronary arteries have been shown to have a uniformly good prognosis for both survival and absence of cardiac events.[6] As noted above, no single unifying diagnosis is responsible for pain in most patients with this syndrome. Occasionally, as in the case above, a specific diagnosis can be made which leads to useful therapy.

## Variant Angina—Coronary Artery Spasm

The smooth muscle of epicardial coronary arteries is capable of producing a wide range of coronary arterial narrowing, including total occlusion. Coronary artery spasm may occur in the presence or absence of fixed atherosclerotic disease. *Variant angina* occurs when there is transient complete occlusion of a coronary artery causing chest pain and ST-segment elevation in the ECG leads that most closely monitor the area of myocardium that has become ischemic (e.g., inferior ECG leads for right coronary artery spasm or precordial leads for left anterior descending coronary artery spasm). In 1959 Myron Prinzmetal suggested that the association of these ECG changes with reversible, rest, ischemic chest pain was secondary to changes in coronary artery "tonus".[13] Since that time angiographic demonstration of this phenomenon has been commonly observed, and the terms *Prinzmetal's angina* or *variant angina* have become almost synonymous with coronary artery spasm.

Epicardial coronary artery spasm may occur spontaneously in the course of cardiac catheterization and may be demonstrated by coronary cineangiography. Minor changes in diameter may occur even in normal coronary arteries; such changes are often not apparent subjectively and require specialized techniques for their demonstration. More commonly, spasm causes total occlusion of a previously normal or narrowed segment. This phenomenon occurs most frequently in patients with the clinical syndrome of vari-

ant angina. An exception to this rule, however, is local spasm occurring at the tip of a coronary catheter. Although such catheter-induced spasm is seen most often at the ostium of the right coronary artery, it may occur at either coronary orifice with any angiographic catheter. As discussed in Chapter 13, various vasoconstrictor stimuli (e.g., ergonovine maleate) can be used as a diagnostic provocation for coronary artery spasm in patients with suspected variant angina. While normal coronary arteries respond to this pharmacologic stimulus by modest diffuse narrowing, patients with variant angina appear to be particularly sensitive and frequently respond with focal spasm totally occluding the coronary artery. This spasm often occurs at a site of fixed atherosclerotic narrowing which, prior to spasm, may have been mild, moderate, or severe.

Sudden coronary artery occlusion due to epicardial coronary artery spasm not only induces chest pain and ECG changes, but also is responsible for abnormalities which may be detected by scintigraphic techniques and ventriculography. Thallium scanning during an episode of variant angina shows a perfusion defect in the myocardium supplied by the coronary artery with spasm. Coincident with the onset of ischemia, hemodynamic abnormalities may be detected.[14] Appearing first is evidence of diastolic dysfunction, with an increase in left ventricular end diastolic pressure due to impaired relaxation of the ischemic segment. During systole, akinesia or even bulging of the ischemic segment may be demonstrated by left ventriculography. If a papillary muscle becomes ischemic as part of this process, then transient mitral regurgitation may occur with abnormally tall V waves seen in the pulmonary capillar wedge tracing. Regurgitation of contrast material into the left atrium may be seen during left ventriculography if the dye injection is performed during an ischemic episode.

Cardiac catheterization may be unnecessary in some cases of variant angina. This is particularly true when episodes of ischemic pain occur *only* at rest, and the problem responds easily to medical therapy with calcium channel blockers or nitrates. The following case demonstrates a more difficult problem where the diagnosis was obscure and difficulty was encountered with conventional therapy.

**Case 2.** Intermittently over the past 6 months a 36-year-old woman has had substernal chest pressure that radiates to her left shoulder and back. The discomfort typically occurs with exertion or emotional stress but also has occurred at rest and on occasion has awoken her from sleep. In addition, she has had episodes of epigastric discomfort associated with nausea and with dizziness. After a brief syncopal episode she is taken to a local emergency room where the physical examination and ECG are entirely normal. She is free of symptoms in the emergency room and is sent home, but because of concern for these episodes, an exercise stress test is scheduled. Two weeks later she undergoes a graded exercise treadmill test. After 8 minutes of exercise, she experiences precordial substernal chest pressure. Coincident with the onset of this symptom she develops ST-segment elevation in ECG leads V2 through V4. Exercise is terminated, and she is given one sublingual nitroglycerin. Early during the recovery period a 5-beat run of ventricular tachycardia is seen. She is given a second sublingual nitroglycerin, and the pain resolves completely after 6 minutes. When she is pain free, her electrocardiogram shows T inversions in the same precordial leads that had shown ST-segment elevation minutes earlier. She is admitted to the hospital to rule out a myocardial infarction. At the time of admission her physical examination is normal, as is her chest roentgenogram. By the second hospital day her electrocardiogram is normal as well. Cardiac enzymes are normal. Continuous single lead bedside monitoring of cardiac rhythm shows no further ventricular ectopy, but fluctuating T wave changes are seen. On the second hospital day she is placed on diltiazem, 60 mg tid.

Because of her young age and because of electrocardiographic evidence of severe ischemia with exercise, she is referred for cardiac catheterization. Diltiazem is discontinued 36 hours prior to catheterization. All hemodynamic measurements at rest are within normal limits. Left ventriculography reveals normal left ventricular function with synchronous contraction of all left ventricular walls. Coronary angiography shows a normal right coronary artery (Fig. 24-2a), a normal left circumflex coronary artery, and a minor stenosis of the left anterior descending coronary artery (Fig. 24-2b). She is given 0.05 mg of ergonovine maleate intravenously.

Ninety seconds later she notes the onset of both precordial chest discomfort and nausea. The ECG monitor (modified lead V1) shows ST-segment elevation where none had been present previously. Coronary angiography of her right coronary artery now reveals a tapering stenosis (approximately 70%) (Fig. 24-2c). Following injection of contrast medium into the right coronary artery, contrast agent is injected into the left system. This reveals subtotal occlusion of the left anterior descending artery (Fig. 24-2d).

The coronary catheter is passed retrograde into the left ventricle; LVEDP has now risen from 8 to 22 mmHg. Intravenous nitroglycerin (100 $\mu$g) is administered immediately after the recognition of provoked coronary artery spasm. Little change is observed in the patient's symptoms, and two minutes later complete heart block develops with a slow ventricular response. The right heart catheter, which had been inserted via a femoral sheath, is immediately withdrawn and a transvenous pacemaker is inserted in its place and positioned in the right ventricle with ventricular pacing rapidly achieved. Right and left intracoronary injections of nitroglycerin (200 $\mu$g each) are immediately administered. Within 45 seconds the patient begins to note abatement of symptoms, and one minute later sinus rhythm is restored. A continuous infusion of intravenous nitroglycerin is begun, and after a period of stability, the patient is transferred from the Cardiac Catheterization Laboratory to the Coronary Care Unit. Over a period of 48 hours a myocardial infarction is ruled out, and the patient is switched to oral isosorbide dinitrate and diltiazem is restarted.

On the third evening following catheterization the patient's roommate calls for nurse's assistance having observed the patient collapse suddenly following a brief complaint of dizziness. An electrocardiogram reveals complete heart block with marked ST-segment elevation in the inferior leads. Sublingual nitroglycerin and sublingual nifedipine are immediately administered, and the patient regains consciousness within 3 minutes. The diltiazem dose is increased to 90 mg three times daily; nifedipine is given in gradually increasing doses (finally 30 mg every six hours). Additionally, isosorbide dinitrate alternating with nitropaste is given every 4 hours while she is awake. On this regimen no further episodes of chest dis-

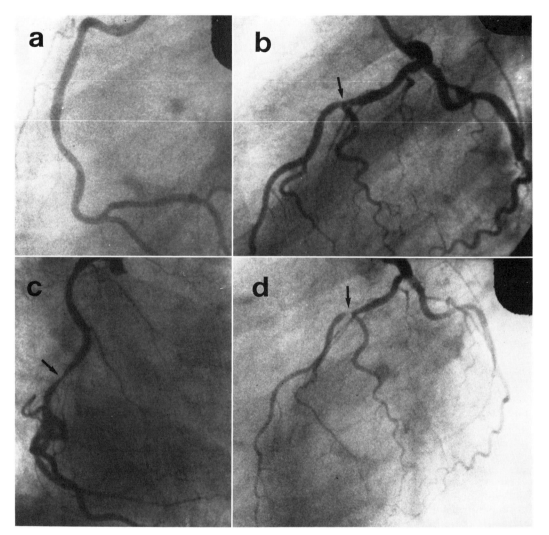

**Fig. 24-2.**   Coronary angiograms in a 36-year-old woman (Case 2) with chest pain and ST segment elevation during exercise. Right (a) and left (b) coronary arteries prior to ergonovine maleate; note the mild stenosis of the mid-left anterior descending artery (arrow, b) while the patient is asymptomatic. Coronary angiograms following the first dose of ergonovine maleate (0.05 mg) demonstrate spasm with tapering stenosis of the right coronary artery (arrow, c) and a high-grade stenosis of the left anterior descending coronary artery (arrow, d) at the site of the previously noted mild stenosis.

comfort, nausea, or heart block occur and the patient is discharged on the eighth hospital day. At follow-up, intermittently over the next 6 months, the patient reports occasional brief episodes of chest discomfort for which she takes a sublingual nitroglycerin, but she notes no prolonged episodes and syncope has not recurred.

***Illustrative Points.***   Although Prinzmetal, in his original series, describes several

patients who, at autopsy, were seen to have high grade atherosclerotic narrowing of at least one epicardial coronary artery,[13] it is recognized now that the syndrome of variant angina may occur in patients with any degree of atherosclerotic narrowing, including those totally free (by coronary angiography) of coronary atherosclerosis.[15] This patient demonstrated spasm at the site of a mild atherosclerotic lesion in her left anterior descending coronary artery. She also demonstrated spasm of an angiographically normal right coronary artery.

Many patients with variant angina have spasm at different sites. Only if the spasm occurs at the site of a severely stenosed artery can coronary bypass surgery be expected to be of benefit.[16] Such patients usually present with both exercise-induced and rest angina. However, as was seen in this case, even patients with normal or nearly normal coronary arteries may have exercise-induced coronary artery spasm. This case also points out the necessity of obtaining coronary angiograms of the entire coronary system when spasm is demonstrated in one portion, since coronary artery spasm may not be limited to a single artery.

Although modest generalized narrowing of the entire coronary arterial system can be seen with ergonovine maleate, particularly at higher doses,[17] severe focal narrowing is the hallmark of variant angina and probably does not occur in the normal population.[18] Even patients with atherosclerotic disease tend not to have focal spasm after ergonovine stimulation unless they also have rest angina. Conversely, the incidence of focal narrowing after ergonovine in patients with rest angina and atherosclerotic fixed narrowing is moderately high.[18]

Although most patients with variant angina respond nicely to the administration of a calcium channel blocker, about 10% of patients with this syndrome require multiple drug therapy. Administration of two different calcium channel blockers in conjunction with intermittent nitrate therapy can control the syndrome in virtually all patients.[19]

## Unstable Angina—Atheroslcerotic Coronary Disease

Many different terms have been used to describe the syndrome now commonly known as unstable angina. The premonitory syndrome, intermediate syndrome, preinfarction angina, crescendo angina, and coronary insufficiency are among the more commonly used ones. In its broadest definition unstable angina includes patients with new angina, increasingly severe angina, and rest angina. Some investigators, however, use the term *unstable angina* in a more limited way

for patients requiring hospital admission because of episodes of rest angina, particularly if such episodes do not respond immediately to medical therapy.

Unstable angina may be present with coronary artery disease of varying severity. Single, double, and triple vessel diseases occur about equally, with left main coronary artery stenosis occurring in about 15% of patients and normal coronary arteries being present in 10%.[20] Although the majority of patients with unstable angina do not go on to develop acute myocardial infarction, an important portion do (10 to 20%).[21,22] At least one study suggests that this clinical progression is frequently associated with angiographic progression of coronary artery stenoses to total occlusions.[23] The role of thrombosis superimposed on fixed atherosclerotic plaques is increasingly recognized in both acute myocardial infarction and unstable angina.[24,25] Additionally, plaque hemorrhage[26] and coronary artery spasm[27] are responsible for some cases of unstable angina.

As with variant angina, during episodes of unstable angina, evidence of systolic and diastolic dysfunction may appear. Once ischemia occurs, heart rate generally increases, mean arterial pressure rises,[27] (unless the quantity of myocardial ischemia is so large that systolic function is severely compromised, in which case blood pressure may fall) and left ventricular end diastolic pressure rises. Mitral and/or tricuspid regurgitation may occur or increase during ischemic episodes. This can be demonstrated by a sudden increase in right- and/or left-sided filling pressures with the presence of a prominent V wave in the pulmonary capillary wedge or right atrial tracings. The height of both the A and the V wave may rise in response to ischemia even when regurgitation across the AV valve is not present. Such a change occurs because ischemia-induced impairment of diastolic relaxation decreases the compliance of the left ventricle so that for the increase in volume occurring with ventricular filling a *greater* increase in pressure is seen than had been present prior to ischemia.

The following two cases are examples of patients with unstable angina. They are chosen to demonstrate both differing pathoanatomy and differing therapeutic options in this syndrome.

***Case 3.*** The patient is a previously

asymptomatic 47-year-old sedentary male executive with moderate hypercholesterolemia and a positive family history for coronary artery disease. He arrives at the emergency room after two days of stressful meetings, reporting an episode of substernal chest pressure that is now waning, but that half an hour earlier had been quite severe. Physical examination reveals blood pressure of 155/98 mmHg, heart rate of 94 beats/min., and otherwise normal findings with the exception of a loud fourth heart sound. His electrocardiogram shows T wave inversion in leads V2 through V6, and inverted T waves in leads II, III, and AVF. He is admitted to the Coronary Care Unit.

Twenty-four hours later his ECG is normal. His cardiac enzymes remain within the normal range, and he is transferred out of Coronary Care Unit. He is placed on long-acting nitrates and a beta-blocker, and an exercise stress test is scheduled. Twelve hours later, before undergoing exercise testing, he complains of mild substernal chest pressure. His ECG reveals biphasic T waves in the anterior leads, clearly abnormal and different from his admission electrocardiogram. The chest discomfort and ECG abnormalities revert promptly after one sublingual nitroglycerin. Because he is continuing to have symptoms at rest, because of strong reluctance on the part of the patient to continue medical therapy indefinitely, and because of his relatively young age, cardiac catheterization is scheduled. He is placed on a calcium channel blocking agent while awaiting catheterization. In the 24 hours prior to angiography, he suffers two further episodes of chest discomfort both relieved by sublingual nitroglycerin.

Cardiac catheterization reveals normal hemodynamics and calculated indices. Left ventriculography, which shows normal ventricular function and no mitral regurgitation, is used for calculation of his left ventricular ejection fraction, which is 0.60. Coronary angiography shows an occluded right coronary artery (Fig 24-3a). The left anterior descending coronary artery has an 85% stenosis proximal to the first septal perforator and to a large diagonal branch (Fig. 24-3b). The left circumflex coronary artery contains no important lesions. The right coronary artery is dominant, with a posterior descending artery, which had originally received antegrade flow via the right coronary artery but now is seen only after contrast injection into the left coronary artery to be filling via collaterals primarily from the distal portion of the left anterior descending coronary artery (Fig. 24-3c). Thus, two-vessel coronary artery disease with an occluded right coronary artery and severe stenosis of the left anterior descending coronary artery is present.

While both lesions could have developed simultaneously, it is more likely that one is old and the other recent. Severe stenosis of a coronary artery, even coronary artery occlusion, may occur silently if extensive collateralization is present to prevent ischemia of the distal myocardial bed. However, once a vessel supplying those collaterals becomes stenosed itself, then flow through the collaterals is compromised and ischemia may occur over a very wide territory.

Percutaneous transluminal coronary angioplasty (PTCA) may be safely and successfully accomplished in selected cases of total coronary artery occlusion.[28] In this case, PTCA was recommended. The right coronary artery occlusion was traversed with a flexible-tipped steerable guide wire (Fig. 24-3d) over which successful angioplasty was performed in the right coronary artery (Fig. 24-3e and f). Then, the left anterior descending coronary artery stenosis was successfully dilated as well (Fig. 24-3g and h).

***Illustrative Points.*** The presence of multiple risk factors in this relatively young man with typical symptoms of ischemia suggested that the probability of atherosclerotic coronary disease was high. Noninvasive testing was not necessary to make this diagnosis (although in a different setting it might have assisted in risk assessment). Thus, coronary angiography was not necessary for diagnosis, but rather for prognostic and management purposes, since his ECG with pain suggested an extensive amount of jeopardized myocardium. Additionally, this busy executive felt strongly opposed to taking medication on a long-term basis, particularly if a relatively safe mechanical alternative was available. In this case, coronary angioplasty could be undertaken and was successful. Despite the risk of restenosis at either of the angioplasty sites, the patient willingly chose that risk.

When inferior and anterior ECG changes are seen simultaneously, such as were present in this case, widespread myocardial ischemia must be considered. It has been ar-

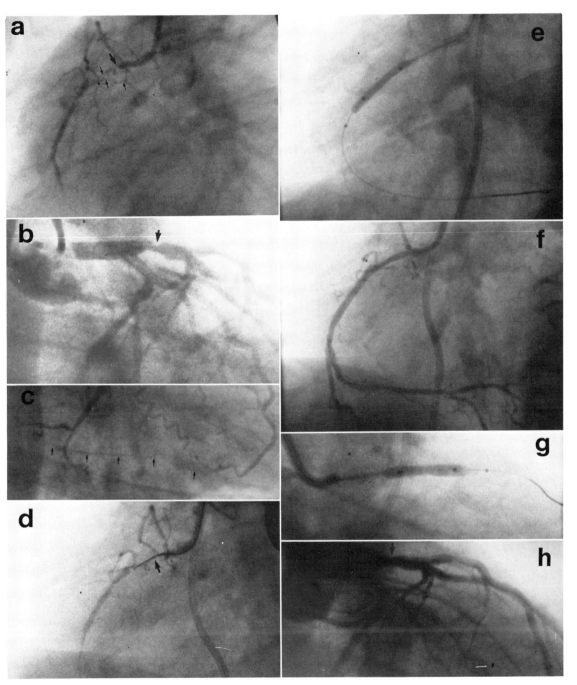

**Fig. 24-3.** (a) Right coronary angiogram in a 47-year-old man with unstable angina (Case 3) demonstrating a proximal total occlusion (large arrow) with bridging collateral vessels (small arrows) and poor distal runoff. There is a high-grade proximal stenosis of the left anterior descending coronary artery (b, arrow). Faintly visualized collateral vessels from the distal left anterior descending artery to the distal right coronary artery (c, arrows) are seen. A guide wire is used to cross the right coronary artery occlusion (d, arrow); this wire is then used to position the angioplasty balloon at the stenotic site where the balloon is inflated (e). Following angioplasty, the right coronary artery is widely patent (f) and excellent antegrade flow is present. Finally, angioplasty of the proximal left anterior descending stenosis is performed (g) and postangioplasty (h) the stenosis (arrow) is considerably reduced.

gued that anatomy such as described in the above case is a *true* "left main equivalent".[29] A high-grade stenosis of the left main coronary artery itself may present a precarious clinical situation. The risk with this defect is probably due to the area of myocardium which becomes ischemic and is thereby threatened by a *single* coronary artery stenosis. Thus, separate left anterior descending coronary artery and left circumflex coronary artery stenoses should not be considered "equivalent" to a left main coronary artery stenosis. However, when a severe stenosis occurs in one vessel that supplies collaterals to a previously occluded second vessel, true left main equivalency may be present (Fig. 24-4). Conversely, as long as the vessel supplying collaterals is not stenosed, extensive collaterals may protect against myocardial ischemia and myocardial infarction. Thus, even in the absence of prior infarction, totally occluded vessels are seen not uncommonly at the time of coronary angiography.

Ischemic ECG changes may persist after symptoms have resolved. It has been suggested that the myocardium remains "stunned" on some occasions following severe ischemia.[30] Persistent ECG changes may reflect metabolic abnormalities that can be present for as long as 7 days.

Case 3 demonstrates the fact that rest angina with relatively severe coronary stenoses may appear as the first manifestation of coronary artery disease. Although typical exertional angina occurs in many patients with similar coronary pathoanatomy, the first manifestation in some may be unstable angina or acute myocardial infarction. Myocardial ischemia and even infarction may occur silently in as many as a third of all patients with coronary artery disease.[31] Additionally, many patients with angina pectoris have frequent episodes of ischemia (as evidenced by transient ECG changes on ambulatory monitoring) in the absence of perceptible symptoms.[32] Thus, the duration, timing, and severity of symptoms are relatively poor predictors of the *extent* of coronary artery disease present.

*Case 4.* A 57-year-old insurance salesman noted precordial chest discomfort while jogging. The symptom had been present for 5 months, provoked by progressively less exertion. Over the last 2 weeks chest discomfort occurred with walking and modest exercise.

The patient seeks medical attention and an exercise stress test is performed prior to planned medical therapy. A standard exercise protocol is utilized and the patient complains of moderately severe precordial pressure 4 minutes after beginning exercise. At that point, 3 mm of ST-segment depression is noted in leads V1 through V5, and the patient's systolic blood pressure, which had been 140 mmHg prior to exercise, has fallen to 115 mmHg. Because of the strongly positive stress test with angina, marked ST-segment depression, and a fall in blood pressure, all at a low work load, the patient is referred for cardiac catheterization.

Prior to angiography, all hemodynamic measurements are normal. Left ventriculography is normal, with a calculated ejection fraction of 0.65. Cineangiography of the right coronary artery reveals no focal lesions. In the left coronary artery system a 90% stenosis of the left main coronary artery is present (Fig. 24-5a) with a 70% stenosis of the left anterior descending coronary artery and a total occlusion of the circumflex artery immediately after the origin of its large first marginal branch (Fig. 24-5b). The distal circumflex territory is supplied by collaterals from the right coronary artery. Shortly after the second contrast injection of the left system, the patient begins to complain of precordial chest pressure. The ECG monitor lead shows ST-segment depression. Pulmonary capillary wedge pressure has risen from normal to 18 mmHg. Repeat contrast injection of the left coronary artery system shows no change in the previously visualized stenoses and no focal spasm. The patient is given sublingual nitroglycerin which briefly diminishes his precordial chest pain, but the discomfort returns within 15 minutes. An intravenous nitroglycerin infusion, sublingual nifedipine, and 4 mg of intravenous propranolol (given slowly over 10 minutes) fail to completely relieve the patient's chest discomfort or return his ST-segment depression to baseline.

Thirty minutes after the onset of chest pain, the coronary angiographic catheter is exchanged, over a guide wire, first for a dialator with a larger diameter, and then for a percutaneously introduced intraaortic balloon. Counterpulsation with the intraaortic balloon pump is rapidly instituted, and within several minutes the patient's precor-

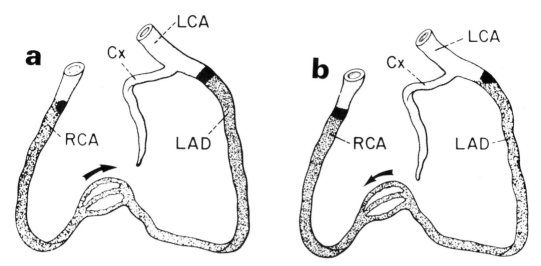

**Fig. 24-4.** Two examples of possible left main "equivalency." Two-vessel coronary disease with an occluded left anterior descending coronary artery (LAD) and myocardium jeopardized by a right coronary artery (RCA) stenosis (a) or an occluded RCA and myocardium jeopardized by a stenotic LAD (b). LCA = left coronary artery; Cx = circumflex coronary artery. (From Hutter AM Jr: Is there a left main equivalent? Circulation 62:207, 1980.)

dial chest discomfort is entirely abolished. A 12-lead ECG taken at that time is unchanged from the precatheterization tracing.

The patient remains stable without evidence of myocardial necrosis over a period of 24 hours. On the day following catheterization, coronary artery bypass graft surgery is performed with grafts placed to the left anterior descending artery and both first and second large left circumflex marginal arteries.

***Illustrative Points.*** While a trial of medical therapy is appropriate for most patients with angina pectoris, occasionally it is useful to perform cardiac catheterization early in the course of the disease. A strongly positive exercise stress test, as was present in this case, is considered by many clinicians an indication for early angiography. Although the exercise stress test was not necessary for the diagnosis of coronary disease in this case, it was useful for prognostic purposes and did lead to a surgical intervention in precisely the kind of case (left main disease) where surgery has been shown to be of benefit when compared with medical therapy.[33] Percutaneous transluminal coronary angioplasty is not usually recommended for left main coronary artery stenosis.[34] Although the risk of acute occlusion with angioplasty is relatively small (probably less than

10%), the consequences of such an event at the site of a left main stenosis could be catastrophic.

Intraaortic balloon counterpulsation is of great value in refractory unstable angina.[35] Control of ischemia may often be achieved even when all pharmacologic modalities have been applied maximally and failed. In controlling ischemia with normal ventricular function, the primary mechanism by which the balloon pump exerts its effect is through the reduction of afterload. By diminishing left ventricular systolic pressure, myocardial oxygen demand is decreased. Although it has been suggested that diastolic augmentation increases coronary flow to the ischemic myocardium, this has not yet been demonstrated unequivocally in the clinical setting. In recent years the availability of intraaortic balloon catheters which may be inserted percutaneously, rather than surgically, has brought this procedure out of the operating room and into the cardiac catheterization laboratory.[36] However, percutaneous insertion has probably not lowered the risk of this procedure, and like any other invasive procedure, its potential benefit must be weighed against known risks before making the decision to proceed with its insertion. Medically refractory ischemia in the setting of left main coronary stenosis, with surgically operable

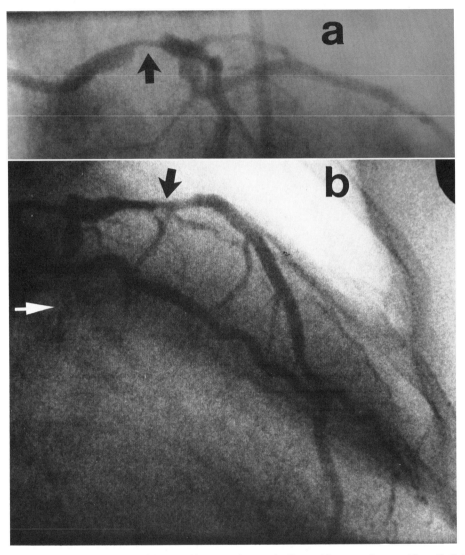

**Fig. 24-5.** Coronary angiogram in a 57-year-old man with a markedly positive exercise test (Case 4). Selective view of the left main coronary artery (a) showing a severe eccentric stenosis (arrow). Angiogram of the entire left coronary artery system (b) in a right anterior oblique view demonstrating proximal left anterior descending disease (large arrow) and a total occlusion of the circumflex system (small arrow) distal to its first large marginal artery. The distal circumflex artery is only faintly visible in the lower left corner of panel b.

disease, is an ideal circumstance in which to consider intraaortic balloon pumping.

## Multivessel Coronary Disease and Left Ventricular Dysfunction

Necrosis of 40% or more of the left ventricle generally leads to cardiogenic shock, and survival in that situation is rare.[37] Less extensive myocardial infarction may produce varying degrees of systolic and diastolic dysfunction. The extent of hemodynamic compromise is based on both the area of muscle damaged and its location. For example, extensive damage of the right ventricle may occur with only modest necrosis of the left ventricle. In this circumstance, signs or symptoms of right-sided congestive failure, such as marked peripheral edema, may occur without pulmonary congestion and without clinical evidence of low forward cardiac output. In another example, a small infarction involving a papillary muscle and myocardium supporting that papillary muscle may be responsible for intermittent episodes of pulmonary edema due to mitral regurgitation induced by the papillary muscle dysfunction. Thus, assessment of coronary pathoanatomy in conjunction with evaluation of left ventricular function and hemodynamics can be exceedingly important in the management of patients with a wide variety of ischemic syndromes and clinical evidence of ventricular dysfunction. The following case demonstrates that symptoms of congestive heart failure and myocardial ischemia cannot be viewed independently of one another.

*Case 5.* The patient is a 62-year-old salesman with 10 years of insulin requiring diabetes mellitus, hyperlipidemia, and a positive family history for premature coronary disease. He suffered an inferior wall myocardial infarction 15 years ago and a moderately large anterior wall myocardial infarction 6 months ago. Although the latter infarction was not associated with acute complications, he developed basilar rales, and diuretic therapy with furosemide was instituted prior to his discharge. At present he reports throat tightness after walking two blocks. The symptom is associated with modest shortness of breath. He has two-pillow orthopnea but no paroxysmal nocturnal dyspnea. His current therapeutic regimen includes furosemide, nitroglycerin ointment, and low-dose metroprolol (decreased from higher doses because of his exertional dyspnea, but continued at a low dose because, in its absence, resting tachycardia had been present).

Physical examination reveals a blood pressure of 105/70 mmHg and a regular pulse of 64 beats/min. Jugular venous pressure is approximately 8 cm of water; carotid upstrokes are normal. Lung examination reveals rales at the left base. The cardiac apex is displaced laterally 2 cm. The first heart sound is normal; the second heart sound is split paradoxically. A loud fourth heart sound is present and a Grade 1/6 murmur is audible at the apex, with radiation to the base. Peripherally, bilateral trace ankle edema is present and pulses are intact. The electrocardiogram reveals sinus rhythm with

left atrial enlargement, left bundle branch block, and inferior and anterior Q waves with diffuse ST and T wave abnormalities. An exercise stress test is performed with thallium imaging. Throat tightness and some precordial discomfort occur in association with shortness of breath, all beginning at 5 minutes of exercise. Electrocardiogaphic changes are seen but are uninterpretable due to the presence of the preexisting left bundle branch block. Thallium imaging during stress reveals defects of the inferior apical, septal, anterior, and posterior lateral walls. Images obtained four hours after exercise show no change in the anterior and septal defects, but dimunution in size of the inferior-apical defect and almost complete disappearance of the posterior-lateral defect. A radionuclide ventriculogram reveals a left ventricular ejection fraction of 0.32.

Because of the patient's activity limitation, with symptoms and evidence by thallium scans of reversible ischemia, despite the presence of congestive heart failure and a depressed ejection fraction, cardiac catheterization is undertaken. That study reveals the following hemodynamics at rest:

Pressures: mmHg

| | |
|---|---|
| Right atrium, mean | 8 |
| Right ventricle | 33/9 |
| Pulmonary artery | 33/20, $\overline{25}$ |
| Pulmonary capillary wedge, mean | 16 |
| Left ventricle | 106/25 |
| Aorta | 106/60 |
| Cardiac output, L/min | 5.2 |
| Cardiac index, L/min/m$^2$ | 2.8 |
| Systemic vascular resistance, dynes-sec-cm$^{-5}$ | 1108 |
| LV end diastolic volume index | 90 |
| LV end systolic volume index | 53 |
| LV ejection fraction | 0.36 |

Left ventriculography revealed multiple localized wall motion abnormalities with anterior akinesis and inferior-apical hypokinesis (Fig. 24-6a and b). Only trace mitral regurgitation is present. Coronary angiography shows extensive, multivessel disease with a near total occlusion of the right coronary artery (Fig. 24-6c), a high-grade stenosis of the left anterior descending coronary artery (perhaps representing recannulized thrombus), a stenoses of the proximal left circum-

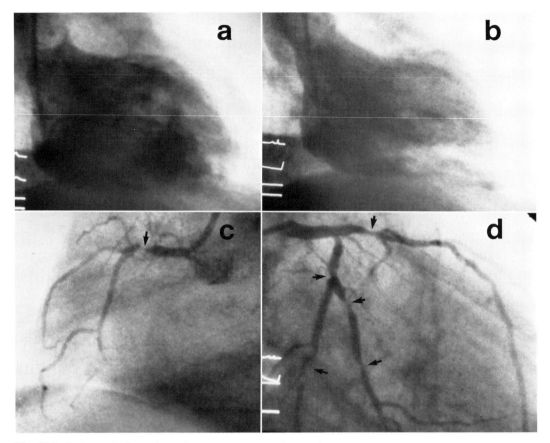

**Fig. 24-6.** Left ventriculography and coronary angiography in a 62-year-old diabetic man with prior myocardial infarction (Case 5). Diastolic (a) and systolic (b) frames from a left ventriculogram show anterior akinesis and inferior and apical hypokinesis. Coronary angiography reveals a near total occlusion of the proximal right coronary artery (c, arrow), and multiple lesions of the left coronary system (d, arrows).

flex coronary artery, and severe stenoses of the first and second obtuse marginal branches of that artery (Fig. 24-6d).

Coronary artery bypass surgery is recommended, and the patient accepts this recommendation despite a slight increase in risk related to impaired left ventricular function. The patient undergoes four vessel bypass graft surgery and recovers uneventfully. Two months following surgery, a repeat exercise stress test with thallium is markedly improved, with the patient exercising for 9 minutes before stopping due to exertional dyspnea. No throat tightness occurs. Thallium scintigraphy demonstrates continued presence of the previously seen persistent defects, but absence of the previously shown reversible posterior-lateral defect.

*Illustrative Points.* In this case, symp-

toms of ischemia and congestion occurred nearly simultaneously. This may not always be the case; sometimes symptoms of congestive heart failure may obscure clinical evidence of reversible ischemia. Noninvasive testing may be exceedingly useful in this situation. Exercise-induced ischemia may be apparent from thallium scintigraphy and the effect of ischemia on ventricular function may be demonstrated by exercise radionuclide ventriculography.[38] When such studies demonstrate the presence of *both* ventricular dysfunction and active myocardial ischemia, proceeding to invasive examination may be appropriate regardless of the fact that ventricular function is moderately or even severely compromised. The Coronary Artery Surgery Study (CASS) has demonstrated that surgical therapy may be of benefit in asymptomatic patients or those with mild symptoms of ischemia when three-vessel coronary artery disease and left ventricular dysfunction (ejection fraction 0.35 to 0.50) are present.[39] In an earlier era of coronary artery bypass graft surgery, operating on patients with depressed ventricular function was often considered too risky. However, with improved surgical techniques, including better methods for intraoperative myocardial preservation, depressed left ventricular function has a less important impact on operative survival. Although the primary purpose of cardiac catheterization in these cases remains the delineation of coronary pathoanatomy for possible bypass surgery in order to control angina, evidence is accumulating that the ventricular function may be improved in some patients, particularly during exertion.[40]

In the future, control of even modest ischemia by mechanical procedures such as coronary artery bypass graft surgery or coronary angioplasty may be appropriate in patients with congestive heart failure so that newer inotropic agents may be utilized. Patients previously considered inoperable because of severe ventricular dysfunction may become appropriate candidates for cardiac catheterization when mechanical procedures to control their ischemia can be combined with the administration of more powerful inotropic agents to improve cardiac function.

## Acute Myocardial Infarction—Interventional Therapy

Until relatively recently cardiac catheterization was not generally performed on patients during an acute myocardial infarction or early after one. The procedure was avoided both because of a presumed increase in risk and because the diagnostic information obtained from that study was of little use *during* acute myocardial infarction. Advances in our understanding of the pathophysiology of infarction and the availabililty of newer therapeutic modalities have led to more frequent cardiac catheterization in the early hours of myocardial infarction. It is recognized that vasospasm is responsible for some cases of myocardial infarction, and in occasional cases the infusion of intracoronary nitroglycerin via an angiographic cathe-

ter can open a previously occluded coronary artery.[41] Within minutes ST-segments may revert to baseline and chest discomfort may resolve. Investigators in Spokane, Washington, have demonstrated that cardiac catheterization can be performed safely in the early hours of acute myocardial infarction for the purpose of selecting vessels for acute surgical revascularization.[24] In this group's hands early coronary artery bypass surgery for acute myocardial infarction has been demonstrated to be possible with a very low incidence of complications. While this approach has not been shown to be more beneficial than medical therapy in a randomized controlled trial, the studies of the Spokane group have contributed importantly in other ways. In addition to demonstrating the safety of cardiac catheterization and bypass surgery in acute myocardial infarction, data on the coronary artery pathoanatomy became available from the earliest hours of the infarction process. Coronary artery thrombosis was seen in the vast majority of cases, and the incidence of this finding was greater the earlier a patient was studied.[24] Thus, the importance of thrombosis in the infarction process has received increasingly careful attention.

The recognition that a thrombus is present in the majority of coronary artery occlusions with acute myocardial infarction has led to mechanical and pharmacologic attempts to improve flow by disrupting or lysing the clot.[42] Mechanical attempts at recanalization have included the use of a soft tipped guidewire[43] and the angioplasty balloon catheter.[44] Pharmacologic interventions have included the use of the fibrinolytic agents streptokinase, urokinase, and more recently, tissue plasminogen activator.[42] While it has been demonstrated that flow can be restored in the majority of patients, it remains to be proven that this restoration of flow is of long-term benefit. Although individual cases of myocardial salvage certainly have occurred, the widespread efficacy of these techniques to preserve myocardium remains controversial. Additionally, it is not clear that mechanical or pharmacologic recanalization decreases the incidence of future ischemic events or prolongs survival. The following case is chosen to demonstrate the paradox of angiographic improvement without obvious preservation of myocardial function.

***Case 6.*** The patient is a 34-year-old taxi

driver with a positive family history of coronary disease and a history of heavy cigarette smoking. Forty-five minutes after the onset of substernal chest pressure, he drives his taxi to the Emergency Room where he reports that his precordial discomfort is extremely severe. He is noted to be quite diaphoretic, his blood pressure is 190/110 mmHg, and his heart rate is 100 beats/min. His chest is clear, the cardiac examination is normal, with the exception of a fourth heart sound, and the remainder of his physical examination is within normal limits. The electrocardiogram reveals 3 to 5 mm of ST-segment elevation in leads V1 through V5. The team responsible for administrating intracoronary streptokinase is notified 15 minutes after the patient's arrival in the Emergency Room (1 hour after the onset of chest pain). Within an additional 15 minutes the decision is made to take the patient to the Cardiac Catheterization Laboratory. However, because another procedure is being performed in the laboratory, the patient waits in the Emergency Room (where he receives nitrates, morphine, and a beta-blocker) for an additional 1 hour and 15 minutes.

Two and one-half hours after the onset of symptoms, the patient enters the Cardiac Catheterization Laboratory, where angiography of the right coronary artery reveals a normal, dominant vessel. The left coronary artery system is visualized, revealing total occlusion of the left anterior descending coronary artery in its proximal portion (Fig. 24-7a). No collaterals to the distal left anterior descending artery are visible on either the right or left coronary contrast injections. After injection of intracoronary nitroglycerin (which fails to open the occlusion), an infusion of intracoronary streptokinase is begun via the coronary angiographic catheter. Angiography 10 minutes after the initiation of this infusion shows no change, but at 20 minutes, faint distal opacification of the left anterior descending artery is visualized. Ten minutes later brisk flow is seen through a moderately stenosed proximal left anterior descending artery. Complete opacification of the distal artery is now seen (Fig. 24-7b). Left ventriculography reveals a large area of anterior wall akinesis (Fig. 24-8). Hyperkinesis of the noninfarcted walls is present. The calculated ejection fraction is 0.42. The patient experiences no further signs or symptoms of myocardial ischemia.

Catheterization is repeated two weeks later and reveals further improvement of the previously seen left anterior descending artery stenosis. The patient's left ventricular end diastolic pressure, which was 26 mmHg at the end of the previous procedure, has fallen slightly to 20 mmHg. There is no improvement in his left ventriculogram (Fig. 24-8c and d); in fact, with less vigorous contraction of the noninfarcted segments, his ejection fraction has fallen to 0.33.

Six months later, the patient notes progressively worsening exertional dyspnea. After treatment with digoxin and diuretics there is a slight improvement in symptoms. A radionuclide ventriculogram obtained at this time reveals marked left ventricular dilatation, a large anterior apical dyskinetic segment, and an ejection fraction of 0.30.

***Illustrative Points.*** Time is clearly critical in the salvage of ischemic myocardium.[45] Both myocardial oxygen demand and oxygen supply are important in determining the timing of progression from reversible ischemia to necrosis. This case demonstrates the all too frequent practical problems involved in delivering an *intracoronary* thrombolytic agent. Obviously, 3 hours and 20 minutes was too long a period of ischemia in this young man who presented with hypertension and tachycardia, and who had no evidence of collateral circulation to the territory supplied by the occluded vessel. Had recanalization been achieved earlier, had myocardial oxygen demand been lower, or had adequate collaterals been present, thrombolytic therapy might have salvaged some or all of this individual's left ventricular anterior wall. Administration of thrombolytic agents *intravenously* permits earlier thrombolysis. However, systemic therapy may be accompanied by more frequent bleeding complications. Newer, clot-specific agents, such as tissue plasminogen activator, may be ideal for intravenous administration. This agent appears to achieve coronary thrombolysis without undue risk and with greater success than that achieved with intravenous streptokinase.[46]

Profoundly ischemic muscle may demonstrate hypoactive function and metabolic abnormalities as long as 10 days after the ischemia is relieved.[30] Thus, left ventriculography in the early hours after successful recanalization should not necessarily be expected to show improvement in ventricular function. By two weeks, however, the ef-

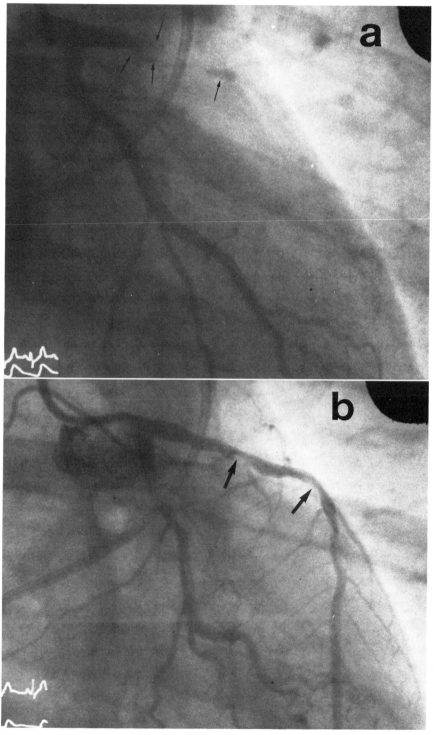

**Fig. 24-7.** Coronary angiogram of the left coronary system in a 34-year-old man with an acute anterior myocardial infarction (Case 6) before (a) recanalization of the left anterior descending coronary artery occlusion with intracoronary streptokinase. The intracoronary thrombosis is outlined by slight angiographic "staining" (arrows). After recanalization (b) only moderately stenotic lesions are visible (arrows) and excellent antegrade flow is restored.

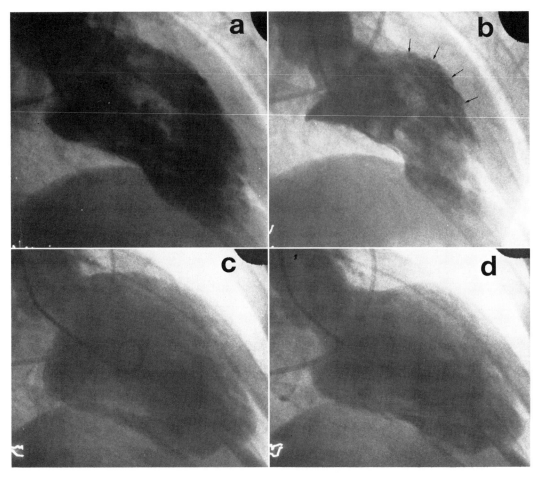

**Fig. 24-8.** Left ventriculography in Case 6. Diastolic (a) and systolic (b) frames from the left ventriculogram obtained minutes after the successful thrombolysis demonstrated in Figure 24-7. Note anterior akinesis (arrows, b) with apical hypokinesis and vigorous contraction of the remaining perimeter. Two weeks later the diastolic volume has increased slightly (c) and anterior wall motion is unimproved (d); contraction of the remaining perimeter is less vigorous than that present on the earlier angiogram.

fects of reversible ischemia should no longer be present, and thus the left ventriculogram performed in this patient 14 days after his first procedure provides an accurate picture of myocardial salvage (or lack of salvage). In the months following acute myocardial infarction, remodeling of the ventricle probably occurs.[47] In some cases actual expansion and thinning of the infarcted area may be present. Bulging of this segment in systole then leads to the characteristic dyskinetic appearance of a ventricular aneurysm. The remaining area of ventricle is forced to "take over" for portions of the ventricle that are no longer functional. This increased load on previously normal myocardium may be functionally similar to the volume load introduced with valvular lesions such as aortic or mitral regurgitation. Recent evidence suggests that this "volume load" introduced by the nonfunctioning myocardium frequently produces dilatation of the ventricle, not only through infarct expansion but also through expansion of the remaining normal perimeter.[47] These observations explain, in part, progressive increases in congestive symptoms due to the rise in left ventricular end diastolic pressure that may occur with dilatation. Although this increase in volume and pressure may be adaptive in terms of maintaining forward flow, diastolic function is compromised, producing symptoms of congestion.

# REFERENCES

1. Johnson RA, Daggett WM Jr: Heart failure resulting from coronary artery disease. *In* Johnson RA, Haber E, Austen WG (eds): The Practice of Cardiology. Boston, Little, Brown, 1980, pp. 339–342.
2. Proudfit WJ, et al: Fifteen year survival study of patients with obstructive coronary artery disease. Circulation 68:986, 1983.
3. Harris PJ, et al: Survival in medically treated coronary artery disease. Circulation 60:1259, 1979.
4. Mock MB, et al: Survival of medically treated patients in the coronary artery surgery study (CASS) registry. Circulation 66:562, 1982.
5. Kennedy JW: Complications associated with cardiac catheterization and angiography. Cathet Cardiovasc Diagn 8:5, 1982.
6. Pasternak RC, et al: Chest pain with angiographically insignificant coronary arterial obstruction. Clinical presentation and long-term follow-up. Am J Med 68:813, 1980.
7. Nakhjavan FK, Natarajan G, Seshachary P, Goldberg H: The relationship between prolapsing mitral leaflet syndrome and angina and normal coronary arteriograms. Chest 70:706, 1976.
8. Opherk D, et al: Reduced coronary dilatory capacity and ultrastructural changes of the myocardium in patients with angina pectoris but normal coronary arteriograms. Circulation 63:817, 1981.
9. Herman MV, Cohen PF, Gorlin R: Angina-like chest pain without identifiable cause. Ann Intern Med 79:445, 1973.
10. James TN: Angina without coronary disease (sic). Circulation 42:189, 1970.
11. Devereux RB, Perloff JK, Reichek N, Josephson ME: Mitral valve prolapse. Circulation 54:3, 1976.
12. Aranda JM, et al: Mitral valve prolapse and coronary artery disease. Clinical, hemodynamic, and angiographic correlations. Circulation 52:245, 1975.
13. Prinzmetal M, et al: Angina pectoris. I. A variant form of angina pectoris. Am J Med 27:375, 1959.
14. Gaasch WH, et al: Prinzmetal's variant angina: Hemodynamic and angiographic observations during pain. Am J Cardiol 35:683, 1975.
15. Luchi RJ, Chahine RA, Raizner AE: Coronary artery spasm. Ann Intern Med 91:441, 1979.
16. Pasternak RC, et al: Variant angina. Clinical spectrum and results of medical and surgical therapy. J Thorac Cardiovasc Surg 78:614, 1979.
17. Cipriano PR, et al: The effects of ergonovine maleate on coronary arterial size. Circulation 59:82, 1979.
18. Schroeder JS, et al: Provocation of coronary spasm with ergonovine maleate. Am J Cardiol 40:487, 1977.
19. Kimura E, Kishida H: Treatment of variant angina with drugs: A survey of 11 cardiology institutes in Japan. Circulation 63:844, 1981.
20. Alison HW, et al: Coronary anatomy and arteriography in patients with unstable angina pectoris. Am J Cardiol 41:204, 1978.
21. Gazes PC, et al: Preinfarctional (unstable) angina—a prospective study—ten year follow-up. Circulation 48:331, 1973.
22. Mulcahy R, et al: Unstable angina: Natural history and determinants of prognosis. Am J Cardiol 48:525, 1981.
23. Neill WA, Wharton TP, Fluri-Lundeen J, Cohen IS: Acute coronary insufficiency-coronary occlusion after intermittent ischemic attacks. N Engl J Med 302:1157, 1980.
24. DeWood MA, et al: Prevalence of total coronary occlusion during the early hours of transmural myocardial infarction. N Engl J Med 303:898, 1980.
25. Mandelkorn JB, et al: Intracoronary thrombus in nontransmural myocardial infarction and in unstable angina pectoris. Am J Cardiol 52:1, 1983.
26. Caulfield JB, Gold HK, Leinbach RC: Coronary artery lesions associated with unstable angina (abst). Am J Cardiol 35:126, 1975.
27. Maseri A, et al: Coronary vasospasm as a possible cause of myocardial infarction. A conclusion derived from the study of "preinfarction angina." N Engl J Med 299:1271, 1978.
28. Dervan JP, Baim DS, Cherniles J, Grossman W: Transluminal angioplasty of occluded coronary arteries: Use of a movable guide wire system. Circulation 68:776, 1983.
29. Hutter AM: Is there a left main equivalent? Circulation 62:207, 1980.
30. Braunwald E, Kloner RA: The stunned myocardium: Prolonged, postischemic ventricular dysfunction. Circulation 66:1146, 1982.
31. Medalie JH, Goldbourt MA: Unrecognized myocardial infarction: Five-year incidence, mortality, and risk factors. Ann Intern Med 84:526, 1976.
32. Deanfield JE, et al: Transient ST-segment depression as a marker of myocardial ischemia during daily life. Am J Cardiol 54:1195, 1984.
33. Chaitman BR, et al: Effect of coronary bypass surgery on survival patterns in subsets of patients with left main coronary artery disease. Am J Cardiol 48:765, 1981.
34. Gruntzig AR, Senning A, Siegenthaler WE: Nonoperative dilatation of coronary-artery stenosis. N Engl J Med 301:61, 1979.
35. Weintraub RM, et al: Medically refractory unstable angina pectoris. I. Long-term follow-up of patients undergoing intraaortic balloon counterpulsation and operation. AM J Cardiol 43:877, 1979.
36. Bregman D, et al: Percutaneous intraaortic balloon insertion. Am J Cardiol 46:261, 1980.
37. Page DL, et al: Myocardial changes associated with cardiogenic shock. N Engl J Med 285:133, 1971.
38. Upton MT, et al: Detecting abnormalities in left

ventricular function during exercise before angina and ST-segment depression. Circulation
62:341, 1980.

39. Passamani, E, Davis, KB, Gillespie, MJ, Killip, T,
and CASS principal investigators and their associates: A randomized trial of coronary artery bypass surgery: survival of patients with a low ejection fraction. N Engl J Med 312:1665, 1985.

40. Kronenberg MW, et al. Left ventricular performance after coronary artery bypass surgery. Ann
Intern Med 99:305, 1983.

41. Oliva PB, Breckinridge JC: Arteriographic evidence of coronary arterial spasm in acute myocardial infarction. Circulation 56:366, 1977.

42. Laffel GL, Braunwald E: Thrombolytic therapy. A
new strategy for the treatment of acute myocardial infarction. N Engl J Med 311:710, 770, 1984.

43. Rentrop P, DeVivie ER, Karsch KR, Kreuzer H:
Acute coronary occlusion with impending infarction as an angiographic complication relieved by
a guide-wire recanalization. Clin Cardiol 1:101,
1978.

44. Pepine CJ, et al: Percutaneous transluminal coronary angioplasty in acute myocardial infarction.
Am Heart J 107:820, 1984.

45. Rude RE, Muller JE, Braunwald E: Efforts to limit
the size of myocardial infarcts. Ann Intern Med
95:736, 1981.

46. The TIMI Study Group: The thrombolysis in myocardial infarction (TIMI) trial: Phase I findings. N
Engl J Med 312:932, 1985.

47. McKay R, et al: Left ventricular remodelling following myocardial infarction—a corollary to infarct expansion (abst). Circulation 70 (II):II, 1984.

## chapter twenty five

# Profiles in Pulmonary Embolism

JOSEPH R. BENOTTI *and* WILLIAM GROSSMAN

P ULMONARY embolism usually manifests itself as one or more clinically and hemodynamically distinct syndromes: acute unexplained dyspnea, pulmonary infarction syndrome, cardiogenic shock and cor pulmonale, or chronic pulmonary hypertension with right ventricular failure resulting from persistent or unresolved pulmonary embolism. These syndromes often have somewhat distinct hemodynamic profiles that support the diagnosis and exclude other conditions that would require alternate therapeutic strategies.

## DIAGNOSIS

The clinical manifestations of pulmonary embolism are often nonspecific. In previously healthy persons pulmonary embolism may mimic pneumonia or viral pleurisy;[1] in older patients with underlying cardiopulmonary disease it may present as worsening heart failure or an acute exacerbation of chronic obstructive lung disease.[2] No laboratory tests are sufficiently sensitive or specific to be useful in diagnosing pulmonary embolism.[3] At one time, arterial hypoxemia in a patient breathing room air was believed to be sufficiently sensitive to be of value as a screening test for diagnosing pulmonary embolism; however, at least one study has found that approximately 13% of patients with pulmonary embolism have an arterial

oxygen tension exceeding 80 mmHg while breathing room air.[4] Normal arterial oxygenation in these patients may be related to a compensatory decline in regional ventilation that complements the reduction in regional perfusion resulting from pulmonary embolism. The end result could be minimal or no ventilation perfusion mismatch and arterial normoxia, which has been reported even in occasional patients with massive pulmonary embolism.[5] Normal arterial blood oxygen saturation is more likely in the younger patient without underlying cardiopulmonary disease who sustains a small pulmonary embolus.[6]

Other patients may have fever, hemoptysis, pleurisy, and parenchymal lung infiltrates resulting from a small to moderate size pulmonary embolism—the so-called pulmonary infarction syndrome.[7] Massive pulmonary embolism may present as syncope and shock. Unresolved pulmonary embolism may manifest itself as pulmonary hypertension and right heart failure.

***EKG Findings.*** Electrocardiographic abnormalities associated with pulmonary embolism are relatively insensitive and nonspecific.[8] Sinus tachycardia, the most common abnormality, is not present with sufficient frequency to be useful for screening and has no specificity. EKG findings that are more suggestive of pulmonary embolism include the $S_1Q_3T_3$ pattern (S wave in lead I, Q wave and inverted T wave in lead III),[9] complete or incomplete right bundle branch

403

block of new onset, and other manifestations of acute right ventricular strain. Unfortunately, these findings are very uncommon in pulmonary embolism,[10] and occur primarily in patients with massive embolism.

***Femoral Venography.*** Previous investigations have emphasized the pathophysiologic role of deep venous thrombosis involving the veins above the knee in the genesis of pulmonary embolism. Approximately 90% of patients presenting with pulmonary embolism have evidence of deep venous thrombosis involving the thigh by objective testing using impedance plethysmography or contrast venography.[11] These latter tests are felt by some to be useful as screening procedures for pulmonary embolism. That is, in a patient with a clinical presentation compatible with pulmonary embolism, but with an indeterminate or nondiagnostic ventilation–perfusion lung scan, if concomitant evidence of deep venous thrombosis in the thigh is not demonstrable by objecting testing, the diagnosis of pulmonary embolism is highly unlikely. Conversely objective evidence of deep venous thrombosis complementing a compatible clinical story enhances the likelihood of pulmonary embolism. However, the utility of this approach to the diagnosis of pulmonary embolism has been called into serious question. Hull et al have demonstrated that approximately 30% of patients with angiographically-proven pulmonary embolism have no evidence of deep venous thrombosis by contrast venography.[12] This finding suggests that in some patients all clot embolized from the thigh veins to the lungs at the same time, or that the pulmonary emboli did not originate in the leg veins, perhaps coming from the pelvic veins, the upper extremity veins, or the right atrium.

Though the importance of deep venous thrombosis of the thigh as the major factor predisposing to pulmonary embolism is incontrovertible, it is often difficult to diagnose deep venous thrombosis or pulmonary embolism by clinical criteria alone.[13–14] Thus, in the individual patient, the diagnosis of pulmonary embolism cannot be reliably substantiated or ruled out by confirming or excluding concomitant deep venous thrombosis. It is important to recognize that approximately 50% of patients with deep venous thrombosis of the thigh established by contrast venography have no suggestive clinical findings (swelling, a palpable chord, tenderness, or erythema).[11,13] Also noteworthy is the observation that approximately 50% of patients with deep venous thrombosis have objective evidence of pulmonary embolism as shown by defects on the perfusion lung scan at the time that the diagnosis of deep venous thrombosis is established.

***Lung Scan.*** The perfusion lung scan is an invaluable screening procedure for pulmonary embolism. In a patient with a suggestive clinical story a normal six-view perfusion lung scan reliably excludes the diagnosis of pulmonary embolism with a certainty approaching 100%.[15,16] However, in many patients in whom pulmonary embolism is suspected there may be an underlying cardiopulmonary disorder that results in an abnormal perfusion lung scan even in the absence of pulmonary embolism. Such conditions include pneumonia, emphysema, pulmonary blebs, atelectasis, and congestive heart failure.[17] Though careful review of the chest roentgenogram and performance of a simultaneous ventilation lung scan frequently enhances the specificity of the perfusion lung scan in diagnosing pulmonary embolism, many patients with acute cardiopulmonary decompensation compatible with pulmonary embolism have underlying pulmonary parenchymal abnormalities that result in an "indeterminate" ventilation–perfusion lung scan, a study that does little to enhance the clinician's diagnostic certainty in confirming or excluding pulmonary embolism.[18]

## SYNDROMES OF PULMONARY EMBOLISM (TABLE 25-1)

Though the clinical and laboratory findings are usually nonspecific, pulmonary embolism frequently presents as one of four hemodynamically and clinically distinct syndromes. These include acute unexplained dyspnea, pulmonary infarction syndrome, acute cardiogenic shock with cor pulmonale, or chronic right ventricular failure with systemic congestion (from multiple unresolved pulmonary emboli.)

### Acute Unexplained Dyspnea

Acute unexplained dyspnea occurs characteristically in the young or middle-aged

**TABLE 25-1.**  *Syndromes of Pulmonary Embolism*

I.   Acute pulmonary embolism
    A.   Unexplained dyspnea
    B.   Pulmonary infarction syndrome
    C.   Acute cor pulmonale and/or cardiogenic shock
II.  Chronic pulmonary embolism
    A.   Right ventricular failure from multiple unresolved pulmonary emboli

patient with one or more predispositions to venous thromboembolic disease. Such predispositions include proscribed bed rest as a result of medical or surgical illness, underlying malignancy, use of estrogen-containing preparations (e.g., oral contraceptives), and trauma to the lower extremity.[19] The clinical presentation almost always involves dyspnea and tachypnea of an abrupt onset. However, after careful clinical evaluation no obvious underlying cardiopulmonary disorder (e.g., congestive heart failure, pneumonia, atelectasis, pleural effusion, or pneumothorax) is readily identified to account for this presentation.

The pathophysiology of dyspnea resulting from pulmonary embolism has not been clearly established. However, approximately 87% of patients with pulmonary embolism and no evidence of prior cardiopulmonary disease have an arterial oxygen tension below 80 mmHg while breathing room air.[4] The mechanism primarily responsible for the development of arterial hypoxia following pulmonary embolism is ventilation/perfusion imbalance with an effective right-to-left shunt within the lungs.

The patient free of chronic cardiopulmonary disease but with acute unexplained dyspnea as the primary manifestation of pulmonary embolism usually demonstrates no reduction in cardiac output, no significant pulmonary hypertension, and no right ventricular failure as a result of the pulmonary embolism. Indeed, the severity of embolic pulmonary artery cross-sectional obstruction is usually less than 50%, the mean pulmonary artery pressure rarely exceeds 20 to 25 mmHg, and the cardiac index is usually elevated (rather than reduced) as a result of the tachycardia resulting from hypoxemia-induced stimulation of the sympathetic nervous system.[20]

## Pulmonary Infarction Syndrome

Pathologically, pulmonary infarction represents necrosis of interalveolar septae, with dense alveolar hemorrhage. Fibrosis is prominent in the healing process, and resolution is accompanied by organization and scar formation. Clinically, the pulmonary infarction syndrome is manifest by fever, hemoptysis, pleurisy (with or without an audible pleural friction rub), rales, leukocytosis, and pulmonary infiltrate(s) on chest roentgenogram. Hemoptysis, rales, and the radiologic infiltrate(s) result from intraalveolar hemorrhage. The pleural effusion is usually blood-tinged to frankly hemorrhagic and exudative in chemical composition. In the patient free of underlying cardiopulmonary disease, when the embolus resolves promptly and alveolar hemorrhage is not associated with necrosis of alveolar septae, healing is usually accompanied by complete resolution with no radiologic or pathologic evidence of scar formation. This is the picture of the so-called incomplete pulmonary infarction. If there is underlying cardiopulmonary disease, it is more likely that healing will be accompanied by scar formation.[21]

The pulmonary infarction syndrome probably results from embolic occlusion of small to moderate sized pulmonary arteries proximal to the insertion of bronchial-artery-to-pulmonary-artery anastomoses. Sudden occlusion of such a vessel allows unimpeded inflow of blood at high pressure from the bronchial arterial anastomoses into the smaller pulmonary arteries distal to the site of embolic occlusion. Sudden inflow of blood at high pressure probably disrupts the small, thin-walled pulmonary arterial branches and results in alveolar hemorrhage.[7,22]

Hemodynamic findings in the pulmonary infarction syndrome include tachycardia with little or no pulmonary hypertension. This is not surprising, since the emboli to medium-sized vessels causing the pulmonary infarction syndrome usually obstruct less than 50% of the total pulmonary vascular cross-sectional area. Tachycardia and an increased cardiac output result from increased sympathetic outflow, which may be due to hypoxia and/or pleuritic chest pain. The cardiac output may also be elevated because of increased sympathetic stimulation.

Figure 25-1 illustrates the left lower lobe pulmonary angiogram in a woman who de-

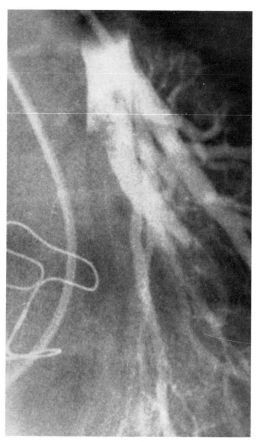

**Fig. 25-1.** Frame from a pulmonary cineangiogram performed by the technique of balloon occlusion in a woman who developed the pulmonary infarction syndrome following mitral valve replacement and coronary artery bypass surgery. The tip of the catheter is positioned in the most proximal segment of the artery to the left lower lobe, and the balloon has been inflated to a volume of 1.5 cc to occlude arterial inflow. The vessel is selectively opacified by a hand-powered injection of 7 ml of radiographic contrast agent. Multiple vessel cutoffs and intralumenal filling defects diagnostic of pulmonary embolism are visualized.

veloped pleuritic chest pain, hemoptysis, and a left pleural effusion 8 days following surgery for myocardial revascularization and mitral valve replacement. There are vessel cut-offs and intraluminal filling defects, diagnostic of pulmonary embolism, in several medium-sized branches of the artery to the left lower lobe. Her clinical presentation illustrates the *pulmonary infarction syndrome*.

## Cardiogenic Shock and Cor Pulmonale

The *hemodynamic consequences* of pulmonary embolism are determined primarily by the size of the pulmonary embolus and whether or not the patient has underlying cardiopulmonary disease. In a patient previously free of cardiopulmonary disease, the hemodynamic impact of pulmonary embolism is related directly to the severity of pulmonary vascular cross-sectional obstruction engendered by the embolus.[6,27] Significant pulmonary hypertension (mean pulmonary artery pressure exceeding 25 mmHg) does not usually develop in such patients unless emboli obstruct at least 50% of the pulmonary vascular cross-sectional area. When 50 to 75% of the pulmonary arterial tree is obstructed, there is usually mild to moderate pulmonary hypertension (mean pulmonary artery pressure in the range of 25 to 40 mmHg), a normal to reduced pulmonary capillary wedge pressure, a normal or increased cardiac index, mild to moderate elevation in pulmonary vascular resistance (180 to 300 dynes-sec-cm$^{-5}$), and a normal mean right atrial pressure (<8 mmHg).

With *massive pulmonary embolism* (obstruction of the pulmonary arterial circulation in excess of 75%) and *acute cor pulmonale*, there is sinus tachycardia and the pulmonary artery mean pressure approaches 40 to 45 mmHg. The previously normal right ventricle cannot pump effectively against a pulmonary artery mean pressure elevated acutely to a level exceeding 40 to 45 mmHg. Instead, severe embolic obstruction of this magnitude is usually accompanied by right ventricular dilatation and failure with an increase in mean right atrial pressure to ≥10 mmHg. There is usually a precipitous reduction in stroke output; cardiac output is reduced as well, but to a lesser extent because of compensatory tachycardia. Mean arterial pressure is usually preserved through an adrenergically-mediated reflex increase in systemic vascular resistance. If the patient demonstrates evidence of impaired organ perfusion (confusion or agitation, cool diaphoretic skin, oliguria with elaboration of urine reduced in sodium concentration), the cardiac index is usually below 1.8 to 2L/min/m$^2$, the systolic pressure is usually reduced, and the arterial pulse pressure is narrowed.

Figure 25-2 illustrates the pulmonary arteriogram of a patient with acute cor pulmonale. The patient was a 36-year-old man with phlebitis of the right leg, who fainted while having a bowel movement. The right pulmonary artery cineangiogram (Fig. 25-2) demonstrates intraluminal filling defects in the right middle and right upper lobe branches. Two proximal branches originating from the right lower lobe artery are nearly flush-occluded at their origins. Similar thrombi were present throughout the left lung. At the time of pulmonary angiography the patient had markedly elevated right atrial (15 mmHg) and pulmonary artery pressures (65/35 mmHg). The mean pulmonary artery pressure was 45 mmHg. The cardiac index was severely depressed at 1.8 L/min/m$^2$, but systemic arterial blood pressure was preserved. This case exemplifies massive pulmonary embolism with acute right ventricular failure, a situation where survival following another pulmonary embolism would be unlikely. Accordingly, he was treated with a thrombolytic agent to promote prompt resolution of the embolic pulmonary artery obstruction.[24] Later, a Kim-Ray inferior vena cava filter was inserted to prevent subsequent pulmonary embolism.

*Cardiogenic shock* resulting from massive pulmonary embolism is manifest hemodynamically by tachycardia, a normal to reduced pulmonary capillary wedge pressure ($\leq$12 mmHg), a pulmonary artery mean pressure between 35 and 45 mmHg, an elevated pulmonary vascular resistance (above 500 dynes sec cm$^{-5}$), an elevated systemic vascular resistance ($>$1600 dynes sec cm$^{-5}$), right atrial pressure in excess of 10 mmHg, and arterial hypotension, or at least a tendency toward this, with narrowing of the arterial pulse pressure ($<$30 mmHg). Cardiac output is very much reduced, and pulmonary arterial blood oxygen saturation is usually $\leq$50%.

The clinical manifestations of cardiogenic shock from pulmonary embolism include severe dyspnea and syncope or light-headedness. There may be chest pain, not necessarily of a pleuritic nature but of a more oppressive retrosternal quality. Objective findings include hypotension, tachycardia, cool, moist skin, central cyanosis, oliguria, mental clouding, jugular venous distention, and a thready arterial pulse. The cardiac examination may be surprisingly unremarkable; however, one should anticipate evidence of pulmonary hypertension. A widely but physiologically split second heart sound (resulting from prolonged right ventricular ejection) with the pulmonic component increased in intensity, a systolic ejection murmur at the base (due to dilatation of the pulmonary trunk) and a left parasternal lift (resulting from pressure overload of the right ventricle with right ventricular dilatation and failure) are commonly present.

The differential diagnosis of cardiogenic shock with an elevated central venous pressure includes cardiac tamponade[25,26] and right ventricular infarction,[27,28] in addition to

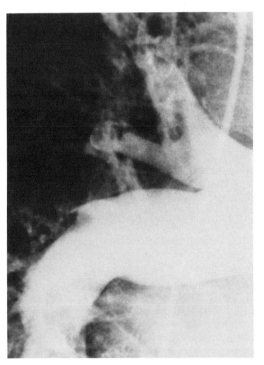

**Fig. 25-2.** A frame from a right pulmonary artery cineangiogram performed in a 36-year-old man with syncope from massive pulmonary embolism. The tip of an Eppendorf catheter has been positioned 2 to 3 cm proximal to the origin of the artery to the right upper lobe. Intralumenal filling defects diagnostic of pulmonary embolism are visualized in the proximal segments of the right upper and right middle lobe vessels. Though the proximal segment of the right lower lobe artery itself is free of thrombi, several of its proximal branches do not opacify because they are cut off by totally occlusive emboli.

pulmonary embolism. *Cardiac tamponade* is characterized by pulsus paradox and a right atrial pressure in excess of 12 to 16 mmHg with near equalization of the right atrial, right ventricular diastolic, and pulmonary capillary wedge pressures. The pulmonary artery systolic pressure usually exceeds the right ventricular diastolic pressure by no more than 10 mmHg. *Right ventricular infarction* with shock is characterized by a depressed cardiac index ($<1.8L/min/m^2$), a right atrial mean pressure in excess of 10 mmHg, arterial hypotension, and a mean pulmonary artery and pulmonary artery wedge pressure that usually exceeds right atrial pressure by less than 3 to 5 mmHg. An important hemodynamic differential point is that,with cardiac tamponade or right ventricular infarction, the mean pulmonary artery pressure is usually less than 25 mmHg; however, with massive pulmonary embolism the mean pulmonary artery pressure usually exceeds 35 to 40 mmHg.

Though pulsus paradox is characteristic of cardiac tamponade, occurring in over 90% of patients, it has also been reported in patients with massive pulmonary embolism.[29] A helpful differential point between pulmonary embolism and tamponade is found on the echocardiogram, which almost always demonstrates an anterior and posterior clear space in cardiac tamponade suggestive of a large pericardial effusion. Also, the echocardiogram shows a decrease in the right ventricular end-diastolic dimension during the inspiratory phase of the respiratory cycle in cardiac tamponade due to cardiac compression. These findings are not present in pulmonary embolism, where the right ventricular chamber is usually dilated.

The findings on bedside hemodynamic monitoring may be somewhat confusing in patients with massive pulmonary embolism, particularly regarding the pulmonary artery phasic pressure as monitored by a flow-directed balloon-tipped catheter. The catheter tip may occasionally engage the soft gelatinous surface of the pulmonary embolus with intermittent damping or loss of the phasic pulmonary artery pressure wave form. Should the catheter intermittently record a very damped pulmonary artery pressure corresponding reasonably well to the previously measured mean pulmonary pressure and catheter manipulation or vigorous flushing restore a more physiologic phasic pulmonary

arterial pressure, one should consider intermittent catheter obstruction by in-situ thrombus or pulmonary embolus. If the distal thermistor electrode of a thermodilution catheter in the pulmonary artery is intermittently embedded in the thrombus, it will be partially insulated from the injectate bolus delivered to measure cardiac output, and thermodilution cardiac output measurements may be falsely elevated, fluctuating, and inconsistent with other measures of cardiac output (e.g., pulmonary artery blood oxygen saturation).

## Unresolved Pulmonary Embolism

Though in an earlier series, it was noted that less than 1 to 3% of patients fail to demonstrate hemodynamic and angiographic resolution of abnormalities following acute pulmonary embolism,[23] there have been more recent[30,31] reports of chronic pulmonary hypertension and cor pulmonale resulting from chronic and unresolved pulmonary embolism. The clinical manifestations usually suggest pulmonary hypertension. Findings may include dyspnea, orthopnea, cardiomegaly with right ventricular dilatation and failure, distended neck veins, pleural effusions, edema and ascites, and a history compatible with previous thrombophlebitis or pulmonary embolism. The chest roentgenograms usually demonstrate cardiomegaly, dilatation of one or more proximal pulmonary arteries, and pleural effusions. In patients with clinically manifest right ventricular failure, the electrocardiogram almost always demonstrates right ventricular hypertrophy. The perfusion lung scan characteristically reveals segmental, lobar, or whole lung perfusion defects suggesting obstruction in the most proximal segments of at least two or three pulmonary arteries.[32] Though this syndrome is uncommon, it is an important consideration in the evaluation of patients with unexplained pulmonary hypertension, since thromboembolectomy with pulmonary endarterectomy often can be successful in such cases.[30,31]

Table 25-2 depicts the hemodynamic findings at rest and during supine bicycle exercise in a patient with chronic bilateral pulmonary embolism before and after pulmonary embolectomy. Though the mean

**TABLE 25-2.** *Hemodynamic Findings in a Patient with Unresolved Pulmonary Embolism*

|  |  | RA | PA | PCW | CO/CI | PVR |
|---|---|---|---|---|---|---|
| Before | Rest | 4 | 38/14 (22) | 9 | 3.7/1.8 | 281 |
| Embolectomy | Exercise | 15 | 101/32 (55) | 15 | 7.2/3.5 | 444 |
| After | Rest | 1 | 26/8 (16) | 8 | 4.1/2.0 | 156 |
| Embolectomy | Exercise | 6 | 65/20 (40) | 21 | 8.6/4.1 | 177 |

RA = mean right atrial pressure (mmHg): PA = pulmonary artery pressure (mmHg), systolic/diastolic (mean); PCW = mean pulmonary artery wedge pressure (mmHg): CO = cardiac output (L/min); CI = cardiac index (L/min/M$^2$); PVR = pulmonary vascular resistance (dynes-sec-cm$^{-5}$).

pulmonary artery pressure at rest was only minimally elevated, it more than doubled with exercise, and the mean right atrial pressure rose to 15 mmHg. Following pulmonary embolectomy, the patient's dyspnea resolved. The pulmonary artery pressure and pulmonary vascular resistance were reduced at rest and during exercise, compatible with partial relief of the embolic pulmonary vascular obstruction. Figure 25-3 demonstrates the perfusion lung scans and angiograms in this patient before and after embolectomy of a right pulmonary artery thromboembolism. Embolectomy resulted in improved perfusion to the right lung, though segmental defects persisted in the right middle lobe and apex. The postembolectomy pulmonary angiogram demonstrates absence of thrombus in the right main pulmonary artery and improved flow to the right middle, right lower, and left lower lobe arteries.

## HEMODYNAMICS OF PULMONARY EMBOLISM IN PATIENTS WITH UNDERLYING CARDIOPULMONARY DISEASE

The hemodynamic impact of pulmonary embolism in patients with underlying cardiopulmonary disease is somewhat different from the effects of pulmonary embolism in patients with normal underlying cardiopulmonary reserve. Patients with underlying cardiopulmonary disease (whether due to chronic left atrial hypertension from coronary mitral, or aortic valve disease or as a result of pulmonary parenchymal destruction from chronic obstructive lung disease) usually have a reduction in pulmonary vascular cross-sectional area. That is, with any increase in pulmonary blood flow (e.g., with exercise) or with any further reduction in pulmonary cross-sectional area (e.g., due to pulmonary embolism or hypoxia-induced pulmonary vasoconstriction) pulmonary hypertension will develop because pulmonary vascular reserve has been exhausted by the underlying disease process. Such patients may develop severe pulmonary hypertension during exercise, even when the pulmonary artery pressure is normal with the patient at rest. Exercise-induced pulmonary hypertension may also result in some degree of right ventricular hypertrophy in the patient with underlying prior cardiopulmonary disease so that superimposed acute pulmonary embolism is likely to evoke more severe pulmonary hypertension than pulmonary embolism of similar size in the patient without prior cardiopulmonary disease.

Because of the development of right ventricular hypertrophy as a result of exercise-induced pulmonary hypertension, the patient with underlying cardiopulmonary disease usually is able to develop a mean pulmonary artery pressure well in excess of 40 to 45 mmHg without developing right ventricular dilatation and failure. Thus, a patient with pulmonary embolism demonstrating a mean pulmonary artery pressure exceeding 50 mmHg likely has underlying chronic cardiopulmonary disease that has already resulted in intermittent pulmonary hypertension with consequent right ventricular hypertrophy prior to the acute event.

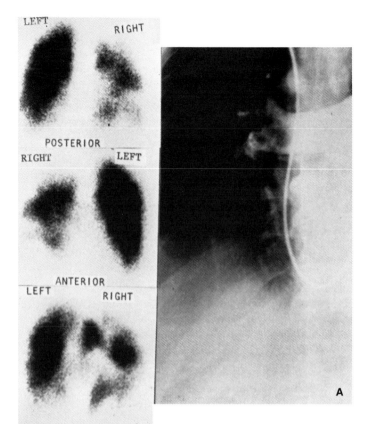

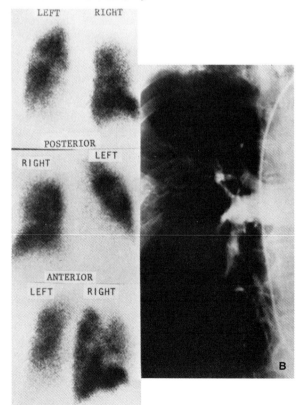

Fig. 25-3(A). Pre-embolectomy perfusion scan (left) and right pulmonary artery angiogram (right) in a patient with severe dyspnea on exertion and unresolved pulmonary embolism. The lung scan reveals several segmental and lobar perfusion defects, more prominent in the right lung. The pulmonary angiogram demonstrates virtually absent flow to the right lung. The hemodynamic findings in this patient are depicted in Table 25-2. (B) Perfusion lung scan (left) and pulmonary angiogram (right) in the same patient, following pulmonary thrombectomy and endarterectomy. The lung scan demonstrates improved perfusion to the right lung though segmental defects persist in the right middle lobe and apex. The pulmonary angiogram reveals that the right main pulmonary artery embolus is no longer present and the arteries to the right middle and right lower lobes are better opacified.

# REFERENCES

1. Stein PD, Willis PW III, DeMeto DL: History and physical examination in acute pulmonary embolism in patients without prior cardiopulmonary disease. Am J Cardiol 47:218, 1981.
2. Lippman M, Fein A: Pulmonary embolism in the patient with chronic obstructive pulmonary disease. Chest 79:38, 1981.
3. Szucs MM, et al: Diagnostic sensitivity of laboratory findings in acute pulmonary embolism. Ann Intern Med 74:171, 1971.
4. Dantzker DR, Bower JS: Alterations in gas exchange following pulmonary thromboembolism. Chest 81:485, 1982.
5. Jardin F, et al: Hemodynamic factors influencing arterial hypoxemia in massive pulmonary embolism with circulatory failure. Circulation 59:909, 1978.
6. McIntyre KM, Sasahara AA: The hemodynamic response to pulmonary embolism in patients without prior cardiopulmonary disease. Am J Cardiol 28:288, 1971.
7. Dalen JE, et al: Pulmonary embolism; pulmonary hemorrhage and pulmonary infarction. N Engl J Med 296:1431, 1977.
8. Stein PD, et al: The electrocardiogram in acute pulmonary embolism. Prog Cardiovasc Dis 17:247, 1975.
9. McGinn S, White PD: Acute cor pulmonale resulting from pulmonary embolism. JAMA 104:1473, 1935.
10. Smith M, Ray CT: Electrocardiographic signs of early right ventricular enlargement in acute pulmonary embolism. Chest 58:205, 1970.
11. Sasahara AA, Sharma GVRK, Parisi AF: New developments in the detection and prevention of venous thromboembolism. Am J Cardiol 43:1214, 1979.
12. Hull RD, et al: Pulmonary angiography, ventilation lung scanning and venography for clinically suspected pulmonary embolism with abnormal perfusion lung scan. Ann Intern Med 98:891, 1983.
13. Jeffrey PC, Immelman EJ, Benatar SR: Deep-vein thrombosis and pulmonary embolism—an assessment of the accuracy of clinical diagnosis. S Afr Med 57:643, 1980.
14. Moser KM, Lemoine JR: Is embolic risk conditioned by location of deep venous thrombosis? Ann Intern Med 94:438, 1981.
15. Caride VJ, et al: The usefulness of the posterior oblique views in perfusion lung imaging. Radiology 12:669, 1976.
16. Nielsen PE, Kirchner PT, Gerber GH: Oblique views in lung perfusion scanning. Clinical utility and limitations. J Nucl Med 18:969, 1977.
17. Newman GE, et al: Scintigraphic perfusion patterns in patients with diffuse lung disease. Radiology 143:227, 1982.
18. Polak JF, McNeil BJ: Pulmonary scintigraphy and the diagnosis of pulmonary embolism. *In* Clinics in Chest Medicine, Hyers TH, (ed): Philadelphia, W.B. Saunders Co., 1984, 457–464.
19. Coon WW: Venous thromboembolism; prevalence, risk factors, and prevention. *In* Symposium on Pulmonary Embolism and Hypertension. Hyers Th (ed)., Philadelphia, W.B. Saunders Co., 1984, 391–402.
20. A National Cooperative Study: Urokinase pulmonary embolism trial. Circulation 47, April 1973. 47(Suppl. II):1–108, 1973.
21. Hampton AO, Castleman B: Correlation of postmortem chest teleroentgenograms with autopsy findings with special reference to pulmonary embolism and infarction. Am J. Roentgenol 43:305, 1940.
22. Roach HO, Laufman H: Relationship between pulmonary embolism and infarction. Surg Forum 5:214, 1955.
23. Dalen JE, Banas JS, Brooks HL, et al: Resolution rate of acute pulmonary embolism in man. N Engl J Med 280:1194, 1969.
24. Volgesang GB, Bell WR: Treatment of pulmonary embolism and deep vein thrombosis with thrombolytic therapy. *In* Symposium on Pulmonary Embolism and Hypertension: Clinics in Chest Medicine, Hyers TM (ed): Philadelphia, W.B. Saunders Co., 1984, 487–494.
25. Shabetai R, Fowler NO, Guntheroth WG: The hemodynamics of cardiac tamponade and constrictive pericarditis. Am J Cardiol 26:480, 1970.
26. Reddy PS, et al: Cardiac tamponade: hemodynamic observations in man. Circulation 58:265, 1978.
27. Cohn JN, Guiha NH, Broder MI et al: Right ventricular infarction. Am J Cardiol 33:209, 1974.
28. Lorell B, et al: Right ventricular infarction: clinical diagnosis and differentiation from pericardial tamponade and constriction. Am J Cardiol 43:465, 1979.
29. Cohen SI, et al: Pulsus paradox and Kussmaul's sign in acute pulmonary embolism. Am J Cardiol 32:271, 1973.
30. Benotti JR, Ockene IS, Alpert JS, Dalen JE: The clinical profile of unresolved pulmonary embolism. Chest 84:669, 1983.
31. Utley JR, et al: Pulmonary endarectomy for chronic obstruction: recent surgical experience. Surgery 92:1096, 1982.
32. Fishman AJ, Moser KM, Fedullo PF: Perfusion lung scans vs. pulmonary angiography in evaluation of suspected primary pulmonary hypertension. Chest 54:678, 1983.

## chapter twenty six

# Profiles in Dilated (Congestive) and Hypertrophic Cardiomyopathies

WILLIAM GROSSMAN

C ARDIOMYOPATHIES are primary disorders of heart muscle. While the term cardiomyopathy is sometimes restricted to refer to cardiac muscle disorders of unknown etiology, most cardiologists include both disorders of unknown and known etiology. For example, the cardiac muscle disorder associated with long-standing ingestion of excessive quantities of ethanol is generally termed alcoholic cardiomyopathy, and that disorder resulting from high-dose doxorubicin therapy for malignancy is called doxorubicin or adriamycin cardiomyopathy.

In general, cardiomyopathies are classified descriptively,[1] as listed in Table 26-1. In this chapter, I shall discuss only the first two types of cardiomyopathy listed in Table 26-1. Restrictive cardiomyopathy is discussed in Chapter 27, along with constrictive pericarditis with which it is often confused. Obliterative cardiomyopathy is extremely rare in the United States and is beyond the scope of this book.

## DILATED (CONGESTIVE) CARDIOMYOPATHY

The clinical syndrome of dilated cardiomyopathy represents a collection of disorders and is also called congestive cardiomyopathy. The term *congestive cardiomyopathy* was introduced initially by Goodwin[2] because the clinical presentation is marked primarily by peripheral and pulmonary edema. More recently, Goodwin and associates have preferred the term *dilated cardiomyopathy*, since with newer diagnostic techniques (echocardiography, radionuclide ventriculography) it has become possible to diagnose this syndrome prior to the onset of clinical signs and symptoms of congestion. Also, with effective diuretic and vasodilator management, the congestive component may be eliminated and ventricular filling pressures may be returned to normal. However, the ventricular chambers remain *dilated*, with increased end-systolic and end-diastolic volumes and reduced myocardial contractility.

## Cardiac Catheterization Protocol

Study of the patient who is suspected of having dilated cardiomyopathy should include right and left heart catheterization with measurement of pressures, cardiac output, and resistances. As is our routine for right heart catheterization (Chapters 4 and 5), oxygen saturation is measured routinely in blood taken from the superior vena cava and pulmonary artery to detect unsuspected

412

**TABLE 26-1.** *Descriptive Classification of Cardiomyopathies*

I. *Dilated (Congestive) Cardiomyopathy:* dilated ventricular chambers with increased end-diastolic and end-systolic volumes and decreased myocardial contractility
   A. Idiopathic
   B. Post-myocarditis
   C. Toxic; 2° to ethanol, doxorubicin, uremia
   D. Peripartum
   E. Chronic overload (e.g., long-standing severe volume overload, untreated hypertension)
   F. Congenital
   G. Miscellaneous (diabetes, autoimmune disease, sarcoid)

II. *Hypertrophic Cardiomyopathy:* hypertrophic ventricular chambers with normal volumes and generally normal contractile function
   A. Asymmetric septal hypertrophy
   B. Apical hypertrophic cardiomyopathy
   C. Diffuse symmetrical hypertrophy

III. *Restrictive Cardiomyopathy:* normal ventricular volumes and contractile function, but increased resistance to diastolic filling
   A. Infiltrative type: amyloidosis, hemochromatosis, Fabry's disease
   B. Idiopathic
   C. Diffuse fibrosis (e.g., post-myocarditis, diffuse nontransmural myocardial infarction)

IV. *Obliterative Cardiomyopathy*
   A. Eosinophilic endomyocardial fibroelastosis

right to left shunting. Angiographic studies will need to be tailored to the individual case, but left ventriculography and coronary angiography are commonly done as a part of the study in such patients.

**Hemodynamic Findings.** In the symptomatic patient with dilated cardiomyopathy referred for cardiac catheterization, *left and right ventricular filling pressures* are usually elevated. However, as mentioned, it is possible that the ventricular filling pressures at rest may be normal; this finding is particularly likely in the asymptomatic patient detected early in the course of his disease by noninvasive screening. Also, the patient who has been intensively treated with diuretics (e.g., furosemide and spironolactone) and who is receiving a potent vasodilator (e.g., captopril) may show little or no elevation in resting filling pressures. In general, increases in left and right ventricular filling pressures can be easily induced in such patients by *supine bicycle exercise*, performed as outlined in Chapter 17. With 6 minutes of supine bicycle exercise, pulmonary capillary wedge pressure will commonly rise from 10 mmHg to 25 to 40 mmHg, and right atrial pressure

will increase from 6 mmHg to 15 to 20 mmHg. Supine bicycle exercise provides an acute volume and pressure load on the ventricular myocardium and easily brings out underlying loss of contractile reserve.

*Cardiac output* is generally reduced in the patient with dilated cardiomyopathy. In the milder cases, the cardiac index may be normal or only slightly reduced and may range from 2.4 to 3.0 L/min/M². In patients with NYHA Class III or IV symptoms from dilated cardiomyopathy, it is common to find the cardiac index depressed more severely. Thus, a cardiac index of 1.6 to 2.3 L/min/M² can be expected in the usual symptomatic patient presenting with dilated cardiomyopathy, and a cardiac index of ≤1.5 L/min/M² indicates an advanced depression of myocardial function and a poor prognosis.

The *left ventricular pressure tracing* is typically quite abnormal in patients with dilated cardiomyopathy. Both the rate of rise and the rate of fall of left ventricular pressure are quite slow, and this is usually visible to the naked eye (Fig. 26–1). Slowing of the left ventricular pressure upstroke and downstroke gives a *triangular appearance* to the

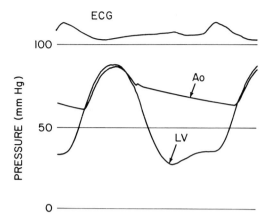

**Fig. 26-1.** Left ventricular (LV) micromanometer and aortic (Ao) pressure tracings in a 68-year-old woman with advanced dilated cardiomyopathy. Marked slowing of the rates of left ventricular pressure rise and fall give the LV pressure tracing a triangular appearance. Also, the minimal value for left ventricular diastolic pressure is markedly elevated.

pressure tracing, with the peak systolic pressure representing the apex of the triangle; end-diastolic and minimal (early)-diastolic left ventricular pressures define the triangle's base. This deformity accounts for the brief duration of systolic ejection in dilated cardiomyopathy and contrasts to the trapezoidal, almost square-wave appearance of left ventricular pressure in a normal, vigorous heart. A corollary of the triangular waveform of left ventricular pressure in dilated cardiomyopathy is a normal or low peak systolic pressure.

A second abnormality of the left ventricular pressure tracing in dilated cardiomyopathy is elevation in the minimal value for left ventricular diastolic pressure (Fig. 26-1). Normally the left ventricular pressure declines briskly following aortic valve closure, reaching a nadir close to 0 mmHg shortly after mitral valve opening. This reflects the normal pattern of rapid myocardial relaxation, acting together with *restoring forces* generated by a vigorous systolic contraction, with end systolic elastic compression and torsion force being released during early diastolic filling. In the experimental laboratory under conditions of extremely vigorous contraction (e.g., isoproterenol infusion), or hypovolemia (e.g., hemorrhage) the left ventricular diastolic pressure may actually become

negative early in diastole, a phenomenon known as *diastolic suction*. In dilated cardiomyopathy, diastolic relaxation generally is slow and incomplete,[3] and restoring forces produced by the weakened systolic contraction are minimal. These factors militate against a normal low value for left ventricular minimal diastolic pressure. In addition, end-systolic volume is increased in patients with dilated cardiomyopathy, and this abnormality tends to elevate diastolic volume and pressure above normal.

To appreciate these abnormalities in the left ventricular pressure waveform in dilated cardiomyopathy, one must have pressure tracings of good quality with careful attention to the details discussed in Chapter 9. Micromanometer catheters are not necessary to achieve such high quality tracings, as can be seen in Figure 26-2, where fluid-filled and micromanometer tracings are superimposed.

The left ventricular pressure tracing abnormalities just described can be corrected substantially by acute administration of an inotropic drug.[4-6] Figures 26-2 and 26-3 illustrate the effects of a phosphodiesterase inhibitor (milrinone) and a beta-adrenergic agonist (prenalterol) on the left ventricular pressure contour in patients with dilated cardiomyopathy. As can be seen, early diastolic relaxation is more rapid and more complete following administration of these drugs, as reflected by the steep decline in left ventricular pressure to a value near zero in early diastole.

Patients with dilated cardiomyopathy often have elevations in pulmonary and systemic vascular resistance. It is common to find pulmonary vascular resistance increased to 150–300 dynes-sec-cm,$^{-5}$ and patients with values >400 dynes-sec-cm$^{-5}$ are not rare. These increases in pulmonary vascular resistance result in pulmonary hypertension with mean pulmonary artery pressure commonly 30 to 50 mmHg. Systemic vascular resistance is usually $\geqq 1500$ dynes-sec-cm$^{-5}$ in untreated patients with advanced dilated cardiomyopathy, probably representing a response to combined elevations in serum levels of angiotensin, vasopressin, and norepinephrine. Since cardiac output is reduced, modest increases in systemic vascular resistance do not result in actual elevation of arterial blood pressure, but rather tend to preserve arterial pres-

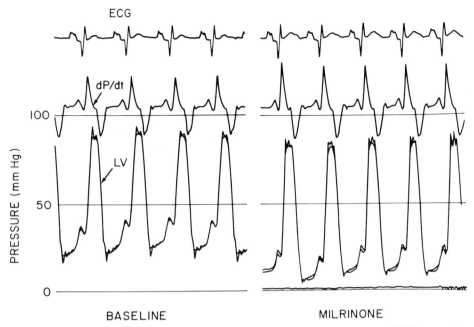

**Fig. 26-2.** Left ventricular (LV) micromanometer pressure and its first derivative (dP/dt) in a patient with dilated cardiomyopathy before (left) and after (right) intravenous infusion of milrinone. Positive and negative dP/dt have increased without increase in arterial pressure and with a decline in preload, suggesting increased myocardial contractility and relaxation. Left ventricular minimal diastolic pressure is now closer to zero, as is normal. Fluid-filled and micromanometer pressures are displayed simultaneously, indicating the excellent fidelity that can be achieved with fluid-filled systems utilizing the principles described in Chapter 9. (Reproduced with permission from Baim DS, et al: Evaluation of a new bipyridine inotropic agent—milrinone—in patients with severe congestive heart failure. N Engl J Med 309:748, 1983.)

sure at a normal or only slightly reduced level.

Reduction of systemic and pulmonary vascular resistances to normal by administration of vasodilator agents often results in a striking increase in cardiac output and a simultaneous reduction in left and right ventricular filling pressures. As shown in Figure 26-4 acute administration of sodium nitroprusside[7,8] or captopril[9–11] results in an upward and leftward displacement of the left ventricular filling pressure-stroke volume relationship, since heart rate is affected minimally by these agents in the setting of chronic heart failure.

During cardiac catheterization in patients with dilated cardiomyopathy, it is often wise to test responsiveness to a vasodilator in the laboratory. In my own practice, I do this routinely using the following protocol. After measurement of cardiac output and resting hemodynamics and prior to angiography, if filling pressures are elevated significantly

(e.g., pulmonary capillary wedge pressure ≧16 mmHg) and cardiac output is depressed (e.g., pulmonary artery blood $O_2$ saturation ≦65%), I begin an infusion of sodium nitroprusside as long as arterial systolic pressure is >90 mmHg and has been stable. The starting dose is 15 micrograms/min through a secure, free-flowing intravenous line, and the infusion rate is increased every 3 to 5 minutes to doses of 25, 50, 75, 100, 150, 200, and 300 micrograms/min, if needed, until arterial mean pressure has fallen 10 to 20 mmHg or wedge pressure has fallen by ≧50%, or pulmonary artery $O_2$ saturation has increased to ≧75%. Usually, one of these three end points is achieved at a dose of sodium nitroprusside ≦200 micrograms/min; however, I have had occasional patients in whom >300 micrograms/min were required. If the patient is feeling well during the vasodilator infusion (as is generally the case), I continue the infusion during left ventriculography and coronary angiography, as a prophylactic measure

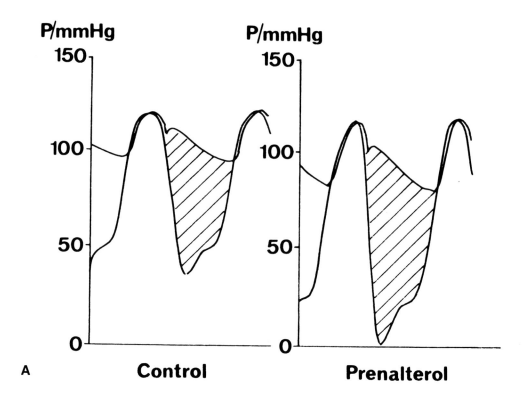

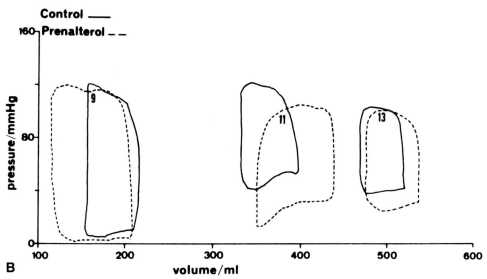

**Fig. 26-3.** Effects of the beta agonist prenalterol on left ventricular and aortic pressure (A) and left ventricular pressure-volume plots (B) in patients with idiopathic dilated cardiomyopathy. The tracings illustrate the restoration of a normal low value for the left ventricular diastolic pressure nadir, as well as a downward shift in the diastolic pressure volume relationship. (Reproduced with permission from Erbel R, et al: Hemodynamic effects of prenalterol in patients with ischemic heart disease and congestive cardiomyopathy. Circulation 66:361, 1982.)

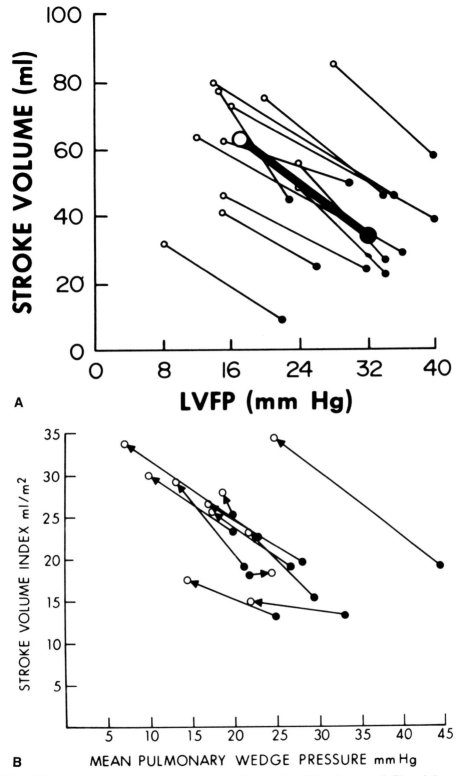

**Fig. 26-4.** Effects of acute administration of sodium nitroprusside (A) and captopril (B) on left ventricular filling pressure-stroke volume relationships in patients with advanced heart failure. Some of these patients had heart failure on the basis of idiopathic dilated cardiomyopathy, and some had ischemic heart disease. Responses were similar and appeared to be independent of etiology. See text for discussion. (Reproduced with permission from Guiha NH, et al: Treatment of refractory heart failure with infusion of nitroprusside. N Engl J Med 291:587, 1974. (A); and Davis R, et al: Treatment of chronic congestive heart failure with captopril, an oral inhibitor of angiotensin-converting enzyme. N Engl J Med 301:117, 1979 (B).)

to protect against pulmonary edema. The dose may need to be reduced if the arterial systolic pressure is $\leqq 80$ mmHg. A favorable response to sodium nitroprusside in the cardiac catheterization laboratory is not only an aid to the safety of the procedure, but also predicts a favorable response to an oral vasodilator (e.g., captopril) in the patient's long-term management.

***Angiographic Studies.*** Left ventriculography in patients with dilated cardiomyopathy classically reveals extensive hypokinesis. This is usually diffuse in nature, but commonly there are regional wall motion abnormalities that suggest a heterogeneity of the myocardial injury and mimic coronary artery disease. This may represent the consequence of asymmetric injury initially, and in this regard it is of interest that myocarditis may be quite focal in its inflammatory effects. We have seen several patients in whom biopsy-proven acute myocarditis mimicked regional ischemia and infarction, with left ventriculography showing discrete areas of akinesis or even focal aneurysm formation. These areas of regional dysfunction could also represent the result of coronary emboli from mural thrombus, since the occurrence of left ventricular mural thrombus is increased in patients with dilated cardiomyopathy.

Kreulen et al described the angiographic abnormalities associated with dilated cardiomyopathy and pointed out that the dilatation is associated with loss of the normal eccentric shape of the left ventricle.[12] Normally, the ratio of long axis (L) to minor axis (M) is $2:1$ for the left ventricular chamber at end-diastole. In dilated cardiomyopathy, L/M approaches $1:1$. This change will tend to increase meridional wall stress (see Chapter 19) but will have an unpredictable effect on longitudinal wall stress, depending on the extent of associated ventricular hypertrophy. In this regard, left ventricular hypertrophy is common in patients with dilated cardiomyopathy.[13] Some authors have reported a substantial beneficial effect of hypertrophy on survival in patients with dilated cardiomyopathy and have suggested that protection against increasing wall stress might have a protective role for these patients.[13,14]

***Endomyocardial Biopsy.*** Enthusiasm for obtaining endomyocardial biopsy as a part of the diagnostic work-up in patients with suspected dilated cardiomyopathy has been increasing, and at our institution we have shared this enthusiasm. Endomyocardial biopsy is done almost routinely in our laboratory as part of the diagnostic study in patients with advanced heart failure. We have done over 100 endomyocardial biopsies in nontransplant patients over the past two years and have found specific heart muscle disorders (inflammatory myocarditis, amyloidosis, hemochromatosis) in approximately 15% of cases. The technique of endomyocardial biopsy and additional specific diseases it can detect is described in detail in Chapter 32. In one study of 100 consecutive endomyocardial biopsies carried out to evaluate heart failure of uncertain etiology,[15] the pathologic information obtained was judged to be clinically useful in 54 patients and not useful in 46 patients. Specific diagnoses that could be made from histologic examination of the biopsy material included inflammatory myocarditis, amyloidosis, sarcoidosis, scleroderma, endomyocardial fibrosis with eosinophilia, doxorubicin cardiomyopathy, radiation-induced cardiomyopathy, and vasculitis[15.]

In summary, a variety of hemodynamic, angiographic, and histologic features can be defined precisely in the course of a single diagnostic cardiac catheterization procedure in patients with suspected dilated cardiomyopathy. Findings from such a study yield valuable information about prognosis[13-17] and will help direct appropriate therapy.

# HYPERTROPHIC CARDIOMYOPATHY

Cardiac hypertrophy develops to some extent in a wide variety of cardiac diseases. However, in hypertrophic cardiomyopathy the development of cardiac hypertrophy proceeds without an obvious inciting stimulus or develops out of proportion to the magnitude of the stimulus or stimuli that can be identified.[1,18] While it is commonly regarded as a genetic disorder,[1] many cases appear to be sporadic. Most authors distinguish between obstructive and nonobstructive forms of the disorder, based on the presence or absence of a resting (unprovoked) systolic pressure gradient within the left ventricle,[18] and the presence of a gradient has caused this disorder to be called idiopathic hypertrophic subaortic stenosis (IHSS) or muscular subaortic stenosis (MSS). There remains a great deal of controversy as to whether true "obstruction" occurs in this condition,[1,19] since there is some evidence that most of the left ventricular stroke volume has been ejected prior to the development of a significant gradient. However, there is general agreement that the pressure gradient, when present, has several adverse consequences, including increased systolic wall stress in cardiac muscle proximal to the site of septal-mitral leaflet contact and increased myocardial oxygen consumption.

Hypertrophic cardiomyopathy may be diffuse and symmetrical, involving all regions of the left ventricle equally, or it may be *asymmetric*. Asymmetric hypertrophic cardiomyopathy commonly involves the high interventricular septum which is disproportionately hypertrophied so that the ratio of thickness of the diastolic septal wall to thickness of the free (lateral or posterior) left ventricular wall is >1.3. Another form of asymmetric hypertrophic cardiomyopathy, which has been reported from Japan,[20] involves massive apical hypertrophy of the left ventricle. A characteristic electrocardiographic feature is the presence of giant negative T waves in the precordial leads. The apical form of hypertrophic cardiomyopathy has now been recognized to occur in Europe and the United States.[21]

### Hemodynamic Findings.

As in the patient with suspected dilated cardiomyopathy, cardiac catheterization in the patient being evaluated for hypertrophic cardiomyopathy should include right and left heart study. Right atrial and right ventricular pressures are usually normal in patients with hypertrophic cardiomyopathy. Rarely, involvement of the right ventricle is said to result in a systolic gradient within the right ventricular chamber, although I have never seen such a case personally. If the hypertrophic process involves the right ventricle, or if the pulmonary capillary wedge pressure is substantially elevated, right ventricular diastolic pressures may be elevated.

Left ventricular end diastolic pressure may be normal in patients with hypertrophic cardiomyopathy but is usually elevated,[18–20,23] reflecting decreased left ventricular diastolic distensibility. The decreased diastolic distensibility in hypertrophic cardiomyopathy is due to both increased passive stiffness of the thick-walled left ventricular chamber and decreased rate and extent of myocardial relaxation.[1,22–28] Pulmonary capillary wedge pressure may be elevated, particularly if there is mitral regurgitation, a common finding in patients with hypertrophic cardiomyopathy.[29]

Cardiac output is usually normal or increased in patients with hypertrophic cardiomyopathy, except in the late stages of the disease where contractility decreases.[22]

The most dramatic hemodynamic features of hypertrophic cardiomyopathy are those related to the systolic intraventricular pressure gradient. As seen in Figure 26-5, the pressure gradient is present between the body and the outflow tract of the left ventricle. A key feature of this systolic gradient and of most of the associated findings is their variability. The majority of patients with hypertrophic cardiomyopathy do not have a systolic pressure gradient at rest, but may develop one with appropriate provocative maneuvers as listed in Table 26-2.

It should be emphasized that the presence of a systolic gradient at rest or following provocation is a hallmark of only one variety of hypertrophic cardiomyopathy: that form with asymmetric septal hypertrophy. The diffuse hypertrophic variety and the variety associated with massive apical hypertrophy do not exhibit systolic gradients at rest or with provocation.[20]

An interesting aspect of the systolic gradient is an associated deformity that develops in the aortic pressure waveform. This deformity consists of an initial rapid rise in aortic pressure to give a spike early in ejection, followed by a dip in pressure and a secondary rounded or dome-shaped tidal wave prior to the dicrotic notch. This spike-and-dome configuration is seen in the central aortic pressure and is transmitted to the carotid pulse and peripheral arterial tracings. It is

**TABLE 26-2.** *Provocative Maneuvers for Development of Systolic Pressure Gradient in Hypertrophic Cardiomyopathy*

1. Valsalva maneuver
2. Amyl nitrite inhalation
3. Postextrasystolic potentiation
4. Isoproterenol
5. Exercise

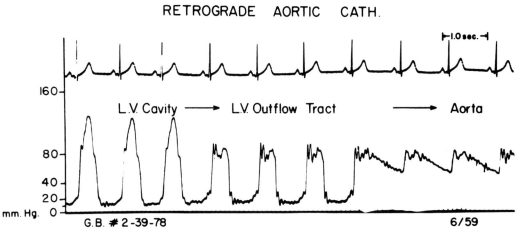

**Fig. 26-5.** Left ventricular (LV) catheter pullback to the aorta in a patient with hypertrophic cardiomyopathy. There is a significant systolic gradient within the left ventricular cavity, and the LV outflow tract and aortic pressure waveforms exhibit a spike-and-dome contour. (Reproduced with permission from Braunwald E, et al: Idiopathic hypertrophic subaortic stenosis. A description based on an analysis of 65 patients. Circulation 30 (Suppl 4):3, 1964.)

most evident following an extrasystolic contraction (Fig. 26-6) but is also seen during Valsalva maneuver (Fig. 26-7) and at other times (Fig. 26-8). The mechanism for this spike-and-dome configuration may be related to blending of an initial hyperdynamic ejection velocity leading to the development of a Venturi effect that sucks the anterior mitral leaflet into the outflow tract, thereby impeding mid and late diastolic ejection velocity.

In addition to developing a spike-and-dome pattern, the aortic pulse pressure fails to widen in a postextrasystolic potentiated beat.[18] Normally, a potentiated left ventricular contraction has a larger stroke volume than the preceding sinus beats, and this increased stroke volume is reflected in an increased aortic pulse pressure. However, patients with hypertrophic cardiomyopathy develop a spike-and-dome configuration in which pulse pressure is unchanged or actually reduced following an extrasystolic beat (Fig. 26-6). This sign, which was described by Brockenbrough, Braunwald, and Morrow in 1961,[30] is believed to reflect worsening of obstruction of the left ventricular outflow tract during the potentiated beat, with diminished stroke volume and aortic pulse pressure.

The impaired left ventricular diastolic relaxation seen in hypertrophic cardiomyopathy [22–28] can be dramatic and can affect the contour of the left ventricular diastolic pressure tracing (Fig. 26-9). The patient illustrated in Figure 26-9 was a 55-year-old woman with a family history of hypertrophic cardiomyopathy, who presented with advanced congestive heart failure manifested by paroxysmal nocturnal dyspnea, marked fatigue, and peripheral edema. Echocardiogram showed asymmetric septal hypertrophy. At cardiac catheterization there was no outflow tract gradient at rest or with provocation. Right atrial mean pressure was increased (11 mmHg), reflecting pulmonary hypertension (60/30, 40 mmHg), which in turn reflected a markedly increased mean pulmonary capillary wedge pressure (32 mmHg). Arteriovenous $O_2$ difference was wide (71 ml $O_2$/liter), and cardiac index was depressed (2.0 L/min/$M^2$). Left ventricular ejection fraction was reduced at 41%, a finding sometimes seen in late-stage hypertrophic cardiomyopathy. As seen in Figure 26-9, the left ventricular diastolic pressure did not exhibit its normal rapid decline to a nadir near zero. Instead, early left ventricular diastolic pressure was increased at approximately 35 mmHg and continued to decline

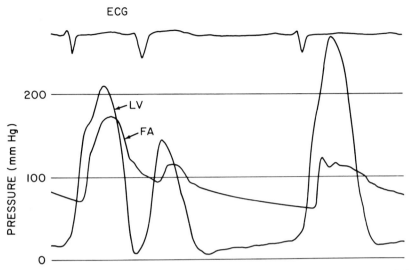

**Fig. 26-6.** Left ventricular (LV) and femoral artery (FA) pressure tracings in a woman with hypertrophic cardiomyopathy and asymmetric septal hypertrophy, illustrating the increase in gradient and development of a spike-and-dome configuration in the arterial pressure waveform following an extrasystolic beat. Also, arterial pulse pressure clearly narrows in the postextrasystolic beat compared to the control value in the beat prior to the extrasystole. This narrowing of pulse pressure is known as the Brockenbrough-Braunwald sign.

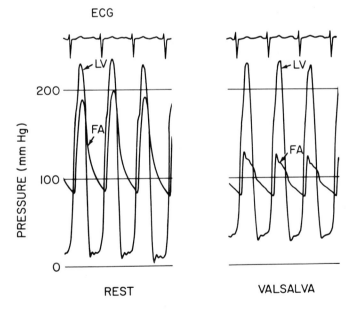

**Fig. 26-7.** Left ventricular (LV) and femoral artery (FA) pressure tracings in the patient illustrated in Figure 26-6. Valsalva maneuver produces a marked increase in the gradient, as well as a change in the femoral arterial pressure waveform to a spike-and-dome configuration.

after mitral valve opening until atrial systole produced a diastolic pressure rise coincident with the "a" wave. This striking diastolic relaxation abnormality was largely corrected with nifedipine,[22] as seen in Figure 26-10.

The diastolic abnormalities of hypertrophic cardiomyopathy are improved by calcium channel blockade,[22-24,31-33] although occasional serious adverse effects have been seen with verapamil.[34]

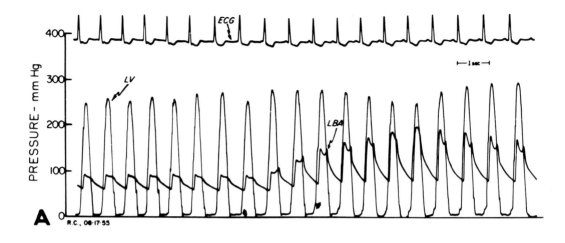

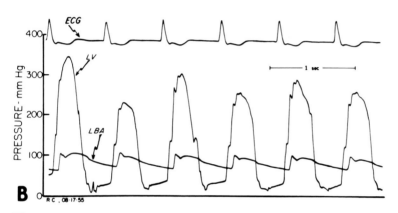

**Fig. 26-8.**  Left ventricular (LV) and left brachial artery (LBA) pressure tracings in a 64-year-old woman with hypertrophic cardiomyopathy. (A) The effect of a spontaneous change from nodal rhythm to sinus rhythm. The short arrows show LV end-diastolic pressure. With restoration of sinus rhythm and a presumed decrease in the obstruction, LV stroke volume increases as reflected in the improved LBA pulse pressure. Also, the loss of atrial kick in patients with a stiff ventricle leads to an acute reduction in cardiac output. (B) Following a premature contraction (not shown) there is LV pulsus alternans. A spike-and-dome pattern is clearly seen in the LBA tracing. (Reproduced with permission from Glancy L, et al: The dynamic nature of left ventricular outflow obstruction in idiopathic hypertrophic subaortic stenosis. Ann Intern Med 75:589, 1971.)

***Angiographic Findings.***  The angiographic findings in hypertrophic cardiomyopathy are rather unique and help to explain some (but not all) of the unusual hemodynamic features just described. In hypertrophic cardiomyopathy with asymmetric septal hypertrophy, left ventriculography shows a thickened intraventricular septum bulging into the left ventricular outflow tract in diastole and systole. In addition to this abnormality, patients with hypertrophic car-

diomyopathy in whom a systolic gradient is present within the left ventricular chamber generally show systolic anterior movement (SAM) of the mitral valve's anterior leaflet (Fig. 26-11). The anterior leaflet is believed to appose the interventricular septum due to suction from a Venturi effect, caused in turn by the very high outflow tract velocity of ejected blood.

In contrast to hypertrophic cardiomyopathy with asymmetric septal hypertrophy, the

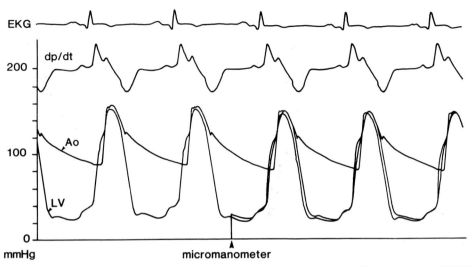

**Fig. 26-9.** Left ventricular (LV) and aortic (Ao) pressure tracings and rate of LV pressure rise (dP/dt) in a 55-year-old woman with hypertrophic cardiomyopathy. There is no resting pressure gradient. LV diastolic pressure waveform is very abnormal, suggesting marked impairment in myocardial relaxation. Fluid-filled and micromanometer LV tracings are both shown.

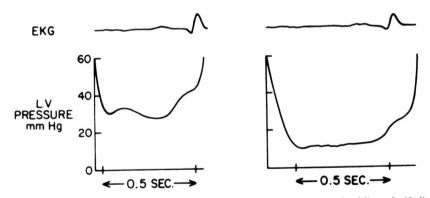

**Fig 26-10.** LV diastolic pressure before (left) and after (right) administration of sublingual nifedipine in the patient illustrated in Figure 26-9. There is a lowering of LV diastolic pressure toward normal, as well as a striking improvement in the abnormal relaxation pattern. (Reproduced with permission from Lorell BH, et al: Improved diastolic function and systolic performance in hypertrophic cardiomyopathy after nifedipine. N Engl J Med 303:801, 1980.)

patient with asymmetric *apical* hypertrophy does not show systolic anterior motion of the mitral leaflet. In patients with apical hypertrophic cardiomyopathy, the left ventricle shows marked thickening of its anteroapical wall, giving the ventricle a spade-shaped appearance (Fig. 26-12).

Patients with *asymmetric septal hypertrophy* have a distortion of the left ventricle that in the right anterior oblique view often resembles a banana. The banana-shaped left ventricle results in part from the large papillary muscles, which appear as filling defects.

In addition to abnormal shapes (spade,

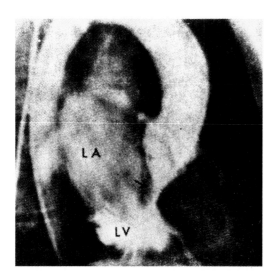

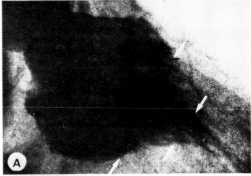

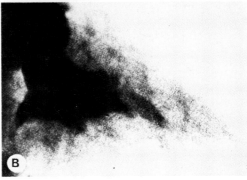

**Fig. 26-11.** Left ventricular (LV) angiogram in the lateral position in patient with hypertrophic cardiomyopathy with obstruction. The anterior leaflet of the mitral valve moves toward the interventricular septum in systole (arrow) producing marked narrowing of the LV outflow tract. Mitral regurgitation into the left atrium (LA) is present. (Reproduced with permission from Braunwald E, et al: Idiopathic hypertrophic subaortic stenosis. A description based on an analysis of 65 patients. Circulation 30 (Suppl 4):3, 1964.)

**Fig. 26-12.** Left ventriculogram at end-diastole (A) and end-systole (B) in a patient with apical hypertrophic cardiomyopathy. There is a spadelike configuration at end-diastole with a marked increase in free wall thickness. There is an extremely vigorous contraction with almost total cavity obliteration at end-systole. (Reproduced with permission from Yamaguchi H, et al: Hypertrophic non-obstructive cardiomyopathy with giant negative T waves (apical hypertrophy): ventriculographic and echocardiographic features in 30 patients. Am J Cardiol 44:401, 1979.)

banana) and systolic anterior movement of the mitral valve, patients with hypertrophic cardiomyopathy often exhibit mitral regurgitation on left ventriculography. This is usually mild but may progress to become hemodynamically significant. Coronary angiography may show characteristic abnormalities in hypertrophic cardiomyopathy, with marked systolic compression of septal branches of the left anterior descending artery.[35] In addition, a "sawfish" systolic narrowing of the left anterior descending artery has been reported by Brugada et al[36] and is illustrated in Figure 26-13. The indentations

of the left anterior descending artery associated with systolic narrowing of the vessel may represent the effect of contracting hypertrophied and disorganized muscle fiber bundles in the vicinity of the coronary artery.[36]

## REFERENCES

1. Goodwin JF: The frontiers of cardiomyopathy. Br Heart J 48:1, 1982.
2. Goodwin JF, Gordon H, Hollman A, Bishop MB: Clinical aspects of cardiomyopathy. Br Med J 1:69, 1961.
3. Grossman W, McLaurin LP, Rolett EL: Alterations in left ventricular relaxation and diastolic compliance in congestive cardiomyopathy. Cardiovasc Res 13:514, 1979.
4. Baim DS, et al: Evaluation of a new bipyridine

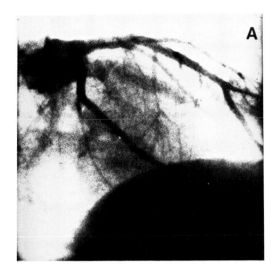

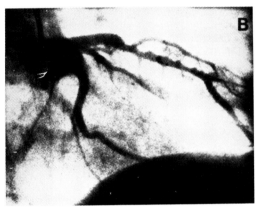

**Fig. 26-13.** Left coronary angiogram in right anterior oblique projection with caudocranial angulation. Diastolic (A) and systolic (B) frames are shown. A "sawfish" appearance of the left anterior descending artery is seen in association with systolic compression of septal branches in this patient with hypertrophic cardiomyopathy. (Reproduced with permission from Brugada P, et al: "Sawfish" narrowing of the left anterior descending coronary artery: an angiographic sign of hypertrophic cardiomyopathy. Circulation 66:800, 1982.)

inotropic agent—milrinone—in patients with severe congestive heart failure. N Engl J Med 309:748, 1983.

5. Monrad ES, et al: Improvement in indices of diastolic performance in patients with congestive heart failure treated with milrinone. Circulation 70:1030, 1984.

6. Erbel R, et al: Hemodynamic effects of prenalterol in patients with ischemic heart disease and congestive cardiomyopathy. Circulation 66:361, 1982.

7. Harshaw CW, Munro AB, McLaurin LP, Grossman W. Reduced systemic vascular resistance as therapy for severe mitral regurgitation of valvular origin. Ann Intern Med 83:312, 1975.

8. Guiha NH, et al: Treatment of refractory heart failure with infusion of nitroprusside. N Engl J Med 291:587, 1974.

9. Davis R, et al: Treatment of chronic congestive heart failure with captopril, an oral inhibitor of angiotensin-converting enzyme. N Engl J Med 301:117, 1979.

10. Dzau VJ, et al: Sustained effectiveness of converting-enzyme inhibition in patients with severe congestive heart failure. N Engl J Med 302:1373, 1980.

11. Ader R, et al: Immediate and sustained hemodynamic and clinical improvement in chronic heart failure by an oral angiotensin-converting enzyme inhibitor. Circulation 61:931, 1980.

12. Kreulen TH, Gorlin R, Herman MV: Ventriculographic patterns and hemodynamics in primary myocardial disease. Circulation 47:299, 1973.

13. Benjamin HJ, Schuster EH, Bulkley BH: Cardiac hypertrophy in idiopathic dilated congestive cardiomyopathy: a clinicopathologic study. Circulation 64:442, 1981.

14. Feild BJ, et al: Left ventricular function and hypertrophy in cardiomyopathy with depressed ejection fraction. Circulation 47:1022, 1973.

15. Parrillo JE, et al: The results of transvenous endomyocardial biopsy can frequently be used to diagnose myocardial disease in patients with idiopathic heart failure. Circulation 69:93, 1984.

16. Unverferth DV, et al: Factors influencing the one-year mortality of dilated cardiomyopathy. Am J Cardiol 54:147, 1984.

17. Fuster V, et al: The natural history of idiopathic dilated cardiomyopathy. Am J Cardiol 54:525, 1981.

18. Braunwald E, et al: Idiopathic hypertrophic subaortic stenosis. A description based on an analysis of 65 patients. Circulation 30(Suppl 4):3, 1964.

19. Murgo JP, et al: Dynamics of left ventricular ejection in obstructive and nonobstructive hypertrophic cardiomyopathy. J Clin Invest 66:1369, 1980.

20. Yamaguchi H, et al: Hypertrophic nonobstructive cardiomyopathy with giant negative T waves (apical hypertrophy): ventriculographic and echocardigraphic features in 30 patients. Am J Cardiol 44:401, 1979.

21. Shapiro LM, McKenna WJ: Distribution of left ventricular hypertrophy in hypertrophic cardiomyopathy: a two-dimensional echocardiographic study. J Am Coll Cardiol 2:437, 1983.

22. Lorell BH, et al: Improved diastolic function and systolic performance in hypertrophic cardiomy-

opathy after nifedipine. N Engl J Med 303:801, 1980.

23. Lorell BH, et al: Modification of abnormal left ventricular diastolic properties by nifedipine in patients with hypertrophic cardiomyopathy. Circulation 64:499, 1982.

24. Hanrath P, et al: Effect of verapamil on left ventricular isovolumic relaxation time and regional left ventricular filling in hypertrophic cardiomyopathy. Am J Cardiol 45:1258, 1980.

25. Sanderson JE, et al: Left ventricular relaxation and filling in hypertrophic cardiomyopathy. An echocardiographic study. Br Heart J 40:596, 1978.

26. St. John Sutton MG, et al: Echocardiographic assessment of left ventricular filling and septal and posterior wall dynamics in idiopathic hypertrophic subaortic stenosis. Circulation 57:512, 1978.

27. Hanrath P, Mathey DG, Siegert R, Bleifeld W: Left ventricular relaxation and filling pattern in different forms of left ventricular hypertrophy. An echocardiographic study. Am J Cardiol 45:15, 1980.

28. Stewart S, Mason DT, Braunwald E: Impaired rate of left ventricular filling in IHSS and valvular aortic stenosis. Circulation 37:8, 1968.

29. Dinsmore RE, Sanders CA, Harthorne JW: Mitral regurgitation in idiopathic hypertrophic subaortic stenosis. N Engl J Med 275:1225, 1966.

30. Brockenbrough EC, Braunwald E, Morrow AG: A hemodynamic technic for the detection of hypertrophic subaortic stenosis. Circulation 23:189, 1961.

31. Paulus WJ, et al: Comparison of the effects of nitroprusside and nifedipine on diastolic properties in patients with hypertrophic cardiomyopathy: Altered left ventricular loading or improved muscle inactivation? J Am Coll Cardiol 2:879, 1983.

32. Lorell BH: Use of calcium channel blockers in hypertrophic cardiomyopathy. Am J Med 78 (suppl 2B):43, 1985.

33. Bonow RO, et al: Effects of verapamil on left ventricular systolic function and diastolic filling in patients with hypertrophic cardiomyopathy. Circulation 64:787, 1981.

34. Epstein SE, Rosing DR: Verapamil: its potential for causing serious complications in patients with hypertrophic cardiomyopathy. Circulation 64:437, 1981.

35. Pichard AD, et al: Septal perforation compression (narrowing) in idiopathic hypertrophic subaortic stenosis. Am J Cardiol 40:310, 1977.

36. Brugada P et al: "Sawfish" systolic narrowing of the left anterior descending artery: an angiographic sign of hypertrophic cardiomyopathy. Circulation 66:800, 1982.

## chapter twenty seven

# Profiles in Constrictive Pericarditis, Restrictive Cardiomyopathy, and Cardiac Tamponade

BEVERLY H. LORELL *and* WILLIAM GROSSMAN

ERICARDITIS of any etiology can be followed by three hemodynamic complications: (1) a pericardial effusion under pressure resulting in cardiac tamponade; (2) progressive pericardial fibrosis and scarring causing constrictive physiology; (3) the combination of both an effusion under pressure and pericardial constriction. A common feature of each is the presence of diastolic dysfunction due to external compression of the heart which prevents adequate diastolic filling, elevates right and left heart diastolic pressures, and results ultimately in reduced stroke volume due to inadequate preload. However, the diastolic filling pattern during each cardiac cycle and the response to respiration differ such that distinctive hemodynamic profiles of constrictive pericarditis, cardiac tamponade, and effusive-constrictive pericarditis can usually be identified in the cardiac catheterization laboratory. The hemodynamic and angiographic evaluation must also include consideration of the presence of restrictive cardio-

myopathy in which features of impaired diastolic filling with preserved systolic contractile function may simulate constrictive pericarditis.[1]

## CONSTRICTIVE PERICARDITIS

***Clinical Features.*** Constrictive pericarditis is a symmetrical process in which there is scarring of both the parietal and visceral pericardial layers affecting all chambers of the heart. Localized constriction which may simulate valvular stenosis is extremely rare. In the chronic stage, pericardial calcification may develop, but it may be absent in earlier stages despite severe hemodynamic compromise. Tuberculosis was previously the leading cause of constrictive pericarditis. Today, more common causes of subacute or chronic constrictive pericarditis include recurrent idiopathic or viral pericarditis, chronic renal failure, neoplastic pericardial involvement, and connective tissue disorders such as rheumatoid arthritis and progressive systemic sclerosis. An increasingly recognized etiology is high dose mediastinal irradiation for malignancy, which may cause severe constrictive pericarditis many years after therapy.[2] Constrictive physiology may develop rapidly following cardiac surgery or trauma due to deposition of fibrin and thrombus adjacent to the heart.[3]

The clinical features of constrictive pericarditis reflect the gradual and often insidious development of systemic and pulmonary venous hypertension. In patients in whom right and left atrial pressures are modestly elevated in the range of 10 to 18 mmHg, symptoms and signs of systemic venous congestion predominate, including leg edema postprandial discomfort, hepatic congestion, and ascites. As right and left heart filling pressures become elevated to a level of 18 to 30 mmHg, exertional dyspnea and orthopnea appear, and pleural effusions often develop. The impairment of diastolic filling results initially in an inability to augment stroke volume in response to stress and may cause symptoms of exertional fatigue or hemodynamic instability during dialysis in the uremic patient. As resting cardiac output falls, severe lethargy and cardiac cachexia supervene. The electrocardiogram usually shows reduced voltage, nonspecific ST-T wave abnormalities, and atrial fibrillation. The chest roentgenogram may show a small, normal, or modestly enlarged silhouette with redistribution of pulmonary blood flow, and the useful marker of pericardial calcification may be present. Advanced tuberculous constrictive pericarditis is associated commonly with dense pericardial calcification, which has been termed "panzerherz" in the German literature, and "concretia cordis" in Latin. Echocardiography can be extremely helpful in suggesting the presence of constrictive pericarditis if a pattern of pericardial thickening, abrupt posterior motion of the interventricular septum in early diastole, and reduced motion of the left ventricular posterior wall is seen. Because of the vague and insidious nature of the symptoms, constrictive pericarditis is often mistaken for primary hepatic disease, intraabdominal malignancy, or nephrotic syndrome.

Constrictive pericarditis should be suspected in any patient with unexplained jugular venous distension, systemic edema, and hepatomegaly. Constrictive pericarditis should also be considered in the postoperative heart surgery patient who has unexplained tachycardia, low cardiac output, and venous congestion within the first 2 to 3 months following surgery. Right and left heart cardiac catheterization and angiography should be performed in every patient with this potentially curable disease to: (1) confirm the presence of constrictive physiology and assess its severity prior to consideration of pericardiectomy; (2) assist in the differentiation of pericardial disease from restrictive cardiomyopathy; (3) exclude coexisting causes of right atrial hypertension; (4) exclude the rare instances of localized constricting bands either within the atrioventricular groove simulating valvular stenosis or causing external stenosis of the coronary arteries.

***Hemodynamic and Angiographic Profile.*** The symmetrical constricting effect of the pericardium usually impairs diastolic filling of all chambers of the heart such that right and left ventricular diastolic pressures are elevated and equal within 5 mmHg or less. Although right and left *ventricular* diastolic pressures are equal in constrictive pericarditis, right and left *atrial* (pulmonary capillary wedge) pressures may differ if coexisting mitral or tricuspid regurgitation is present associated with a large A or V wave in either atrium. For this reason, it is critical to record right and left ventricular pressures simultaneously, using equisensitive gains. Care should be taken to calibrate the transducers simultaneously to a column of mercury, and the transducers should be leveled to precisely the same height. Severe pulmonary hypertension is usually absent in constrictive pericarditis unless coexisting heart disease is present, and the pulmonary artery and right ventricular systolic pressures are usually between 35 and 45 mmHg.

The major determinant of the filling pressures is the degree of constriction. Moderate constriction is associated with filling pressures between 12 and 15 mmHg, and severe constriction is associated with filling pressures between 20 and 25 mmHg. However, hypovolemia may lower these pressures so that it is important to know if the patient has been treated intensively with diuretics and to avoid excessive diuresis immediately prior to catheterization. In this regard, an entity of "occult" pericardial constriction has been described in which patients with nondescript

chest pain who had normal baseline hemodynamics were shown to develop elevation
and equilibration of diastolic pressures suggestive of pericardial constriction after rapid
infusion of 1000 ml of normal saline solution.[4] Many of these patients subsequently
underwent pericardiectomy, following which
their symptoms improved. A word of caution
is in order, however, since the sensitivity and
specificity of this volume-challenge test in
patients with atypical chest pain is as yet
poorly defined and there is potential for
doing harm with a massive volume infusion.

The constricting pericardium causes virtually all ventricular filling to occur in early
diastole. In severe constrictive pericarditis,
in which the heart is encased in a rigid and
adherent fibrotic shell, the end-systolic volume is usually less than that defined by the
pericardium. Therefore, early diastolic filling
is unimpeded and abnormally rapid due to
the elevation of venous pressure, but filling
halts abruptly in early diastole when total
cardiac volume expands to the volume set by
the stiff pericardium.[5] This pattern of virtually all ventricular filling occurring in early
diastole is reflected in the early diastolic dip-
and-plateau pattern in the right and left ven-

tricular waveforms. Since right atrial and
right ventricular pressures are equilibrated
in diastole, the right atrial waveform typically shows a prominent and rapid diastolic
Y descent, which indicates that right atrial
emptying after tricuspid valve opening is
rapid and unimpeded. The Y descent is followed by a steep "a" wave and X descent,
since the atrium is attempting to eject blood
into a right ventricle that is already filled to
its capacity. The steep X and Y descents im-
part to the pressure waveform its characteristic M or W configuration[6] (Fig. 27-1). It is
important to avoid an underdamped pressure-transducer system, since this causes
overshoot in the pressure tracing which may
artifactually produce this sign. Conversely,
the presence of tachycardia with a shortened
diastole may obscure the presence of the
plateau component of the ventricular waveform (Fig. 27-2).

In severe pericardial constriction, negative
intrathoracic pressure during inspiration is
not communicated to the intrapericardial
space and right heart. In contrast to what is
seen in normal subjects, systemic venous
and right atrial pressures do not fall, and
venous flow to the right atrium does not ac-

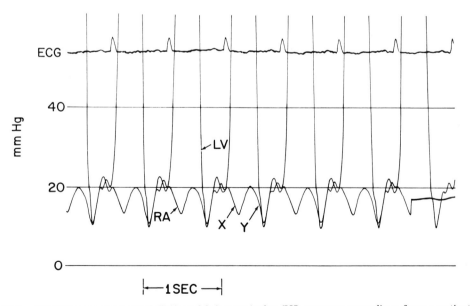

**Fig. 27-1.** Simultaneous right atrial (RA) and left ventricular (LV) pressure recordings from a patient with
constrictive pericarditis, illustrating that both pressures are elevated and equal throughout diastole. Note the
prominent Y descent in the right atrial waveform which indicates that right atrial emptying is rapid and unimpeded in early diastole. The prominent X and Y descents give the right atrial waveform its characteristic M- or
W-shaped appearance in constrictive pericarditis.

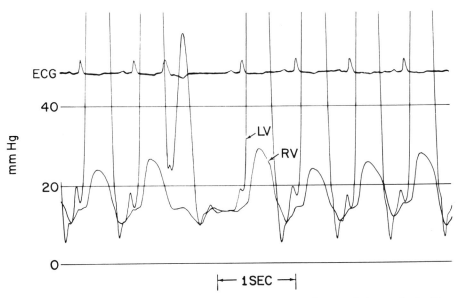

**Fig. 27-2.**  Left (LV) and right (RV) ventricular pressures recorded simultaneously in a patient with surgically confirmed constrictive pericarditis illustrate technical pitfalls in evaluation of pressure tracings. The presence of resting tachycardia partially obscures evaluation of the diastolic waveforms, and underdamping of the left ventricular pressure-transducer system accentuates an undershoot of left ventricular pressure in early diastole and an overshoot during atrial contraction. A long diastole following a premature beat permits the recognition of equilibration of left and right ventricular diastolic pressures and the appreciation of a dip and plateau component of the ventricular waveforms.

celerate during inspiration in patients with severe constrictive pericarditis. As illustrated in Fig. 27-3, in extreme cases, systemic venous pressure may increase during inspiration (Kussmaul's sign).[7] The lack of phasic augmentation of right heart filling during inspiration accounts for the fact that pulsus paradoxus is less prominent in constrictive pericarditis than in cardiac tamponade, in which right heart filling is exaggerated during inspiration at the expense of left heart filling.

Stroke volume is almost always reduced in patients with constrictive pericarditis, but resting cardiac output may be preserved because of tachycardia. Supine dynamic exercise usually causes only a slight rise in cardiac filling pressures, but cardiac output fails to rise appropriately relative to the increase in systemic oxygen consumption. In these patients, enhanced oxygen demand is met almost entirely by increased oxygen extraction and widening of the arteriovenous oxygen difference. In severe cases, resting cardiac index is depressed in association with systemic arterial vasoconstriction and arterial hypotension.

The combination of low stroke volume, low stroke work, and increased ventricular filling pressure indicates failure of cardiac pump function. However, pump failure in constrictive pericarditis is due to reduced chamber compliance and diminished myocardial fiber stretch or preload rather than myocardial systolic failure. In the absence of coexisting cardiac disease, left ventricular angiography usually shows that left ventricular volume is moderately-to-severely reduced. Left ventricular end-systolic volume is small, and left ventricular ejection fraction is normal-to-increased. In the absence of myocardial inflammation or fibrosis, both isovolumic and ejection phase indices of systolic contractile function (e.g., peak dP/dt) are normal.[8,9] Superior vena caval angiography can be helpful in selected patients with neoplastic disease to exclude coexisting superior vena caval compression. In patients with constrictive pericarditis, venous angiography may demonstrate dilatation of the superior vena cava, straightening of the right heart border, and pericardial thickening. Coronary angiography should be considered in older patients at increased risk of coro-

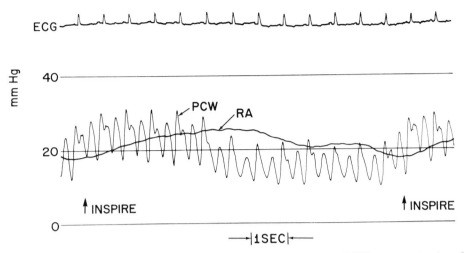

**Fig. 27-3.** Right atrial (mean, RA) and pulmonary capillary wedge (phasic, PCW) pressure tracings from a patient with constrictive pericarditis. An arrow marks the beginning of the inspiratory phase of each respiratory cycle. Note that mean right atrial pressure increases during inspiration (Kussmaul's sign). The pulmonary capillary wedge pressure is out of phase with right atrial pressure and begins to fall during inspiration as right atrial pressure is rising.

nary atherosclerosis prior to open heart operation for extensive pericardiectomy. Coronary angiography is also indicated in all patients with constrictive pericarditis and angina-like chest pain, since the pericardial scarring process can rarely cause external pinching or compression of the coronary arteries.[10]

The hemodynamic and angiographic findings may differ somewhat in patients with subacute noncalcific pericarditis of less than one year's duration, in whom the pericardium is characterized by an adherent fluid-fibrin layer in the process of organization rather than a rigid scarred shell. Hancock has compared this relatively *elastic form of constrictive pericarditis* to encircling the heart tightly with rubber bands.[11] In this elastic form of fibroelastic pericardial disease, cardiac compression is present throughout the cardiac cycle, and the patterns of ventricular filling and pressure waveforms are more like those of cardiac tamponade.

## RESTRICTIVE CARDIOMYOPATHY

***Clinical Features.*** The differentiation between constrictive pericarditis and restrictive cardiomyopathy is often difficult at the bedside and in the catheterization laboratory. In restrictive cardiomyopathy, the restrictive element resides in the myocardium itself such that the ventricular walls resist stretch abnormally during cardiac filling. Therefore, the clinical features of patients with restrictive cardiomyopathy due to idiopathic etiology, metabolic storage diseases, amyloidosis, or hemochromatosis are often similar to constrictive pericarditis. In both disorders, ventricular diastolic filling is impaired, ventricular filling pressures are elevated, stroke volume is fixed or reduced, and systolic contractile function is essentially normal.

***Hemodynamic and Angiographic Profile.*** In most cases, careful attention to hemodynamics does permit identification of the patient with restrictive cardiomyopathy. Diastolic pressure in the left ventricle is usually higher than in the right ventricule when both are recorded simultaneously.[1,12] (Fig. 27-4). Furthermore, exercise will generally increase left ventricular diastolic pressure more than right ventricular diastolic pressure. Pulmonary hypertension is usually more severe in restrictive cardiomyopathy than in constrictive pericarditis, and pulmonary systolic pressures in excess of 50 mmHg are commonly found. In constrictive pericarditis, this degree of pulmonary hypertension is rare, and diastolic plateau

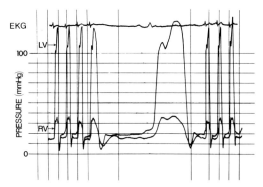

**Fig. 27-4.** Right and left ventricular (RV and LV) pressure tracings in a 43-year-old woman with idiopathic restrictive cardiomyopathy. A dip and plateau pattern is seen in both ventricles and diastolic pressures are increased. However, the plateaus are at different absolute levels, approximately 16 mmHg for the RV and 20 mmHg for the LV. In this patient, both RV and LV diastolic pressures increased simultaneously with exercise, and final confirmation of the diagnosis of restrictive cardiomyopathy (versus constrictive pericarditis) was made by thoracotomy. (From Benotti JR, Grossman W, Cohn PF: The clinical profile of restrictive cardiomyopathy. Circulation 61:1206, 1980, by permission of the American Heart Association, Inc.)

pressure usually exceeds one third of the right ventricular systolic pressure.[7] Published data regarding myocardial contractile function are few, but isovolumic and ejection phase indices are often normal.[13,14] In some cases of cardiac amyloidosis, the picture of restrictive cardiomyopathy is absent, and impaired indices of contractile function are present.[12]

In 9 patients with restrictive cardiomyopathy and symptoms of either congestive heart failure or chest pain studied at Peter Bent Brigham Hospital, left ventricular ejection fraction was 63 ± 8%, suggestive of normal myocardial contractile function.[15] In these patients, left ventricular end-diastolic pressure (23 ± 6 mmHg) was substantially higher than right ventricular end-diastolic pressure (16 ± 5 mmHg) and moderate elevation of pulmonary artery systolic pressure was present (49 ± 21 mmHg).

However, the hemodynamic findings in some patients with restrictive cardiomyopathy are virtually indistinguishable from those of constrictive pericarditis.[13,16] Frame-by-frame angiographic analysis of left ventricular filling has been proposed as a method of distinguishing between these two conditions, since early diastolic filling tends to be slower than normal in restrictive cardiomyopathy, but is excessively rapid in constrictive pericarditis.[17] However, the predictive value of this approach has not been established in the patient with suspected restrictive myopathy who has a dip-and-plateau ventricular waveform which itself suggests that early diastolic filling is excessively rapid and abruptly attenuated in mid-diastole. Myocardial biopsy can be helpful in documenting the presence of amyloid in some patients in whom cardiac catheterization findings do not differentiate between constrictive pericarditis and restrictive cardiomyopathy.[14] However, it must be kept in mind that amyloid may infiltrate both the myocardium and the pericardium.[16] Furthermore, in many cases no specific pathologic finding can be identified by biopsy to explain the hemodynamic findings.[15] Thus, in selected patients, exploratory thoracotomy with careful histologic examination of pericardium and myocardium is justified to differentiate the surgically correctable condition of constrictive pericarditis from restrictive cardiomyopathy.

## OTHER CONDITIONS ASSOCIATED WITH CONSTRICTIVE PHYSIOLOGY

The normal pericardium provides a substantial restraining effect on cardiac dilatation in conditions in which pericardium has not hypertrophied or stretched to accommodate an increase in cardiac volume. Acute and massive right ventricular infarction with right ventricular dilatation may cause constrictive physiology with elevation and equilibration of right and left ventricular pressures and dip-and-plateau ventricular waveforms.[18] These hemodynamic findings have been shown in animal models of experimental right ventricular infarction to be due to increased intrapericardial pressure.[19] Similarly, volume overload due to subacute tricuspid regurgitation in the presence of an intact pericardium may cause marked elevation and equilibration of ventricular diastolic pressures (Fig. 27-5).

Just as acute volume overload of the right ventricle (as in right ventricular infarction or

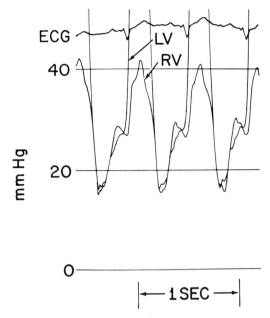

**Fig. 27-5.** Simultaneous right (RV) and left (LV) ventricular pressure tracings recorded in a patient with several weeks' history of severe tricuspid insufficiency. Note that right and left ventricular end-diastolic pressures are markedly elevated (approximately 28 mmHg) with virtual identity of pressures throughout diastole. Right ventricular systolic pressure is minimally increased, indication that the elevation of right ventricular diastolic pressure is not primarily due to pulmonary hypertension. These findings are suggestive of a restraining effect of the intact pericardium in the presence of subacute volume overload of the right ventricle.

severe tricuspid regurgitation) can compress the left ventricle by displacement of the elastic shared interventricular septum, overload of the left ventricle can adversely affect right ventricular filling. Bartle and Hermann reported evidence that acute mitral regurgitation in man can present a striking hemodynamic pattern highly suggestive of pericardial restriction.[20] In this instance, significant pulmonary hypertension will be an obligatory part of the hemodynamic pattern (Fig. 27-6). This feature allows distinction from the findings in primary right ventricular volume overload (Fig. 27-5) where pulmonary hypertension will often be absent. Acute massive pulmonary embolism may present with an intermediate picture, where pulmonary hypertension causes acute right

ventricular failure and dilatation, and this may cause some compression of the left ventricle.

## CARDIAC TAMPONADE

***Clinical Features.*** The development of an increase in intrapericardial pressure and the restriction of cardiac filling from a pericardial effusion depend on several factors: (1) the rate of fluid accumulation; (2) the actual volume of fluid; (3) the distensibility of the pericardium; and (4) the underlying distensibility of the ventricular chambers. The normal unstretched pericardium usually contains less then 50 ml of fluid and can accommodate mild fluctuations in intrapericardial volume with little change in intrapericardial pressure. However, the rapid accumulation of greater than about 150 ml of fluid is associated with a steep rise in intrapericardial pressure. Intracardiac diastolic pressures also rise so that the transmural difference between ventricular diastolic pressure and

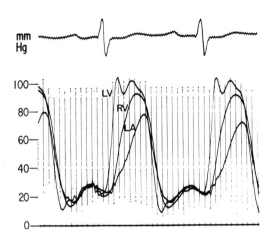

**Fig. 27-6.** Left and right ventricular (LV, RV) and left atrial (LA) pressure tracings in a 60-year-old man with acute, severe mitral regurgitation. The acute LV and LA volume overloads result in a constrictive physiology, with equalization of LV and RV diastolic pressures, since the pericardium has not yet grown sufficiently to accommodate the increased chamber volumes. (Reproduced with permission from Bartle SH, Hermann HJ: Acute mitral regurgitation in man. Hemodynamic evidence and observations indicating an early role for the pericardium. Circulation 36:839, 1967.)

intrapericardial pressure falls; when equilibration of pericardial and ventricular diastolic pressures occurs, transmural distending pressure falls to zero, and stroke volume falls precipitously.[21] Cardiac output and blood pressure are maintained initially by reflex vasoconstriction and tachycardia, but as the impairment of cardiac filling becomes more severe, hypotension and shock ensue.

Cardiac tamponade from acute intrapericardial hemorrhage due to cardiac trauma may occur when an effusion of less than 200 ml of fluid is sufficient to cause an abrupt rise in intrapericardial pressure to a level above 20 mmHg. These patients exhibit the classic clinical triad described by Claude S. Beck:[22] (1) elevation of systemic venous pressure; (2) systemic arterial hypotension; (3) a small, quiet heart. Patients with the acute development of cardiac tamponade are typically agitated and confused and exhibit tachycardia, tachypnea, and profound systemic arterial hypotension. However, the cardiologist in the catheterization laboratory should recognize that medical patients with chronic pericardial inflammation due to viral pericarditis, uremia, neoplasm, radiation injury, or collagen vascular disease may slowly accumulate large volumes of fluid up to 1 to 2 liters before intrapericardial pressure rises. The clinical picture of slowly developing cardiac tamponade differs from that of acute tamponade due to cardiac trauma or rupture.[23]

This clinical picture may be further altered in patients with "low-pressure cardiac tamponade" (Fig. 27-7) in whom the development of a pericardial effusion in the setting of severe hypovolemia results in compromised ventricular filling and stroke volume when intrapericardial and right atrial pressures rise and equilibrate at a level of only 5 to 15 mmHg.[24] Low pressure tamponade usually is associated with severe dehydration and has been reported in neoplastic and tuberculous pericarditis.

In patients with gradual development of cardiac tamponade, the major complaint is usually dyspnea on exertion accompanied by the insidious appearance of systemic problems such as anorexia, edema and weight loss. In this setting, clinical findings usually include jugular venous distension, moderate tachycardia, pulsus paradoxus, and hepatomegaly, but the classic findings of agitation, severe hypotension, and distant heart sounds

("the small quiet heart") are typically absent.[23]

Depending on the volume of intrapericardial fluid, the cardiac silhouette on the chest roentgenogram may be normal or increased in size. The development of electrical alternation on the electrocardiogram usually reflects pendular, periodic swinging of the heart within the fluid-filled pericardium, but this finding is not specific and may occur in other conditions such as severe heart failure and tension pneumothorax.

In virtually every case of cardiac tamponade, with the possible exception of a moribund patient with an obvious diagnosis (e.g., stab wound of the heart with distended neck veins and marked pulsus paradoxus), an *echocardiogram*, preferably two-dimensional, should be obtained prior to pericardiocentesis. First, it documents the presence and size of effusion; in this regard, the lack of evidence of an effusion on a good quality echocardiographic study essentially excludes the presence of cardiac tamponade (with the exception of postoperative localized hematoma) and contraindicates needle pericardiocentesis. Secondly, the probability of success and safety of pericardiocentesis is related to the size of the effusion, since it has been shown that the procedure is likely to be uncomplicated if both anterior and posterior echo-free spaces (greater than 10 mm) are present.[25,26]

### Combined Cardiac Catheterization and Pericardiocentesis.

We recommend a combined procedure of cardiac catheterization and percutaneous catheter pericardiocentesis since (1) it is the only reliable way to determine the hemodynamic significance of a pericardial effusion; (2) it excludes other important coexisting causes of right atrial hypertension, which may be present in as many as 40% of medical patients with cardiac tamponade;[26] (3) it permits complete drainage of nonloculated pericardial fluid; (4) it allows assessment of adequacy or inadequacy of relieving tamponade physiology; and (5) hemodynamic monitoring and fluoroscopic guidance substantially increase the safety of the procedure. There is rarely justification today for performing blind needle pericardiocentesis at the bedside without hemodynamic monitoring. Percutaneous pericardiocentesis should be attempted only as a temporizing measure in the patient with hemorrhagic traumatic cardiac tamponade

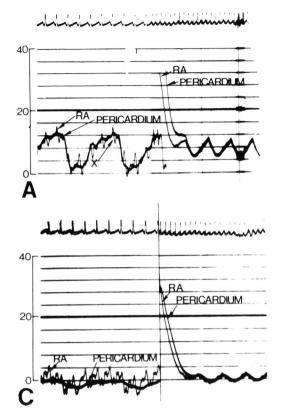

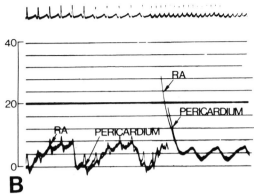

**Fig. 27-7** Simultaneous pericardial and right atrial (RA) pressure tracings in a 76-year-old man with "low pressure cardiac tamponade" due to tuberculous pericardial effusion in the setting of fever and dehydration. The patient had hypotension and pulsus paradoxus, at a mean right atrial pressure of only 8 mmHg (A). Blood pressure improved and pulsus paradoxus disappeared after removal of 200 ml (B) and 600 ml (C) of pericardial fluid. Initially, there is only an X descent in the RA tracing (A). (Reproduced from Antman EM, Cargill V, Grossman W: Low-pressure cardiac tamponade. Ann Intern Med 91:403, 1979.)

and may be difficult or impossible in patients who have (1) a loculated effusion, (2) localized clot and/or fibrin post cardiac surgery, or (3) absence of an anterior effusion greater than 200 ml in size by echocardiography. Cardiology trainees should probably confine their initial taps to patients with clear-cut echocardiographic evidence of large anterior and posterior effusions.

The combined procedure of cardiac catheterization and percutaneous catheter pericardiocentesis is performed in the cardiac catheterization laboratory with hemodynamic and fluoroscopic monitoring. Prior to the procedure in high-risk patients, the cardiac surgical team may be alerted and the patient's blood should be typed and cross-matched. The pressure transducers for measurement of left heart, right heart, intrapericardial, and arterial pressures are prepared to avoid underdamping and assure equisensitive pressure measurements (see Chapter 9). The transducer that will be used to record intrapericardial pressure should be con-

nected via a short length of fluid-filling tubing to the side of a 3-way stopcock. The male end of the stopcock is attached to a long (8-inch), thin-walled, 18-gauge hollow pointed needle (BD Longdwell, Becton-Dickenson, NJ). The needle with its stopcock is then attached to a hand-held syringe filled with 1 or 2% lidocaine (Fig. 27-8). The metal needle hub may be attached by sterile connector to the V lead of an electrocardiographic recorder, but equipotential grounding of the apparatus must be assured to avoid a current leak that could cause ventricular fibrillation.

It is important to measure systemic arterial pressure directly with an intraarterial catheter or cannula during pericardiocentesis. Right heart catheterization should be carried out with right atrial, ventricular, pulmonary artery and pulmonary capillary wedge pressures measured and recorded. Pulmonary artery and systemic arterial blood samples are then drawn for oxygen determination, and cardiac output is measured. Before beginning pericardiocentesis,

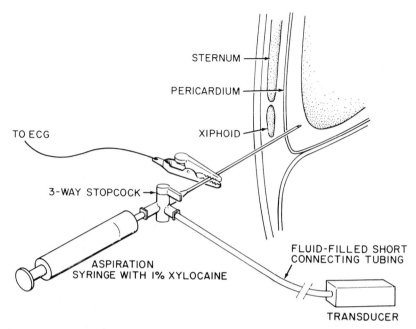

**Fig. 27-8.** Schematic diagram showing the subxiphoid approach to pericardiocentesis. A hollow, thin-walled, 18-gauge needle is connected via a 3-way stopcock to an aspiration syringe filled with 1% or 2% lidocaine and to a short length of fluid-filled tubing to a pressure transducer. A sterile V lead of an electrocardiographic recorder is attached to the metal needle hub. The needle is advanced until pericardial fluid is aspirated or an injury current appears on the V lead monitor recording. Once fluid is aspirated, the stopcock is turned so that needle-tip pressure is displayed against simultaneously measured right atrial pressure from a right heart catheter. When needle tip position within the pericardial space is thus confirmed, a J-tipped guide wire is passed through the needle into the pericardial space. The needle is then removed, and a catheter with end and side holes is advanced over the guide wire and subsequently connected via the 3-way stopcock to both its transducer and its syringe. This permits thorough drainage of the pericardial effusion using a catheter with multiple side holes rather than a sharp needle, and documentation that tamponade physiology is relieved when right atrial pressure falls and intrapericardial pressure is restored to a level at or below zero.

the right heart catheter should be repositioned in the right atrium.

Pericardiocentesis is then performed with the patient's head and thorax propped up with a wedge *so that the patient is sitting at 30-degree or 45-degree elevation,* to promote anterior and inferior pooling of the effusion. *It is critical for the safety of the procedure that the patient be sitting up, at least partially.* We prefer to use the subxiphoid approach which avoids the major epicardial coronary and internal mammary arteries. The skin is shaved and prepared in aseptic fashion, and both skin and subcutaneous tissues are anesthetized with 1 or 2% lidocaine. The skin is then pierced with a No. 11 blade, about 0.5 cm below and to the left of the xiphoid process, and the subcutaneous tissues are separated with a small mosquito clamp.

The needle, which is connected via its 3-way stopcock to both the xylocaine-filled syringe and to a transducer (Fig. 27-8), is advanced posteriorly until its tip is posterior to the bony rib cage. The hub of the needle is then flattened toward the abdomen, and the needle is advanced cephalad toward the patient's head or either shoulder with approximately a 15-degree posterior tilt. As the needle is slowly advanced, the syringe is aspirated repeatedly (to determine if a fluid-filled space has been entered) and lidocaine is injected frequently to provide adequate anesthesia and to keep the needle clear. The needle is advanced until either the pericardial membrane is felt to give and fluid is freely aspirated, or until an injury current of ST elevation is observed on the lead monitored from the needle. If an injury current is obtained before the fluid can be aspirated, the needle is withdrawn slowly with gentle syringe suction, after first clearing the tip with lidocaine. The needle may then be redirected (preferably with echocardiographic guidance) and advanced once more.

When fluid is freely aspirated, the stopcock is turned into its transducer (Fig. 27-8), and needle tip and right atrial pressures are simultaneously displayed and recorded. If the needle tip is in the pericardial space, and if tamponade is present, intrapericardial and right atrial pressures should be equal and elevated with virtually identical waveforms. If hemorrhagic fluid is aspirated, the pressure waveforms usually enable differentiation of pericardial from right ventricular position of the needle tip. In occasional cases where it is not immediately obvious from the pressure waveforms whether or not the needle tip is in the pericardial space, a few milliliters of contrast medium can be injected under fluoroscopic observation. If the contrast medium immediately swirls and disappears, the needle is most likely within the right or left ventricle; sluggish layering of contrast medium inferiorly indicates that the needle is within the pericardial space.

Once the needle tip's position within the pericardial space is confirmed, a floppy-tip 0.038 inch guide wire is passed through the needle into the pericardial space, and "wrapped" around the heart as confirmed by fluoroscopy. The needle is removed and a soft tapered catheter with end and side holes (we usually use a 6F or 7F Teflon Gensini catheter*) is advanced over the guide wire, the guide wire is removed, and the catheter hub is connected via the 3-way stopcock attached to its transducer and to the syringe.

Pressure in the pericardium is now recorded simultaneously with right atrial pressure. As mentioned, if cardiac tamponade is present, right atrial and pericardial mean pressures will be equal, as seen in Figures 27-7 and 27-9. On occasion, the pressures will differ by several millimeters of mercury due to unequal heights of the right atrial and pericardial catheter tips in a patient who is sitting at 30° to 45° of elevation. This gravitational effect may obscure the presence of tamponade physiology. It may be minimized or eliminated by either returning the patient to a supine position (this is safe once the pericardial space has been successfully catheterized) or by checking under fluoroscopy (lateral view) to adjust the catheter tip positions so that both right atrial and pericardial catheter tips are at the same horizontal level, and that the pressure transducers are zeroed at this level.

After pericardial and right atrial pressures (properly zeroed) are recorded, samples of pericardial fluid are aspirated and sent for chemical, bacteriologic, cytologic, and immunologic examination. As fluid is then gradually removed, intermittent recording of simultaneous pericardial and right atrial pressures and systematic arterial pressure is done (Fig. 27-9).

Tamponade physiology is relieved when right atrial and intrapericardial pressures have separated such that (1) intrapericardial pressure has fallen to a mean value of zero and exhibits a negative pressure during inspiration; (2) the right atrial pressure has fallen to a normal level; (3) the right atrial waveform has changed to a normal configuration with reappearance of the diastolic Y descent (Figs. 27-7 and 27-9). Systemic arterial pressure usually rises, and pulsus paradoxus disappears unless respiratory distress from a coexisting pulmonary process is present. Failure of intrapericardial pressure to fall to a level of 0 to −2 mmHg indicates that pericardial fluid (free or loculated) under pressure is still present. Failure of right atrial pressure to fall to a normal level below 8 mmHg indicates that a coexisting cause of right atrial hypertension is present. *Persistent elevation of right atrial pressure with the appearance of a prominent Y descent suggests the presence of effusive-constrictive physiology.* The jugular veins should also be examined. Continued jugular venous distension after relief of tamponade in patients with suspected neoplastic pericarditis mandates exclusion of co-existing superior vena caval obstruction. Special attention should be given to right and/or left atrial pressure in patients with cardiac trauma in whom continued pressure elevation can be present due to traumatic rupture of the atrioventricular valves.

The pericardial pressure-volume curve has a steep slope, such that removal of a small amount of fluid may restore intrapericardial pressure to zero and completely relieve tamponade physiology. However, it is very important to realize that a large volume (1 to 2 liters in chronic tamponade) may still be present in the pericardial space! The operator should attempt to remove all fluid that can be aspirated so that reaccumulation of a small volume of fluid will not again cause tamponade. We have found that extremely thorough drainage can be accomplished reliably by removing the attached syringe from the stopcock and connecting the intrapericardial catheter via sterile tubing to a stoppered sterile glass bottle with a vacuum. This should only be done *only when a soft catheter is in the pericardial space* as vacuum suction would be very hazardous with sharp needle drainage. The patient may be gently tilted to either side to facilitate complete drainage. Complete drainage is usually present when no further fluid can be aspirated; at this point, some patients note the appearance of mild pleuritic chest pain consistent with the apposition of inflamed visceral and parietal pericardial surfaces. Systemic arterial, complete right heart pressures, and cardiac output should be recorded at completion of the procedure to assess the effectiveness of the pericardiocentesis and the presence or absence of other cardiac abnormality.

The pericardial catheter may be left in place safely for 24 hours and attached securely to a closed drainage system using gravity and not a vacuum for suction. Ordinarily, the catheter should not be left in place for longer than 24 hours due to the hazard of introducing an iatrogenic pericardial infection, and it should be rinsed frequently with 1 to 2 ml of fluid. We no longer routinely inject air or carbon dioxide into the pericardium at the end of the procedure. In general, this procedure is of little value in identifying tumor masses.[26] Presently, two-dimensional echocardiography is a readily available and more accurate method for assessing reaccumulation of an effusion and detecting masses adjacent to the heart. We find that it is often helpful to obtain an echocardiogram immediately following pericardiocentesis, for future comparison. Following pericardiocentesis, most patients should be observed for about 24 hours in an intensive care setting with the flow-directed right heart catheter left in place to monitor for recurrent tamponade, which will be manifest by a progressive increase in right atrial pressure.

### Hemodynamic and Angiographic Profile.

Although cardiac tamponade and constrictive pericarditis are both characterized by elevation of intracardiac pressures, progressive reduction of diastolic filling, and

reduction of stroke volume, there are several important differences between these conditions which can be identified in the catheterization laboratory. Unlike pericardial constriction, *cardiac tamponade causes continuous compression of the heart throughout the cardiac cycle* which prevents rapid emptying of the right atrium into the right ventricle when the tricuspid valve opens. Thus, cardiac tamponade is not characterized by the constrictive pattern of excessively rapid ventricular filling in early diastole. A second important physiologic difference is that in cardiac tamponade, unlike constriction, *negative intrathoracic pressure is transmitted to the fluid-filled intrapericardial space and right atrium during inspiration, associated with an inspiratory increase in right ventricular filling* and stroke volume at the expense of that of the left ventricle. Thus, as will be discussed below, patients with cardiac tamponade differ from patients with constriction in that they show: (1) lack of an early diastolic dip-and-plateau or "square root" pattern in the ventricular wave forms; (2) an attenuated or absent early diastolic Y descent in the right atrial waveform; (3) a fall of right atrial and intrapericardial pressure with inspiration, i.e., absence of Kussmaul's sign; (4) striking pulsus paradoxus due to inspiratory augmentation of right ventricular filling at the expense of left ventricular filling.

In the normal individual, intrapericardial pressure is zero or actually slightly negative and is identical to fluctuations in intrathoracic pressure.[7] During cardiac tamponade, simultaneous recording of intrapericardial, right, and left heart pressures on equisensitive gain usually shows that intrapericardial, right atrial, and right and left ventricular diastolic pressures are virtually identical and elevated, generally to 15 mmHg or more (Fig. 27-9). In patients with severe hypovolemia, intrapericardial and right atrial pressures may be equal but only modestly elevated. Usually, the pulmonary capillary wedge and left ventricular diastolic pressures are elevated and identical to right atrial and intrapericardial pressure. It is important to appreciate that in patients with preexisting marked elevation of left ventricular diastolic pressure, cardiac tamponade can be present when intrapericardial and right heart pressures are elevated and equal, but lower than left ventricular diastolic pressure.[27] This underscores the importance of measuring the intrapericardial pressure in addition to right and left heart filling pressures in the patient with suspected cardiac tamponade. Pulmonary artery and right ventricular systolic pressures are generally less than 50 mmHg with a narrow pulse pressure reflecting the depressed stroke volume. When tamponade is moderately severe, right ventricular end diastolic pressure equals or exceeds the right ventricular pulse pressure in magnitude. In extremely severe cardiac tamponade, right ventricular systolic pressure may be only minimally higher than right ventricular diastolic pressure.

Since the heart is continuously compressed by fluid under pressure during cardiac tamponade, right ventricular pressure does not fall to near zero in early diastole, as it normally does; consequently, the right atrium cannot empty rapidly into the right ventricle in early diastole. Thus, unlike constrictive pericarditis, the right ventricular waveform has an attenuated fall of pressure in early diastole and does not show a dip and plateau.[7] The right atrial wave form is distinctive in that the prominent early diastolic Y descent characteristic of constriction is absent or, indeed, replaced by a positive wave[6] (Fig. 27-9).

*Pulsus paradoxus* is easily recorded from systemic arterial pressure measurements; in severe cases, peak systolic arterial pressure declines by more than 15–20 mmHg during inspiration. The decline in diastolic arterial pressure is less, so that the arterial pulse pressure decreases during inspiration.[6,28] The predominant mechanism of pulsus paradoxus in cardiac tamponade has been elegantly studied by Shabetai and co-workers[29] who showed that when experimental cardiac tamponade was produced in dogs, *pulsus paradoxus depended on the inspiratory expansion of right heart volume at the expense of left heart filling within the heart compressed by fluid.* Other factors that may contribute to the striking inspiratory fall in left ventricular stroke volume and systemic arterial pressure include inspiratory pooling of pulmonary venous blood, an inspiratory rise in transmural aortic pressure causing an increase in left ventricular afterload, and the fact that the underfilled left ventricle is operating on the steep ascending limb of the Starling curve such that any inspiratory reduction of left

heart filling elicits a striking fall in left ventricular stroke volume.[30,31]

These physiologic effects of respiration in cardiac tamponade result in an inspiratory increase of right ventricular stroke volume. As a result, respiratory variation in systolic pulmonary arterial and right ventricular pressures is out of phase by two or three beats with the inspiratory fluctuation in systemic arterial pressure. Pulsus paradoxus may be *absent* with coexisting atrial septal defect because the inspiratory increase in venous return is distributed between the right and left atria,[32] and in conditions such as aortic regurgitation where there is a major contribution to ventricular filling independent of respiration. This is an important consideration when tamponade due to aortic dissection is evaluated. Pulsus paradoxus may also be absent if cardiac compression is due to localized collections of fluid or thrombus around the heart, as in the postoperative heart patient. In severe cases of tamponade, in which compensatory mechanism of sinus tachycardia and an increased systemic resistance are inadequate, systemic hypotension is found.

Aspiration of intrapericardial fluid is accompanied by an initial parallel fall in intrapericardial and right atrial pressures. Further aspiration causes intrapericardial pressure to fall to zero or become negative. Systemic arterial pressure and stroke volume increase, and the magnitude of pulsus paradoxus falls progressively during initial aspirations; these parameters do not change further after pericardial pressure falls below right atrial pressure.

Angiographic studies are rarely indicated if echocardiographic and hemodynamic studies indicate the presence of a pericardial effusion and the physiology of cardiac tamponade. During simple fluoroscopy, as the catheter is advanced to the lateral wall of the right atrium, it is typically not possible to position the catheter tip immediately adjacent to the cardiac silhouette's border, and the catheter tip will appear to pulsate while the cardiac silhouette's border appears immobile. The rapid injection of contrast medium into the superior vena cava will show a separation between the opacified right atrium and the right and outer border of the heart due to the presence of nonopacified pericardial fluid. The normal convexity of the right heart border is replaced by a

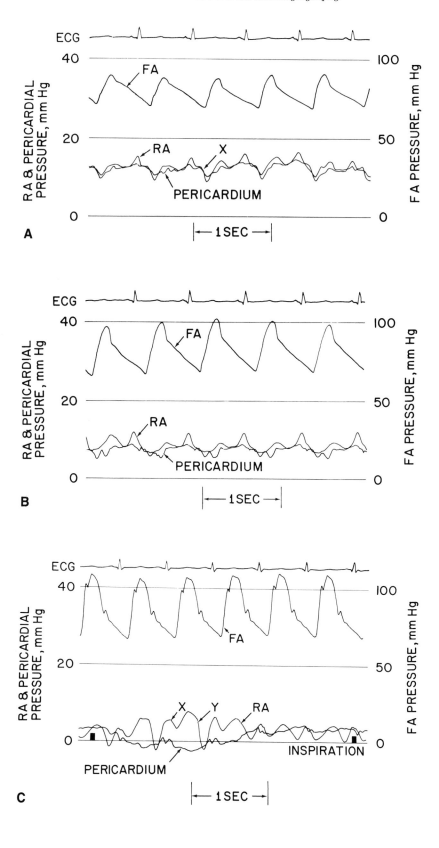

straight or, in more severe cases, a concave right atrial border. In traumatic hemopericardium in which only 100 to 200 ml of fluid may cause cardiac tamponade, the contour of the right atrial border will show characteristic features of tamponade, but the separation of the outer pericardial border from the heart itself may not be evident. The technique of introducing carbon dioxide into the right atrium to document the presence of pericardial effusion by providing negative contrast between the outer border of the cardiac silhouette and right atrium is now largely obsolete.

Left ventriculography is usually not useful in evaluation of cardiac tamponade unless there is a suspicion of coexisting left ventricular dysfunction or valvular heart disease. In cardiac tamponade, as in constrictive pericarditis, the fall in stroke volume due to limitation of diastolic filling is accompanied by a reflex increase in heart rate and contractility from enhanced autonomic tone.[33] Thus, left and right ventricular diastolic volumes are small,[28,34] but the ejection fraction is high, end-systolic volume is small, and isovolumic contractility indices are normal or supranormal due to enhanced cardiac contractility.[28] When cardiac tamponade is extremely advanced and cardiac output falls, coronary hypoperfusion[35] may reverse these effects followed by the development of profound sinus bradycardia and electromechanical dissociation.

## EFFUSIVE-CONSTRICTIVE PERICARDITIS

An intermediate stage in the development of constrictive pericarditis can exist in which a pericardial effusion under pressure is present as well as a constricting visceral pericardium.[36–38] Hancock called this condition effusive-constrictive pericarditis and emphasized that *its hallmark is the continued elevation of right atrial pressure after pericardial fluid aspiration has restored intrapericardial pressure to zero.*[39] Diagnosis of this common cause of pericardial compression requires simultaneous recording of intrapericardial pressure and cardiac filling pressures during combined pericardiocentesis and cardiac catheterization.[39,40] Initially, intrapericardial, right atrial, right ventricular diastolic, left atrial, and left ventricular diastolic pressures are elevated and equal. Prior to pericardiocentesis, the hemodynamic features are those of cardiac tamponade. Pulsus paradoxus is usually present, and the right atrial waveform shows a reduced or absent diastolic Y descent indicating that cardiac compression is present throughout the cardiac cycle, including early diastole. Aspiration of pericardial fluid restores intrapericardial pressure to zero and pulsus paradoxus is relieved. However, right atrial pressure remains elevated, and the right atrial waveform acquires the configuration of constriction with a prominent Y descent and diminished respiratory fluctuation, as shown in Fig. 27-10. Similarly, the right ventricular waveform changes from that of tamponade in which early diastolic pressure fall is attenuated, to that of constrictive pericarditis with an early diastolic dip-and-plateau configuration. The latter indicates that cardiac compression by the visceral pericardium does not impede ventricular filling until mid-diastole.

Effusive-constrictive pericarditis is usually associated with tuberculosis, mediastinal irradiation, or neoplastic pericardial infiltration.[39] It is extremely important to recognize

---

**Fig. 27-9.** Simultaneous right atrial (RA) and intrapericardial pressure (scale 0 to 40 mmHg) and femoral artery (FA) pressure (scale 0 to 100 mmHg) recorded in a patient with cardiac tamponade. (A) Recordings prior to pericardiocentesis show the presence of systemic hypotension, and the elevation and equalization of right atrial and intrapericardial pressures. Note that a systolic X descent is present, but the diastolic Y descent is absent, suggesting that right atrial emptying in early diastole is impeded due to cardiac compression by the pericardial effusion. (B) After aspiration of 100 ml of pericardial fluid, right atrial and intrapericardial pressures have fallen and are beginning to separate, and systolic arterial hypotension has improved compared with baseline. (C) After aspiration of a total of 300 ml of pericardial fluid, tamponade physiology is relieved as evidenced by: (1) restoration of intrapericardial pressure to zero; (2) restoration of right atrial pressure to a normal level; (3) reappearance of the diastolic Y descent in the right atrial wave form, indicative of the relief of cardiac compression in early diastole. Note the negative fluctuation in intrapericardial pressure during inspiration which is accompanied by an increased steepness in the fall of right atrial pressure during the X and Y descents. Although this degree of fluid aspiration completely relieved tamponade physiology, an additional 1500 ml of fluid was removed from the pericardial space.

## A. BEFORE PERICARDIOCENTESIS

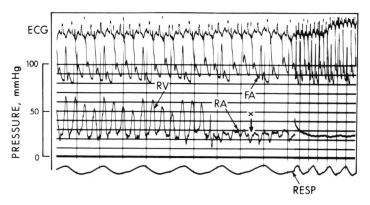

## B. AFTER PERICARDIOCENTESIS

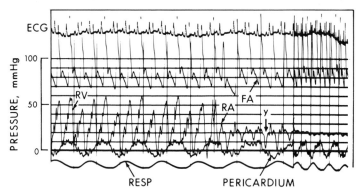

**Fig. 27-10.** Femoral arterial (FA) and right ventricular (RV) to right atrial (RA) pull-back pressure tracings before (A) and after (B) pericardiocentesis in a patient with effusive-constrictive pericarditis secondary to carcinoma of the lung. After pericardiocentesis and return of pericardial pressure to normal levels (B), there is a loss of the abnormal pulsus paradoxus, but the RV end-diastolic and RA mean pressures remain elevated. Note that a diastolic Y descent is absent in the right atrial waveform before pericardiocentesis (A) while a steep Y descent is the prominent feature of the waveform after pericardiocentesis (B). Time lines are 1 second; a respiratory trace (RESP) is seen with inspiration indicated by a positive (upward) deflection. (From Mann T et al: Effusive-constrictive hemodynamic pattern due to neoplastic involvement of the pericardium. Am J Cardiol 41:781, 1978.)

and diagnose accurately during cardiac catheterization. In such patients, the initial pericardiocentesis may improve cardiac output and relieve hypotension. However, subsequent long-term relief of cardiac compression requires total visceral and parietal pericardiectomy,[41] rather than repeated pericardiocentesis or a limited subxiphoid pericardial window.

## OTHER CAUSES OF CARDIAC COMPRESSION

Compression of the heart by masses extrinsic to the pericardium may cause the pathophysiologic abnormalities of cardiac tamponade. Acute compression of the heart by an organizing mediastinal hematoma is an increasingly recognized complication in the postoperative heart patient even when the pericardium is left open.[42,43] In these patients true fibrotic constrictive pericarditis may gradually develop in association with an organized hematoma.[44]

Wynne and co-workers have reported extrinsic compression of the heart by tumor simulating cardiac tamponade.[45] As shown in Fig. 27-11, a massive posterior sarcoma displaced the heart anteriorly and superiorly causing increased right and left atrial pressures. Constriction may also be caused by massive neoplastic involvement with tumor encircling the heart (cor en cuirasse).

## ANOMALIES OF THE PERICARDIUM

Anomalies of the pericardium may cause confusion during cardiac catheterization and angiography unless their characteristic features are recognized. Pericardial cysts, which are filled with clear fluid, are usually located at the right costophrenic angle and come to attention as an unexplained enlargement of the right heart border on the chest roentgenogram.[46] They rarely may be associated with atypical chest pain suggestive of angina or pericarditis. Contrast angiography is occasionally required to differentiate a cyst from cardiac aneurysm. Although most patients can be managed conservatively, large pericardial cysts located at the right costophrenic angle can be decompressed in the catheterization laboratory by percutaneous aspiration under fluoroscopic guidance.[47]

Total absence of the pericardium is extremely rare and is usually not associated with symptoms. *Absence of the left side of the pericardium* is more common. Such patients may come to cardiac catheterization because of chest pain, palpitations, or dyspnea in association with widened splitting of the second heart sound, a systolic murmur at the upper left sternal border, and electrocardiographic abnormalities of right axis deviation and clockwise displacement of the precordial transition zone due to levoposition of the heart. The chest roentgenogram typically

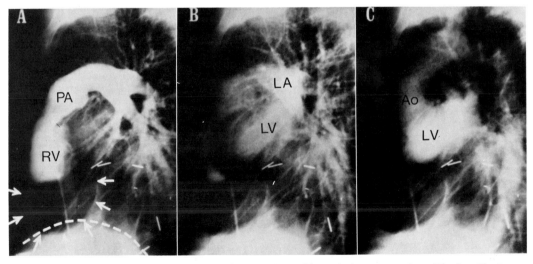

**Fig. 27-11.** Right ventriculogram (lateral view) in a patient with extrinsic compression of the heart by tumor masquerading as cardiac tamponade. (A) Right ventricular (RV) ejection phase with filling of the pulmonary arteries (PA), and subsequent (B) early and (C) late levo-phase, demonstrating left atrium (LA), left ventricle (LV), and aorta (Ao). Note displacement of both ventricles superiorly and anteriorly by a large radiolucent mass (arrows) interposed between the diaphragm (broken line) and inferior surface of the heart. Metal clips are from the patient's original tumor resection surgery and reflect the location of known persistent tumor mass. (From Wynne J, Markis, JE, and Grossman, W.: Extrinsic compression of the heart by tumor masquerading as cardiac tamponade. Cathet Cardiovasc Diagn 4:81, 1978.)

shows leftward position of the heart and a prominent pulmonary artery, and this condition may be confused with other conditions such as pulmonic stenosis or atrial septal defect.[48] Findings at cardiac catheterization are usually normal and cardiac angiography with diagnostic left pneumothorax to outline the pericardium is indicated rarely today to make the diagnosis if typical clinical and radiologic features are present. However, in patients with *partial left-sided pericardial defects*, angiography can be helpful. Such patients frequently complain of chest pain and syncope and are at risk for sudden death related to herniation and strangulation of the heart through the defect.[49] A definitive diagnosis can be made by pulmonary artery angiography with follow-through to the left heart by showing herniation of the left atrium or its appendage beyond the heart border. Partial right-sided pericardial defect can be complicated by severe pleuritic or pericarditis-like chest pain due to inspiratory herniation of the right atrium through the defect.[50] In this condition, right atrial contrast angiography in the left anterior oblique projection shows herniation of the right atrium (and sometimes, the right ventricle) through the defect.

# REFERENCES

1. Shabetai R, Fowler NO, Fenton JC: Restrictive cardiac disease. Pericarditis and the myocardiopathies. Am Heart J 69:271, 1965.
2. Applefeld MM, et al: Delayed pericardial disease after radiotherapy. Am J Cardiol 47:210, 1981.
3. Cohen MV, Greenburg MA: Constrictive pericarditis: Early and late complication of cardiac surgery. Am J Cardiol 43:657, 1979.
4. Bush CA, Stang JM, Wooley CF, Kilman JW: Occult constrictive pericardial disease: Diagnosis by rapid volume expansion and correction by pericardiectomy. Circulation 56:924, 1977.
5. Tyberg TI, Goodyer AVN, Langou RA: Genesis of pericardial knock in constrictive pericarditis. Am J Cardiol 46:570, 1980.
6. Hansen AT, Eskildsen P, Gotzsche H: Pressure curves from the right auricle and right ventricle in constrictive pericarditis. Circulation 3:881, 1951.
7. Shabetai R, Fowler NO, Guntheroth WG: The hemodynamics of cardiac tamponade and constrictive pericarditis. Am J Cardiol 26:480, 1970.
8. Lewis BS, Gotsman MS: Left ventricular function in systole and diastole in constrictive pericarditis. Am Heart J 86:23, 1973.
9. Gaasch WH, Peterson KL, Shabetai R: Left ventricular function in chronic constrictive pericarditis. Am J Cardiol 34:107, 1974.
10. Goldberg E, Stein J, Berger M, Berdoff RL: Diastolic segmental coronary artery obliteration in constrictive pericarditis. Cathet Cardiovasc Diagn 7:197, 1981.
11. Hancock EW: On the elastic and rigid forms of constrictive pericarditis. Am Heart J 100:917, 1980.
12. Chew C, Ziady GM, Raphael MJ, Oakley CM: The functional defect in amyloid heart disease. The "stiff heart" syndrome. Am J Cardiol 36:438, 1975.
13. Meaney E, et al: Cardiac amyloidosis, constrictive pericarditis and restrictive cardiomyopathy. Am J Cardiol 38:547, 1976.
14. Swanton RH, et al: Systolic and diastolic ventricular function in cardiac amyloidosis. Studies in six cases diagnosed with endomyocardial biopsies. Am J Cardiol 39:658, 1977.
15. Benotti JR, Grossman W, Cohn PF: The clinical profile of restrictive cardiomyopathy. Circulation 61:1206; 1980.
16. Kern MJ, Lorell BH, Grossman W: Cardiac amyloidosis masquerading as constrictive pericarditis. Cathet Cardiovasc Diagn 8:629, 1982.
17. Tyberg TI, et al: Left ventricular filling in differentiating restrictive amyloid cardiomyopathy and constrictive pericarditis. Am J Cardiol 47:791, 1981.
18. Lorell BH, et al: Right ventricular infarction. Am J Cardiol 43:465, 1979.
19. Goldstein JA, et al: The role of right ventricular systolic dysfunction and elevated intrapericardial pressure in the genesis of low output in experimental right ventricular infarction. Circulation 65;513, 1982.
20. Bartle SH, Hermann HJ: Acute mitral regurgitation in man. Hemodynamic evidence and observations indicating an early role for the pericardium. Circulation 36;839, 1967.
21. Fowler NO: Physiology of cardiac tamponade and pulsus paradoxus. II. Physiologic, circulatory, and pharmacologic responses in cardiac tamponade. Mod Concepts Cardiovasc Dis 47:115, 1978.
22. Beck, CS: Two cardiac compression triads. JAMA 104:714, 1935.
23. Guberman BA, et al: Cardiac tamponade in medical patients. Circulation 64:633, 1981.

24. Antman EM, Cargill V, Grossman W: Low-pressure cardiac tamponade. Ann Intern Med 91:403, 1979.

25. Wong B, et al: The risk of pericardiocentesis. Am J Cardiol 44:1110, 1979.

26. Krikorian JG, Hancock EW: Pericardiocentesis. Am J Med 65:808, 1978.

27. Reddy PS, Curtiss EI, O'Toole JD, Shaver JA: Cardiac tamponade: Hemodynamic observations in man. Circulation 58:265, 1978.

28. Shabetai R: The pathophysiology of cardiac tamponade and constriction. Cardiovasc Clin 7:67, 1976.

29. Shabetei R, Fowler NO, Fenton JC, Massangkay M: Pulsus paradoxus. J Clin Invest 44:1882, 1965.

30. Fowler NO: Physiology of cardiac tamponade and pulsus paradoxus. I. Mechanisms of pulsus paradoxus in cardiac tamponade. Mod Concepts Cardiov Dis 47:109, 1978.

31. Friedman HS, Sakurai H, Lajam F: Pulsus paradoxus: a manifestation of a marked reduction in left ventricular end-diastolic volume in cardiac tamponade. J Thorac Cardiovasc Surg 79:74, 1980.

32. Winer HE, Kronzon I: Absence of pulsus paradoxus in patients with cardiac tamponade and atrial septal defects. Am J Cardiol 44:378, 1979.

33. Friedman HS, et al: Effect of autonomic blockade on the hemodynamic findings in acute cardiac tamponade. Am J Physiol 232:H5, 1977.

34. Craig RJ, Whalen RE, Behar VS, McIntosh HD: Pressure and volume changes of the left ventricle in acute pericardial tamponade. Am J Cardiol 22:65, 1968.

35. Jarmakani JM, McHale PA, Greenfield JC, Jr.: The effect of cardiac tamponade on coronary hemodynamics in the awake dog. Cardiovasc Res 9:112, 1975.

36. Spodick DH, Kumar S: Subacute constrictive pericarditis with cardiac tamponade. Dis Chest 54:62, 1968.

37. Gonin A, Froment R, Gravier J: Les epicardopericardites tuberculeuses a evolution constrictive subaigue. J Med Lyon 32:1049, 1951.

38. Soulie P, Chiche P, Acar J: Pericardites chronique et constriction pericardique. Presse Med 66:579, 1958.

39. Hancock EW, Subacute effusive-constrictive pericarditis. Circulation 43:183, 1971.

40. Mann T, Brodie BR, Grossman W, McLaurin LP: Effusive-constrictive hemodynamic pattern due to neoplastic involvement of the pericardium. Am J Cardiol 41:781, 1978.

41. Walsh TJ, Baughman KL, Gardner TJ, Bulkley BH: Constrictive epicarditis as a cause of delayed or absent response to pericardiectomy. J Thorac Cardiovasc Surg 83:126, 1982.

42. Geis WP, Johnson CF, Zajtchuk R, Kittle CF: Extrapericardial (mediastinal) cardiac tamponade. Arch Surg 100:305, 1970.

43. Little WC, Primm RK, Karp RB, Hood WP: Clotted hemopericardium with the hemodynamic characteristics of constrictive pericarditis. Am J Cardiol 45:386, 1980.

44. Kutcher MA et al: Constrictive pericarditis as a complication of cardiac surgery: Recognition of an entity. Am J Cardiol 50:742, 1982.

45. Wynne J, Markis JE, Grossman W: Extrinsic compression of the heart by tumor masquerading as cardiac tamponade. Cathet Cardiovasc Diagn 4:81, 1978.

46. Unverferth DV, Wooley CF: The differential diagnosis of paracardiac lesions: Pericardial cysts. Cathet Cardiovasc Diagn 5:31, 1979.

47. Peterson DT, Zatz LM, Popp RL: Pericardial cyst ten years after acute pericarditis. Chest 67:719, 1975.

48. Nasser WK: Congenital absence of the left pericardium. Am J Cardiol 26:466, 1970.

49. Saito R, Hotta F: Congenital pericardial defect associated with cardiac incarceration. Am Heart J 100:866, 1980.

50. Minocha GK, Falicov RE, Nijensohn E: Partial right-sided congenital pericardial defect with herniation of right atrium and right ventricle. Chest 76:484, 1979.

*chapter twenty eight*

# Profiles in Congenital Heart Disease

MICHAEL D. FREED *and* JOHN F. KEANE

P EDIATRIC cardiology has made great strides in the diagnosis, management, and correction of complex congenital malformations in the past two decades. The foundation of these advances is a more precise understanding of the physiology and anatomy of complex lesions that has been obtained from cardiac catheterization and angiography. The techniques for catheterization of infants and children have been discussed in Chapter 6. This chapter will focus on brief profiles of some of the more important congenital abnormalities.

The incidence cited in the discussion of each abnormality pertains to a population comprised of children and adults referred to The Children's Hospital Medical Center and Peter Bent Brigham Hospital, respectively, for evaluation of congenital heart disease. (See Table 28-1.)

The discussion of each lesion is necessarily cursory; those interested in a more in-depth view are advised to consult one of the standard texts of pediatric cardiology.[1-3]

## ATRIAL SEPTAL DEFECTS

Atrial septal defects (ASD) occurred in about 6% of children and 46% of adults with congenital heart disease in the population under study[4] (Table 28-1).

Anatomically, there are three types of atrial septal defect. The ostium primum de-

fect, associated with a superior counterclockwise loop on the frontal plane of the electrocardiogram, is found low in the atrial septum. Embryologically, it is due to a lack of fusion of the septum primum and endocardial cushion tissue of the atrioventricular canal and may be associated with defects in the ventricular septum or abnormalities in the mitral or, less frequently, the tricuspid valve. The secundum atrial defect, by far the most common, is found midway in the atrial septum under the superior limbic band and results from a failure of the septum secundum to completely cover the ostium secundum.

The sinus venosus defect occurs posteriorly in the atrial septum near the entrance of the superior vena cava. It is the rarest form of atrial defect and is often associated with anomalous pulmonary venous return of the right upper pulmonary vein into the superior vena cava or right atrium.

The magnitude of shunting through an atrial defect is a function not only of the size of the hole, but also of the relative compliance of the two ventricles, which in turn is influenced by the afterload they face. In childhood, when the right ventricle is more compliant than the left and its afterload is less, the left-to-right shunt may be large. If the pulmonary vascular resistance increases and pulmonary artery hypertension ensues, the RV afterload is increased and its compliance is decreased. The left-to-right shunt

**TABLE 28-1.** *Incidence of Congenital Heart Disease in Children and Adults*

| | CHMC (Total)* 1973–84 | | CHMC (cath)† 1973–84 | | PBBH 1960–70 | |
|---|---|---|---|---|---|---|
| | No. | % | No. | % | No. | % |
| Ventricular septal defect | 2071 | 20.0 | 700 | 15.4 | 36 | 23.0 |
| Tetralogy of Fallot | 1030 | 10.0 | 738 | 16.3 | 3 | 1.9 |
| Pulmonic stenosis | 1011 | 9.8 | 395 | 8.7 | 23 | 14.7 |
| Aortic stenosis | 784 | 7.6 | 408 | 9.0 | ‡ | — |
| Atrial septal defect | 645 | 6.2 | 197 | 4.3 | 72 | 46.1 |
| Patent ductus arteriosus | 550 | 5.3 | 84 | 1.9 | 9 | 5.8 |
| Coarctation of the aorta | 525 | 5.1 | 255 | 5.6 | 5 | 3.2 |
| D-Transposition | 493 | 4.8 | 344 | 7.6 | — | — |
| Endocardial cushion defect | 483 | 4.7 | 280 | 6.2 | — | — |
| Mitral regurgitation stenosis | 382 | 3.7 | 117 | 2.6 | — | — |
| Single ventricle | 200 | 1.9 | 153 | 3.4 | — | — |
| Double outlet right ventricle | 191 | 1.8 | 143 | 3.2 | — | — |
| Other | 1985 | 19.2 | 745 | 15.8 | — | — |
| | 10350 | 100. | 4529 | 100. | 156 | 100. |

*Diagnosis based on surgery 4622, catheterization 1720, clinical 4008.
†Most recent diagnosis used for patients with more than one catheterization.
‡Aortic stenosis not classified as congenital.
CHMC = The Children's Hospital Medical Center; PBBH = Peter Bent Brigham Hospital.

diminishes, and eventually right-to-left shunting and cyanosis may develop.

Occasionally, associated congenital anomalies affecting the right side of the heart (e.g., pulmonary stenosis or tetralogy of Fallot) also alter RV afterload and compliance and may reduce left-to-right shunting and mask the presence of an ASD. Conversely, with normal pulmonary vascular resistance, anything that increases left ventricular (LV) afterload (e.g., systemic hypertension) or decreases LV diastolic compliance (e.g., coronary artery disease) may increase the left-to-right shunt.

In a child with the typical physical examination, roentgenogram, ECG, and two-dimensional echocardiogram cardiac catheterization may be unnecessary and operation may be recommended purely on clinical grounds.[5] In adults this is less likely to be the case.

*Catheterization Technique.* The recognition and characterization of atrial defects is facilitated by catheterization from below. By advancing the catheter from the inferior vena cava into the right atrium posteriorly, it is almost always possible to cross the atrial defect and enter the left atrium. Failure to enter the left heart readily suggests the presence of a sinus venosus defect.

Often, when manipulating the catheter in the right atrium, the catheter may cross from the right side of the cardiac silhouette into a right pulmonary vein, but it is difficult to be certain by catheter position alone whether the veins are draining anomalously into the right atrium or a large secundum defect has been crossed. Fortunately, since the advent of cardiopulmonary bypass, this differentiation is rarely important, since the cardiac surgeon can see the anomalous veins at the time of open heart surgery and modify the operation accordingly.

Finally, merely crossing the atrial septum into the left heart does not prove the presence of an atrial septal defect. Most children and a few adults will have a probe (or catheter) patent foramen ovale. Proof of a significant defect depends on saturation and pressure data in conjunction with angiography or indicator dilution studies.

*Saturation.* The characteristic finding in atrial septal defects without pulmonary hypertension is an increase in the oxygen saturation (or content) in the right atrium compared to the superior vena cava (Fig. 28-1). On the basis of our studies in *children*, we regard an increase of 10% in a single observation or 8% on multiple observations to be significant.[6] As discussed in Chapter 12,

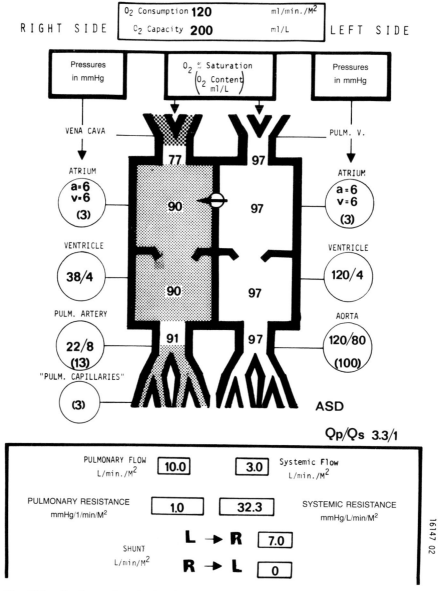

**Fig. 28-1.** Cardiac catheterization findings in a patient with atrial septal defect. Note the left-to-right shunt at the atrial level and the flow gradient across the pulmonary valve.

studies in *adults* have generally used oxygen saturation from superior and inferior vena cavae, according to Flamm's formula, and have found that an increase of 11% in a single observation or 7% using the average of multiple samples is significant. We have not found inferior vena caval samples helpful because of variation due to incomplete mixing of hepatic, renal, and iliac streams.

A high saturation ($\geq$85%) in the superior vena cava suggests the presence of anomalous drainage of some or all of the right pulmonary veins into the superior vena cava. If this is a possibility, two samples taken from the superior vena cava, one high, near the junction of the innominate vein, and another low, near the junction of the right atrium, may be helpful. Occasionally an ostium primum defect that occurs low in the atrial septum will not be evident by a rise in saturation until the right ventricle owing to incomplete mixing in the right atrium.

The calculated pulmonary blood flow and pulmonary-to-systemic flow ratio (Chapter 12) may be inaccurate in patients with ASDs, in part due to the difficulty in obtaining an accurate mixed systemic venous sample, and in part due to inaccuracies in the pulmonary flow when high pulmonary artery saturations narrow the pulmonary arteriovenous oxygen difference.

When the pulmonary vascular resistance begins to rise, the right ventricular afterload increases, right ventricular compliance decreases, and the left-to-right shunting is reduced. Eventually there may be right-to-left shunting, with a decrease in the saturation between the pulmonary veins and the left atrium. Often bidirectional shunting is present before the shunt becomes exclusively right to left.

Other causes of a left-to-right shunt at the atrial level are listed in Table 28-2.

***Pressures.*** With large atrial defects, the a and v waves in the right atrial tracing become equal. The mean pressures in the two atria are equal and, in the usual case, normal. The right ventricular systolic pressure is often slightly elevated (30 to 40 mmHg), and gradients of 10 to 15 mmHg are found across the right ventricular outflow tract, presumably related to increased flow. Pulmonary arterial pressure is usually normal, as are pulmonary venous, left atrial, left ventricular, and aortic pressures. As the pulmonary vascular resistance begins to rise, the pulmonary artery and right ventricular systolic pressures increase, becoming higher than

systemic arterial pressure in severe pulmonary vascular obstructive disease.

When congestive failure intervenes, the diastolic pressures in the right and left ventricles as well as atrial pressures are elevated. In the adult population, "congestive failure" with increased right and left atrial pressures is a manifestation of *left ventricular failure*, with the right ventricular output in such patients tending to increase as left ventricular failure worsens.

***Angiography.*** In the presence of the "classic" physiologic findings of an atrial defect, angiography is often unnecessary. The defect can be visualized on the levophase of a right ventricular or pulmonary artery angiogram by the loss of definition of the rightward and inferior portion of the left atrium, and by the appearance of contrast material in the right atrium and often in the inferior vena cava. Direct visualization of the defect can be accomplished by injection of contrast medium into a right pulmonary vein (or the left atrium), with angulation of the camera (or patient) into a position that puts the atrial septum perpendicular to the x-ray beam—about 70 degrees left anterior oblique with 25 degrees cranial angulation (Fig. 28-2).[7]

In patients in whom an ostium primum defect is suspected by the characteristic ECG, a left ventricular angiogram in the hepatoclavicular view (45 degrees of cranial

**TABLE 28-2.** *Causes of Increased Oxygen Saturation at the Atrial Level*

1. Atrial septal defects
2. Partial anomalous pulmonary venous return
3. Left ventricular-right atrial shunt
4. Ruptured sinus of Valsalva fistula to right atrium
5. Coronary AV fistula draining into right atrium
6. Tricuspid regurgitation associated with VSD

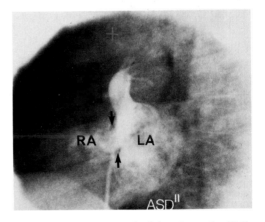

**Fig. 28-2.** Angiogram in the left atrium using 70 degrees of left anterior obliquity and 25 degrees of cranial angulation. The secundum atrial septal defect (arrows) is seen midway in the atrial septum. LA = left atrium, RA = right atrium, ASD$^{II}$ = atrial septal defect, secundum type.

angulation and 39 degrees of left anterior obliquity)[8,9] should be obtained to rule out an associated ventricular septal defect and/or mitral regurgitation. In primum defects, the characteristic left ventriculogram shows a goose- (or swan's) neck deformity of the left ventricular outflow tract formed by the attachments of the anterior leaflet of the mitral valve to the ventricular septum (Fig. 28-3). Visualization of the goose- or swan's neck deformity is perhaps best when the left ventriculogram is done in the AP projection.

## VENTRICULAR SEPTAL DEFECTS

Ventricular septal defects (VSD) are the most common form of congenital heart disease, occurring in 20% of the children and 23% of the adults with congenital heart disease in the population under study. Defects can occur almost anywhere in the ventricular septum, but the most common site is the membranous portion at the junction of the embryologic conal septum and muscular septum. High defects (subpulmonic), above the crista supraventricularis, and low de-

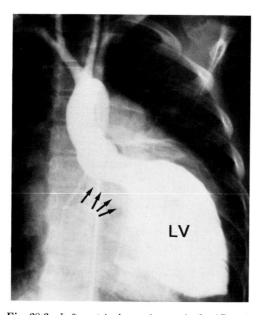

**Fig. 28-3.** Left ventricular angiogram in the AP position in a patient with a primum atrial septal defect. LV = left ventricle. Note the Swan's neck deformity of the LV outflow tract.

fects, in the muscular septum (muscular or atrioventricular canal type), are found less frequently. Occasionally two or more defects may be present.

The flow through a VSD is a function of the size of the hole and, if the defect is large (greater than one half of the aortic orifice), of the ratio of pulmonary to systemic vascular resistance. In infancy, beyond the neonatal period, and in childhood, when the pulmonary resistance is low, torrential left to right shunts may be present. In older children and adults, the shunts usually decrease as the defects spontaneously become smaller or as the pulmonary resistance increases.

Often VSDs are associated with other congenital cardiac anomalies, such as atrial defects, patent ductus arteriosus, or as part of the complete atrioventricular canal complex. They also may be associated with pulmonic stenosis (tetralogy of Fallot), transposition of the great arteries, or coarctation of the aorta. Seven percent of children with isolated VSDs develop aortic regurgitation.

At present we catheterize all children suspected of having a VSD, except those with a defect that is obviously insignificant (based on the absence of either symptoms or a mitral flow rumble on physical examination, and on the presence of a normal roentgenogram and electrocardiogram).

***Catheterization Technique.*** The catheterization protocol in patients with a VSD usually follows the procedure outlined in Chapter 6. With large high-placed defects, it is possible to cross from right ventricle to left ventricle or aorta with the venous catheter by exerting a sharp clockwise rotation to the catheter in the right ventricle just beyond the tricuspid valve. In children, the venous catheter will often cross the atrial septum through an atrial defect or patent foramen ovale and allow left ventriculography by way of a venous approach.

***Saturation.*** An increase in oxygen saturation between the right atrium and right ventricle of 10% on one run or 5% on two runs is usually considered diagnostic of VSD,[6] although no rise may be found in small defects, and a rise of 20% or 30% is not uncommon in sick infants (Fig. 28-4). Occasionally in patients with large defects, the rise in oxygen saturation may be detected at the atrial level, owing to shunting through a valve-incompetent foramen ovale secondary

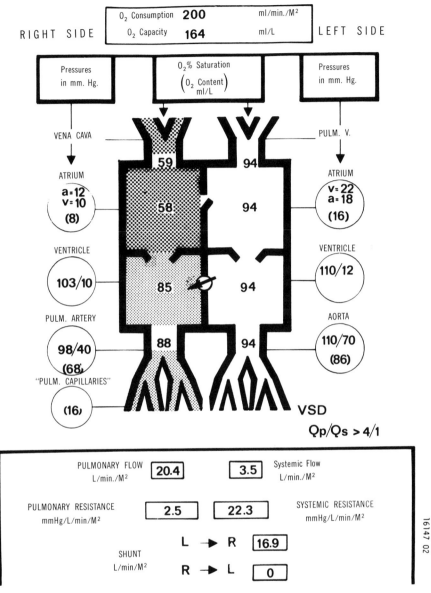

**Fig. 28-4.** Cardiac catheterization findings in a patient with a large ventricular septal defect. Note the left-to-right shunt at the ventricular level. There is hyperkinetic pulmonary hypertension with nearly normal pulmonary vascular resistance. Left ventricular filling pressure is increased, reflecting a combination of increased flow and volume decreased compliance, and perhaps early myocardial failure.

to left atrial dilatation, associated tricuspid regurgitation, or an LV to RA shunt. In supracristal VSDs, the rise in oxygen saturation may not be apparent until the great vessel level.

The systemic arterial saturation is usually normal, but hypoxemia may be present in infants and young children because of pulmonary edema or pneumonia, and in older children and adults because of right-to-left shunting at the ventricular level secondary to increased pulmonary vascular resistance (Eisenmenger syndrome).

Because of the high saturation of blood in

the pulmonary artery in patients with a large VSD with pulmonary artery hypertension, the presence of an associated patent ductus arteriosus is impossible to evaluate by saturation data alone, and aortic angiography is necessary. The differential diagnosis of left to right shunts at the ventricular level is listed in Table 28-3.

*Pressures.* With small ventricular defects, the intracardiac pressures are usually normal. With moderate defects the right ventricular and pulmonary artery systolic pressures are mildly elevated, but the diastolic pressures are normal. Left atrial pressure and left ventricular end-diastolic pressure may also be mildly elevated.

If the hole is as large as one half the cross-sectional area of the aorta, systolic pressures in the right and left ventricle are equalized. The systolic pressures in the aorta and pulmonary artery are also equal, but the diastolic and mean pressures in the PA are lower than those in the aorta because of the large run-off. With a large left-to-right shunt, the left atrial mean and left ventricular end-diastolic pressures are usually elevated, often to 10 to 15 mmHg. Flow gradients of 20 to 30 mmHg across the pulmonary valve and up to 5 mmHg across the mitral valve may be present without structural abnormality. As the pulmonary resistance rises, the left to right shunt decreases and the left atrial and left ventricular end-diastolic pressures fall. Pulmonary diastolic pressure is increased, eventually becoming equal to aortic diastolic pressure.

*Angiography.* Angiography in patients with this lesion is necessary to determine the size, number, and location of the defect(s) (Fig. 28-5) and to rule out associated cardiac anomalies. It is best performed by contrast

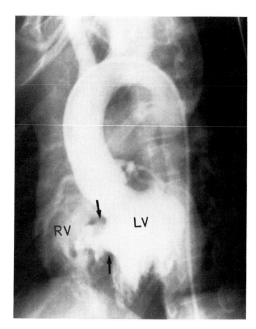

**Fig. 28-5.** Left ventricular angiogram in left anterior oblique position. A rather large, low muscular defect is outlined. LV = left ventricle, RV = right ventricle.

injection in the left ventricle, using oblique views for filming. Defects in the subaortic and anterior muscular portion of the septum are best visualized with a 70-degree left anterior oblique projection and about 20 degrees of cranial angulation. Defects in the posterior septum are better viewed with a lesser degree of left obliquity (30 degrees) with approximately 45 degrees of cranial angulation, (hepatoclavicular view of Bargeron).[8,9] All children and adults with high pulmonary artery pressures should have an aortogram as well, to exclude a coexistent patent ductus arteriosus. An aortogram with supravalvular injection will also allow the diagnosis of coexistent aortic insufficiency, which may develop due to prolapse of an unsupported aortic valve cusp or secondary to a bicuspid aortic valve.

**TABLE 28-3.** *Causes of Increased Oxygen Saturation at the Ventricular Level*

1. Ventricular septal defect
2. Ruptured sinus of Valsalva aneurysm to right ventricle
3. Coronary AV fistula draining into right ventricle
4. Low atrial septal defect
5. Left-to-right shunt into pulmonary artery with pulmonary regurgitation

## PATENT DUCTUS ARTERIOSUS

Persistence of a ductus arteriosus (PDA) is not uncommon. It occurred in approximately 5% of children and 6% of adults in the study population. Premature infants have a high incidence of PDA, up to 40% in those with a birth weight of less than 1000 grams. Although the exact mechanism of normal closure is uncertain, it is clear that prostaglandins play a significant role, since it has been shown that PGE$_1$ will maintain patency of the ductus in neonates with cyanotic heart disease,[10] and prostaglandin synthetase inhibitors will promote closure of the ductus in a high proportion of premature infants.[11]

In most children the diagnosis of a patent ductus arteriosus is based on the presence of a characteristic continuous machinery murmur, best heard just below the left clavicle. Catheterization is reserved for those in whom the clinical findings are atypical or other congenital defects are present or pulmonary artery hypertension is suspected.

***Catheterization Technique.*** In the majority of patients the catheter can be manipulated from the pulmonary artery across the ductus arteriosus into the descending aorta by probing the region near the origin of the left pulmonary artery (Fig. 28-6).

***Saturation.*** A rise in oxygen saturation of at least 3% to 5% between right ventricle and pulmonary artery is typical.[6] With a small PDA there may be no detectable shunt by oximetry, but a large PDA may lead to an increase of as much as 20% to 30% in oxygen saturation of pulmonary artery blood. The oxygen saturation of blood in the left pulmonary artery is usually higher than that in the main or right pulmonary arteries because of preferential streaming through the ductus, and thus accurate calculations of pulmonary flow by the Fick method are impossible because of the difficulty in obtaining true mixed pulmonary artery blood for determination of oxygen saturation (Fig. 28-7).

The systemic arterial saturation is usually normal, but may be low for the reasons previously mentioned for ventricular septal defects. In the presence of severe pulmonary vascular disease, the saturation may be lower in the descending aorta than in the ascending aorta (differential cyanosis) because of right-to-left shunting through the ductus. The various conditions associated with left-to-right shunts at the great vessel level are listed in Table 28-4.

***Pressures.*** With a small PDA, all pressures are usually normal. As the left-to-right shunt increases in magnitude, the systolic pressures in the right ventricle and pulmonary artery, mean pressure in the left atrium,

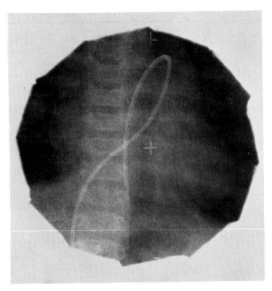

**Fig. 28-6.** Catheter course in the AP projection in a child with a patent ductus arteriosus. The venous catheter goes from the inferior vena cava to the right atrium, right ventricle, and main pulmonary artery through the ductus arteriosus and into the descending aorta.

and end-diastolic pressure in the LV may become elevated. Diastolic pressure in the aorta usually falls and the pulse pressure widens because of the large run-off into the pulmonary artery. With a large PDA, the systolic pressures in both ventricles and both great vessels are equal, as are the diastolic pressures in the aorta and pulmonary artery.

As the pulmonary vascular resistance increases, the left-to-right shunt decreases, and while the systolic pressures in the aorta and pulmonary artery remain the same, the diastolic pressures rise and pulse pressures narrow. Left atrial and left ventricular end-diastolic pressures return to normal.

**TABLE 28-4.** *Causes of Increased Oxygen Saturation at the Great Vessel Level*

1. Patent ductus arteriosus
2. Aortopulmonary window
3. Coronary AV fistula draining into pulmonary artery
4. Anomalous coronary artery arising from pulmonary artery
5. Supracristal (subpulmonary) VSD

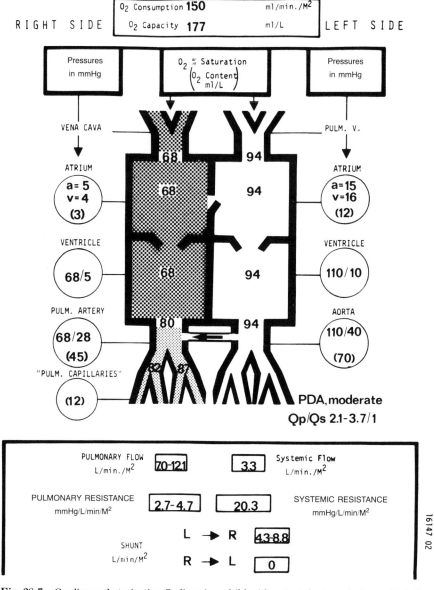

**Fig. 28-7.** Cardiac catheterization findings in a child with patent ductus arteriosus. Note the left-to-right shunt at the great vessel level, with moderate pulmonary artery hypertension. The pulmonary flow can only be approximated in this case because the different saturations in the left and right pulmonary arteries make it impossible to determine the pulmonary arteriovenous oxygen difference.

***Angiography.*** Angiography is often unnecessary in the patient with uncomplicated patent ductus arteriosus, but may be necessary to rule out associated cardiac anomalies and to confirm the diagnosis in patients with elevated pulmonary vascular resistance.

The best projection for visualization of the ductus arteriosus is a steep (70 degrees) left anterior oblique, which "opens up" the aortic arch. Injection should be made in the ascending aorta or aortic arch in the usual case, or in the pulmonary artery if elevated pulmonary vascular resistance and right-to-left shunting are present.

# AORTIC STENOSIS

Congenital aortic stenosis (AS) has been present in 7.6% of children referred for cardiac evaluation at Children's Hospital Medical Center in Boston. The incidence in adults is more difficult to evaluate, since many adults who develop "acquired" calcific aortic stenosis probably have a congenital bicuspid valve that became calcified and fibrotic later in life. In fact, bicuspid aortic valve may be the most common congenital cardiac anomaly.

In about 75% of children with AS, the abnormality is at the valvular level. Subvalvular (subaortic) stenosis (20%) is usually due to a fibromuscular ring encircling the left ventricular outflow tract, 0.5 to 2.0 cm below the valve, but occasionally it may be due to a thin membranous diaphragm that exists immediately below the valve. On auscultation, children with subaortic obstruction rarely have a systolic ejection click, whereas a systolic ejection click is almost invariably present in those with valvular AS. Muscular subaortic obstruction associated with idiopathic hypertrophic subaortic stenosis is occasionally seen in children, and it is not significantly different from the disease as it appears in adults. Supravalvular AS may be due to a fibrous ring or diaphragm that occurs above the valve or, less commonly, it may be part of a diffuse hypoplasia of the ascending aorta and may be associated with the Williams syndrome of mental retardation, elfin facies, and hypercalcemia of infancy.

Because of the notorious difficulty in clinically assessing the severity of aortic stenosis, we catheterize children with any one of the following: symptoms of chest pain, angina, or syncope; grade 4/6 murmurs at the right upper sternal border; ST-T changes on the electrocardiogram at rest or exercise; an estimated LV pressure of more than 160 mmHg by the Frank vectorcardiogram or an estimated gradient of 50 mmHg or more by Doppler echocardiography. Similarly, because of the difficulties in evaluating residual aortic stenosis postoperatively, we recatheterize all children operated on for this lesion at one year after operation.

Since catheterization techniques for children with AS differ little from those for adults previously described in Chapter 23, only a few abbreviated comments will be made.

***Catheterization Technique.***   Usually the aortic valve can be crossed retrograde from the ascending aorta, but if after 10 to 20 minutes of fluoroscopy this proves impossible, we do a transseptal puncture (using biplane fluoroscopy) for access to the left side of the heart (see Chapter 5). Once in the left ventricle, it is important to advance the catheter to the apex of the chamber, because if the catheter is passed only to the outflow portion, subaortic obstruction may be missed.

***Saturation.***   No significant oxygen rise is noted on the right side of the heart. Cardiac index is usually normal or slightly elevated in children with AS.

***Pressures.***   In evaluating the gradient across the left ventricular outflow tract, either a pull-back tracing or simultaneous left ventricular and ascending aortic pressures may be used. If the left ventricular and femoral artery pressures are used, the gradient will be systematically underestimated because of the reflected wave effect in the femoral artery. Often it is possible to determine the site of obstruction if a slow pull-back from the left ventricular apex to the ascending aorta is obtained with an end-hole catheter. Cardiac output is always measured, and should be used in the calculation of valve area (see Chapter 11). The right-sided pressures are usually normal in children with aortic stenosis.

***Angiography.***   Left ventricular angiography is always performed to identify precisely the area of obstruction and to evaluate left ventricular function. The best view to see the aortic valve and supravalvular region is the left anterior oblique projection. If about 25 degrees of cranial angulation are added, the area immediately below the valve is elongated and discrete subaortic obstruction is more clearly visualized.

A supravalvular aortic injection is sometimes helpful to outline the anatomy of the valve and to evaluate the degree of aortic regurgitation.

# PULMONIC STENOSIS

Pulmonic stenosis (PS) is often associated with other congenital cardiac anomalies, but as an isolated lesion it accounted for almost 10% of children and 15% of adults with congenital heart disease in the population under study. Obstruction is at the valvular level in more than 80% of the cases, but it may be subvalvular (infundibular, anomalous muscle bundles, or double-chamber right ventricle), supravalvular, or in the peripheral pulmonary artery branches.

We catheterize all children in whom we suspect the stenosis to be severe, including those with cyanosis, severe right ventricular hypertrophy (RVH) on the ECG or auscultatory or echo-Doppler evidence of severe right ventricular outflow obstruction.

In the past we have recommended routine postoperative catheterizations approximately four years after pulmonary valvotomy. Since the natural history study of congenital defects[12] confirmed the impression that significant residual obstruction after valvotomy is unusual, we now recatheterize only those in whom we suspect a less than optimal repair. For children with valvular stenosis, relief of the obstruction is now frequently obtained by balloon dilatation of the stenotic valve in the catheterization laboratory (see Chapter 6).

*Catheterization Technique.* The foramen ovale is usually patent, allowing access to the left heart. In infants with severe PS and cyanosis, obstruction of the pulmonary lumen by the catheter has been reported,[13] so we do not attempt to cross the pulmonary valve in such patients.

*Saturations.* In the usual case, no left-to-right shunt is present and the arterial saturation is normal. With severe stenosis, a right-to-left shunt at the atrial level may be present, through either a patent foramen ovale or an atrial septal defect, resulting in cyanosis (Fig. 28-8). Occasionally in those patients with full oxygen saturation at rest, mild degrees of cyanosis may appear with exercise.

*Pressures.* (Fig. 28-8). In mild PS, the right atrial pressure is usually normal, but when the right ventricular pressure exceeds 50 mmHg, the a wave in the right atrium is usually increased. The right ventricular pressure varies with the degree of stenosis; with mild PS, the right ventricular pressure may

be 25 to 30 mmHg, but with severe stenosis, peak systolic pressures as high as 250 or 300 mmHg are found. By slow withdrawal from branch pulmonary arteries to the right ventricle using an end-hole catheter, it is usually possible to localize the site of obstruction to either the branch pulmonary artery, the valvular or subvalvular level. In patients with severe PS, the pulmonary artery mean pressure is decreased, with the instantaneous pressure actually becoming negative early in systole secondary to a Venturi effect from the jet across the valve. Left sided pressures are usually normal.

*Angiograms.* The most useful angiogram is a biplane right ventriculogram in the AP and lateral projections (Fig. 28-9). In patients with severe valvular stenosis, the valve is usually domed and thickened, and a central, or rarely, an eccentric, jet of contrast material can be seen. Occasionally the valve annulus may be small or dysplastic. The infundibulum usually becomes quite narrow in systole but opens widely during diastole. Subvalvular stenosis due to obstructing muscle bundles in the right ventricle may be of two types—a high obstruction a few centimeters under the valve, or a lower diagonal hypertrophied moderator band that bisects the ventricle into two almost equal triangles. Many children with subvalvular PS have an associated VSD. Supravalvular and pulmonary branch stenoses are best seen using about 40 degrees of cranial angulation, with some left or right obliquity, depending on the branch that is to be visualized. If there is any question about the possibility of an associated ventricular defect, a left ventriculogram in the left anterior oblique position should be performed.

# COARCTATION OF THE AORTA

Coarctation of the aorta is a relatively common anomaly; in our study group, it occurred in 5% of children and 3.2% of adults with congenital heart disease. The complex coarctation involving hypoplasia of the aortic arch and a ventricular septal defect, the so-called preductal coarctation, usually presents with severe congestive heart failure in the first few weeks of life and is beyond the scope of this discussion. Simple or discrete coarctation is probably a postnatally ac-

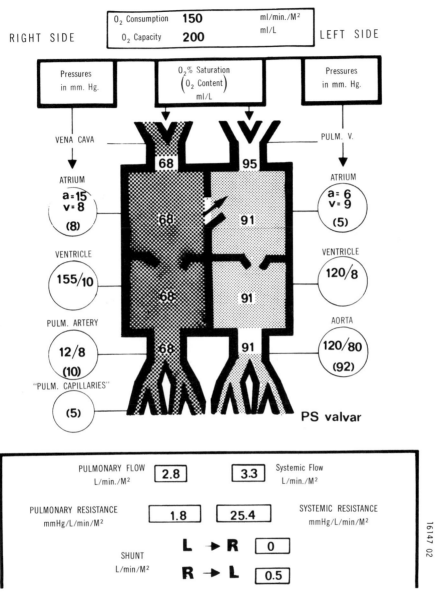

**Fig. 28-8.** Catheterization findings in a patient with valvar pulmonic stenosis. There is a 142-mmHg peak systolic gradient across the pulmonic valve and some right-to-left shunting at the atrial level through a patent foramen ovale.

quired disease that occurs with ductal closure, although the exact mechanism is still a topic of lively debate.

In older children and adults, large collateral vessels may develop from the subclavian artery and its branches to the intercostal arteries below the obstruction to give the classic appearance of rib notching on the chest roentgenogram. Many patients, up to 80% in some series, have a bicuspid aortic valve, and approximately 6% have mitral valve abnormalities.

We do not routinely catheterize children with coarctation of the aorta unless we suspect the presence of associated abnormalities, such as aortic stenosis or mitral valve

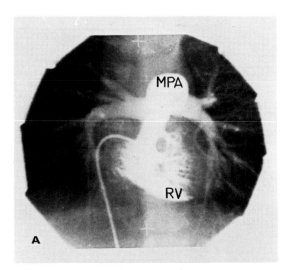

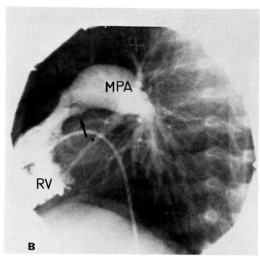

**Figure 28-9.** Biplane cineangiogram in the (A) AP and (B) lateral projections in a child with valvar pulmonic stenosis. Note the domed and thickened pulmonic valve (arrows) and the poststenotic dilatation in the main pulmonary artery (MPA). RV = right ventricle.

before percutaneous puncture. Passing the catheter across the coarctation can usually be accomplished by advancing the soft end of a guide wire out the end of the catheter, but if this does not succeed, an angiogram should be performed, since occasionally there is complete atresia of the aorta distal to the left subclavian artery. If a right arm approach is contemplated, an esophagogram with barium is recommended to exclude an anomalous origin of the right subclavian artery, since such an anomaly makes passage of the catheter into the ascending aorta difficult.

*Saturation.* In the usual case no shunts are present, and the aortic blood is fully saturated.

*Pressures.* Right heart pressures are usually normal, but the wedge pressure is occasionally elevated. The systolic pressures in the left ventricle and the ascending aorta may be normal in mild cases, but are increased in most. The systolic and mean pressures in the descending aorta are diminished, and a systolic and a mean gradient are present across the coarctation. The diastolic pressure in the ascending and descending aorta is usually normal in children but is often elevated in adults. The systolic gradient alone may be a poor reflection of the severity of the coarctation, since it depends on the degree of collateral vessels. Exercise usually increases both the systolic pressure in the ascending aorta and the gradient.

*Angiocardiography.* The area of coarctation appears optimally on the AP, lateral, or left anterior oblique views. Radiopaque contrast agent can be injected in the left ventricle, ascending aorta, or at the aortic isthmus, depending on which associated lesions need to be excluded. Large tortuous collateral vessels are usually seen; their absence should alert one to the possibility that the coarctation is not as severe as suspected.

disease, or suspect that the coarctation may be positioned abdominally rather than in its usual position just distal to the take-off of the left subclavian artery.

*Catheterization Techniques.* Although some have favored the brachial artery approach for retrograde studies, we have had good success from the femoral artery. If the pulse is not palpable in the groin, a Doppler probe is useful to locate the artery

## TETRALOGY OF FALLOT

Tetralogy of Fallot (TOF) is the most common cyanotic congenital heart lesion in children who survive past infancy and has become the most common lesion studied in our catheterization laboratory (16.3%) in the past 10 years. It is not unexpectedly a rare lesion (2%) in adults. The term *tetralogy* is a misnomer, since the four components may all be the result of a single embryologic defect: underdevelopment of the subpulmonary infundibulum with displacement of the parietal band, which obstructs the right ventricular outflow tract, leaving a defect at the normal position of the attachment site to the septal band.[14] The infundibular pulmonary stenosis, a large, nonrestrictive ventricular septal defect, right ventricular hypertrophy, and overriding aortic valve, probably all result from this one defect.

In the presence of a large ventricular septal defect, the degree of intracardiac shunting and therefore cyanosis is a function of the relative resistances to right and left ventricular ejection. If the pulmonary stenosis is mild and the total pulmonary resistance is less than systemic, a net left-to-right shunt will be present with little if any cyanosis (the so-called pink tetralogy). Conversely, with severe pulmonary stenosis (or pulmonary atresia as an extreme) the right-to-left shunt may lead to profound arterial hypoxemia and cyanosis. Large collateral vessels from the descending aorta may augment pulmonary flow, especially in those with severe pulmonary stenosis or atresia. Often, other cardiovascular anomalies coexist with TOF, especially ASD (about 15%), right aortic arch (25%), bicuspid aortic valve occasionally with aortic regurgitation (10%), and anomalies of the coronary arteries (5%).

We catheterize all cyanotic children to establish an accurate anatomic diagnosis and to gain some idea of the prognosis.

Since children with tetralogy of Fallot depend on maintaining systemic resistance for pulmonary blood flow, and since our usual premedication (Demerol Compound) reduces systemic resistance, we use morphine 0.1 mg/kg IM as premedication in patients with this lesion. Cyanotic spells in the catheterization laboratory continue to be a rare but potentially lethal problem.

### Catheterization Technique.
In children and adults it is usually possible to pass the catheter from the right ventricle through the ventricular septal defect into the ascending aorta by applying a clockwise rotation to the catheter in the right ventricle, as if one were attempting to enter the pulmonary artery but directing the catheter a little more medially than normal.

In severely cyanotic children we do not attempt to manipulate the catheter into the pulmonary artery, as this will often precipitate a "cyanotic spell." The foramen ovale is often patent allowing access to the left heart.

### Saturation.
In those with severe pulmonary obstruction, no left-to-right shunt will be present, and the pulmonary artery saturation will be equal to that in the superior vena cava (Fig. 28-10). A small amount of right-to-left shunting may be present at the atrial level through an atrial defect or a patent foramen ovale, with left atrial saturation being less than the pulmonary venous values (Fig. 28-10). Left ventricular saturation usually reflects the left atrial level. The saturation in the ascending aorta is less than that in the left ventricle, reflecting right-to-left shunt from the right ventricle into the aorta. If a patent ductus arteriosus or a Blalock-Taussig, Waterston, or Potts shunt is present, the pulmonary artery saturation will be higher than that of the right ventricle.

With lesser degrees of pulmonary stenosis the arterial saturation may be normal, and a net left-to-right shunt at the ventricular level may be present. Occasionally large variations in the arterial and venous saturations may occur if the child is restless or crying, thus changing the relative resistances in the pulmonary and systemic circuits.

### Pressures.
(Fig. 28-10). The right atrial pressure is usually normal, but the a wave may be slightly elevated. Right ventricular systolic pressure is equal to that in the left ventricle and aorta. The pulmonary artery pressure is normal if the stenosis is mild, but usually it is decreased with a narrow pulse pressure (mean value of 6 to 10 mmHg) when the stenosis is moderate to severe. A careful pull-back with an end-hole catheter can often detect the site or sites of obstruction at the supravalvular, valvular, or subvalvular levels, but angiography is necessary for accurate delineation of the stenosis. Occasionally the pulmonary artery pressure and/or pulmonary vascular resistance may be elevated in those with long-standing large surgical shunts (Potts, Waterston, Blalock) in older children, or adults with severe hypoxemia and polycythemia. The left heart pressures are usually normal, but the left atrial a wave and mean pressures may be less than the right atrial values.

### Angiography.
High resolution angiography is essential for the differential diagnosis and accurate delineation of the abnormal anatomy. Right ventricular biplane cineangi-

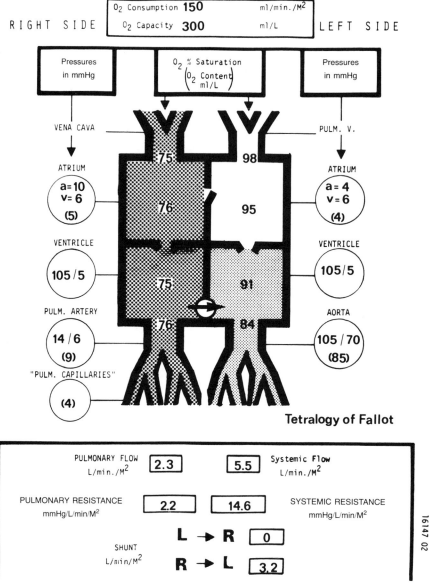

RIGHT SIDE

| O₂ Consumption **150** | ml/min./M² |
| O₂ Capacity **300** | ml/L |

LEFT SIDE

Pressures in mmHg

O₂ % Saturation
$\left(\begin{array}{c} O_2 \text{ Content} \\ ml/L \end{array}\right)$

Pressures in mmHg

VENA CAVA                     PULM. V.

ATRIUM          75      98      ATRIUM
a=10                            a=4
v=6      76      95      v=6
(5)                             (4)

VENTRICLE                       VENTRICLE
105/5      75      91      105/5

PULM. ARTERY      76      84      AORTA
14/6                            105/70
(9)                             (85)

"PULM. CAPILLARIES"
(4)

**Tetralogy of Fallot**

| PULMONARY FLOW L/min./M² | 2.3 | 5.5 | Systemic Flow L/min./M² |
| PULMONARY RESISTANCE mmHg/L/min/M² | 2.2 | 14.6 | SYSTEMIC RESISTANCE mmHg/L/min/M² |
| SHUNT L/min/M² | **L → R** 0 | | |
| | **R → L** 3.2 | | |

16147 02

**Fig. 28-10.** Catheterization findings in a patient with tetralogy of Fallot. There is right-to-left shunting at the ventricular level with arterial desaturation. The pressures in both ventricles are equal and there is a 91-mmHg peak systolic gradient across the pulmonary outflow tract. We normally do not attempt to enter the pulmonary arteries in children with tetralogy of Fallot with right-to-left shunts.

ography in the AP and lateral projections with 40 degrees of cranial angulation (Fig. 28-11) will outline the sites of stenosis at infundibular, annular, or supravalvular levels on AP projection while identifying the location of the VSD on the lateral view. A left ventricular angiogram in the LAO projection will delineate the site(s) of the VSD and determine if multiple defects are present. A supravalvular aortic angiogram through an antegrade or retrograde catheter is necessary to outline the coronary arteries, to ex-

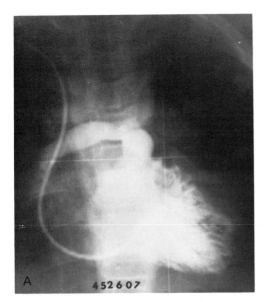
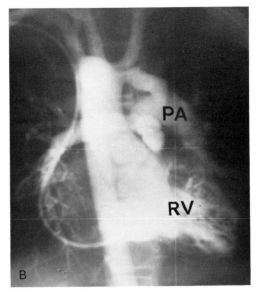

**Fig. 28-11.** Right ventricular injection in the AP projection (A) and with about 25 degrees of cranial angulation (B) in a patient with tetralogy of Fallot. There is infundibular, valvar, and supravalvar pulmonic stenosis. The aorta fills through a VSD. There is a right aortic arch and left Blalock-Taussig anastomosis. RV = right ventricle, PA = pulmonary artery. Note the elongation of the main pulmonary artery with cranial angulation with better visualization of the origin of the right and left pulmonary arteries.

clude *anomalous origin of the anterior descending artery from the right coronary artery* (and thus crossing the right ventricular outflow tract), to evaluate the degree of aortic insufficiency, if any, and to visualize any previously created surgical shunts. If the collateral vessels from the descending aorta are unusually large, or if the pulmonary arteries are not well visualized from a right ventricular angiogram, an angiogram in the descending aorta or selective injections of the collateral vessels may be necessary.

## TRANSPOSITION OF THE GREAT ARTERIES

Transposition of the great arteries occurred in about 5% to 10% of all children with congenital heart disease in our study group, and it is the most common cause of cyanotic heart disease seen in the first year of life. Untreated, the natural history is dismal, with 90% of such children dying before their first birthday. With palliation in the neonatal period and "correction" before one year of age,

an increasing number of these children are expected to survive into adulthood.

The structural abnormality in transposition is that the aorta arises anteriorly from the right ventricle and the pulmonary artery posteriorly from the left ventricle. The circulations are arranged in parallel rather than in series; that is, systemic venous blood from the cavae traverses the right atrium and ventricle and is ejected into the aorta, while oxygenated blood from the pulmonary veins, after passing through the left heart chambers, returns via the pulmonary artery to the lungs. A communication at the atrial, ventricular, or great vessel level is necessary for survival. Associated lesions are common, especially VSD and PS or pulmonary atresia. Mitral or tricuspid atresia, overriding or common atrioventricular valves, and single ventricle are also occasionally seen. In this section we will discuss only the most common form, D-transposition of the great arteries (DTGA)—that is, the aorta is "dextro" or to the right of the pulmonary artery—without a VSD or PS and with an atrial septal defect or patent foramen ovale. Infants with this defect are often hypoxic and occasionally acidotic soon after birth, and catheterization is done as an emergency procedure in the first days of life. Elective catheterization may be performed again at six to nine months of age prior to corrective surgery. A few centers, including our own, have started to correct most infants in the neonatal period without prior palliation. Those who seek a more in-depth discussion of DTGA are referred to one of the standard texts of pediatric cardiology.[1-3]

### Catheterization Technique.

Catheterization from the femoral vessels is recommended to facilitate crossing the atrial septum into the left side of the heart. Studies via the umbilical artery and/or vein are occasionally possible in the first few days of life. The venous catheter can be advanced into the aorta from the right ventricle, but this is not diagnostic of DTGA, since in children with normally related great vessels, the aorta may occasionally be entered by crossing into the left ventricle through a VSD. A variety of methods have been used to enter the pulmonary artery from the left ventricle: In the younger infants we prefer to use a soft balloon catheter, and in older infants we use a balloon catheter or, less commonly now, a standard angiographic catheter with a spring guide wire to make a "J" curve at the tip of the catheter, which will help to turn it up into the left ventricular outflow tract after passing through the mitral valve.

In 1966, Rashkind and Miller[15] described a procedure to enlarge the foramen ovale and improve mixing of blood in neonates with DTGA by tearing a portion of the atrial septum with a balloon catheter. Briefly, a specially constructed no. 5 French catheter is inserted through the umbilical or femoral vein into the left atrium under fluoroscopic control. After its location in the left atrium is established, the balloon is inflated with dilute angiographic contrast material and then rapidly withdrawn across the atrial septum with an abrupt, short tug. The catheter is then advanced rapidly into the mid-right atrium and deflated. This procedure is repeated several times. If the septum primum flap valve of the fossa ovalis is torn, little resistance should be felt on the second attempt.

### Saturation.

(Fig. 28-12). With poor mixing between the two circuits, the superior vena cava saturation may be quite low, even in the mid-20s. Even in the presence of good mixing, the SVC saturation is low, usually in the mid-50s.

There is usually a step-up between the SVC and right atrium due to left-to-right shunting at the atrial level (Fig. 28-12). The saturations in the right ventricle and aorta are similar to that in the right atrium. The pulmonary veins are fully saturated in the absence of lung disease. The left atrium is usually mildly desaturated due to right-to-left shunting at the atrial level. The left ventricular and pulmonary artery oxygen saturations are similar to the left atrial saturation. Because of a high pulmonary artery saturation and a narrow atrioventricular oxygen difference between pulmonary artery and pulmonary venous blood, calculation of the pulmonary blood flow may be subject to considerable error. The amount of left-to-right shunting must equal the right-to-left shunt over the long run to avoid one of the parallel circuits from becoming overloaded.

### Pressures.

(Fig. 28-12). Since the right-to-left and left-to-right shunts must be equal, the atrial mean pressures are also usually equal in the absence of a VSD or PDA. Occasionally, aorta-to-pulmonary artery shunting through bronchial collaterals must be balanced by left-to-right shunting at the atrial level, and in this case, left atrial pressure may be slightly higher than right atrial pressure. A large gradient suggests the presence of a significant VSD or great vessel shunt. Interestingly, in spite of the fact that the right ventricle is the systemic ventricle and the left ventricle is the pulmonary ventricle, the atrial pressure contours are normal; that is, the a wave in the right atrium predominates, as does the V wave in the left atrium. The right ventricular systolic pressure is at normal systemic arterial level. The left (pulmonary) ventricular systolic pressure is low (except in the newborn), usually 25 to 40 mmHg, and a 10 to 20 mmHg systolic gradient is often present across an anatomically normal pulmonary valve, probably due to subpulmonic obstruction due to apposition of the anterior leaflet of the mitral valve against the posteriorly bowed interventricular septum. The pulmonary artery pressure is normal in the absence of pulmonary vascular obstructive disease.

### Angiography.

As with most forms of complicated heart disease, angiography is essential for the diagnosis and surgical treatment of transposition (Fig. 28-13). A left ven-

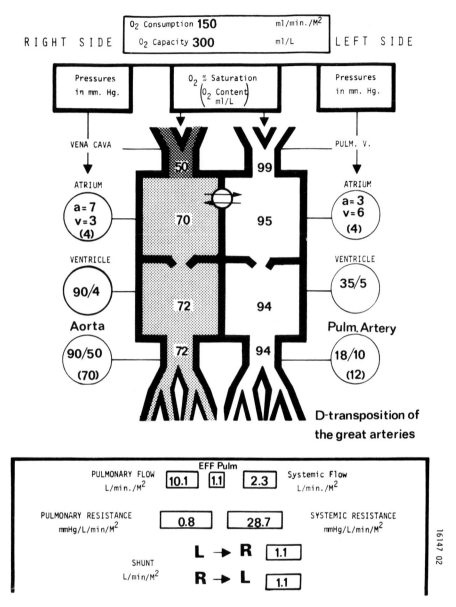

**Fig. 28-12.** Catheterization findings in an infant with transposition of the great arteries and an atrial septal defect. Note the bidirectional shunting at the atrial level and the arterial hypoxemia. There is a small systolic pressure gradient across the left ventricular outflow tract.

triculogram in the left anterior oblique projection with axial angulation will outline mitral-pulmonary continuity as well as the left ventricular outflow tract, and will rule out a ventricular septal defect and subpulmonic obstruction. A right ventriculogram will evaluate right ventricular function and rule out tricuspid regurgitation, ventricular septal defects, and patent ductus arteriosus. The coronary artery pattern is unusual, with the left circumflex artery often arising from the right coronary artery on the posterior surface of the heart.

***Operative Repair.*** Repair of tranposition can be accomplished by switching the great vessels and moving the coronary ar-

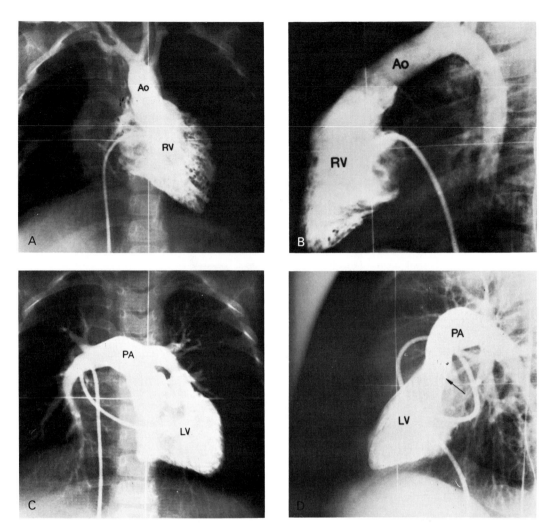

**Fig. 28-13.** AP (A) and lateral (B) views of a right ventricular angiogram, and AP (C) and lateral (D) views of a left ventricular (LV) angiogram in a child with D-transposition of the great arteries. The aorta (Ao) arises from the right ventricle (RV) and is anterior and to the right of the pulmonary artery (PA). CS = conal septum. Mitral-pulmonary continuity is shown by the arrow (D).

teries so that the right ventricle ejects into the pulmonary artery and the left ventricle ejects into the aorta. Postoperative catheterization is performed in the usual fashion, making sure the aortic, pulmonic, and coronary artery anastomoses are unobstructed. An alternative method for correction involves insertion of an atrial baffle so that systemic venous blood from the cava is diverted through the mitral valve into the left ventricle and pulmonary artery, and pulmonary venous blood is diverted through the tricuspid valve into the right ventricle and aorta. Postoperative catheterization assess-

ment involves evaluating the integrity of the intraatrial baffle and ventricular function, and ruling out systemic and pulmonary venous obstruction by the baffle.

An approach from the femoral artery facilitates passing the catheter from the left ventricle to the pulmonary artery, but we have occasionally used a brachial artery approach. The same techniques used to enter the pulmonary artery before corrective procedures are used after the intraatrial baffle repair. It is often possible to advance a retrograde arterial catheter from the aorta to the right ventricle and then through the tricuspid valve into the new left atrium and pulmonary veins if the aortic valve is crossed with a small loop. No intracardiac shunting should be present, but occasionally a left-to-right shunt at the atrial level may be present due to leaks around the baffle. There may be mild arterial desaturation, since the coronary sinus is often left on the pulmonary venous side of the baffle.

A comparison between both the superior and inferior vena cava and right atrial pressures must be made, since obstructions at the superior and inferior aspects of the atrial baffle are not uncommon. The left ventricular pressure is often mildly elevated, with a small gradient persisting across the left ventricular outflow tract. The pulmonary artery pressure is usually normal. Gradients between the pulmonary capillary wedge pressure and right ventricular end-diastolic pressure suggest obstruction across the pulmonary venous portion of the atrial baffle.

Angiography in the right ventricle is necessary to evaluate systemic ventricular function (since many patients have increased right ventricular end-diastolic volume and decreased ejection fraction) and to assess the degree of tricuspid regurgitation, if any. Left ventricular angiography is useful to evaluate the left ventricular outflow tract and to visualize the pulmonary venous atrium on the levo phase. Angiograms in the superior or inferior vena cava should also be performed if there is a suggestion of systemic venous obstruction.

# TRICUSPID ATRESIA

Tricuspid atresia is an uncommon form of cyanotic congenital heart disease, occurring in less than 2% of children with cardiac anomalies in the population under study. In the past, few such children lived into adulthood, but in view of advances in palliative surgery, survival will undoubtedly increase in the future.

In tricuspid atresia there is agenesis of the tricuspid valve, with no connection between the right atrium and right ventricle. An interatrial communication and a communication between the systemic and pulmonary circuits, usually a VSD, is invariably present. The embryologic defect is unknown, but current theory suggests that it is due to a malalignment between the ventricular loop and the atrium. Several classifications are available; we prefer a modification of that of Edwards and Burchell,[16] which divides the group into three types: normally related great arteries (I); D-transposition of the great arteries (II); and L-transposition of the great arteries (III). Each type may have an intact ventricular septum and pulmonary atresia (a), a small VSD with PS (b), or a large VSD without PS (c). Type Ib, that is, with normally related great arteries and a small VSD with PS, is the most common and represents about two thirds of the cases at our hospital. Type IIc is the second most common, and represents about 15% to 20% of cases in most series. Presenting symptoms, associated lesions, catheterization findings, and prognosis vary considerably depending on the presence or absence of transposition, the size of the VSD, and the degree of PS. Since type Ib is the most common and currently has the best survival rate, the remainder of this section will deal with that lesion.

***Catheterization Techniques.*** An approach from the groin is preferred. Since the tricuspid valve is atretic, the venous catheter crosses the atrial defect (invariably present) into the left atrium. Usually, the catheter is easily advanced into the left ventricle. If pulmonary flow is substantial, the catheter usually can be advanced across a VSD into the hypoplastic right ventricle and the pulmonary artery. A balloon catheter facilitates this maneuver. Occasionally, a retrograde aortic catheter will enter the pulmonary artery through a previously created systemic-to-pulmonary artery shunt (Blalock, Waterston or Potts anastomosis) and, less frequently, from the left ventricle through the VSD into the right ventricle and then to the pulmonary artery.

***Saturation.*** The oxygen saturation of blood in the superior vena cava and right atrium is usually low because of a normal AV oxygen difference with low arterial saturation, low cardiac output, or both. Pulmonary venous saturation is normal in the absence of pulmonary disease. Since all right atrial blood passes into the left atrium, there is complete mixing at the left atrial level with similar saturations in the left atrium, left ventricle, aorta, right ventricle, and pulmonary artery (Fig. 28-14). Systemic arterial hypoxemia is invariably present, and the degree of hypoxemia is a function of the pulmonary

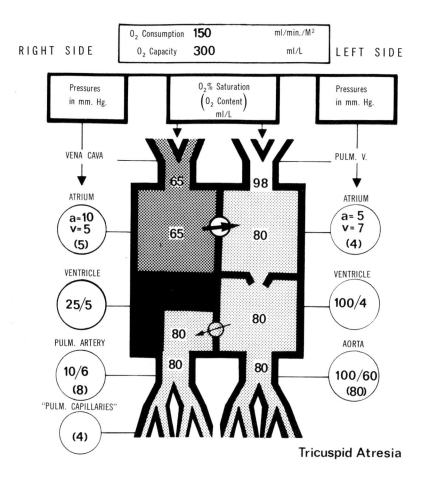

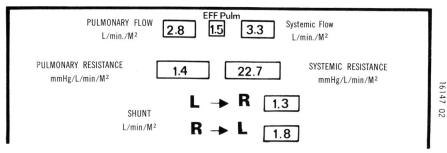

**Fig. 28-14.** Catheterization findings in a patient with tricuspid atresia, a small ventricular septal defect, and pulmonic stenosis. There is complete mixing of blood in the left atrium with similar saturations in LA, LV, aorta and PA. A small intra-atrial pressure gradient is present.

flow and pulmonary-to-systemic flow ratio. If the oxygen consumption is measured, the pulmonary flow can be calculated even in the absence of a pulmonary blood sample, since in the presence of complete mixing, the pulmonary saturation can be assumed to be the same as the arterial or left ventricular saturation.

***Pressures.*** Right atrial pressure is usually elevated. The a wave may be increased, especially if the atrial defect is restrictive. The left atrial pressure is usually normal, with a small gradient across the atrial septum (right atrium greater than the left atrium). The left ventricular and arterial pressures are normal. The pulmonary artery pressure is usually normal due to a restrictive ventricular septal defect, valvular or infundibular pulmonic stenosis, or both.

***Angiograms.*** The diagnosis of tricuspid atresia is angiographic. Injection of contrast agent into the inferior vena cava or right atrium in the left anterior oblique projection shows a dilated chamber with all contrast material crossing the atrial septum into the left atrium. In the simultaneous right anterior oblique projection, there is a negative shadow on the floor of the right atrium created by the absence of a tricuspid valve and right ventricular sinus (Fig. 28-15). A left ventriculogram in the hepatoclavicular position is essential to determine the size and site of the ventricular defect(s) and the size of the hypoplastic right ventricle, and to assess the pulmonary arteries. A right ventriculogram (again hepatoclavicular) is helpful if the catheter can be manipulated into this chamber. An aortogram may be necessary to delineate the patency of previously performed operative shunts.

***Postoperative Catheterization.*** The corrective surgery most commonly used for tricuspid atresia, the Fontan procedure[17] involves connecting the right atrium either directly or with a conduit to the hypoplastic right ventricle or pulmonary artery with closure of the VSD and ASD. Postoperatively, catheterization is usually facilitated by a balloon catheter. No residual intracardiac shunting should be present, although there may be a right-to-left shunt from a leak around the ASD patch or a left-to-right shunt from a residual ventricular defect. The right atrial mean pressure is elevated to 8 to 15 mmHg since venous pressure must overcome pulmonary resistance as the right atrium serves the right heart pump function. A gradient may be present at the anastomotic sites in the right atrium, right ventricle, or pulmonary artery, or in the conduit. The right ventricular and pulmonary artery pressures may be normal, although the high a wave from the right atrium may be transmitted to the tracings in end-diastole. Left heart pressures are usually normal. Angiography in

the right ventricle may be helpful to visualize the anastomosis or valved conduit and pulmonary arteries, and to evaluate left heart function in the levophase.

## EBSTEIN'S ANOMALY

Ebstein's anomaly is a rare form of congenital heart disease; it occurred in about 0.5% of children with cardiac anomalies whom we studied. The characteristic features are a redundancy of tricuspid valve tissue with adherence of a variable portion of the septal leaflet to the right ventricular wall, so that the origin of the free portion of the cusp is displaced downward below the atrioventricular junction. The portion of the right ventricle between the atrioventricular junction and the downward displaced tricuspid valve origin forms a common chamber with the right atrium. The degree of impairment of right ventricular function depends upon the extent of this "atrialized" portion and the degree of tricuspid regurgitation, stenosis, or both. Similarly, the clinical presentation is highly variable, with some children in the neonatal period having right heart failure and profound hypoxemia due to right-to-left

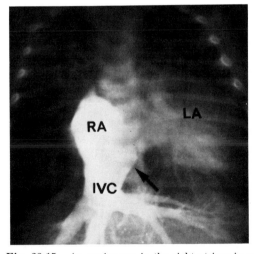

**Fig. 28-15.** An angiogram in the right atrium in a child with tricuspid atresia. Note the absence of tricuspid valve (arrow) with contrast, crossing the ASD into LA.

shunting at the atrial level, and others first being diagnosed at time of routine roentgenography as adolescents or young adults.

Cardiac catheterization previously was thought to be hazardous in Ebstein's anomaly because of a high incidence of atrial arrythmias, especially paroxysmal atrial tachycardia. With more experience and improved catheterization techniques, the indications and risks of cardiac catheterization associated with this anomaly do not seem to differ from those associated with other forms of congenital heart disease.

***Catheterization Technique.*** A primary purpose of the diagnostic procedure is demonstrating the "atrialized" portion of the right ventricle. The preferred method, first demonstrated by Hernandez,[18] utilizes an electrode catheter with a lumen. By slowly withdrawing the catheter from the right ventricle to the right atrium, one initially demonstrates a ventricular electrogram with a ventricular pressure tracing in the distal right ventricle, followed by a ventricular electrogram with an atrial pressure in the "atrialized" portion of the right ventricle, and finally

an atrial electrogram with an atrial pressure in the true right atrium (Fig. 28-16). In those with a large atrialized portion of the right atrium, this may be easy. In milder cases in which the atrialized chamber is small or when severe tricuspid regurgitation is present, the classic tracings may be more difficult to obtain. The right atrium is usually large. The right ventricle can usually be entered, although there may be some difficulty because of tricuspid regurgitation. The right ventricular pressure tracing is usually encountered to the left of its usual position. The catheter often enters the left atrium through a patent foramen ovale.

***Saturations.*** Arterial hypoxemia may be present from right-to-left shunting at the atrial level due to a noncompliant right ventricle with an atrial septal defect or patent foramen ovale. Equal saturation would then be present in the left atrium, left ventricle, and aorta. The pulmonary veins are fully saturated.

***Pressures.*** The pressure measurements depend on whether there is tricuspid regurgitation, tricuspid stenosis, or both. With tri-

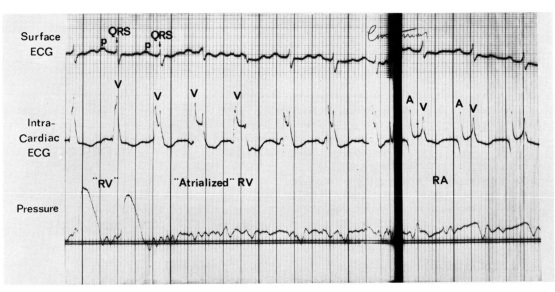

**Fig. 28-16.** Surface ECG, intracardiac ECG, and pressure recording in a 15-year-old girl with Ebstein's disease. As catheter is withdrawn from right ventricle (RV) (left) to right atrium (right), one sees an RV electrogram with RV pressure in the body of the RV, and RV electrogram with atrial pressures in the "atrialized" portion of the RV, and an atrial electrogram with atrial pressures in the true right atrium. V and A refer to ventricular and atrial depolarization, respectively.

cuspid regurgitation, there will be a large C-V wave in the right atrium; with tricuspid stenosis, there would be a large a wave with a diastolic gradient across the tricuspid valve. The right ventricular and pulmonary artery pressures are usually normal, but may have the a wave of the right atrium tracing prominent in end-diastole. Left heart pressures are usually normal.

*Angiography.* The diagnosis is usually clear from a selective right ventricular angiogram. The right atrium, atrialized portion of the right ventricle, and the right ventricular outflow tract will be visualized and one can appreciate downward displacement of the septal leaflet of the tricuspid valve, the size of the right ventricle, and the degree of tricuspid regurgitation (Fig. 28-17). If a right-to-left shunt at the atrial level is present, the left heart chambers will also be opacified.

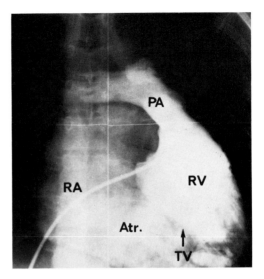

**Fig. 28-17.** Right ventricular (RV) angiogram in the AP projection in a patient with Ebstein's disease. Note the atrialized (Atr.) portion of the RV and right atrium (RA) opacified because of the tricuspid regurgitation. The downward displacement of the septal leaflet of the tricuspid valve (TV) is well visualized.

# REFERENCES

1. Nadas AS, Fyler DC: Pediatric Cardiology. Philadelphia, WB Saunders, 1972.
2. Rudolph AM: Congenital Diseases of the Heart. Chicago, Yearbook Medical Publishers, 1974.
3. Adams FH, Emmanouilides CC: Heart Disease in Infants, Children and Adolescents. Baltimore, Williams & Wilkins, 1983.
4. Alpert J, Dexter L: Personal communications, 1978.
5. Freed MD, Nadas AS, Norwood WI, Castaneda AR: Is routine pre-operative cardiac catheterization necessary before repair of secundum and sinus venosus atrial septal defects. JACC 4:333, 1984.
6. Freed MD, Miettinen OS, Nadas AS: Oximetric detection of intracardiac left-to-right shunts. Br Heart J 42 690, 1979.
7. Fellows KE, Keane JF, Freed MD: Angled views in cineangiocardiography of congenital heart disease. Circulation 56:485, 1977.
8. Bargeron LM Jr. et al: Axial cineangiography in congenital heart disease: section I, concept, technical and anatomic considerations. Circulation 56:1075, 1977.
9. Elliott LP, et al: Axial cineangiography in congenital heart disease: section II, specific lesions. Circulation 56:1084, 1977.
10. Freed MD, et al: Prostaglandin E. in infants with ductus arteriosus dependent congenital heart disease. Circulation 64:899, 1981.
11. Gersony WM, et al: Effects of indomethacin in premature infants with patent ductus arteriosus: Results of a national collaborative study. J Pediatr 102:895, 1983.
12. Nadas AS (ed): Report from the Joint Study on the Natural History of Congenital Heart Defects. Circulation 56 (Suppl I), 1977.
13. Paul MH, Rudolph AM: Pulmonary valve obstruction during cardiac catheterization. Circulation 18:53, 1958.
14. Van Praagh R, et al: Tetralogy of Fallot: underdevelopment of the pulmonary infundibulum and its sequelae: report of a case with cor triatriatum and pulmonary sequestration. Am J Cardiol 26:25, 1970.
15. Rashkind WJ, Miller WW: Creation of an atrial septal defect without thoracotomy. JAMA 196:991, 1966.
16. Edwards JE, Burchell, HR: Congenital tricuspid atresia: a classification. Med Clin North Am 33:1177, 1949.
17. Fontan F, Bandet E: Surgical repair of tricuspid atresia. Thorax 26:240, 1971.
18. Hernandez FA, Rochkind R, Cooper HR: The intracavitary electrogram in the diagnosis of Ebstein's anomaly. Am J Cardiol. 1:181, 1958.

# PART VII
*Special Catheter Techniques*

## chapter twenty nine

# Coronary Angioplasty

DONALD S. BAIM *and* DAVID P. FAXON

---

TRANSLUMINAL angioplasty—enlargement of the lumen of a stenotic vessel using an intravascular catheter—was conceived and initially reported by Dotter and Judkins in 1964.[1] They developed a technique in which a guide wire was advanced through an atherosclerotic arterial stenosis, allowing the subsequent advancement of serially larger rigid dilators until an improvement in luminal caliber was evident. Although this technique was clearly effective in peripheral arteries, the need to pass large-caliber rigid dilators through an arterial puncture and the high shear forces applied to the atherosclerotic plaque limited its clinical application. In 1974, Gruentzig modified this technique, replacing the rigid dilator with an inflatable nonelastomeric balloon mounted on a comparatively smaller catheter shaft.[2] This device could be introduced with minimal trauma, advanced easily across a vascular stenosis, and then inflated with sufficient force to enlarge the stenotic lumen. In 1977, following a series of experiments in animals, cadavers, and patients undergoing coronary artery bypass surgery, Gruentzig and co-workers extended the technique of percutaneous balloon angioplasty to the coronary arteries in conscious man.[3] Subsequent further improvements in equipment and technique have resulted in the dramatic growth of percutaneous transluminal coronary angioplasty (PTCA) over the last seven years, with performance of an estimated 50,000 procedures during 1984,[4] compared to only 1,000 procedures in 1980.[5] With current techniques, as many as 40% of patients with coronary artery disease and medically refractory, stable angina may benefit from PTCA as an alternative to bypass surgery, and angioplasty promises to play an increasingly important role in the management of unstable angina and acute myocardial infarction.

## EQUIPMENT

A coronary angioplasty system consists of three components: (1) a guiding catheter, which provides stable access to the coronary ostium and allows advancement of the dilatation equipment, (2) a nonelastomeric balloon dilatation catheter filled with liquid contrast medium, and (3) a leading guide wire (Fig. 29-1).

*Catheters.* Guiding catheters remain a crucial component in PTCA. The typical catheter has an outer diameter or 8 or 9 Fr (2.7 or 3 mm), a nontapered tip, and a Teflon-lined lumen with a diameter of 0.071 to 0.077 inches (1.7 to 2 mm). Current guiding catheters are available in shapes similar to conventional Judkins and Amplatz curves, as well as a woven Dacron configuration designed to be used from the brachial approach. To function adequately, the guiding catheter must be able to selectively engage the ostium of the involved vessel without occluding arterial inflow. Although this is

473

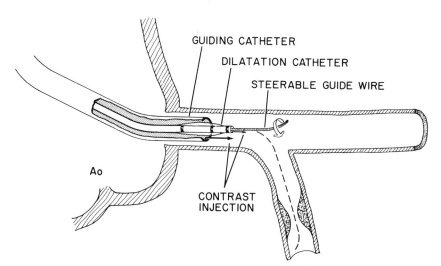

**Fig. 29-1.** Schematic diagram showing the three components used in coronary angioplasty: guiding catheter positioned in ostium of coronary artery, dilatation catheter positioned in left main artery ready to be advanced over the guide wire, and soft-tip, shapeable guide wire which can be steered to enter the desired vessel and advanced gently across the target stenosis.

routinely possible in the left coronary artery, ostial damping has been a vexing problem in the right coronary artery until the recent introduction of a Judkins-type catheter equipped with side holes to allow ongoing perfusion despite wedged engagement of the right coronary ostium. In the hands of some operators, the guiding catheter is also used to deliver small boluses of contrast medium into the involved vessel to visualize vascular side-branches and the target lesion for angioplasty. The most important function of the guiding catheter, however, is to provide adequate support for the advancement of the dilatation catheter across the target stenosis. This support derives from the intrinsic stiffness of the guiding catheter material, buttressing of the catheter against the opposite aortic wall, and/or deep engagement of the guiding catheter into the coronary ostium. In the patient with a short left main coronary artery, correct choice of the shape and size of the guiding catheter may also facilitate direction of the dilatation system to the left anterior descending or circumflex coronary artery, as required. A slightly shorter catheter (i.e., a JL 3.5 rather than a JL 4) or an out-of-plane catheter with anterior deflection of the tip will help to orient the dilatation system toward the left anterior descending; a slightly longer catheter (i.e., JL 4.5) or a

posterior out-of-plane tip orientation will help to direct the system toward the circumflex artery.[6] On the other hand, new steerable guide wires have made vessel selection quite easy and have reduced the risk that overzealous manipulation of the guiding catheter may lead to dissection of the coronary ostium.

The dilatation catheters for coronary angioplasty have undergone radical evolution since 1977. Whereas the original Gruentzig catheters were designed with a short segment of guide wire permanently affixed to the catheter tip, virtually all dilatation catheters since 1982 employ the feature of an independently movable and/or steerable guide wire extending the entire length of the dilatation catheter, as described by Simpson and co-workers.[7] (see Guide Wires, below). The dilatation catheter must have a central lumen of sufficient caliber to allow free movement of the guide wire, measurement of distal coronary arterial pressure from the tip of the dilatation catheter,[8] and in some designs the injection of small boluses of contrast material to visualize the distal coronary arterial lumen. A second important feature of the dilatation catheter is its "profile," defined as the smallest diameter opening through which the deflated balloon can be passed. Although current standard balloons have a substantially lower profile (approximately 0.050 inch, 1.25 mm) than the original Gruentzig design, specialized devices with profiles as small as 0.030 inch (0.75 mm) are currently being tested. A third feature is the ability of the balloon to bend so as to permit advancement through tortuous vascular segments, while retaining enough shaft stiffness to force it through the stenosis. The final important characteristic of the dilatation catheter is its ability to inflate to a precisely defined diameter despite application of pressures as high as 10 atm (150 psi). This is essential to permit the delivery of adequate distending forces to fibrotic stenoses without overdistending the adjacent normal vessel. Dilatation catheters that meet these design specifications are currently available with inflated diameters of 2.0, 2.5, 3.0, 3.5, and 4.0 mm to match the size of coronary artery in which the stenosis is located.

***Guide Wires.*** The original movable guide wire system designed by Simpson employed a standard 0.018-inch Teflon coated wire, which moved freely through the dilatation catheter and could be directed past branches by removal from the dilatation catheter, reshaping of its tip, and reintroduction.[7] In contrast, the guide wires used in modern angioplasty are specially designed devices that combine tip softness, radiographic visibility, and precise torque control, so that the guide wire can be steered past vascular side branches and through tortuous stenotic segments.[4] These features are now obtainable in guide wires with diameters ranging from 0.014 to 0.018 inch (0.3 to 0.5 mm). Exchange length (300 cm) angioplasty wires are also available to allow the serial advancement of different sized dilatation catheters (i.e., use of an initial low profile balloon to cross and partially dilate a severe stenosis, followed by a full-sized balloon to complete the dilatation) without the risk of subintimal passage of the second guide wire and balloon catheter as it crosses the partially dilated segment.[9] The movable guide wire concept and the current highly sophisticated steerable guide wires have simplified, shortened, and improved the success rate of coronary angioplasty. Even with these sophisticated devices, however, it is important to heed the advice of Dotter and Judkins that "the guide wire is passed across the atheromatous block more by the application of judgement than of force."[1]

## PROCEDURE

Although the angioplasty procedure bears a superficial resemblance to diagnostic cardiac catheterization in that catheters are introduced under local anesthesia, the procedure is a great deal more complicated and entails a 3 to 5% risk of abrupt vessel "reclosure" (the development of complete coronary occlusion during attempted PTCA of a stenotic vessel) or severe myocardial ischemia requiring emergency bypass. Angioplasty should thus be attempted only by experienced personnel in a setting where full cardiac surgical and anesthetic support is available. The patient is prepared as for cardiac surgery with an antiseptic soap shower, cross matching of blood, and proscription of oral intake after midnight on the evening prior to the procedure. In our current regimen, calcium channel blockers and antiplatelet therapy (usually aspirin 325 mg/day and dipyridamole 200 mg/day) are begun 24 hours before angioplasty and continued for 6 months after the procedure, to prevent vessel spasm and to diminish platelet adhesion to the disrupted endothelium at the PTCA site. Intravenous heparin (10,000 to 15,000 units) is administered during the procedure, but most centers have discontinued the concurrent use of low molecular weight dextran due to lack of experimental efficacy and side effects including increased blood loss, volume overload, and allergic reactions.

Angioplasty may be done by either the femoral or brachial approach.[10] In either case, right heart catheterization is usually performed for the measurement of baseline filling pressures and/or standby ventricular pacing. Baseline angiograms are obtained of one or both coronary arteries, using either standard diagnostic catheters or the angioplasty guiding catheter. If the guiding catheter is used for angiography, it must be manipulated carefully, since the large diameter, nontapered tip, and relative stiffness of the guiding catheter increase the risk of ostial injury. Coronary injections should be repeated after the administration of 200 mcg of intracoronary nitroglycerin, to demonstrate that spasm is not a significant component of the target stenosis and to minimize the occurrence of coronary spasm during the subsequent angioplasty. Intravenous verapamil or sublingual nifedipine may be administered in addition to nitroglycerin. Baseline angiography also serves to evaluate any potential changes in angiographic appearance (interval development of total occlusion, thrombus formation) since the prior diagnostic catheterization and to permit the selection of angiographic views which allow optimal visualization of the coronary stenoses and their surrounding branch vessels.

Following baseline angiography, the appropriate guiding catheter is introduced and positioned in the coronary ostium. The dilatation catheter and leading guide wire are then advanced into the guiding catheter through a sidearm device, which permits continued monitoring of pressure within and injection of contrast medium through the guiding catheter lumen. While the dilatation catheter remains within the tip of the guiding catheter, the steerable guide wire is advanced into the involved coronary artery, through the target stenosis, and into the distal vessel. Its position relative to vessel branches and lesions is evaluated by a series of contrast injections through either the guiding catheter or the dilatation catheter. This guide wire then serves as a track permitting safe advancement of the dilatation catheter through the lesion.

Once the dilatation catheter has been positioned within the target stenosis, the balloon segment is inflated progressively until it assumes its full cylindrical profile. In most cases this is associated with a transient "hourglass" constriction of the balloon by the coronary stenosis, which resolves abruptly once adequate distending pressure is developed. With current balloon catheters able to tolerate inflation pressures of 10 to 12 atmospheres (150 to 180 psi),[11] full cylindrical inflation of the balloon is almost always possible. In elastic stenoses, however, the arterial wall tends to recoil partially once the balloon is deflated. Depending on the angiographic appearance of the dilated segment, the residual transstenotic pressure gradient measured between the guiding catheter and the tip of the dilatation catheter positioned beyond the stenosis,[12] and the clinical condition of the patient, it may be necessary to repeat or prolong inflations (up to one minute in duration[13]) or to exchange the initial balloon for a larger-sized device, in order to achieve the desired result. While polyethylene balloons tend to maintain their specified inflated diameter at pressures between 6 and 10 atmospheres (90 to 150 psi),

polyvinyl chloride balloons tend to expand further (up to 20% over specified diameter) at high pressures, allowing some operators to use higher pressure inflations to more fully dilate elastic stenoses. By using one or more of these techniques, it is usually possible to reduce the severity of the stenosis by at least 20% and to reduce the transstenotic gradient to less than 20 mmHg. While most operators rely heavily on the transstenotic gradient as an index of dilatation adequacy, actual measurement of the gradient is complicated by the presence of the dilatation catheter within the stenosis and the small size of the dilatation catheter lumen.[8,12] Similarly, angiographic evaluation of the residual stenosis may be difficult, owing to eccentricity or poor definition of the lumen after angioplasty.[14] While complete normalization of the vessel lumen is the ideal end result of coronary angioplasty, the operator must bear in mind that the use of excessively large balloon sizes or inflation pressures in the pursuit of this goal may lead to extensive coronary dissection and vessel closure. As our surgical colleagues often remark: "The enemy of good is better."

Once adequate dilatation is achieved, the balloon catheter is withdrawn into the guiding catheter. It is common practice in our laboratory to leave the guide wire across the dilated segment for an initial period of up to 15 minutes while observing the vessel for angiographic deterioration in a situation where readvancement of the balloon over the guide wire would provide easy access to the dilated segment. If the dilated segment remains stable, the guide wire is withdrawn and other significant lesions are dilated similarly, or the patient is transferred to a recovery area.

Although most laboratories initially reversed the heparin administered during PTCA and removed the femoral sheaths in the catheterization laboratory at the end of the procedure, it is now common practice to leave the sheaths in place until the heparin wears off spontaneously (usually 4 hours) or overnight during continuous heparin infusion if substantial intimal dissection is evident on the post-PTCA films.[15] In addition to the benefit of continued anticoagulation, this approach allows rapid reintroduction of catheters for the evaluation and management of the occasional patient who develops chest pain of electrocardiographic evidence of myocardial ischemia during the several hours following angioplasty. If the sheath is left in place it is important to perfuse its lumen adequately (20 ml/hr) and to monitor closely for limb ischemia.

The patient typically remains at bed rest for 18 to 24 hours after removal of the femoral sheath, then ambulates prior to discharge. The postangioplasty physiologic state should be evaluated by a maximal exercise test just before discharge, or within the week following discharge. The patient is discharged from hospital on aspirin, dipyridamole, a calcium channel blocker, and frequently a long-acting nitrate preparation. The latter two drugs are usually discontinued between six weeks and three months after the procedure, and dipyridamole is usually discontinued at six months after angioplasty. The patient is encouraged to return to full activity as soon as the femoral puncture site has healed and should expect to have no anginal symptoms. Return of anginal symptoms or deterioration in follow-up exercise test findings suggests restenosis of the dilated segment (see Immediate and Longterm Efficacy, below).

## MECHANISM OF PTCA

According to the original explanation advanced by Dotter[1] and by Gruentzig,[3] the enlargement of the vessel lumen following angioplasty was ascribed to compression of the atheromatous plaque. In fact, compression accounts for only about 5% of the improvement.[16,17] Extrusion of liquid components from the plaque accounts for some improvement in soft plaques but contributes minimally to improvement in more fibrotic lesions, even when balloon inflation is prolonged to one minute.[13] The bulk of the improvement following PTCA seems to result from controlled overstretching of the vessel by the PTCA balloon, leading to fracture of the intimal plaque, partial disruption of the media and adventitia, and enlargement of the overall caliber of the vessel[17,18] (Fig. 29-2). This localized vessel trauma is apparent in the post-PTCA angiogram,[19] and histologic examination of animal and cadaveric angioplasty specimens.[20] Fortunately, dislodgment and distal embolization of plaque fragments seems to be an infrequent event in both experimental studies[21] and clinical an-

gioplasty procedures, although it has been described in one patient undergoing dilatation of a saphenous vein bypass graft[22] and several patients with intracoronary thrombus adherent to the dilated lesion.

## IMMEDIATE AND LONGTERM EFFICACY OF PTCA

Most published data on coronary angioplasty derive from the NHLBI Angioplasty Registry, which collected all procedures performed between 1977 and September 1981.[5] These 3000 patients have been the subject of reports on clinical success and complications, and a full and excellent review of this experience has been published recently.[23] Although case selection in the Registry focused on "ideal" PTCA candidates—those with proximal, discrete, concentric, subtotal, noncalcified stenoses of a single vessel—the primary success rate of 63% would be considered disappointing by current standards. The main explanations for the low primary success rate in the registry were failure to cross the lesion with the dilatation system (29% of cases) and failure to dilate the lesion adequately once having crossed (12% of cases).[5] These failures were due to two factors: (1) the relative lack of experience of operators contributing cases to the Registry (the "learning curve") and (2) the use of original Gruentzig fixed-wire dilatation catheters with limited maneuverability, a comparatively high deflated balloon profile, and a low peak inflation pressure.[6] By comparison, centers with a large volume of angioplasties (20 to 100 cases/month) are now reporting a primary success rate above 90% despite the selection of anatomically more difficult lesions. Failure to cross the lesion now occurs in less than 10% of cases, and failure to dilate a lesion that has been crossed occurs in less than 5% of cases, owing to improved operator skill and recent improvements in angioplasty equipment.[4,24] In patients undergoing angiographically successful PTCA, anatomic improvement correlates with elimination of anginal symptoms and improved function at atrial pacing[25] or conventional exercise testing.[26,27] Recent studies using thermodilution[25] and videodensitometric techniques[28] have shown restoration of nearly normal coronary flow

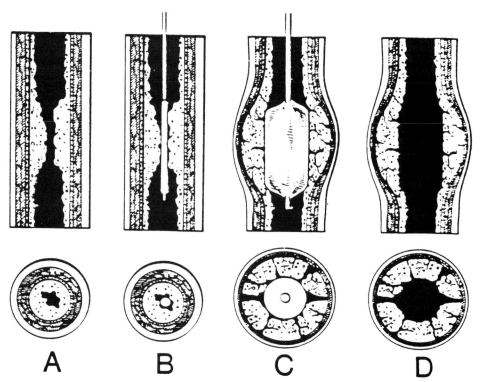

**Fig. 29-2.** Proposed mechanism of angioplasty. Inflation of the balloon catheter within the stenotic segment leads to cracking of the intimal plaque, stretching of the media and adventitia, and expansion of the outer diameter of the vessel. In contrast, compression of the plaque material and extrusion of liquid plaque components appear to contribute only slightly to the improvement in luminal diameter. (From Castaneda-Zuniga WR, et al: The mechanism of balloon angioplasty. Radiology 135:565, 1980.)

reserve following successful coronary angioplasty.

These improvements are generally well maintained during follow up ranging over several years,[29] but approximately 20% of patients redevelop anginal symptoms or exercise test evidence of ischemia as the result of restenosis of the dilated segment during the 1.5 to 6 months after successful PTCA. An additional 10% of patients will have angiographic evidence of partial restenosis despite lack of symptoms and a negative exercise test.[23,24] Restenosis appears to be the result of several factors, including elastic recoil of the dilated segment, platelet adhesion or thrombosis formation, and localized proliferation and lipid uptake by smooth muscle at the site of PTCA-induced intimal damage[24,30,31] (Fig. 29-3). Although restenosis is more likely if the initial angioplasty was incomplete, it is clear that rapid restenosis can follow technically ideal angioplasty

procedures as well (Fig. 29-4). Restenotic lesions may progress more rapidly than native atherosclerosis, which should be borne in mind when evaluating the patient with recurrent angina after angioplasty; progression to an unstable pattern and myocardial infarction may occur if corrective action (repeat angioplasty or bypass surgery) is not undertaken promptly.

In part, the high incidence of restenosis following coronary angioplasty reflects our limited understanding of the healing phase following arterial injury and its optimal pharmacologic manipulation, since restenosis occurs despite the current use of antiplatelet and calcium-channel blocking agents.[32,33] While future refinements in drug treatment may reduce the incidence of restenosis, most patients with symptomatic restenosis are currently managed by the repeat angioplasty, which can be accomplished with a lower complication rate than the primary proce-

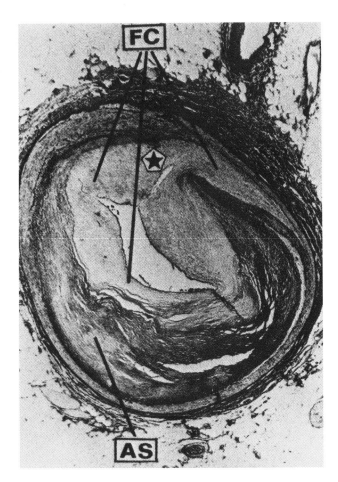

**Fig. 29-3.** Proposed mechanism of restenosis: cross section of a restenotic lesion in the left anterior descending artery 5 months after initial coronary angioplasty shows the original atherosclerotic plaque (AS), the crack in the medial layer induced by the original procedure (star), and the proliferation of fibrocellular tissues (FC) which constitutes the restenotic lesion. While this may represent in part organization of an early platelet-fibrin thrombus, smooth muscle cell proliferation stimulated by the release of platelet derived growth factor appears to be a more important contributor to restenosis. (From Serruys PW, et al: Assessment of percutaneous transluminal coronary angioplasty by quantitative coronary angiography: diameter versus videodensitometric area measurements. Am J Cardiol 54:482, 1984.)

dure and generally effects a permanent improvement.[24] Serial restenoses occur in some patients, however, and up to 5 angioplasty procedures have been performed on the same recurrent lesion. On the other hand, if restenosis is not evident by 6 months after angioplasty procedure, it is unlikely to develop during further follow-up.

Two other causes of recurrent symptoms after apparently successful coronary angioplasty should be mentioned. The first is coronary artery spasm, which may be exacerbated within the first six weeks after the procedure.[34] Most groups are now employing calcium-channel blockers and nitrates during this period, particularly given the suggestion that uncontrolled spasm may increase the chance of organic restenosis.[35] The second cause of recurrent symptoms

after several months is progression of disease in undilated segments.[6] Whereas cardiac surgeons routinely bypass all significant stenoses at the time of surgery, most angioplasty operators confine their efforts to the severe (greater than 70%) stenoses, leaving behind moderate lesions that are unlikely to cause persistent symptoms. The rationale for this approach is that dilatation of these milder lesions requires additional time and administration of contrast medium, exposes the patient to additional hazards of abrupt vessel closure, and may initiate progressive restenosis leading to a more severe lesion than was present initially.[36] If recurrent symptoms are the result of progressive disease in a previously undilated segment, they can usually be abated by angioplasty of the offending lesion (Fig. 29-5).

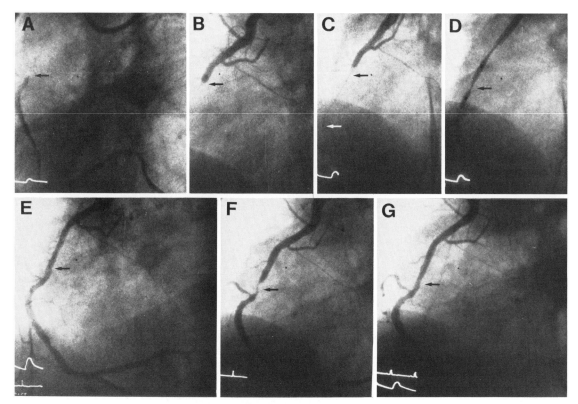

**Fig. 29-4.** Clinical restenosis. (A to D) A totally occluded right coronary artery with filling of the distal vessel via left to right collaterals. (E) The essentially normal appearance of the right coronary artery following successful angioplasty. (F) The appearance six weeks later when angina had recurred. (G) The appearance following successful re-PTCA. Restenosis developed again six weeks following the second PTCA, but the patient is now asymptomatic more than two years after a third PTCA procedure. (From Dervan JP, Baim DS,Cherniles J, Grossman W: Transluminal angioplasty of occluded coronary arteries: use of a moveable guide wire system. Circulation 68:776, 1983.)

## COMPLICATIONS

As a specialized form of cardiac catheterization, coronary angioplasty is attended by the usual risks relating to vessel trauma at the catheter insertion site. The large-caliber angioplasty guiding catheter is more likely to result in damage to the proximal coronary artery than conventional coronary angiographic catheters, and subselective advancement of guide wires and dilatation catheters may lead to vessel injury if they are manipulated too aggressively. The most common complications of coronary angioplasty, however, relate to local injury at the dilatation site.[37]

*Coronary Artery Dissection.* Although plaque dissection may be caused by overly

vigorous attempts to pass the guide wire through a tortuous stenotic lumen, most dissections are the result of the "controlled injury" induced intentionally by inflation of the dilatation catheter.[17] In fact, localized dissections can be found routinely in animal or cadaveric models of angioplasty[18,20] and are evident angiographically in approximately one half of patients immediately after angioplasty.[19] When these dissections are small and nonprogressive and do not interfere with antegrade flow in the distal vessel, they have no clinical consequence other than transient mild pleuritic chest discomfort. Follow-up angiography as soon as six weeks after the angioplasty procedure will usually demonstrate complete healing of the dissected segment[4] (Fig. 29-6), although occasional localized formation of aneurysms has been described at the site of dissection[38] (Fig. 29-7).

In contrast, large progressive dissections may interfere with antegrade flow and lead to total occlusion of the dilated segment within 30 minutes of final balloon inflation (Fig. 29-8). This may be the result of compression of the true lumen by the dissection flap, although superimposed thrombus formation, platelet adhesion, or vessel spasm may contribute. While this process can be reversed in up to one half of the patients with abrupt vessel reclosure by administration of intracoronary nitroglycerin or readvancement of the balloon dilitation catheter to "tack up" the dissection via repeated or prolonged balloon inflations,[15] failure to reopen the occluded vessel and the resultant severe myocardial ischemia mandate emer-

gency coronary artery bypass surgery in 3 to 5% of patients in whom angioplasty is attempted. This makes it desirable to observe the patient both clinically and angiographically in the cardiac catheterization laboratory for 15 to 30 minutes after the dilatation and to perform elective coronary angioplasty only in a setting where the resources for prompt emergency bypass surgery are available. Most centers report an elapsed time of approximately two hours between the occurrence of an angioplasty-related vessel occlusion in the cardiac catheterization laboratory and the re-establishment of coronary perfusion (cross-clamp release) at the completion of an emergency bypass procedure.[39] With this surgical procedure, significant transmural myocardial infarction can usually be averted, and postoperative recovery is similar to that seen following elective bypass

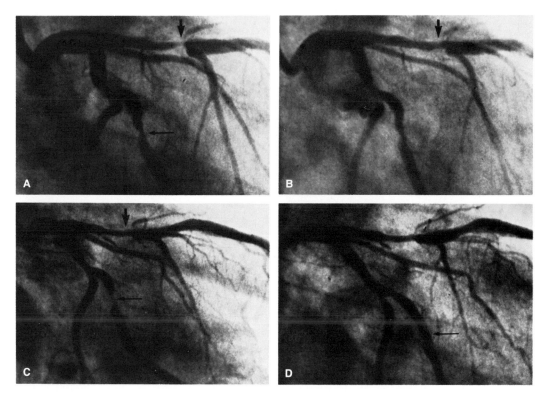

**Fig. 29-5.** Recurrent angina due to progressive disease in a nondilated segment. Left coronary artery in RAO projection before (A) and after (B) successful dilatation of the middle left anterior descending artery. Despite the presence of a moderate lesion in the circumflex marginal branch, this patient had an entirely normal exercise tolerance test until the recurrence of symptoms one year later. (C, D) Preserved patency of the LAD, but interval progression of the circumflex stenosis, which was then dilated successfully to restore an asymptomatic status. (From Baim, DS: Percutaneous transluminal coronary angioplasty—analysis of unsuccessful procedures as a guide toward improved results. Cardiovasc Intervent Radiol 5:186,1982.)

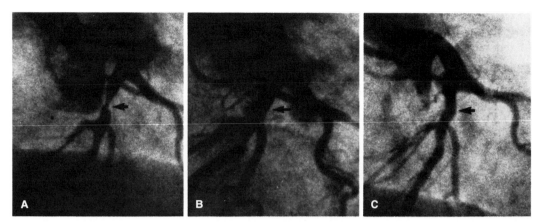

**Fig. 29-6.** Normal healing of PTCA-related coronary dissection. Compared to the baseline angiogram (A), the immediate post-PTCA angiogram (B) shows enlargement of the LAD lumen with two small filling defects typical of an uncomplicated coronary dissection. Follow-up angiogram 3 months later (C) shows preservation of luminal caliber with complete healing of the localized dissection. (From Baim DS: Percutaneous transluminal coronary angioplasty. *In* Braunwald E (ed): Harrison's Principles of Internal Medicine: Update VI, New York, McGraw Hill, 1985.)

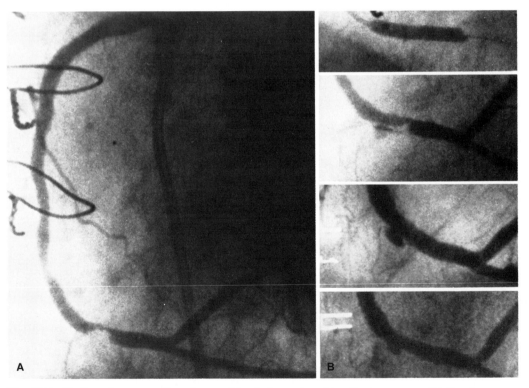

**Fig. 29-7.** Healing of coronary dissection resulting in formation of localized aneurysm. (A) Baseline appearance of a distal right coronary stenosis in a patient with prior left coronary bypass. (B) (Top to bottom) The inflated 3.0 mm balloon within the stenosis, the appearance of a localized dissection immediately following PTCA, a localized coronary artery aneurysm 6 weeks after procedure, and partial normalization of this aneurysm 6 months after procedure.

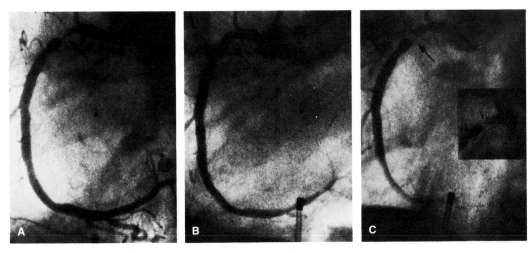

**Fig. 29-8** Coronary dissection leading to abrupt reclosure. The appearance of a right coronary stenosis prior to (A), and immediately following (B) coronary angioplasty, with an evident localized dissection. Within 15 minutes following removal of the dilatation catheter, the patient experienced chest pain associated with inferior ST segment elevation and angiographic evidence of progressive dissection with impeded antegrade flow (C). Although current practice would be to attempt to recross the lesion and "tack down" the dissection, standard management in 1980 consisted of emergency bypass surgery which was accomplished without complication. (From Baim DS: Percutaneous transluminal angioplasty—analysis of unsuccessful procedures as a guide toward improved results. Cardiovasc Intervent Radiol 5:186, 1982.)

procedures.[40] It must be pointed out, however, that some patients with ischemic events precipitated by coronary angioplasty do sustain major infarctions or become hemodynamically unstable during preparations for or recovery from emergency operation and that most large angioplasty series report a procedure-related mortality of 0.2 to 1%. In certain subgroups—those with extensive prior myocardial damage in other territories, a large myocardial territory perfused by the target stenosis, or prior coronary bypass surgery—procedure-related mortality may be as high as 2 to 3%,[23] requiring the most vigilant surgical standby and the immediate availability of intraaortic balloon counterpulsation. Some centers are currently constructing dual function procedure rooms (combination catheterization laboratory and cardiac operating room) for the safe performance of angioplasty on such high risk-patients, and work is proceeding on a variety of catheter techniques to maintain myocardial perfusion during the interval between vessel occlusion and the initiation of cardiopulmonary bypass.

**Other Complications.** A variety of other complications have been described as the result of coronary angioplasty. *Embolization of plaque constituents* is fortunately very rare,[22] but embolization of large thrombi that are adherent to the stenosis may occur and should be taken into account during angioplasty of patients with unstable angina or acute myocardial infarction (see below).

*Occlusion of branch vessels* originating from within the stenosed segment occurs in 14% of vessels at risk during angioplasty of the main vessel, according to what has been termed the "snowplow effect"[41] (Fig. 29-9). If the branch vessel is small, this event usually has no significant clinical sequelae and should not discourage attempted angioplasty. On the other hand, if a large branch vessel originates from within the stenosed segment, simultaneous dilatation of the main vessel and the involved branch with two separate dilatation systems (the "kissing balloon" or dual guide wire technique) may be required for preservation of both vessels.[42]

*Perforation of the coronary artery* with a stiff guide wire occurs rarely and does not necessarily have dire consequences. *Frank rupture of the coronary artery* due to use of too large a dilatation catheter leading to rapid tamponade death has been de-

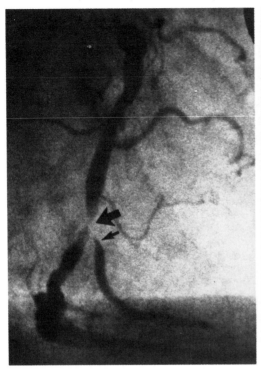 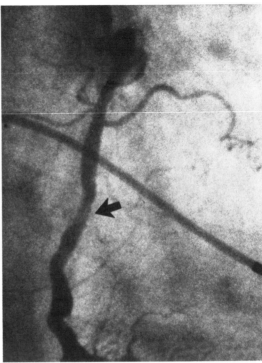

**Fig. 29-9** The "snowplow" effect. Dilatation of mid-right coronary stenosis resulting in occlusion of a diseased right ventricular branch which originated from within the stenotic segment. There were no clinical sequelae. Approximately 14% of involved branches will suffer a similar fate. If the branch is quite large, use of a multiple guide wire technique (simultaneous advancement of one guide wire down the main artery and one guide wire down the diseased branch) should be considered as a means of preserving the patency of both vessels. (From Baim DS: Percutaneous transluminal angioplasty. In Braunwald E (ed): Harrison's Principles of Internal Medicine: Update VI. New York, McGraw-Hill, 1985.)

scribed.[43] Tamponade may also result from perforation of the right atrium or right ventricle during placement of temporary pacemaker electrode catheters, particularly in angioplasty patients who are receiving antiplatelet therapy in addition to full heparinization.

*Ventricular fibrillation* occurs in approximately 1% of angioplasty procedures, usually as the result of prolonged ischemia during balloon advancement. Finally, the operator must be careful to limit the amount of contrast material administered (usually to 3 or at most 4 ml/kg) to avoid renal toxicity, particularly during complex or multivessel procedures.

## CURRENT INDICATIONS

***Single-Vessel Coronary Disease.*** When the NHLBI Registry was formed in 1979, pa-tients were considered to be candidates for coronary angioplasty if they had medically refractory angina, objective evidence of myocardial ischemia, and single-vessel coronary disease accessible to then-current angioplasty equipment.[5,23] Lesions considered appropriate for angioplasty were usually proximal, discrete, subtotal, concentric, and noncalcified. Although these criteria continue to identify patients with a high likelihood of success, major improvement in equipment and technique have permitted the safe and effective application of coronary angioplasty in patients with less ideal anatomy. Steerable guide wires and dilatation catheters with smaller deflated profile have allowed most operators to attempt dilatation of more distal and diffusely diseased segments. The routine use of prolonged inflations at low pressure (50 to 60 psi) has allowed dilatation of eccentric stenoses or those located within curved vessel segments, although such segments appear to be more prone to dissection.[44]

***Total Coronary Occlusion.*** It is also now clear that many totally occluded vessels can be dilated successfully in patients with ongoing ischemic symptoms due to inadequate collateral flow[45,46] (Fig. 29-10). To avoid vascular dissection or perforation, the guide wire must be used to gently probe the stump of the occlusion until the latent vascular channel is entered. Once the guide wire has been passed into the distal vessel and contrast injection confirms an intravascular wire position, the lesion can be crossed and dilated in the usual manner. The success rate of angioplasty in totally occluded vessels is clearly lower than in conventional stenotic vessels (60% versus 90% in our experience), with most unsuccessful procedures resulting from inability to advance the guide wire transluminally into the distal vessel. Success is favored by the presence of a "funnel" entry to the total occlusion, a short totally occluded segment, and comparatively recent occlusion. Patients in whom coronary stenosis progresses to total occlusion in the interval between diagnostic angiography and electively scheduled angioplasty,[47] which include up to 20% of patients whose initial diagnostic study shows a severe stenosis and slow antegrade flow competing with collaterals, comprise a particularly favorable subgroup, although chronic total occlusions of several years' duration have been dilated successfully as well. Total coronary occlusions in the setting of acute myocardial infarction are also amenable to coronary angioplasty (see below), with the caveat that the mass of associated thrombus is usually larger than that seen in established total occlusions and the risk of distal embolization may therefore be increased.[45]

***Multivessel Coronary Disease.*** With the improved success rate in single-vessel coronary angioplasty, extension of the technique to patients with multivessel disease seems natural. In fact, many patients in the NHLBI Registry underwent single-vessel an-

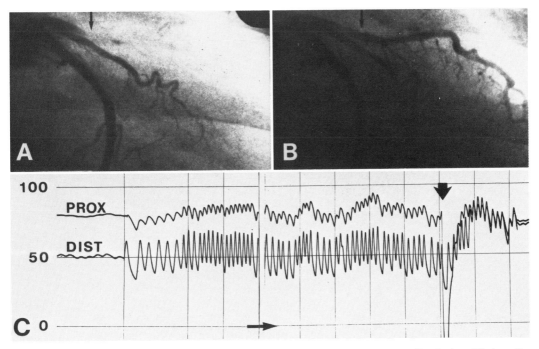

**Fig. 29-10** Angioplasty of a totally occluded left anterior descending coronary artery. Panels A and B show the artery before and after angioplasty, and panel C shows the proximal (PROX) and distal (DIST) left anterior descending artery presence. This patient had normal anterior wall motion due to the presence of right to left collaterals capable of maintaining a distal occluded left anterior descending pressure of nearly 50 mmHg, but not capable of meeting flow requirements during exertion. (From Dervan JP, Baim DS, Cherniles J, Grossman W: Transluminal angioplasty of occluded coronary arteries: use of a movable guide wire system. Circulation 68:776, 1983.)

gioplasty in the setting of multivessel disease, with the hope that correction of the single most severe lesion would control ischemic symptoms, even though milder lesions in other vessels remained untreated mechanically.[5,23] Although it is possible to attempt angioplasty on these *milder* residual lesions, experience has shown that these dilatations carry a significant risk of acute vessel occlusion and may initiate the restenosis process resulting in the formation of a severe stenosis within a matter of months.[36] In contrast, patients with *severe* stenosis of two or even all three coronary arteries are increasingly being considered for true multivessel angioplasty.[23,48] Such procedures are technically more demanding than single vessel angioplasty and carry a higher risk of complication should vessel occlusion occur. One possible exception is the "boot-strap" two-vessel procedure, in which a totally occluded artery is collateralized by a second vessel with a severe stenosis (Fig. 29-11). In this sit-

uation, the total occlusion can be dilated first without risk, thereby providing retrograde collateral flow to the stenotic vessel to improve the safety of the second dilatation. Except in the most aggressive centers, or for patients with major contraindications to bypass surgery, angioplasty of diffuse three-vessel disease or left main stenosis is still considered investigational.

**Stable Angina.** The largest group of patients who are candidates for coronary angioplasty are patients with stable but medically refractory angina pectoris and suitable coronary anatomy. Occasional patients with milder symptoms and ideal anatomy are candidates, if they willingly accept the 3 to 5% risk that angioplasty will lead to emergency bypass surgery. Patients with prior bypass surgery are candidates for angioplasty of the bypass conduit itself (Fig. 29-12) or of a native coronary artery (if supplied by an occluded graft or if narrowed by progressive disease since the time of operation (Fig.

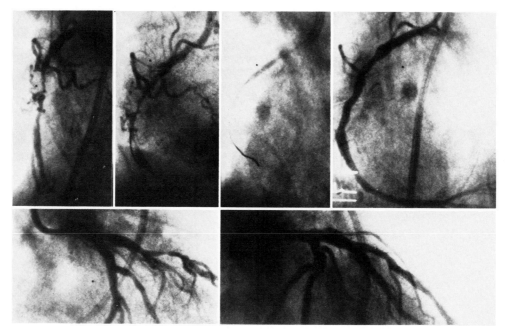

**Fig. 29-11.** "Boot-strap" two-vessel coronary angioplasty. Dilatation of a subtotally occluded right coronary (top) which received collaterals from a severely stenotic left anterior descending artery. Because the right coronary artery was protected by the left-to-right collaterals, it could be dilated at low risk. Once the right coronary was dilated, it served as a source of collateral flow to protect the left anterior descending artery during subsequent angioplasty of that vessel (bottom). Angioplasty of these two vessels in the opposite order (LAD first) would have carried significantly greater risk due to simultaneous jeopardy of both territories.

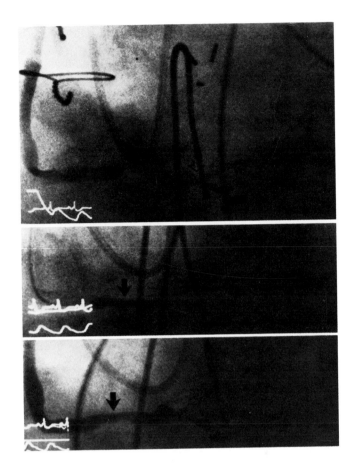

**Fig. 29-12.** Angioplasty of a stenotic right coronary saphenous vein bypass graft in a high-risk patient with unstable angina and poor left ventricular function seven years after bypass surgery for cardiogenic shock. (From Baim DS: Percutaneous transluminal angioplasty. *In* Braunwald, E (ed): Harrison's Principles of Internal Medicine: Update VI. New York, McGraw-Hill, 1985.)

29-7) but may be at greater risk due to mediastinal fibrosis if emergency surgery is required.[31,49,50]

***Unstable Angina and Myocardial Infarction.*** At the other extreme are patients with unstable angina or acute myocardial infarction.[23] Patients with new onset angina (within 90 days) have nearly a 50% likelihood of having single-vessel coronary artery disease and are considered candidates for a combined diagnostic coronary angiogram and coronary angioplasty at our institutions, with a success rate comparable to that in stable angina patients.[4,23,51] Similar findings have been described in patients with ongoing angina following a subendocardial myocardial infarction, in whom the angiogram shows subtotal occlusion or collateralized total occlusion of a single vessel. Patients with acute myocardial infarction have also been treated with coronary angioplasty in several situations.[4,23] The most common situation occurs in the patient with a high-grade residual stenosis following intracoronary or intravenous thrombolysis,[52] in whom successful angioplasty reduces the residual stenosis and hopefully the probability of vessel reocclusion or continued angina pectoris. The second situation is seen in the patient with an acute infarction in whom angioplasty is used as the primary therapy. This is our treatment of choice in the patient who has any faint antegrade flow and is a viable option in the patient who has a total occlusion without a large mass of associated thrombus, or in whom thrombolytic therapy has failed to recanalize the vessel (Fig. 29-13). In the patient with significant thrombus, however, there is a distinct possibility that angioplasty will dislodge the thrombus into the distal vessel and that subsequent thrombolysis will be required. While these situations are among the most dramatic in coronary angioplasty and can be of clear benefit to individ-

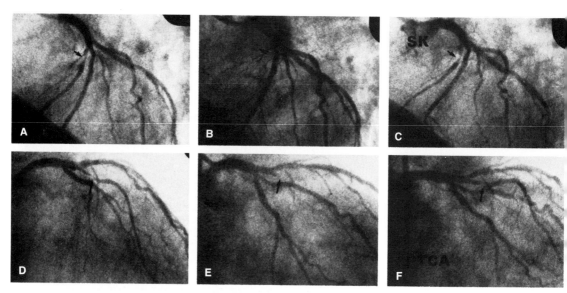

**Fig. 29-13.** Angioplasty following thrombolytic therapy. (A, B) Severe left anterior descending stenosis in a patient with unstable angina. (C, D) Spontaneous occlusion at the site of stenosis, which was refractory to intracoronary treatment with nitroglycerin and sublingual nifedipine. (E, F) Restoration of antegrade flow by administration of intracoronary streptokinase and treatment of the underlying coronary stenosis by acute coronary angioplasty. Despite ST elevation during the period of occlusion, this patient demonstrated no CPK elevation after procedure and continues to be asymptomatic more than 2 years later.

ual patients, their role in patient care depends on the skill and experience of the operator. Controlled studies of safety and efficacy will be required before acute angioplasty can be endorsed for general application in myocardial infarction or unstable angina.

## FINANCIAL AND REGULATORY CONSIDERATIONS

Since coronary angioplasty is performed in a cardiac catheterization laboratory under local anesthesia, it is attended by substantially lower direct costs than coronary bypass surgery. One multicenter study found combined hospital and professional costs for angioplasty to be $5,315 versus $15,580 for conventional bypass surgery.[23] Assuming an 80% primary success rate, this would represent a savings of $7,149 for each patient treated by angioplasty, not including the savings to the gross national product which would accrue by virtue of the more rapid return to work of the postangioplasty patient. While this does not include the hidden costs

of maintaining surgical standby and treating coronary restenosis (versus reoperation for graft closure), it seems clear that angioplasty affords the potential for a decrease in health care cost as well as patient morbidity when compared to bypass surgery. The ultimate savings will depend on subsequent revisions in institutional and professional reimbursement as coronary angioplasty continues to mature from a completely investigational to an established therapeutic modality.

Another consideration in the creation of a large-volume angioplasty program is that the radiation dose to the operator is at least twice that encountered during a routine diagnostic catheterization, as a result of the need for intricate manipulation of the guide wire and dilatation catheter under fluoroscopic control[53] and may exceed reasonable safety limits if large numbers of complex procedures are performed.

Finally, formal training standards have yet to be developed for angioplasty operators. Once the original Gruentzig catheter was licensed by the Food and Drug Administration in March 1980, operators have been able to purchase equipment and begin angioplasty programs at their own centers at their own discretion. Most have learned the general technique by observing procedures in active laboratories or by attending one of several demonstration courses. However, there is some concern that this approach may lead to overutilization of the technique, particularly since the same cardiologist frequently both determines the need for angioplasty and performs the procedure. The proliferation of angioplasty programs may also contribute to poor results due to an inadequate number of procedures per operator. The Executive Committee of the NHLBI Registry has thus recommended that patients be referred to regional centers with larger angioplasty volume unless the local operators have adequate training, fluoroscopic equipment, and case load to permit satisfactory results.[54] On the other hand, improvements in angioplasty equipment and case volume, and the provision of formal angioplasty training experience for senior cardiovascular fellows, make it likely that angioplasty will continue to dif-fuse to hospitals in which both a cardiac catheterization laboratory and cardiac surgical program are present.

While the chief application of coronary angioplasty has been in the catheterization laboratory, the technique has also been applied during conventional bypass surgery as a means of improving distal runoff beyond the graft insertion site.[55] Fogarty has developed an ingenious "linear extrusion" balloon for intraoperative use without fluoroscopy,[16,56] although conventional balloon catheters are also employed. The application of angioplasty in other vessels continues to develop in parallel with coronary angioplasty. The technique is in widespread use in the peripheral[57-60] and renal arterial beds[61] (Fig. 29-14). Preliminary work is in progress on angioplasty in the cerebral circulation, variety of congenital cardiac conditions (coarctation of the aorta[62,63]), pulmonary vascular or valvular stenoses,[64-66] and stenosis of surgical baffles.[67]

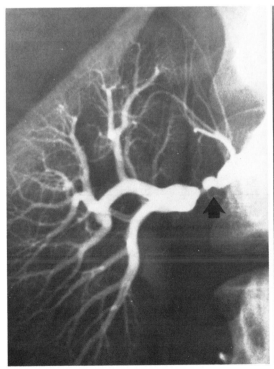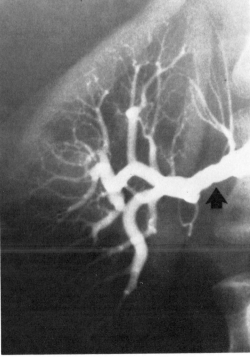

**Fig. 29-14.** Dilatation of right renal artery stenosed by fibromuscular dysplasia in a young woman with medically refractory hypertension. Following dilatation of both the left and right renal arteries with a 4.0 mm balloon, her blood pressure returned to normal off all antihypertensive medications.(Courtesy of Dr. Duck Soo Kim, Beth Israel Hospital, Boston.)

# FUTURE DIRECTIONS

Because of year-by-year improvements in equipment, technique, and success, published data about coronary angioplasty have failed to keep abreast of the current status of this procedure. By 1985 angioplasty has become the treatment of choice for most patients with symptomatically limiting single-vessel coronary artery disease and selected patients with multivessel disease, with an expected primary success rate in excess of 90% and an emergency surgical rate of 2 to 3%.[68] While further improvements in equipment can be expected to increase the success rate further, the biggest changes in coronary angioplasty over the next several years are likely to concern safe application of the technique to a progressively larger percentage of the current bypass population and to patients with unstable ischemic syndromes, definition of improved medical regimens for the prevention of coronary restenosis, and the development of alternative technologies to deal with the problem of abrupt reclosure. Fusion of mechanical angioplasty with laser[69,70] or thermal techniques to allow refractory dissections to be tacked down or shunt catheters that can be placed in the damaged vessel to allow more elective bypass operations may be advantageous in the management of abrupt reclosure.

# REFERENCES

1. Dotter CT, Judkins MP: Transluminal treatment of arteriosclerotic obstruction: description of a new technique and a preliminary report of its application. Circulation 30:654, 1964.
2. Gruentzig A, Kumpe DA: Technique of percutaneous transluminal angioplasty with the Gruentzig balloon catheter. Am J Radiol 132:547, 1979.
3. Gruentzig AR, Senning A, Siegenthaler WE: Nonoperative dilatation of coronary artery stenosis—percutaneous transluminal coronary angioplasty. N Engl J Med 301:61, 1979.
4. Baim DS: Percutaneous transluminal angioplasty. *In* Braunwald E (ed): Harrison's Principles of Internal Medicine: Update VI. New York, McGraw-Hill, 1985 pp. 133–146.
5. Kent KM, et al: Percutaneous transluminal coronary angioplasty: report from the registry of the National Heart, Lung, and Blood Institute. Am J Cardiol 49:2011, 1982.
6. Baim DS: Percutaneous transluminal coronary angioplasty—analysis of unsuccessful procedures as a guide toward improved results. Cardiovasc Intervent Radiol 5:186, 1982.
7. Simpson JB, Baim DS, Robert EW, Harrison DC: A new catheter system for coronary angioplasty. Am J Cardiol 49:1216, 1982.
8. Busch UW, Sebening H, Beeretz R, Heinze R: Reliability of pressure recordings via catheters used for transluminal angioplasty. Tex Heart Inst 11:160, 1984.
9. Dervan JP, McKay RG, Baim DS: The use of an exchange wire in coronary angioplasty. Cathet Cardiovasc Diagn 11:207, 1985.
10. Dorros G, et al: The brachial artery method to transluminal coronary angioplasty. Cathet Cardiovasc Diagn 8:233, 1982.
11. Abele J: Balloon catheters and transluminal dilatation: technical considerations. Am J Radiol 135:901, 1980.
12. Liboff R, et al: Determinants of trans-stenotic gradients observed during angioplasty: an experimental model. Am J Cardiol 52:1311, 1983.
13. Kaltenbach M, et al: Prolonged application of pressure in transluminal angioplasty. Cathet Cardiovasc Diagn 10:213, 1984.
14. Serruys PW, et al: Assessment of percutaneous transluminal coronary angioplasty by quantitative coronary angiography: diameter versus videodensitometric area measurements. Am J Cardiol 54:482, 1984.
15. Hollman J, et al: Acute occlusion after percutaneous transluminal angioplasty—a new approach. Circulation 68:725, 1983.
16. Fogarty TJ, Kinney TB: A new approach to transluminal angioplasty. Vasc Diagn & Therap Jan/Feb 1984.
17. Castaneda-Zuniga WR, et al: The mechanism of balloon angioplasty. Radiology 135:565, 1980.
18. Sanborn TA, et al: The mechanism of transluminal angioplasty: evidence for formation of aneurysms in experimental atherosclerosis. Circulation 68:1136, 1983.
19. Holmes DR, et al: Angiographic changes produced by percutaneous transluminal coronary angioplasty. Am J Cardiol 51:676, 1983.
20. Block PC, Baughman KL, Pasternak RC, Fallon

JT: Transluminal angioplasty: correlation of morphologic and angiographic findings in an experimental model. Circulation 61:778, 1980.

21. Sanborn TA, et al: Transluminal angioplasty in experimental atherosclerosis: analysis for embolization using an in vitro perfusion system. Circulation 66:917, 1982.

22. Aueron F, Gruentzig A: Distal embolization of a coronary artery bypass graft atheroma during percutaneous transluminal coronary angioplasty. Am J Cardiol 53:953, 1984.

23. Proceedings of the National Heart, Lung, and Blood Institute workshop on the outcome of percutaneous transluminal angioplasty (June 7-8, 1983), Kent KM, Mullin SM, Passamani ER (eds.). Am J Cardiol 53:1C, 1984.

24. Meier B, et al: Repeat coronary angioplasty. J Am Coll Cardiol 4:463, 1984.

25. Williams DO, Riley RS, Singh AK, Most AS: Restoration of normal coronary hemodynamics and myocardial metabolism after percutaneous transluminal coronary angioplasty. Circulation 62:653, 1980.

26. Kent KM, et al: Improved myocardial function during exercise after successful percutaneous transluminal coronary angioplasty. N Engl J Med 306:441, 1982.

27. Hirzel HO, Neusch K, Gruentzig AR, Luetolf UM: Short- and long-term changes in myocardial perfusion after percutaneous transluminal coronary angioplasty assessed by thallium-201 exercise scintigraphy. Circulation 63:1001, 1981.

28. O'Neill WW, et al: Criteria for successful coronary angioplasty as assessed by alterations in coronary vasodilatory reserve. J Am Coll Cardiol 3:382, 1984.

29. Meier B, Gruentzig AR, Siegenthaler WE, Schlumpf M: Long-term exercise performance after percutaneous transluminal coronary angioplasty and coronary artery bypass grafting. Circulation 68:796, 1983.

30. Essed CE, Van Den Brand M, Becker AE: Transluminal coronary angioplasty and early restenosis—fibrocellular occlusion after wall laceration. Br Heart J 49:393, 1983.

31. Waller BF, et al: Morphologic observations after percutaneous transluminal balloon angioplasty of early and late aortocoronary saphenous vein bypass grafts. J Am Coll Cardiol 4:784, 1984.

32. O'Gara PT, et al: Effect of dextran and aspirin on platelet adherence after transluminal angioplasty of normal canine coronary arteries. Am J Cardiol 53:1695, 1984.

33. Faxon DP, Sanborn TA: Restenosis following transluminal angioplasty in experimental atherosclerosis. Arteriosclerosis 4:189, 1984.

34. Holman J, et al: Coronary artery spasm at the site of angioplasty in the first two months after successful percutaneous transluminal coronary angioplasty. J Am Coll Cardiol 2:1039, 1983.

35. David PR, et al: Percutaneous transluminal angioplasty in patients with variant angina. Circulation 66:695, 1982.

36. Ischinger T, et al: Should coronary arteries with less than 60% diameter stenosis be treated by angioplasty? Circulation 68:148, 1983.

37. Dorros G, et al: Percutaneous transluminal coronary angioplasty: report of complications from the National Heart, Lung, and Blood Institute PTCA Registry. Circulation 67:723, 1983.

38. Hill JA, et al: Coronary arterial aneurysm formation after balloon angioplasty. Am J Cardiol 52:261, 1983.

39. Murphy DA, et al: Surgical revascularization following unsuccessful percutaneous transluminal coronary angioplasty. J Thorac Cardiovasc Surg 84:342, 1982.

40. Kabbani SS, et al: Surgical experience following transluminal coronary angioplasty. Tex Heart Inst J 11:112, 1984.

41. Meier B, et al: Risk of side branch occlusion during coronary angioplasty. Am J Cardiol 53:10, 1984.

42. Meier B: Kissing balloon coronary angioplasty. Am J Cardiol 54:918, 1984.

43. Saffitz JE, Rose TE, Oaks JB, Roberts WC: Coronary artery rupture during coronary angioplasty. Am J Cardiol 51:902, 1983.

44. Meier B, et al: Does length or eccentricity of coronary stenoses influence the outcome of transluminal dilatation? Circulation 67:497, 1983.

45. Dervan JP, Baim DS, Cherniles J, Grossman W: Transluminal angioplasty of occluded coronary arteries: use of a movable guide wire system. Circulation 68:776, 1983.

46. Holmes DR, et al: Angioplasty in total coronary artery occlusion. J Am Coll Cardiol 3:845, 1984.

47. Kimbiris D, et al: Rapid progression of coronary stenosis in patients with unstable angina pectoris selected for coronary angioplasty. Cathet Cardiovasc Diagn 10:101, 1984.

48. Vlietstra RE, et al: Balloon angioplasty in multivessel coronary artery disease. Mayo Clin Proc 58:563, 1983.

49. Douglas JS, et al: Percutaneous transluminal coronary angioplasty in patients with prior coronary bypass surgery. J Am Coll Cardiol 2:745, 1983.

50. Block PC, et al: Percutaneous angioplasty of stenoses of bypass grafts or of bypass graft anastomotic sites. Am J Cardiol 53:666, 1984.

51. Roberts KB, et al: The prognosis of patients with new-onset angina who have undergone cardiac catheterization. Circulation 68:970, 1983.

52. Meyer J, et al: Percutaneous transluminal coronary angioplasty immediately after intracoronary streptolysis of transmural myocardial infarction. Circulation 66:905, 1982.

53. Dash H, Leaman DM: Operator radiation expo-

sure during percutaneous transluminal coronary angioplasty. J Am Coll Cardiol 4:725, 1984.

54. Williams DO, et al: Guidelines for the performance of percutaneous transluminal coronary angioplasty. Circulation 66:693,1982.

55. Wallsh E, et al: Transluminal coronary angioplasty during saphenous coronary bypass surgery—a preliminary report. Ann Surg 191:234, 1980.

56. Fogarty TJ, et al: Adjunctive intraoperative arterial dilation. Arch Surg 116:1391, 1981.

57. Gallino A, Mahler F, Probst P, Nachbur B: Percutaneous transluminal angioplasty of the arteries of the lower limbs: a 5 year follow up. Circulation 70:619, 1984.

58. Kadir S, et al: Long-term results of aortoiliac angioplasty. Surgery 94:10, 1983.

59. Spence RK, et al: Long-term results of transluminal angioplasty of the femoral and iliac arteries. Arch Surg 116:1377, 1981.

60. Doubilet P, Abrams HL: The cost of underutilization—percutaneous transluminal angioplasty for peripheral vascular disease. N Engl J Med 310:95, 1984.

61. Sos TA, et al: Percutaneous transluminal renal angioplasty in renovascular hypertension due to atheroma or fibromuscular dysplasia. N Engl J Med 309:274, 1983.

62. Lock JE, et al: Balloon angioplasty of aortic coarctations in infants and children. Circulation 68:109, 1983.

63. Kan JS, et al: Treatment of restenosis of coarctation by percutaneous transluminal angioplasty. Circulation 68:1087, 1983.

64. Lock JE, Castaneda-Zuniga WR, Fuhrman BP, Bass JL: Balloon dilatation of hypoplastic and stenotic pulmonary arteries. Circulation 67:962, 1983.

65. Driscoll DJ, Hesslein PS, Mullins CE: Congenital stenosis of individual pulmonary veins: clinical spectrum and unsuccessful treatment by transvenous balloon dilation. Am J Cardiol 49:1767, 1982.

66. Rocchini AP, et al: Percutaneous balloon valvuloplasty for treatment of congenital pulmonary valvular stenosis in children. J Am Coll Cardiol 3:1005, 1984.

67. Lock JE, et al: Dilatation angioplasty of congenital or operative narrowings of venous channels. Circulation 70:457, 1984.

68. Libow M, Gruentzig AR, Greene L: Percutaneous transluminal coronary angioplasty. Current Problems in in Cardiology. 1:3, 1985.

69. Eldar M, et al: Transluminal carbon dioxide-laser catheter angioplasty for dissolution of atherosclerotic plaques. J Am Coll Cardiol 3:135, 1984.

70. Choy DSJ, Stertzer SH, Myler RK, Fournial G: Human coronary laser recanalization. Clin Cardiol 7:377, 1984.

*chapter thirty*

# Percutaneous Intraaortic Balloon Insertion

JULIAN M. AROESTY

T HE INTRAAORTIC balloon pump (IABP) is
the most commonly used mechanical
cardiac support device. For 20 years
after the conception[1] and initial clinical use[2]
of intraaortic balloon pumping, there were
unavoidable limitations and delays in its utilization because of the requirement that a
vascular surgeon insert and remove the device. This problem was largely eliminated by
the development of the percutaneous insertion technique in 1980.[3]

The intraaortic balloon is a flexible polyurethane bladder which is placed within the
descending thoracic aorta and is inflated
immediately after aortic valve closure with
consequent increase in aortic diastolic pressure. As the aortic valve opens, the balloon
deflates rapidly, producing a decrease in aortic systolic pressure with a consequent decrease in resistance to left ventricular ejection. The balloon is connected to a console
which uses the electrocardiogram for triggering each balloon cycle. However, timing is
adjusted to the arterial pressure tracing.

Balloon inflation occurs during diastole,
when coronary vascular resistance is at its
lowest. The most striking characteristic of
intraaortic balloon use, expansion during
diastole and deflation during systole, is appropriately called *counterpulsation*. This
has, as its major advantage, a decrease in
myocardial oxygen consumption without a
concomitant decrease in coronary perfusion
pressure.

## CONSTRUCTION OF THE IABP

Intraaortic balloon catheters are available
from several manufacturers, at a variety of
specifications. Some of the more widely used
products are listed in Table 30-1.

***Surgically Implanted Catheters.*** The
surgically implanted IABP catheter manufac-
tured by AVCO-Kontron has a three cham-
bered polyurethane balloon utilizing helium
as the inflation gas, whereas that produced
by Datascope is a two-chambered polyurethane balloon inflated by $CO_2$. Although helium is much less viscous than $CO_2$ and
therefore will follow much faster heart rates
at 1:1 counterpulsation, the low solubility of
helium gas in blood requires special fail-safe
mechanisms within the console to detect and
react to balloon rupture in order to prevent
serious gas embolism.

***Percutaneous Catheters.*** Kontron,
Datascope, and Aries all produce a balloon
catheter for percutaneous introduction
which has a single chamber and can be wire
guided. The SMEC Corporation does not
make a wire-guided balloon catheter, but
their balloons are tightly wound around the
catheter shaft at the factory and are very
flexible. The increased flexibility and lower
profile of the SMEC balloons partly compensate for the absence of a guide-wire lumen.
Introducing sheaths and balloon catheters of
different sizes are available to accommodate
arterial systems of different diameters. The

493

**TABLE 30-1.** *Percutaneous Intraaortic Balloons*

| Manufacturer* | Balloon Catheter Size (French) | Volume of Balloon (cc) | Size of Introducer | |
|---|---|---|---|---|
| | | | Internal (French) | External (French) |
| *Datascope* | | | | |
| With central lumen | 10.5 | 40 | 11.4 | 13.2 |
| | 12.0 | 40 | 12.5 | 14.0 |
| | 10.5 | 50 | 11.5 | 13.2 |
| Without central lumen | 8.5 | 40 | 10.0 | 11.5 |
| | 9.5 | 40 | 10.0 | 11.5 |
| *Kontron* | | | | |
| With central lumen | 10.5 | 40 | 11.5 | 13.6 |
| | 12. | 40 | 12.5 | 14.0 |
| Without central lumen | 9.5 | 40 | 11.0 | 12.6 |
| *SMEC* | | | | |
| With central lumen | None | | | |
| Without central lumen | 10.5 | 30 | 10.5 | 12.5 |
| | 11.0 | 40 | 11.0 | 13.0 |
| | 11.5 | 50 | 11.5 | 13.5 |
| | 11.5 | 60 | 11.5 | 13.5 |
| *Aries* | | | | |
| With central lumen | 10.5 | 40 | 11.0 | 12.5 |

*Manufacturers' addresses: Datascope Corp., Paramus, NJ: Kontron Cardiovascular Inc., Everett, MA; SMEC Inc., Cockeville, TN; Aries Medical, Woburn, MA)

various intraaortic balloon catheters are produced both with and without a central lumen (Table 30-1). The central lumen balloon catheters provide the extra safety of guide-wire directed placement as well as the opportunity for reliable arterial pressure monitoring. However, balloon catheters with a central lumen require a larger introducing sheath than those without (Table 30-1).

## INDICATIONS AND CONTRAINDICATIONS

Counterpulsation is most often utilized in medically refractory unstable angina,[4] cardiogenic shock,[5-7] or perioperative hemodynamic instability.[8] Less well-established indications include the limitations of infarction size in patients with uncomplicated acute myocardial infarction,[9] treatment of intractable ventricular tachycardia,[10] or support of patients with recent infarction who require general anesthesia for noncardiac surgical procedures.[11]

Counterpulsation is absolutely contraindicated in the presence of abnormally increased aortic diastolic runoff (e.g., aortic regurgitation or patent ductus arteriosus), since the regurgitation or shunt will be increased by the higher aortic diastolic pressure. Other contraindications include the presence of severe arterial insufficiency of lower limbs, bypass grafting to lower limbs, a marked bleeding diathesis, uncontrolled septicemia, documented cholesterol embolism to abdomen or legs, excessive tachycardia, or marked irregularity of rhythm.

## PREINSERTION

***Planning.*** If an indication for counterpulsation is present prior to selective coronary arteriography, the possibility of intraaortic balloon placement should be discussed with the patient and consent obtained.

Since patients with unstable angina and those with critical left main or multivessel coronary obstructions may require counter-pulsation following coronary angiography, it may be useful to note the anatomy of the distal aorta, iliac arteries, and femoral arteries during the diagnostic coronary angiogram. This need not require power injection through a special catheter. A large amount of information can be obtained from observation of the course taken by guide wire and catheter, and small hand injections with fluoroscopic imaging will demonstrate areas of excessive tortuosity or significant arterial obstruction. Even in the absence of arterial obstruction, peripheral angiography may be helpful in avoiding complications by demonstrating areas of potential problems due to unusual anatomy or tortuosity (Fig. 30-1).

**Evaluation.**   If feasible, a complete blood count, prothrombin time, partial thromboplastin time, bleeding time, and platelet count should be obtained within 24 hours of the planned insertion to insure that there is no serious bleeding problem.

In order to minimize vascular complications, a careful history should be obtained, with specific questioning regarding symptoms of limb ischemia. The strength of bilateral femoral, popliteal, dorsalis pedis, and posterior tibial pulses should be recorded. The abdomen, pelvis, and both legs should be auscultated for the presence of bruits. If there is evidence of possible arterial insufficiency, noninvasive evaluation of limb circulation (Doppler pressures, pulse volume recording) is very helpful in initial evaluation as well as follow-up. All of our percutaneous intraaortic balloon patients are evaluated periodically by the vascular nurse and surgeon before insertion, throughout the course of counterpulsation, and after removal of the balloon catheter. This has been extremely helpful in the prevention and early diagnosis of vascular complications.

## PUNCTURE TECHNIQUE

Prior to intraaortic balloon insertion, both groins should be scrubbed, and sterile drapes should be applied in a fashion that will permit utilization of the opposite groin if the initial site is unsuitable. Since insertion of a balloon catheter introduces a foreign body into the vasculature, meticulous attention should be paid to sterile technique, even during emergency placement.

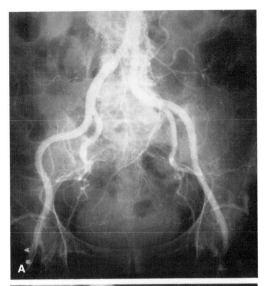

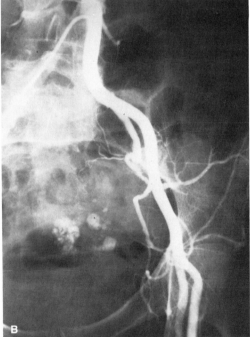

**Fig. 30-1**   (A) Angiography in a 62-year-old woman reveals an unobstructed aorta, iliac, and femoral system with marked tortuosity which is more prominent on the right side. Insertion via the left femoral artery would be preferable. (B) Left iliac arteriography in a 65-year-old female patient without any arterial obstruction but with a very proximal femoral artery bifurcation on the left side. Puncture at the usual site 2 cm below the inguinal ligament would enter a femoral branch with probable limb ischemia. Note the relationship between femoral artery and the head of the femur. The artery usually crosses the femoral head at its medial half.

The most common complications of intra-aortic balloon placement are related to puncture at an improper site or to forceful advancement of the guide wire when it is not within the lumen of the artery. Puncture should be performed within the segment of the common femoral artery between the inguinal ligament and the femoral arterial bifurcation into superficial and deep branches. The optimal puncture site is 2 cm below the inguinal ligament, usually near the level of the inguinal crease. Puncture proximal to this segment might not allow control of bleeding at the time of balloon catheter removal, which might lead to the formation of a false aneurysm. It is much more common for improper puncture to be too distal rather than too proximal. With a distal site, the intraaortic balloon catheter will be inserted into a relatively small artery, either the superficial or profunda branch of the femoral artery, with resultant obstruction to flow producing immediate limb ischemia or thrombosis-induced late ischemia.

For a right-handed operator, insertion of the balloon catheter in the right groin is somewhat easier. Enough time should be spent palpating the femoral artery so that its location and course are well defined. If the thumb of the left hand is placed on the anterior superior iliac spine and the left index finger is placed on the symphysis pubis, the line drawn between the tip of the thumb and the index finger will outline the right inguinal ligament. The femoral artery will usually cross this line at its midpoint. The femoral vein lies within the femoral sheath medial and immediately adjacent to the femoral artery while the femoral nerve is adjacent and lateral.

If the patient is in cardiogenic shock, the femoral artery may not be palpable. Despite this, successful puncture can be performed using fluoroscopy. The femoral artery puncture site lies within the medial half to medial third of the femoral head (Fig. 30-1). If the puncture needle is placed in this position by fluoroscopy and the position is marked on the skin with a sterile marking pen, the artery will be entered by puncturing at the marked position or within 1 or 2 cm medially or laterally. Puncture lateral to the femoral artery may produce a sharp lancinating pain down the leg if the femoral nerve is struck, and puncture too medial may enter the femoral vein. If the latter occurs, a small radiopaque catheter can be inserted within the femoral vein and used as a guide for puncture of the adjacent femoral artery. Even in the presence of severe cardiogenic shock, arterial puncture is usually recognized by the color and pulsation of blood returning through the needle.

A syringe loaded with 1% lidocaine, the Seldinger puncture needle, a 0.035-inch 60-cm or 145-cm guide wire and a French 8 dilator should be within reach of the operator's right hand while the left hand is palpating the femoral artery.

Four fingers of the left hand are placed along the course of the right femoral artery, in a position sufficiently proximal to localize the site of puncture beneath the second finger of the left hand. The subcutaneous fat is compressed sufficiently to permit accurate localization of the artery. Once the artery has been accurately localized, the left hand should not be moved until the artery has been punctured. Over the right femoral artery and distal to the left index finger, a skin bleb is raised with 0.5 ml of anesthetic. Without moving the fingers of the left hand, a #11 scalpel is used to make a 5-mm wide incision by inserting the blade through the skin and subcutaneous fascia while holding the blade parallel to the floor. A hemostat is inserted to spread the skin and subcutaneous fascia sufficiently to permit easy passage of the large sheath and dilator. The arterial puncture needle is placed alongside the puncture site. While the operator continues to maintain the left hand firmly on the femoral artery, the incision is entered with the anesthesia needle. Some physicians prefer to enter the femoral artery with the anesthesia needle; others will try to avoid doing so. I find it helpful to localize the artery with the anesthesia needle, since this step facilitates subsequent puncture and minimizes patient discomfort.

Enter the leg at an angle 45 degrees to the table top and inject 1 to 2 ml of lidocaine followed by suction on the syringe while the needle is advanced ½ cm; another 1 to 2 ml of anesthesia is administered, suction is applied, and needle is advanced until the artery is entered. Many physicians will go through the artery and place 0.5 ml of anesthesia behind it.

The anesthesia syringe is withdrawn, concentrating on the position, angle, and depth that produced successful puncture. Without turning away, slowly advance the arterial puncture needle along the exact same course, at a 45-degree angle, aiming for puncture of the artery beneath the second finger of the left hand. If the artery is large, it may be entered freely without going through its posterior wall. I have found it easier to go through the artery, stopping when the needle tip contacts periosteum. Place the guide wire within its introducer near the needle in a position convenient for insertion. Remove the arterial needle trocar, rest both hands on the patient's leg for stability, grasp the hub of the needle with the thumb and forefinger of each hand, move the arterial needle dorsally until it is nearly parallel to the table, and withdraw the needle very slowly, parallel to the course of the artery, until there is brisk pulsatile arterial flow through the Seldinger needle. If the systemic pressure is normal and there is not a brisk bright red stream of blood exiting the hub of the needle, continue to withdraw slowly until there is good arterial flow or the needle is totally withdrawn. There is little morbidity to a second or third puncture as compared to the problems created by improper advancement of the guide wire with resultant dissection of the artery.

## ADVANCEMENT OF THE GUIDE WIRE

Advancement of the guide wire *should be painless* and should proceed without any sensation of resistance. If resistance, pain, or kinking of the guide wire is observed by fluoroscopy, it must not be forced. A movable core guide with a smaller J tip will occasionally succeed when a standard guide wire cannot be advanced. In that case, advancement of the large introduction sheath may be difficult, and it would be wise to insert a French 5 or 6 end-hole catheter over the guide wire, followed by hand injections of diluted contrast material to define the arterial anatomy and preferable insertion site.

If the passage of the guide wire to the descending thoracic aorta has been uneventful, an 8F dilator is inserted next to predilate the artery. The guide wire is kept in place, and the 8F dilator is then removed and discarded.

Firm pressure is applied over the puncture site to prevent bleeding, the exposed guide wire is wiped clean with a wet lint-free sponge, and the sheath/dilator assembly is inserted with a twisting motion. The incision in the skin and fascia should be sufficiently large to permit easy passage of the sheath. Once the dilator section is beneath the skin, the sheath should be advanced from the distal or hub end of the assembly to prevent the sheath from sliding over the dilator and causing buckling or crimping of the sheath and damage to the femoral artery as the crimped sheath is advanced within the arterial lumen.

Before the operator handles the balloon catheter, powder should be washed off sterile gloves, since it may alter the nonthrombogenic properties of the balloon surface. The balloon should be wrapped according to the instructions of the manufacturer. The details of balloon wrapping and preparation differ for each brand (Kontron, Datascope, SMEC, Aries), as well as each type (noncentral lumen, guide wire-directed central lumen) of balloon catheter.

A clockwise rotation of the wrapping apparatus handle is used to wrap the balloon tightly. It is then lubricated with sterile heparinized flush solution. Passage through the introduction sheath is tested prior to insertion and the balloon is rewrapped if it will not traverse the sheath easily. The central lumen of the balloon catheter is irrigated with heparinized solution. The balloon may be advanced over a guide wire that has been passed to the aortic knob, or the J tip guide wire can be preloaded within the balloon until it is 2 cm from its tip. In the latter case the introduction sheath will be inserted over the shorter (60 cm) 0.035-inch guide wire. I always use the former technique (145 cm J tip guide wire to the aortic knob) if there has been any problem with advancement of the guide wire.

Two centimeters of the introduction sheath are exposed to permit pinching of the sheath for hemostasis after removal of the dilator and short guide wire. If a 0.035" 145-cm guide wire has been used for sheath insertion, it can be left in place while the dilator is removed, and the intraaortic balloon can be passed over the guide wire in a manner analogous to exchanging an arterial catheter over a guide wire. The guide wire is withdrawn gradually until the distal end appears at the distal balloon catheter hub, and then the intraaortic balloon catheter is advanced under fluoroscopy.

The balloon catheter should fit the sheath snugly enough so that there is little bleeding. It should be passed through the sheath with slight *counterclockwise* rotation of the balloon shaft in order to tighten the wrap as it is advanced. Once within the sheath, the guide wire is advanced ahead of the wrapped balloon until it is positioned in the aorta at the level of the left subclavian artery. The wrapped balloon should advance without resistance until its radiopaque tip marker is within the descending thoracic aorta, just below the origin of the left subclavian artery. The guide wire is then removed and discarded. The central lumen of the balloon catheter is aspirated vigorously twice, and the central lumen is irrigated cautiously with heparinized solution. Special care must be taken to avoid inadvertent injection of air bubbles or thrombi. The cuff is advanced to the hub of the introduction sheath to prevent back bleeding. The central lumen is attached to a heparinized transducer and continuous infusion system through a three-way stopcock.

The continuous infusion system is pressurized to 300 mmHg and provides a continuous flow of 3 ml/hr with less than a 2% error in recorded arterial pressures.[12] Since air will pass through this apparatus and may be released into the central aorta, it must be purged completely from the system. Heparin is added to the flush solution at a concentration of 10 IU/ml (5000 IU heparin in a 500-ml bag of flush solution).

Because an embolus from the tip of the catheter would enter the cerebral or coronary circulation, the central lumen must be flushed with extreme care. It should be flushed only with the continuous infusion system (which will run at 1.5 ml/sec while its valve is held open) while the balloon is temporarily turned off. Except during initial insertion, the central lumen should never be flushed manually with a syringe and it should not be used for drawing blood samples. If the central lumen pressure trace becomes damped and the cause is not related to a loose connection in the system, aspiration of the central lumen should be attempted. If there is marked resistance to aspiration of

blood, *DO NOT FLUSH*. The lumen should be considered occluded, and the central aortic pressure line should be capped and discontinued.

## UNWRAPPING THE BALLOON AND STARTING COUNTERPULSATION

The balloon is unwrapped by rotating the wrapping knob counterclockwise until it reaches the stop. Balloon placement may be verified by a cautious 10-ml hand injection of contrast medium through the central lumen, although I prefer to skip this step unless absolutely necessary. The balloon is attached to the appropriate connector for the Datascope, Kontron, SMEC, or Aries console. Following a purge with the helium or $CO_2$ inflation gas, the balloon is *half-filled* and counterpulsation is begun at 1:2.

Fluoroscopy is used to identify the position of the proximal portion of the balloon, to insure that the balloon is fully unwrapped and is inflating without any twist or kink, and that the distal portion of the balloon has fully exited the introduction sheath. If it is necessary to adjust the position of the balloon, it may be moved *within* the sheath but must never be adjusted by advancing the sheath itself, since advancement is likely to produce arterial damage at the distal end of the introduction sheath.

If the half-filled balloon is operating satisfactorily, the balloon is filled to its full volume and pumped at 1:1, using fluoroscopy to verify that the balloon position is appropriate and that the filled balloon has a uniform symmetrical cylindrical shape. The seal is sewn to the skin, betadine ointment is applied to the entrance site, and a sterile dressing is applied.

Aqueous heparin, 5000 IU, is administered intravenously followed by continuous intravenous heparin or dextran. A supine chest roentgenogram is obtained to confirm the presence of satisfactory balloon position.

## BALLOON TIMING

If balloon timing is not adjusted properly, left ventricular systolic emptying may take place during balloon inflation with disastrous consequences in critically ill patients. Timing is adjusted with the console set at 1:2 pumping (i.e., counterpulsation of every other beat) so that arterial pressure tracings can be compared with and without counterpulsation. Use of the aortic pressure tracing from the balloon lumen is preferable to monitoring the radial artery tracing because of the timing delay and change in arterial contour as the pulse wave moves from the central aorta to the periphery. Since there is a 50-msec delay between the central aorta and radial artery pressure wave, balloon inflation timing will have to be adjusted accordingly if the central balloon lumen is not used.

***Inflation.*** While observing a high fidelity central aortic pressure trace of good waveform, the operator should slowly move the inflation knob toward the right (later inflation) until the dicrotic notch is exposed and then back to the left until inflation occurs *on* the central aortic dicrotic notch. This position will also produce maximal height of the augmented diastolic pressure (Fig. 30-2, A).

***Deflation.*** Deflation should take place just before the opening of the aortic valve. The deflation knob is moved to the left (earlier deflation) so that deflation is too early and then slowly moved to the right until there is maximum reduction in the aortic systolic pressure in the beat following balloon deflation, and an end-diastolic dip which is 10 to 15 mmHg below the nonaugmented diastolic pressure (Fig. 30-2, B).

If there is a marked irregularity of cardiac rhythm (e.g., atrial fibrillation with marked variation in cycle length) balloon timing is best adjusted so deflation occurs on the peak of the R wave in order to avoid occasional cycles during which left ventricular ejection may take place against an inflated balloon.

Atrial pacing may also produce difficulty with balloon timing because the balloon console may misinterpret the atrial pacing spike as the peak of the R wave. This error can be corrected by setting the timing by the arterial pressure wave, choosing an EKG lead that magnifies the difference between QRS and atrial pacing spike, or by setting the console to a mode that discriminates between the pacing spike and the R wave by sensing both the height and duration of the signal (Fig. 30-2, C).

## MANAGEMENT DURING COUNTERPULSATION

During counterpulsation, there should be daily evaluation for evidence of sepsis, thrombocytopenia, blood loss, hemolysis-induced anemia, or vascular obstruction caused by the balloon, thrombus, embolus, or dissection. Thrombocytopenia is almost invariable, but the platelet count will often level off at 50,000 to 100,000/ml. Platelet transfusions should be considered if there is serious bleeding, but they are rarely necessary. Following balloon removal, the platelet count returns to normal rapidly.[13]

Aortic dissection, which can be present even in the presence of apparent successful balloon pump function, will usually be accompanied by significant pain in the back, limbs, or pelvis, and must be treated promptly by removal of the balloon and vascular evaluation.

Local sepsis can be minimized by good aseptic insertion technique, careful daily changes of dressings with application of povidone-iodine (Betadine) ointment to the insertion site, and careful technique in changing bottles of flush solution. However, disseminated sepsis is an emergency that may require balloon removal for control. Prophylactic antibiotics are not given routinely but should be used if there is any compromise in sterile technique during insertion.

After balloon insertion, patients must be kept at bed rest. Hip flexion is proscribed, as well as elevation of the head of the bed beyond 30 degrees. The entire bed may be tilted head-up or head-down, however, to treat pulmonary edema or hypotension, respectively. A loose bandage that attaches the involved ankle to the bed will help to maintain appropriate leg position during periods of sleep, confusion, or discomfort.

If cardiac angiography is necessary after balloon insertion, it can be performed by the Sone's technique during continuous counterpulsation.[14] The femoral technique can also be used safely, although the balloon should be turned off while the coronary catheter traverses the area of the balloon and special care must be exercised to avoid damage to the balloon by the tip of the catheter. A J *guide wire* is extended 5 cm beyond the tip of the femoral coronary catheter in the pelvis, the balloon is turned off, and the cathe-

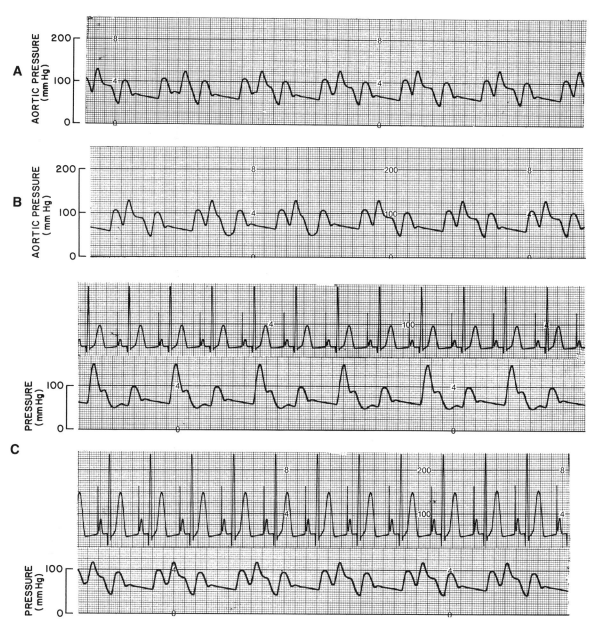

**Fig. 30-2**  (A) The timing of balloon inflation is adjusted until it occurs late in diastole, uncovering the dicrotic notch. Subsequently, inflation timing is moved earlier in the cardiac cycle until the dicrotic notch on the central aortic tracing just disappears (beat #4). The augmented pressure will rise as inflation timing is moved earlier. (B) Deflation knob is moved toward the right (later in the cardiac cycle) until the end diastolic dip is 10 to 15 mmHg below the patient's unassisted diastolic pressure. This will produce a maximal lowering of the patient's unassisted systolic pressure. (C) The balloon console is triggering on an atrial pacing artifact. This is corrected by changing the console to a mode that will discriminate between a pacing spike and an R wave.

ter plus guide wire is advanced as a unit, with the catheter tip pointing away from the balloon, until it is beyond the proximal end of the balloon pump. The guide-wire is removed, the balloon is turned on, and selective angiography is performed in the usual way.

The catheter is then withdrawn to a position above the proximal end of the balloon, a *straight* guide wire is advanced 5 cm beyond the tip of the catheter, the balloon is turned off, and the guide wire plus the catheter is removed as a unit while pointing the tip of the catheter away from the balloon. We have performed several hundred catheter exchanges in this way without any recognized balloon damage.[15]

## BALLOON REMOVAL

Prior to removal of an intraaortic balloon catheter, the patient is weaned from 1:1 mode to 1:2, 1:4, and finally 1:8. Sufficient time should elapse between each stage to insure that the patient will tolerate a progressive decrease in the level of counterpulsation. Anticoagulation should be discontinued prior to balloon removal. At 1:8 pumping, the balloon can be turned off and removed.

A 50-ml syringe is attached via a stopcock to the balloon inflation lumen and a full 50 ml is withdrawn to create a vacuum. The balloon is withdrawn to, *but not into*, the insertion sheath, since the latter maneuver may tear and embolize a portion of the balloon. After the skin ties are cut, the sheath and balloon are withdrawn as a single unit. A small spurt of blood is allowed to escape by compressing the artery distal and then proximal to the insertion site to flush out any thrombus. The site is then compressed firmly by hand or with a mechanical compression device (Compressar, Intromedix, Portland, OR) for 30 to 60 minutes. Distal limb circulation should be checked during and after compression. The patient is kept at bed rest, and hip flexion is not allowed on the involved side for 24 hours.

## RESULTS

In almost all reported series to date, percutaneous balloon insertion has been performed with a 90% success rate. There is a wide variance in reported complication rates, at least partly related to differences in the patient population. The average rate of serious complications is 10 to 20% (mostly due to iliofemoral thrombosis) and is similar to that observed in several large surgical intraaortic balloon series.[13,16–28] The guide-wire technique should produce fewer dangerous arterial lacerations, although the number of local thromboses may be increased.

***Hemodynamic Effect of Counterpulsation.*** The hemodynamic effect of counterpulsation will depend in part on the underlying problem for which it has been applied. When instituted relatively early in the course of cardiogenic shock, counterpulsation produced a 19 to 25% reduction in peak LV wall stress with a concomitant increase in coronary blood flow in dogs.[29] Studies in patients have been performed on relatively small numbers. Often the cardiogenic shock patients described in one paper are not comparable to those studied in another investigation. Seventy percent of patients in cardiogenic shock who were studied 14 hours after IAPB insertion showed no change or a fall in coronary blood flow with counterpulsation and no significant change in myocardial lactate extraction,[30] yet a comparable group of patients studied 4 to 6 hours after initiation of counterpulsation showed an 18% decrease in LV systolic pressure and a 38% increase in cardiac index. Coronary sinus studies in those patients documented a 34% increase in coronary blood flow (reflecting an increase in mean arterial pressure) and a change from 6% lactate production to 15% extraction[31] or an improvement in lactate production toward normal.[32] Using multiple EKG leads in a dog model or in man, counterpulsation produced a marked decrease in the extent and severity of myocardial ischemia (as determined by the sum of ST segment elevation in multiple electrocardiographic leads) if it was applied within 3 hours of coronary occlusion. In addition, IABP reversed the increased myocardial ischemia induced by isoproterenol infusion.[34]

In contrast to the studies of coronary blood flow above, almost all investigators have demonstrated a favorable effect of counterpulsation on the cardiac index, mean arterial pressure, and left ventricular filling pressures of patients with cardiogenic shock[5,7,31,32,34,35] (Fig. 30-3). Although the intraaortic balloon will result in an initial improvement in hemodynamics, after 3 to 4 days there is often recurrent deterioration in hemodynamics unless corrective surgery can be performed.

Patients with medically refractory unstable angina may be improved by counterpulsation but will show only a 7% decrease in peak systolic pressure and a 17% decrease in left ventricular filling pressure (Fig. 30-4). The left ventricular systolic volume, diastolic volume, and ejection fraction are all unchanged during counterpulsation,[36] and there is no improvement in regional coronary flow to the ischemic area.[37] Although the favorable effects of counterpulsation for unstable angina seem to be due largely to its effects on preload and afterload, the addition of intraaortic balloon pumping to a maximal medical program produced marked improvement in 95% of patients.[4] Occasionally it will be necessary to discontinue counterpulsation transiently in order to refill the balloon with helium or carbon dioxide. In unstable patients, even one or two minutes without counterpulsation may result in clinical deterioration (Fig. 30-4).

The variable effect of counterpulsation on coronary blood flow is probably related to the type of patient studied (i.e., cardiogenic shock versus unstable angina), the effect on normally perfused myocardium (which may demonstrate a decrease in regional coronary flow due to a decrease in loading conditions), and the effect on ischemic myocardium (a region with maximal vasodilatation and therefore a marked change in regional coronary blood flow with changes in perfusion pressure).

An example of the effectiveness of intraaortic balloon counterpulsation in cardiogenic shock due to mitral regurgitation is shown in Figures 30-5 and 30-6. These tracings were recorded in a 45-year-old woman who had presented in cardiogenic shock with pulmonary edema from acute ruptured chordae and massive mitral regurgitation. As seen in Figure 30-5, counterpulsation reduced left ventricular diastolic pressure and the V wave in the pulmonary capillary wedge tracing. Figure 30-6 shows pressures during a

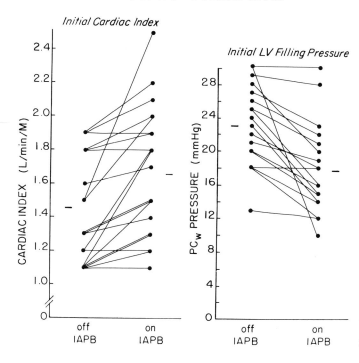

HEMODYNAMIC EFFECT OF IAPB
IN PATIENTS WITH CARDIOGENIC SHOCK

*Initial Cardiac Index*

*Initial LV Filling Pressure*

**Fig. 30-3.** Hemodynamic effects of intraaortic balloon pump (IABP) in cardiogenic shock. Although cardiogenic shock patients sustained an initial improvement in cardiac index and left ventricular filling pressure (PCW), the largest changes were noted in patients with a mechanical defect (ventricular septal defect or mitral regurgitation).

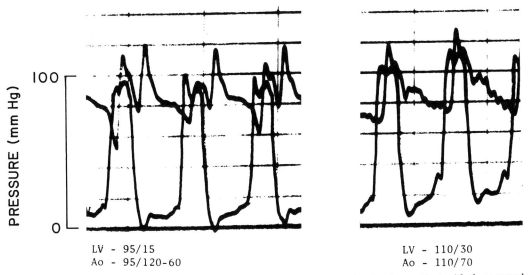

LV - 95/15
Ao - 95/120-60

LV - 110/30
Ao - 110/70

**Fig. 30-4.** One minute following temporary discontinuation of counterpulsation in a patient with three-vessel coronary artery disease, left main coronary artery stenosis, and severe unstable angina, there is a prompt increase in left ventricular systolic and end-diastolic pressure with rapid return of ischemic pain.

pullback of the left heart catheter from the left ventricle to the aorta during balloon counterpulsation. Careful inspection of the tracings and their relation to the simultaneous ECG shows that the major pressure wave in the aorta is occurring during diastole and represents a 30 mmHg effect of counterpulsation. Thus, despite a left ventricular

systolic pressure of 60 to 70 mmHg, the patient's condition stabilized, permitting successful mitral valve surgery.

***Identification of Patients at High Risk.*** Although complications of intraaortic balloon placement are discussed throughout the text of this chapter, some specific comments should be made concerning risk

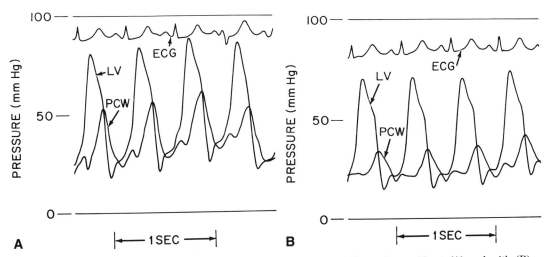

**A**

**B**

**Fig. 30-5.** Left ventricular (LV) and pulmonary capillary wedge (PCW) tracings without (A) and with (B) intraaortic balloon counterpulsation in a 45-year-old woman in cardiogenic shock from ruptured chordae of the mitral valve. See text.

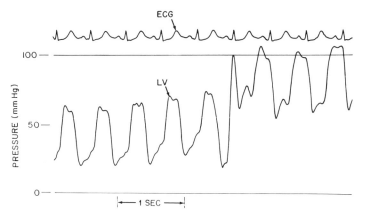

**Fig. 30-6.** Same patient as in Figure 30-5. Tracings during catheter pullback from left ventricle (LV) to central aorta during intraaortic balloon counterpulsation. See text.

factors for complications. This point was examined in a study of 206 consecutive patients undergoing intraaortic balloon placement at Johns Hopkins Hospital.[38] Of these 206 balloon placements, 105 were introduced by percutaneous technique and 101 by surgical implantation. Vascular complications were reported in 42/206 or 20% of patients, and half of these patients required operations for their complications. Multivariate analysis demonstrated that preexisting peripheral vascular disease (evidenced by a history of claudication, presence of femoral bruit, or absence of foot pulses) *and* the use of the percutaneous approach were risk factors for major complications. In patients with previous peripheral vascular disease, the risk for a major vascular complication was 31% with percutaneous technique and

16% when surgical implantation was used.

An interesting additional finding of this study was that in patients without peripheral vascular disease, the risk of a major vascular complication was four times higher in women (15%) then in men (3.5%).[38] Age, duration of counterpulsation, and indication for insertion were not significant risk factors. It should be pointed out that this study was carried out on insertions performed between 1980 and 1982; significant advances in catheter design and insertion technique in recent years may reduce the complication rates to be expected today. Specific complications included vascular injury/perforation, thrombosis, emboli, aortic dissection, limb ischemia, infection, renal failure, cerebrovascular accident, mesenteric infarction, balloon rupture, and death.[38]

# REFERENCES

1. Moulopoulos SD, Topaz S, Kolff WJ: Diastolic balloon pumping (with carbon dioxide) in the aorta—a mechanical assistance to the failing circulation. Am Heart J 63:669, 1962.
2. Kantrowitz A, et al: Initial clinical experience with intraaortic balloon pumping in cardiogenic shock. JAMA 203:113, 1968.
3. Bregman D, Casarella WJ: Percutaneous intraaortic balloon pumping: Initial clinical experience. Ann Thorac Surg 29:153, 1980.
4. Weintraub RM, et al: Medically refractory unstable angina pectoris: Long-term follow-up of patients undergoing intraaortic balloon counterpulsation and operation. Am J Cardiol 43: 877, 1979.
5. Aroesty JM: Cardiogenic shock. *In* Donoso E, Cohen S (eds): Critical Cardiac Care. New York, Stratton Intercontinental Medical Book Corp. 1979, pp. 51–64.
6. Gold HK, et al: Intraaortic balloon pumping for ventricular septal defect or mitral regurgitation complicating acute myocardial infarction. Circulation 47:1191, 1973.
7. Dunkman WB, et al: Clinical and hemodynamic results of intraaortic balloon pumping and surgery for cardiogenic shock. Circulation 46:465, 1972.
8. Sturm et al: Treatment of postoperative low output syndrome with intraaortic ballon pumping:

experience with 419 patients. Am J Cardiol 45:1033, 1980.

9. Leinbach RC, et al: Early intraaortic balloon pumping for anterior myocardial infarction without shock. Circulation 58:204, 1978.

10. Hanson EC, et al: Control of post infarction ventricular irritability with intraaortic balloon pump. Circulation 62 (suppl I): 130, 1980.

11. Cohen S, Weintraub RM: A new application of counterpulsation; safer laparotomy after recent myocardial infarction. Arch Surg 110:116, 1975.

12. Gardner RM, Bond EL, Clark JS: Safety and efficiency of continuous flush systems for arterial and pulmonary artery catheters. Ann Thorac Surg 23:534, 1977.

13. McCabe JC, Abel RM, Subramanian VA, Gay WA: Complications of intra-aortic balloon insertion and counterpulsation. Circulation 57:769, 1978.

14. Leinbach RC, et al: Selective coronary and left ventricular cineangiography during intraaortic balloon pumping for cardiogenic shock. Circulation. 45:845, 1972.

15. Aroesty JM, Schlossman D, Weintraub RM, Paulin S: Transfemoral selective coronary artery catheterization during intra-aortic balloon by-pass pumping. Radiology 111:307, 1974.

16. Isner JM, et al: Complications of the intraaortic counterpulsation device: clinical and morphological observations in 45 necropsy patients. Am J Cardiol 45:260, 1980.

17. Vignola PA, Swaye PS, Gosselin AJ: Guidelines for effective and safe percutaneous intraaortic balloon pump insertion and removal. Am J Cardiol 48:660, 1981.

18. Leinbach RC, et al: Percutaneous wire-guided balloon pumping. Am J Cardiol 49:1707, 1982.

19. Hauser, AM, et al: Percutaneous intraaortic balloon counterpulsation. Clinical effectiveness and hazards. Chest 82:422, 1982.

20. Shahian D, Neptune WB, Ellis FH, Maggs PR: Intraaortic balloon pump morbidity: a comparative analysis of risk factors between percutaneous and surgical techniques. Ann Thor Surg 36:644, 1983.

21. Alcan K, et al: Comparison of wire-guided percutaneous insertion and conventional surgical insertion of intra-aortic balloon pumps in 151 patients. Am J Med 75:24, 1983.

22. Todd G, Bregman D, Voorhees A, Reemtsma K: Vascular complications associated with percutaneous intra-aortic balloon pumping. Arch Surg 118:963, 1983.

23. McEnany MT, et al: Clinical experience with intraaortic balloon pump support in 728 patients. Circulation 57, 58 (Suppl. I):124, 1978.

24. Weintraub RM, Thurer RL: The intra-aortic balloon pump—a ten-year experience. Heart Transpl 3:8, 1983.

25. Bregman D, et al: Percutaneous intraaortic balloon insertion. Am J Cardiol 48:261, 1980.

26. Subramanian VA, et al: Preliminary clinical experience with percutaneous intraaortic balloon pumping. Circulation 62 (Suppl 1):123, 1980.

27. Singh AK, et al: Percutaneous vs. surgical placement of intra-aortic balloon assist. Cathet Cardiovasc Diagn 8:519, 1982.

28. Vignola PA, Swaye PS, Gosselin AJ. Percutaneous intra-aortic balloon pumping: new problems and dilemmas. Cathet Cardiovasc Diagn 9:117, 1983.

29. Braunwald E, Covell JW, Maroko PR, Ross J Jr: Effects of drugs and of counterpulsation on myocardial oxygen consumption. Circulation 39 and 40 (supplement 4):220, 1970.

30. Leinbach RC, et al: Effects of intraaortic balloon pumping on coronary flow and metabolism in man. Circulation 43 and 44 (Suppl 1): 77, 1971.

31. Mueller H, et al: The effects of intra-aortic counterpulsation on cardiac performance and metabolism in shock associated with acute myocardial infarction. J Clin Invest 50:1885, 1971.

32. Mueller H, et al: Effect of isoproterenol, 1-norepinephrine, and intraaortic counterpulsation on hemodynamics and myocardial metabolism in shock following myocardial infarction. Circulation 45:335, 1972.

33. Maroko PR, et al: Effects of intraaortic balloon counterpulsation on the severity of myocardial ischemic injury following acute coronary occlusion. Circulation. 45:1150, 1972.

34. Dilley RB, Ross J, Jr, Bernstein EF: Serial hemodynamics during intra-aortic balloon counterpulsation for cardiogenic shock. Circulation 47 and 48: (Suppl 3):99, 1973.

35. Bardet J, et al: Clinical and hemodynamic results of intraaortic balloon counterpulsation and surgery for cardiogenic shock. Am Heart J 93:280, 1977.

36. Aroesty JM, Weintraub, RM, Paulin S, O'Grady GP: Medically refractory unstable angina pectoris II. Hemodynamic and angiographic effects of intraaortic balloon counterpulsation. Am J Cardiol 43:883, 1979.

37. Williams DO, Korr KS, Dewirtz H, Most AS: The effect of intraaortic balloon counterpulsation on regional myocardial blood flow and oxygen consumption in the presence of coronary artery stenosis in patients with unstable angina. Circulation 66 (3):593, 1982.

38. Gottlieb SO, et al: Identification of patients at high risk for complications of intraaortic balloon counterpulsation: A multivariate risk factor analysis. Am J Cardiol 53:1135, 1984.

## chapter thirty one

# Endomyocardial Biopsy

ROBERT E. FOWLES *and* DONALD S. BAIM

A S THE result of recent improvements in catheter design and pathologic interpretation, transvascular endomyocardial biopsy has become an important component in the invasive evaluation of patients with known or suspected primary myocardial dysfunction.[1] Because significant controversy remains about the definition, frequency, natural history, and optimal treatment of many of these myocardial disorders, however, use of the endomyocardial biopsy in the routine evaluation of patients with myocardial disease varies from center to center. This chapter will focus on the currently available techniques for endomyocardial biopsy and the disease states in which myocardial histology appears most valuable, rather than on a precise listing of current indications for this procedure.

## BIOPSY DEVICES

Cardiac biopsy in the 1950s was initially performed via limited thoracotomy. Subsequent attempts at transthoracic needle biopsy were frustrated by a nearly 10% incidence of major complications, including pneumothorax, tamponade, and coronary laceration.[2,3] Over the past 20 years, these techniques have been replaced by a series of biopsy catheter systems (or bioptomes) which permit rapid and safe transvascular endomyocardial biopsy. There are two basic types of bioptomes: (1) stiff devices which are maneuvered independently through the

506

vasculature, and (2) floppy devices which are positioned with the aid of a long sheath or introducing catheter.

## Independent Bioptomes

*The Konno Bioptome.* In 1962, Sakakibara and Konno developed a biopsy catheter capable of transvascular introduction and procurement of endomyocardial biopsy samples from either the left or the right ventricular chamber.[4] This device consists of a 100-cm catheter shaft with two sharpened cups (diameter either 2.5 or 3.5 mm) at its tip. These cups can be opened or closed under the control of a single wire activated by a sliding assembly attached to the proximal end of the catheter. Because of the large size of the catheter head, it is usually introduced via cutdown on the saphenous or basilic vein or the femoral or brachial artery. The bioptome is maneuvered into the desired ventricle under fluoroscopic guidance and applied to the endocardial surface with its jaws closed. The catheter is then withdrawn slightly, opened, readvanced into contact with the endocardium, reclosed, and withdrawn. While the Konno bioptome is still in use throughout the world, the stiffness of its shaft complicates intravascular and intracardiac manipulation and has led to a variety of other devices based on the same theme.

*The Kawai Bioptome.* Developed by Kawai and Kitaura in 1977, this device has a very flexible tip that can be deflected up to 40 degrees in one direction and up to 10 degrees in the opposite direction by rotation of a knob on the operating handle[5,6] (Fig. 31-1). This allows easy maneuvering through the vasculature and across the aortic or tricuspid valve for right or left ventricular biopsy. Because of its extremely flexible tip, a stylet must be advanced into the catheter shaft prior to excision of an endomyocardial sample.

### The Stanford (Caves-Schulz) Bioptome.

This device, developed as a modification of the Konno bioptome, was designed specifically for right ventricular biopsy via the right internal jugular vein[7,8] (Fig. 31-2) and has wide application in the United States. It consists of a somewhat flexible coil shaft fabricated from stainless steel and coated by clear plastic tubing (Sholten Surgical Supply, Palo Alto, CA). The tip of the catheter has two hemispherical cutting jaws with a combined diameter of 3.0 mm (9 French); one jaw is opened and closed by a stainless steel wire running through the center of the bioptome shaft, and the other jaw is stationary. The control wire is attached to a ratcheting surgical mosquito clamp via a pair of adjustable nuts which allow the operator to set the force applied during opening and closing of the surgical clamp. These nuts should be adjusted so that the two biopsy jaws close just as the two halves of the ratchet mechanism make contact. The distal end of the catheter is equipped with a curve which forms an angle between 45 and 90 degrees (depending on whether the clamp is closed to its first or second click) and lies in the same orientation as the handle of the clamp. With adequate care and cleaning, each such instrument can be used for more than 50 procedures without need for sharpening or service.

The biopsy procedure involves percutaneous entry of the right internal jugular vein. This is performed with the patient lying supine without a pillow and with his or her head turned far to the left. In this position, the operator should be able to identify the sternal notch, the sternal and clavicular heads of the right sternocleidomastoid muscle, and the top of the clavicle (Fig. 31-3). These anatomic features can be defined more easily if the patient is asked to lift his or her head just off the table. With a 25-gauge needle, a small intradermal bleb of 1% xylocaine is injected into the center of the triangle formed by the two muscle heads and the clavicle, at a point approximately two finger breadths above the top of the clavicle.

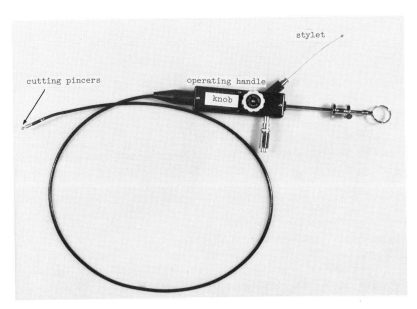

**Fig. 31-1.** The Kawai flexible endomyocardial biopsy catheter. (From Kawai C, Matsumori A, Kawamura K: Myocardial biopsy. Ann Rev Med 31:139, 1980. with permission.)

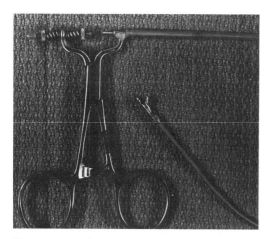

**Fig. 31-2.** Stanford (Caves-Schulz) bioptome. The surgical clamp drives the control wire by way of its connection through the two adjustable nuts, thereby controlling the position of the single mobile jaw.

A skin nick is created with the tip of a No. 11 blade and enlarged with a small mosquito clamp. A 6-ml non-Luer syringe is filled with 2 ml of xylocaine and attached to a 22-gauge, 1.5-inch needle. This needle is advanced through the skin nick at an angle 30 to 40 degrees from vertical, and 20 to 30 degrees right of the sagittal plane. Continuous suction is applied until the vein is entered, usually at a depth of 1 to 2.5 cm below the skin, using the steep angle of entry described above. If desired, small boluses of xylocaine can be injected into the soft tissues along the way, but the total volume injected should be kept under 1 ml to avoid compression of the vein within the carotid sheath. If the vein is not found, the needle should be withdrawn to the skin under continued suction, and puncture should be attempted with a slightly more lateral angulation; if this fails, a more medial angulation may be tried, but this increases the risk of carotid puncture. In patients with normal or low right atrial pressure, jugular venous puncture may be facilitated by elevation of the legs, the Trendelenburg position, or a Valsalva maneuver (Fig. 31-4). Once the vein is entered, we usually leave the "test" needle in place and perform a parallel puncture using a 2¾-inch 18-gauge thin-wall needle (UMI, Universal Medical Instruments, Ballston Spa, NY), through which a 40 cm J guide wire is then advanced into the right atrium. The "test" needle is

now removed, and a 9 French sheath with a side-arm and backbleed-valve (Cordis Corp., Miami, FL) is then advanced over the guide wire and attached to a continuous intravenous drip adjusted to a moderate flow rate.

With the clamp closed on its first click, the bioptome is advanced into the sheath until its tip lies against the lateral right atrial wall in its lower third (Fig. 31-5). The catheter is then rotated counterclockwise into an anteromedial orientation and advanced across the tricuspid valve. As the valve is crossed, counterclockwise rotation is continued until the handle clamp is pointed nearly straight posteriorly, thus directing the tip of the bioptome at the interventricular septum. The bioptome should then appear on fluoroscopy to have its tip across the spine and below the upper margins of the left hemidiaphragm, in contact with the ventricular myocardium (recognized by the lack of further advancement, the occurrence of premature ventricular contractions, and the transmission of ventricular impulses to the operator's hand). This maneuver must be performed with both finesse and assurance. The bioptome is quite stiff and will perforate the heart if advanced too vigorously in the wrong orientation (Fig. 31-6). If there is any doubt about its final position in the right ventricle and against the septum, this can be evaluated further by fluoroscopy in the 30-degree right anterior oblique and 60-degree left anterior oblique views. On occasion these views have disclosed unintentional positioning of the bioptome in the coronary sinus (i.e., in the A-V groove in the RAO projection) or in an infradiaphragmatic vein (i.e., under the heart and beyond the left heart border in the LAO projection). Attempted biopsy in either of these positions would fail to obtain a myocardial sample and might lead to significant complications. The bioptome must be withdrawn into the atrium and repositioned appropriately before sampling. In some patients, correct positioning may be facilitated by closing the handle clamp to its second click, thus increasing the curve of the bioptome to 90 degrees.

Once the biopsy catheter is in the desired position against the septal endocardium, it is withdrawn about 1 cm, the jaws are opened, and the catheter is gently readvanced into contact with the endocardium (Fig. 31-5). The jaws are closed and the catheter is gently withdrawn with its enclosed sample. While there is frequently a slight "tug" on the catheter as the sample is removed from the wall, forceful tugging with multiple premature ventricular contractions and inward retraction of the ventricular wall suggest that the jaws may have trapped a sample that includes the pericardium, in which case the jaws should be opened and the bioptome withdrawn without the sample.

A special 7 French pediatric Stanford bioptome is also available, which may be used from the subclavian vein in adults with difficult jugular venous access. Use of any rigid bioptome from the subclavian vein is more difficult than from the right internal jugular vein, however, and the possibility of using one of the long-sheath techniques from an alternate site should be considered.

## Long-sheath Devices

***The King's Bioptome.*** The King's bioptome is a modification of the stainless steel Olympus bronchoscopic biopsy forceps

(Olympus Corporation of America, New Hyde Park, NY), which is widely used in Europe[9,10] (Fig. 31-7). Its double opening scissor-action jaws are controlled by an inner drive wire which is attached to a proximal control handle. A compression spring on the control handle keeps the jaws in their closed position unless the handle's thumb ring is pushed in. The flexible forceps shaft and closed jaws have an outer diameter of 1.8 mm, allowing the catheter to be introduced into the desired ventricle through a radiopaque 6 or 7 French sheath which has been previously placed within the desired chamber. The sample is retrieved as described for the Stanford bioptome.

Disposable 50- and 104-cm versions of the King's type bioptome are now available (Cordis Corp., Miama, FL), which can be employed for biopsy of either the left or right ventricle. The longer bioptome is introduced through a 7 or 8 French, 98-cm curved Teflon introducing sheath (equipped with a back-bleed valve and side-arm flush mechanism) which has been previously positioned within

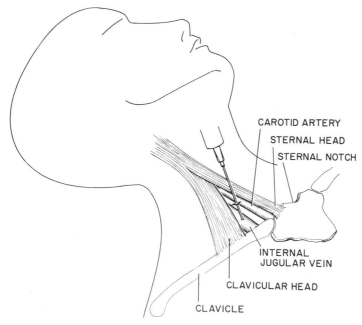

**Fig. 31-3.** Regional anatomy for right internal jugular vein puncture. With the patient's head rotated to the left, the sternal notch, clavicle, and the sternal and clavicular heads of the sternocleidomastoid muscle are identified. A skin nick is made between the two heads of the muscle, two fingerbreadths above the top of the clavicle, and the needle is inserted at an angle of 30 to 40 degrees from vertical and 20 to 30 degrees right of sagittal. This approach leads to reliable puncture of the internal jugular vein, and aims the needle away from the more medially located carotid artery.

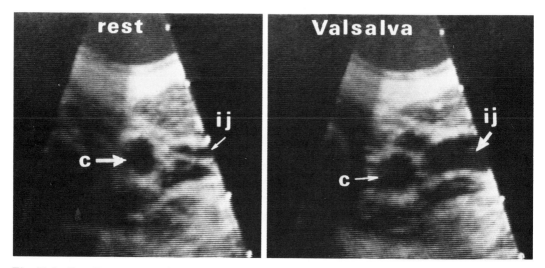

**Fig. 31-4.** Two-dimensional echo of the carotid artery (c) and the internal jugular vein (ij) at rest (left) and during a Valsalva maneuver (right), showing the marked enlargement in jugular venous caliber with increased distending pressure.

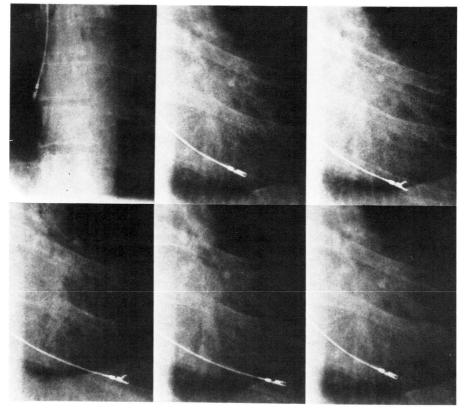

**Fig. 31-5.** Cineangiographic frames obtained during right ventricular endomyocardial biopsy using the Stanford bioptome: From left to right, the bioptome is shown against the lateral right atrial wall, against the ventricular septum, withdrawn slightly with jaws opened, reapplied to the septum with subsequent closure of the jaws, and withdrawn with sample.

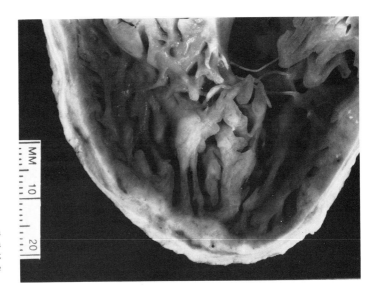

**Fig. 31-6.** Postmortem specimen showing the heavy trabeculation of the interior surface of the right ventricle and the thinness of the right ventricular free wall.

the desired chamber over a conventional cardiac catheter. Once the tip of the sheath is in position, the conventional catheter is withdrawn and the bioptome is introduced. The shorter bioptome is employed for right ventricular biopsy using a 45-cm length sheath inserted via the right internal jugular vein. A similar system has recently been used to permit transseptal catheterization and endomyocardial biopsy of the left ventricle in children.[11]

***The Stanford Left Ventricular Bioptome.*** The original Stanford bioptome has been modified for left ventricular biopsy by doubling its length to 100 cm and reducing its outer diameter to 6 French.[8] With this reduction in shaft diameter, the catheter is no longer capable of independent movement through the vasculature and must be positioned with the aid of a 90-cm curved Teflon sheath which is itself introduced into the desired ventricle over a conventional 100 cm 6.7 French pigtail catheter (Stanford Biopsy Set, Cook Inc., Bloomington, IN. The tip of the sheath is positioned below the mitral apparatus and away from the posterobasal segment (which is more easily perforated than other areas of the left ventricle). The pigtail catheter is then removed, the sheath is flushed, and the bioptome is introduced.

The Stanford left ventricular sheath has recently been modified by Anderson to permit biopsy of the right ventricular septum via the percutaneous femoral venous ap-

proach.[12] The Teflon sheath is heated over a forming wire to create an 8-cm distal semicircular curve with 70-degree posterior angulation of the final 3 cm (Fig. 31-7). When this sheath is placed in the right ventricle over the 6.7 French pigtail catheter (itself heated to form a distal Cournand-like curve), it rests

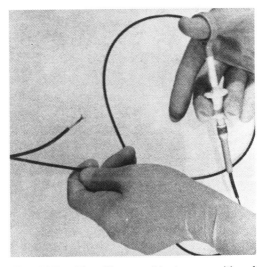

**Fig. 31-7.** The Olympus bioptome positioned through a modified Stanford biopsy sheath. (From Anderson JL, Marshall HW: The femoral venous approach to endomyocardial biopsy: comparison with internal jugular and transarterial approaches. Am J Cardiol 53:833, 1984, with permission.)

against the septum to allow safe biopsy of that structure without risk of free wall perforation (Fig. 31-8).

## COMPLICATIONS

Transvascular endomyocardial biopsy of either the left or right ventricle can be performed safely using any of the techniques described. A worldwide survey of more than 6000 cases showed a procedure-related mortality of only 0.05%.[13]

The main hazard of endomyocardial biopsy (using any of the biopsy techniques) is cardiac perforation, which occurs in 0.3 to 0.5% of cases and rapidly can lead to tamponade and circulatory collapse.[1,13] This risk can be minimized by careful attention to catheter position, suitable caution during catheter advancement, and continuous monitoring of the patient. Biopsy passes associated with chest pain or those producing samples that float in 10% formalin (suggesting the presence of epicardial fat) are of particular concern and should prompt monitoring of the blood pressure, right atrial pressure, and the fluoroscopic appearance of the heart border for at least 10 minutes followng the final biopsy sample. Frank cardiac perforation is usually heralded by sudden bradycardia and hypotension, associated with loss of the normal fluoroscopic motion of the right atrial and left ventricular heart borders. If the diagnosis of perforation with hemopericardium is in question in a hemodynamically stable patient, it may be desirable to confirm the presence of pericardial effusion via a portable echocardiogram in the cardiac catheterization laboratory, but the operator must be prepared to perform pericardiocentesis without hesitation if hemodynamic compromise develops. In most cases, simple aspiration or temporary catheter drainage of the pericardial space allows nonoperative management of biopsy-induced cardiac perforation in a patient with normal coagulation parameters. *We avoid right ventricular biopsy in any patient with a prothrombin time greater than 17 seconds, any patient who is heparinized, or any patient with a clinical coagulapathy.* On the other hand, left ventricular biopsies are generally performed *with* systemic anticoagulation (Heparin 5000 u), which is *not* reversed with protamine at the end of the procedure to minimize the risk of thrombus formation at the biopsy site. Left ventricular biopsies should be avoided in patients with prior myocardial infarction, since local wall thinning or weakness may increase the risk of perforation.

A second hazard of cardiac biopsy is embolization. With continuous flushing of the entry sheath, right sided thromboembolism during cardiac biopsy is rare. Air embolization has been described, however, as the result of the smaller size of the bioptome shaft

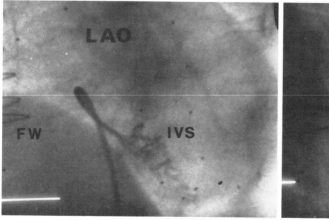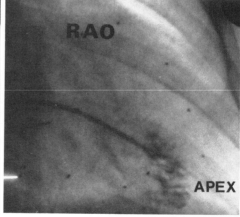

**Fig. 31-8.** Contrast injection in the left anterior oblique (left) and right anterior oblique projections demonstrates correct position of the long sheath against the apical-septal wall. FW = free wall of right ventricle; IVS = interventricular septum.

relative to its head. This allows aspiration of air through any sheath lacking a suitable valve, when used in a patient with a low central venous pressure. The possibility of paradoxical air or thromboembolism constitutes a relative contraindication for right ventricular biopsy in patients with significant right-to-left intracardiac shunting. Of course, thromboembolism poses a greater potential problem during left ventricular biopsy, where cerebral embolization has been reported despite careful technique, systemic angiocoagulation, and avoidance of patients with mural thrombi.[6] Finally, a number of less serious complications of endomyocardial biopsy have been described, including transient arrhythmias and transient or permanent bundle branch block. Since these complications are invariably evident before the patient leaves the catheterization laboratory, we are currently performing serial right ventricular biopsies (in cardiac transplant or myocarditis patients) on an outpatient basis.

## TISSUE PROCESSING

The operator must take responsibility for obtaining an adequate tissue sample and performing the initial preparations that permit subsequent pathologic evaluation. It is usually recommended that 3 to 5 separate specimens be obtained from either the right or the left ventricle to minimize sampling errors. Most myocardial diseases affect both ventricles, so that either chamber may be sampled, depending on operator experience and preference. Selective left ventricular involvement may be present in certain diseases (endomyocardial fibrosis, scleroderma, left heart radiation, and cardiac fibroelastosis of infants and newborns). Left ventricular biopsy should be performed in these conditions or in patients in whom right ventricular biopsy has been unsuccessful or nondiagnostic. In the remaining patients, we generally prefer right rather than left ventricular biopsy because of greater ease, speed, and freedom from morbidity.

The safest and most elegant techniques of endomyocardial biopsy are useless without expert pathologic interpretation. The availability of a cardiac pathologist who is fully trained in the evaluation of biopsy-obtained tissue is mandatory for any biopsy program.

Artifacts such as crushing or contraction bands are frequently present and may be overinterpreted by the inexperienced observer or one used to evaluating only postmortem specimens. The operator may assist the pathologist by appropriate handling of the tissue in the catheterization laboratory. Biopsy specimens should be gently removed from the jaws of the bioptome with a fine needle and placed on moistened filter paper to be transferred immediately to the appropriate fixative—10% formalin for light microscopy, or 2.5% buffered glutaraldehyde for electron microscopy. Frozen specimens may be prepared in the catheterization laboratory by placing samples in a suitable fluid imbedding medium and immersing them in liquid air or a dry ice–isopentane mixture to allow immediate interpretation (as in the case of transplant rejection) or subsequent immunologic staining. Special sample preparation or staining may be indicated for the evaluation of specific disease states (see below).

## FINDINGS IN SPECIFIC DISEASE STATES

### Transplant Rejection

Endomyocardial biopsy has been the cornerstone of monitoring of antirejection therapy in patients with heart or heart-lung transplants.[14] It allows the detection of early rejection before the clinical findings of advanced graft damage (arrhythmias, third heart sound, congestive heart failure) become manifest and confirms the adequacy of pulsed immunosupressive therapy to control each acute rejection episode. Because rejection is a diffuse process, sampling errors are rare. The light-microscopic histologic features of rejection include interstitial edema, inflammatory infiltration, and immunoglobulin deposition. More severe rejection is marked by myocytolysis and even interstitial hemorrhage.

### Adriamycin Cardiotoxicity

Doxorubricin hydrochloride (Adriamycin) is a potent anthracycline antibiotic which is active against many tumors, but whose usefulness is limited by its tendency to cause irreversible dose-related cardiotoxicity. One approach to safe clinical use has been to limit the total cumulative dose to 500 mg/sq m, but this constitutes an unnecessary limitation in patients who can tolerate substantially higher doses without cardiotoxicity and who depend on the drug for tumor control. On the other hand, patients with preexisting heart disease, prior radiotherapy or cyclophosphamide adminstration, or over age 70 may develop cardiac toxicity at substantially lower doses. Because overt impairment of cardiac function is a relatively late finding in adriamycin toxicity, noninvasive testing may fail to disclose whether additional doses of adriamycin can be given safely. Bristow and co-workers have demonstrated, however, that a progressive series of histologic changes (including electron microscopic evidence of myofibrillar loss and cytoplasmic vacuolization) take place during the development of adriamycin cardiotoxicity.[15] The extent of these changes can predict whether a patient is likely to develop clinical cardiotoxicity during the subsequent chemotherapy cycle, permitting maximal yet safe dosing with adriamycin while substantially decreasing the incidence of morbidity and mortality from adriamycin cardiotoxicity.

## Dilated Cardiomyopathy

Approximately 10,000 cases of dilated cardiomyopathy—primary myocardial failure in the absence of underlying coronary, valvular, or pericardial disease—occur in the United States each year.[16–18] Most patients present with well-established cardiac damage, and since the myocardium has a limited number of ways in which to manifest such damage histologically, the majority of patients with dilated cardiomyopathy will display only the monotonous findings of myocyte hypertrophy, interstitial and replacement fibrosis, and endocardial thickening.[19] These findings do not necessarily aid in establishing etiology, long-term prognosis, or appropriate specific therapy. As such, some authorities have suggested that endomyocardial biopsy is of little value in patients with dilated cardiomyopathy.[20,21] On the other hand, recent studies have demonstrated the clinical utility of endomyocardial biopsy in the detection of pa-

tients with active ongoing inflammatory myocarditis or myocardial disorders for which specific therapy may be of value. Since dilated cardiomyopathy carries a substantial 5-year mortality, our approach for any young or middle-aged patient with dilated cardiomyopathy includes an invasive evaluation with endomyocardial biopsy.

## Myocarditis

Epidemiologic studies suggest that approximately 5% of a coxsackie B virus-infected population will show some evidence of cardiac involvement.[16–18] In most cases, these abnormalities do not come to medical attention and subside with the resolution of the acute viral infection. In some patients, however, cardiac inflammation associated with viral, protozoal, metazoal, or bacterial infections may persist, leading to ongoing symptoms of heart failure, chest pain, or arrhythmias. Interestingly, only about 25% of patients with clinically suspected acute myocarditis will have positive biopsies[22–24], but the yield may be increased by prebiopsy screening with a gallium 67 scan.[25]

Several studies suggest that 15 to 30% of patients with established dilated cardiomyopathy, unexplained chest pain, or ventricular arrhythmias may have biopsy evidence of inflammatory myocarditis despite the absence of clinical findings such as fever, leukocytosis, or an elevated erythrocyte sedimentation rate.[24,26,27] Although pathologists may disagree on some aspects of the histologic diagnosis of myocarditis, most would concur with this diagnosis in a patient who has foci of round-cell infiltration in proximity to areas of myocyte damage.[28] Although no controlled trials have been performed to date, up to 60% of patients with inflammatory myocarditis improve when treated with a regimen of prednisone and azothioprine.[8,16] On the other hand, some patients may also improve spontaneously, and death from sepsis and opportunistic infections has been reported in immunosuppressive-treated patients. Conclusive proof of the efficacy of immunosuppressive therapy can only be established by a large-scale randomized trial, and the results of such a trial will be pivotal in establishing the ultimate role of cardiac biopsy in the diagnosis and treatment of myocarditis.

With the exception of patients with inflammatory myocarditis, endomyocardial biopsy in most patients with dilated cardiomyopathy will show simply the nonspecific findings described above. Occasionally, however, specific findings will allow the diagnosis of disorders such as hemochromatosis[29] or sarcoidosis[30,31] for which specific therapy may exist. Other disorders, such as postpartum or alcoholic cardiomyopathy,[32] lack both distinctive histologic features and specific therapy and cannot be separated from idiopathic myocardial failure.

## Restrictive versus Constrictive Disease

Heart failure due to impaired diastolic functioning of a normal-sized or mildly dilated left ventricle is an uncommon but important clinical entity. In some cases, this may be due to pericardial constriction or hypertrophic myopathy, in which cases endomyocardial biopsy would offer no further information.[1] On the other hand, diastolic dysfunction may also be due to one of a series of diseases which can be readily diagnosed with endomyocardial biopsy, thus sparing the patient from inappropriate medical or surgical therapy. These disorders include primary amyloidosis,[33] Loeffler's endomyocardial fibrosis, carcinoidosis, Fabry's disease,[34] and the glycogen storage diseases.[1,17,18]

## FUTURE DIRECTIONS

Based on the increased ease and safety of endomyocardial biopsy, the increased awareness of inflammatory myocarditis, and the proliferation of cardiac pathologists trained to evaluate endomyocardial biopsy samples, endomyocardial biopsy is playing an increasing role in the invasive evaluation of patients with primary myocardial disorders.[35] As further knowledge is gained about the natural history and therapy of the various myocardial disorders, the use of endomyocardial biopsy should continue to expand.

## REFERENCES

1. Fowles RE, Mason JW: Endomyocardial biopsy. Ann Intern Med 97:885, 1982.
2. Shugoll GI: Percutaneous myocardial and pericardial biopsy with the Menghini needle. Am Heart J 85:35, 1973.
3. Shirey EK, Hawk WA, Mukerji D, Effler DB: Percutaneous myocardial biopsy of the left ventricle: experience in 198 patients. Circulation 46:112, 1972.
4. Sakakibara S, Konno S: Endomyocardial biopsy. Jpn Heart J 3:537, 1962.
5. Kawai C, Kitaura Y: New endomyocardial biopsy catheter for the left ventricle. Am J Cardiol 40:63, 1977.
6. Kawai C, Matsumori A, Kawamura K: Myocardial biopsy. Ann Rev Med 31:139, 1980.
7. Caves PK, Stinson EB, Dong E Jr: New instrument for transvenous cardiac biopsy. Am J Cardiol 33:264, 1974.
8. Mason JW: Techniques for right and left ventricular endomyocardial biopsy. Am J Cardiol 41:887, 1978.
9. Richardson PJ: King's endomyocardial bioptome. Lancet 1:660, 1974.
10. Brooksby IAB, et al: Left ventricular endomyocardial biopsy. Lancet 2:1222, 1974.
11. Rios B, Nihill MR, Mullins CE: Left ventricular endomyocardial biopsy in children with the transseptal long sheath technique. Cathet Cardiovasc Diagn 10:417, 1984.
12. Anderson JL, Marshall HW: The femoral venous approach to endomyocardial biopsy: comparison with internal jugular and transarterial approaches. Am J Cardiol 53:833, 1984.
13. Sekiguchi M, Take M: World survey of catheter biopsy of the heart. *In* Sekiguchi M, Olsen EGJ (eds.): Cardiomyopathy. Clinical, Pathological, and Theoretical Aspects. Baltimore, University Park Press, 1980; pp. 217-225.
14. Billingham ME, Mason JW: The role of endomyocardial biosy in the management of acute rejection in cardiac allografts. *In* Fenoglio JJ Jr (ed.): Endomyocardial Biopsy: Techniques and Applications. Boca Raton FL, CRC Press, 1982, pp. 57-64.
15. Bristow MR, Mason JW, Billingham ME, Daniels JR: Doxorubicin cardiotoxicity: evaluation of phonocardiography, endomyocardial biopsy, and cardiac catheterization. Ann Intern Med 88:168, 1978.
16. Kereiakes DJ, Parmley WW: Myocarditis and cardiomyopathy. Am Heart J 108:1318, 1984.
17. Abelmann WH: Classification and natural history

of primary myocardial disease. Prog Cadiovasc Dis 27:73, 1984.

18. Johnson RA, Palacios I: Dilated cardiomyopathies of the adult. N Engl J Med 307:1051, 1119, 1982.

19. Unverferth DV, et al: Human myocardial histologic characteristics in congestive heart failure. Circulation 68:1194, 1983.

20. MacKay EH, Littler WA, Sleight P: Critical assessment of diagnostic value of endomyocardial biopsy. Br Heart J 40:69, 1978.

21. Ferrans VJ, Roberts WC: Myocardial biopsy: a useful diagnostic procedure or only a research tool? Am J Cardiol 41:965, 1978.

22. Mason JW, Billingham ME, Ricci DR: Treatment of acute inflammatory myocarditis assisted by endomyocardial biopsy. Am J Cardiol 45:1037, 1980.

23. Aretz HT, Chapman C, Fallon JJ: Morphologic and immunologic findings in patients with clinically suspected acute myocarditis (abstract). Circulation 68 (Supp III):27, 1983.

24. Parrillo JE, et al: The results of transvenous endomyocardial biopsy can frequently be used to diagnose myocardial diseases in patients with idiopathic heart failure. Circulation 69:93, 1984.

25. O'Connell JB, Robinson JA, Henkin RE, Gunnar RM: Immunosuppressive therapy in patients with congestive cardiomyopathy and myocardial uptake of gallium-67. Circulation 64:780, 1981.

26. Nippoldt TB, et al: Right ventricular endomyocardial biopsy—clinicopathologic correlates in 100 consecutive patients. Mayo Clin Proc 57:407, 1982.

27. Zee-Chung C, et al: High incidence of myocarditis by endomyocardial biopsy in patients with idiopathic congestive cardiomyopathy. J Am Coll Cardiol 3:63, 1984.

28. Fenoglio JJ, et al: Diagnosis and classification of myocarditis by endomyocardial biopsy. N Engl J Med 308:12, 1983.

29. Short EM, Winkle RA, Billingham ME: Myocardial involvement in idiopathic hemochromatosis: morphologic and clinical improvement following venesection. Am J Med 70:1275, 1981.

30. Lorell B. Alderman EL, Mason JW: Cardiac sarcoidosis: diagnosis by transvenous endomyocardial biopsy and treatment with corticosteroids. Am J Cardiol 42:143, 1978.

31. Silverman KJ, Hutchins GM, Bulkley BH: Cardiac sarcoid: a clinicopathologic study of 84 unselected patients with systemic sarcoidosis. Circulation 58:1204, 1978.

32. Rubin E: Alcoholic myopathy in heart and skeletal muscle. N Engl J Med 301:28, 1979.

33. Schroeder JS, Billingham ME, Rider AK: Cardiac amyloidosis: diagnosis by transvenous endomyocardial biopsy. Am J Med 59:269, 1975.

34. Colucci WS, et al: Hypertrophic obstructive cardiomyopathy due to Fabry's disease. N Engl J Med 307:926, 1982.

35. Mason JW: Endomyocardial biopsy: balance of success and failure. Circulation 71:185, 1985.

*chapter thirty two*

# Temporary and Permanent Pacemakers

STAFFORD I. COHEN

D R. PAUL ZOLL made the first serious attempt to accelerate an excessively slow heart rate in man with external cardiac stimulation applied to the chest wall.[1] Although effective in controlling heart action, the electric shock and skeletal muscle stimulation caused discomfort. The transvenous method of pacing followed and was painless,[2] and implantable permanent cardiac pacing proved to be the first reliable long term-method of managing Stokes-Adams attacks.[3] Most of the early workers in the permanent pacemaker field were thoracic surgeons who placed epimyocardial leads directly on the exposed heart. The technically simpler permanent transvenous pacemaker technique aroused the interest of general surgeons and cardiologists with surgical skills.

The evolution of cardiac pacemaker therapy represents an uncommon example of scientific success in restoring reliable rate control to flawed hearts. The effort has required collaboration among cardiac physiologists, biomedical engineers, and the pacemaker industry. Pacemaker technology has advanced so rapidly that it confounds some implanters and is not understood by many physicians and cardiologists who are primarily committed to patient care. A pacemaker certification requirement has been proposed to assure that there are proper indications for implanting a pacemaker and that the se-

lected device is well suited to the patient's special need.[4]

Technologic advance in the design of pacemaker electrodes and generators now permits several options in the selection of a temporary or a permanent pacemaker system. There is single chamber right atrial or right ventricular pacing. There is also dual chamber pacemaker technology, which not only maintains a satisfactory heart rate but does so by simulating physiologic cardiac excitation. The Intersociety Commission for Heart Disease Resources established a *three-letter code* for characterizing pacemaker capability.[5] *The first letter signifies the chamber paced, the second letter the chamber sensed, and the third letter the response of the pacemaker to sensed intrinsic cardiac activity.* Fourth and fifth letters have recently been added to identify programmability and anti-tachycardia characteristics.[5,6] (Table 32-1)

## TEMPORARY PACEMAKER

*Indications.* Table 32-2 lists the indications for temporary pacemaker placement, and Figure 32-1 represents an example of one of these indications. Pacemakers were first used to manage high grade atrioventricular (A-V) block or so-called Stokes-Adams

517

**TABLE 32-1.** *ICHD Five-Position Code of Pacemaker Mode and Function*

| Position of letter | I | II | III | IV | V |
|---|---|---|---|---|---|
| Letter designates | Chamber(s) paced | Chamber(s) sensed | Modes of response(s) | Programmable functions | Special anti-tachyarrhythmia functions |
| Letters used | V—ventricle | V—ventricle | T—triggered | P—programmable rate and/or output | B—bursts |
| | A—atrium | A—atrium | I-inhibited | M-multi-programmable | N—normal rate competition |
| | D—double | D—double | D—double | C—communicating | S—scanning |
| | | O—none | O—none | O—none | E—external |
| | | | R—reverse | | |

**TABLE 32-2.** *Indications for Placement of a Temporary Pacemaker*

Symptomatic Bradycardia
Sinus node dysfunction | arrest
| bradycardia
| S-A block
A-V node dysfunction | second degree block
| third degree block
His-Purkinje dysfunction | Mobitz II block
| trifascicular block
| bifascicular and Wenckebach block
| right and left bundle branch block

Prophylactic Pacemaker Placement
Right heart catheterization in presence of LBBB
Electrical cardioversion in presence of known sick slow sinus
Acute anterior myocardial infarction with new onset bifascicular block (example, Fig. 32-1)

Tachyarrhythmia Control
Convert atrial tachycardia and flutter
Overdrive suppress ventricular ectopy/tachycardia
Accelerate rate in setting of torsade de pointes with long Q-T interval

attacks. The indications for pacemaker placement have expanded to include acute or anticipated bradyarrhythmias from any electrophysiologic mechanism. Although pacemakers are also used to treat or prevent tachyarrhythmias, this chapter will not review antitachycardia principles or devices.

The management of a bradyarrhythmia crisis is usually pharmacologic or mechanical. Atropine, isoproterenol, and epinephrine are generally available and are often effective. The simple act of a chest thump or forceful slap can excite an asystolic heart to contract. Rhythmic chest thumping can sustain life until other methods are substituted.

Electrical methods to accelerate heart rate can be applied if the underlying cause of bradyarrhythmia is not rapidly reversed, if the life-threatening bradyarrhythmia is likely to recur, or if the excessively slow heart rate persists. External electrical stimulation can be applied swiftly, and a recent modification of this historic technique, utilizing prolongation of stimulus duration, permits effective cardiac pacing without pain in most conscious patients.[7] When there is an absolute emergency such as a cardiac arrest requiring cardiopulmonary resuscitation, a transthoracic pacing wire can be placed quickly through an intracardiac needle positioned from a subxyphoid approach. The desperate circumstance of a stubborn asystolic heart justifies potential injury to a coronary artery as the needle passes through the myocardial wall. If the patient survives, a temporary transvenous pacer must be substituted for the transthoracic pacemaker. The placement of a temporary transvenous pacemaker requires preparation and care. Ideally, the procedure is performed on a relatively stable patient.

Temporary pacemakers are indicated whenever there is symptomatic bradycardia from any cause that is not quickly reversed and is expected to continue to recur. Symptoms of bradyarrhythmia usually relate to cerebral insufficiency and consist of frank syncope, dizziness, or light-headed spells. It should be noted that some patients with syncope and a witnessed unconscious state later insist that they were fully alert. Other manifestations of bradycardia include fatigue and heart failure.

***Procedure for Temporary Pacemaker Placement.*** Temporary pacing requires that a catheter be introduced into a vein and advanced to the right atrium or ventricle. There are several options for venous access. The choice should depend upon the expected duration of the bradyarrhythmia, anatomic considerations, and the anticipated need and timing of a permanent pacemaker.

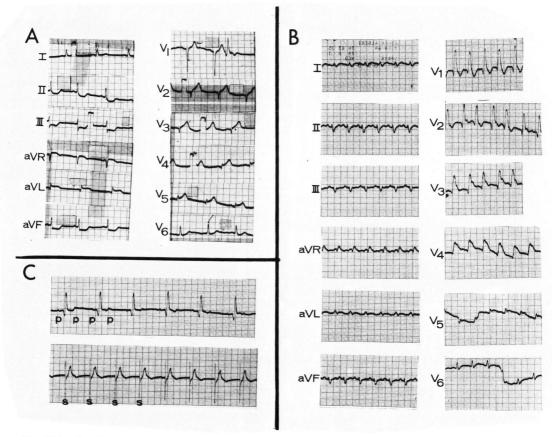

**Fig. 32-1.** Prophylactic temporary pacemaker during acute myocardial infarction. A. Presenting ECG in emergency ward of a patient with crushing chest pain. Poor R wave progression $V_1 - V_4$, ST depression leads II, III, aVF, ST elevation aVL and $V_4$. B. Several hours later, there is a pattern of acute anterior infarction with new onset of right bundle branch block with left axis deviation. A temporary pacemaker is placed because of the likelihood of high grade A-V block. C. High grade heart block: Top, monitor strip reveals 2:1 heart block. Bottom, temporary unipolar pacer is required. S = pacemaker stimulus.

The venous access sites commonly used are internal jugular, external jugular, subclavian, brachial, median basilic, and femoral veins. Percutaneous transvenous introducer techniques can be used to enter each of the major venous routes. Cut-down techniques are often applied to the median basilic, brachial, or external jugular veins. Considerations regarding selection of a venous approach are presented in Table 32-3. Whatever the venous site, placement must be done under aseptic conditions such as those prevailing in a catheterization laboratory or operating room.

The operator must select from several catheter models and several guidance systems that are available to help the operator

direct the catheter from the venous introduction site to the right ventricle. There are three guidance systems: (1) fluoroscopic surveillance, (2) catheter-tip electrogram, and (3) cardiac monitor or electrocardiogram rhythm strip during pacemaker stimulation. Most temporary pacing catheters are bipolar and come in a variety of diameter sizes and have a range of relative flexibility. Some have an inflatable balloon tip, which allows venous flow to direct the catheter tip to the right ventricle.

Fluoroscopy is clearly the best method for assisting the operator to direct the pacing catheter through the venous system and right atrium to a final position in the right ventricle. The availability and location of flu-

**TABLE 32-3.** *Special Considerations When Selecting Vein Access For Temporary Pacing*

| Vein | Consider |
|---|---|
| Internal jugular | Can patient lie flat? <br> Avoid air embolism |
| Subclavian | Avoid preferred side of permanent pacer placement <br> Avoid air embolism |
| External jugular | Can patient lie flat? <br> Avoid preferred side of permanent pacer placement |
| Femoral | Avoid if edema, phlebitis, or varicosities of leg <br> Avoid if ambulation important <br> Not possible if past IVC ligation, clip, or umbrella <br> Requires fluoroscopy |
| Median basilic | Long tortuous course <br> Prone to spasm <br> High displacement rate |

oroscopic equipment and the severity of the arrhythmia dictate the approach and physical location of the pacemaker procedure. Some hospitals have a procedure room within or adjacent to a critical care unit, or there may be radiolucent patient beds and a portable fluoroscope machine, which permits pacemaker placement in any intensive care room. Patients with a failing permanent pacemaker or a Swan-Ganz catheter should have a temporary pacemaker placed under fluoroscopic guidance to avoid entangling or knotting the catheters within the heart.[8] Fluoroscopy is also suggested when the pacemaker is inserted into the femoral vein or when tricuspid regurgitation, a dilated right atrium, and cardiogenic shock or a low flow state are present.

Placement can also be achieved by monitoring the electrogram derived from the pacing catheter's distal electrode.[9] The terminal pin of the distal electrode is connected to the central lead of a standard patient ECG cable after the limb leads have been attached. The ECG lead selector is placed in the V position, and the electrogram is monitored as the pacing catheter is advanced. The pattern of intrinsic atrial excitation will be recognized when the catheter tip is within the right

atrial cavity. Further advancement of the catheter will result in a ventricular intracavity electrogram pattern. When the ventricular pacing and sensing thresholds are satisfactory, a chest roentgenogram should be obtained to confirm the catheter's position and orientation. Catheter placement with electrogram guidance should be used only in an environment that is under strict surveillance for electrical safety. Ventricular fibrillation can result if there is inadequate grounding of equipment, electrical leaks, or improperly functioning wall receptacles. A temporary pacing catheter in the right ventricle is a low resistance pathway from the external environment to the heart. Very low 60-cycle electric current can produce ventricular fibrillation when applied directly to the heart. Also, it is obvious that there must be sustained cardiac excitation to record intracavitary electrical activity; therefore, electrogram guidance is not useful during asystolic cardiac arrest.

The last technique for guiding the pacing catheter to the right ventricle is by using combined sensing and pacing during continuous electrocardiographic monitoring. This approach is necessary when fluoroscopy is unavailable, when the electrograms are not of diagnostic quality, or when the heart is asystolic. After the pacing catheter is introduced into and advanced within the venous system, the bipolar pacemaker's electrode terminal pins are attached with a standard cable to an external pacemaker-generator. If the patient has intrinsic cardiac activity with reasonable rate and rhythm, the pacemaker's sensing circuit is adjusted to its lowest threshold; the energy output and rate are also adjusted to their lowest level. If the intrinsic heart rate is too slow, the pacemaker's rate is set at 60 to 70/min., and the energy output increased to 3.0 volts or 6.0 milliamperes (mA). The pacing catheter is again advanced. If the pacemaker generator indicates sensing of intrinsic cardiac activity, the paced rate is adjusted to a faster rate. The energy output is increased. The cardiac monitor is observed for excitation of the atria or ventricles. If the former occurs, the generator settings are returned to their original position, and the catheter is withdrawn slightly and readvanced with rotation to enter the right ventricle. If the pacing catheter is balloon tipped, the balloon must be deflated each time the catheter is withdrawn. Fragile chordae tendinae have been known to be torn as an inflated balloon is forcefully withdrawn against chordal resistance. After manipulation, the catheter should advance across the tricuspid valve and result in ventricular excitation when the rate and energy settings are properly adjusted. Entry into the right ventricle is usually heralded by ectopy; therefore, the electrocardiographic monitor should be observed carefully during catheter manipulation. If the initial indication for a pacemaker was asystolic arrest, the pacemaker-generator is activated for pacing as the catheter is advanced. Low thresholds for stimulation are desirable. Although a pacing threshold of less than 1.0 mA is ideal, thresholds between 1.0 and 2.0 mA are common.

After satisfactory positioning, the catheter must be secured to prevent inadvertent withdrawal by the patient or medical personnel. The pacing catheter should be secured to the skin by a lock stitch and then arranged with an accessory loop such that a "tug" on the proximal catheter will cause the loop to contract rather than the catheter to be withdrawn from the vein. Antibiotic or iodinated ointment should be applied over the insertion site before the wound is dressed. A chest roentgenogram is then obtained to document the catheter position. The introduction site should be examined at intervals, and the pacing system should be checked for malfunctions, most of which will be discussed in the section of the chapter discussing permanent pacing.

***Need for Temporary Physiologic Pacing.*** A variety of pathologic cardiac conditions have been identified that need the normal sequence of atrial and ventricular activation to maintain a satisfactory cardiac output and blood pressure. Aortic stenosis, mitral stenosis, and obstructive myopathies should alert the operator to the theoretical or actual need of a physiologic pacing system. Other cardiac states that may require physiologic pacing include myocardial infarction, the immediate postoperative period following heart surgery, and left ventricular hypertrophy from any cause. Except in mitral stenosis, there is usually a noncompliant left ventricle in need of the "priming" action of atrial systole.

Atrial pacing alone maintains physiologic chamber activation in the presence of intact A-V conduction. The anatomy of the right atrium does not easily permit a conventional temporary pacing catheter to remain in contact with the atrial wall. On occasion a catheter can be effectively positioned at the atrial in-flow, looped against the lateral wall, or advanced from the femoral vein directly to the atrial appendage. Because of unreliable atrial pacing with conventional catheters, models have been specifically designed for the purpose.

A catheter is relatively secure against displacement while in the coronary sinus or veins.[10] Some catheters have been adapted specifically for coronary sinus pacing by positioning the electrode rings several centimeters proximal to the tip. Other temporary atrial pacing catheters include those that must be positioned in the right atrium through a strategically placed introducer catheter. The end of the atrial pacing catheter may assume a ring-like form with each of the oppositely charged semicircles making contact with opposing sides of the atrial wall.[11] The ends of another atrial catheter design have two electrode prongs, which flare in opposite directions to contact opposing walls of the atrium (Atri-pace I, Mansfield Scientific, Mansfield, MA), and this catheter is discussed in Chapter 18.

Dual chamber temporary pacing is beneficial when there is A-V heart block and need for preservation of physiologic chamber activation. Separate pacing catheters may be required. However, there are pacing catheters designed for dual chamber pacing. Some have multipolar electrodes situated along the atrial and ventricular course of the catheter. Other designs need an introducer through which a single catheter with two sets of flared prongs or two catheters can be passed.

Temporary pacemakers can remain in position for days to weeks. The longer the catheters remain, the greater the risk of infection. Therefore, a permanent pacing system should be placed as soon as the clinical status permits. If placement of a permanent pacemaker is an obvious long-term therapeutic consideration, the preferred veins should be reserved for the permanent pacemaker, and the temporary pacer should be introduced through another approach. In addition, the patient should not have skin electrodes for cardiac monitoring placed near the preferred sites of permanent pacemaker placement. The skin should be free of excoriations and allergic reaction to adhesives, which could result in infection. Anticoagulants and antiplatelet agents should be avoided or adjusted if permanent pacer placement is imminent.

In addition to infection, an important potential complication of a temporary pacemaker is cardiac perforation (Fig. 32-2). This complication is more likely when the pacemaker is placed without fluoroscopic guidance, when stiff pacing catheters are used, and when there is recent right ventricular infarction where the ventricular myocardium is necrotic.

## PERMANENT PACEMAKER

***Preoperative Evaluation.*** Guidelines for permanent cardiac pacemaker implantation have been developed by a task force of cardiologists and surgeons representing the American Heart Association and the American College of Cardiology.[12] The guidelines include three patient categories: those with unqualified need, qualified need, and doubtful need. The categories are listed in Table 32-4.

There are many approaches to permanent pacer implantation.[13-17] The suggestions that follow are personalized and relate to my own experience. Permanent pacemaker implantation is performed under local anesthesia. The patient is awake, and patients who are expected to cooperate need not be sedated.

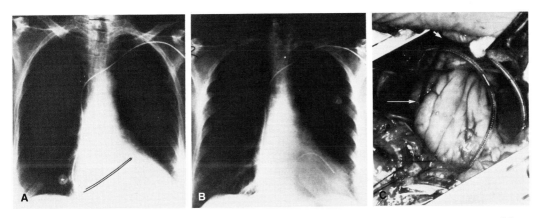

**Fig. 32-2.** Cardiac perforation by temporary pacemaker catheter. A. Temporary pacer catheter inserted from left arm to right ventricular outflow tract. Course of catheter in the right ventricle has been outlined. It is pointing towards the left shoulder. B. Repeat roentgenogram following intermittent failure of capture and rising threshold for pacing. There is myocardial perforation by the catheter which is turning down along the lateral border towards the ventricular apex. C. An epimyocardial permanent pacer system is being placed. Viewing the left ventricular apex, two epicardial leads are curving about the lateral heart border to their fixation position on the diaphragmatic surface. The perforated temporary pacer exits from the base of the right ventricle (large arrow) and is directed superiorly. The small arrow points to the tip electrode. The temporary pacer was withdrawn under direct vision without any bleeding from the site of perforation.

**TABLE 32-4.**  *Indications for Implantation of Permanent Cardiac Pacemakers*

*Group I.*  Conditions under which implantation of a cardiac pacemaker is generally considered acceptable or necessary, provided that the conditions are chronic or recurrent and not due to transient causes such as acute myocardial infarction, drug toxicity, or electrolyte imbalance. In the cases where there is a rhythm disturbance, if the rhythm disturbance is chronic or recurrent, a single episode of a symptom such as syncope or seizure is adequate to establish medical necessity.

1. Acquired complete AV heart block with symptoms (e.g., syncope, seizures, congestive heart failure, dizziness, confusion, or limited exercise tolerance).

2. Congenital complete heart block with severe bradycardia (in relation to age), or significant physiologic deficits or significant symptoms due to the bradycardia.

3. Second degree AV heart block of Mobitz Type II with symptoms attributable to intermittent complete heart block.

4. Second degree AV heart block of Mobitz Type I with significant symptoms due to hemodynamic instability associated with the heart block.

5. Sinus bradycardia associated with major symptoms or substantial sinus bradycardia (heart rate less than 50) associated with dizziness or confusion. The correlation between symptoms and bradycardia must be documented, or the symptoms must be clearly attributable to the bradycardia rather than to some other cause.

6. In selected and few patients, sinus bradycardia of lesser severity (heart rate 50–59) with dizziness or confusion. The correlation between symptoms and bradycardia must be documented, or the symptoms must be clearly attributable to the bradycardia rather than to some other cause.

7. Sinus bradycardia that is the consequence of long-term necessary drug treatment for which there is no acceptable alternative, when accompanied by significant symptoms. The correlation between symptoms and bradycardia must be documented, or the symptoms must be clearly attributable to the bradycardia rather than to some other cause.

8. Sinus node dysfunction with or without tachyarrhythmias or AV conduction block— i.e., the bradycardia-tachycardia syndrome, sinoatrial block, sinus arrest—when accompanied by significant symptoms.

9. Sinus node dysfunction with or without symptoms when there are potentially life-threatening ventricular arrhythmias or tachycardia secondary to the bradycardia.

10. Symptomatic bradycardia associated with supraventricular tachycardia.

11. The occasional patient with hypersensitive carotid sinus syndrome with syncope due to bradycardia and unresponsive to prophylactic medical measures.

*Group II.*  Conditions under which implantation of a cardiac pacemaker may be found acceptable or necessary, provided that the medical history and prognosis of the patient involved can be documented and there is evidence that the pacemaker implantation will assist in the overall management of the patient. As with Group I, the conditions must be present chronically or recurrently and not due to such transient causes as acute myocardial infarction, drug toxicity, or electrolyte imbalance.

1. Acquired complete AV heart block without symptoms.

2. Congenital complete heart block with less severe bradycardia (in relation to age).

3. Bifascicular or trifascicular block accompanied by syncope that is attributed to transient complete heart block after other plausible causes of syncope have been reasonably excluded.

4. Prophylactic pacemaker use following recovery from acute myocardial infarction during which there was temporary complete (third degree) and/or Mobitz Type II second degree AV block.

5. Asymptomatic second degree AV block of Mobitz Type II.

6. Very substantial sinus bradycardia (heart rate less than 45) that is a consequence of long-term necessary drug treatment for which there is no acceptable alternative, when not accompanied by significant symptoms.

7. In patients with recurrent and refractory ventricular tachycardia, "overdrive pacing" (pacing above the basal rate) to prevent ventricular tachycardia.

*Group III:*   Conditions that although used by some physicians as bases for permanent pacemaker implantation, are considered unsupported by adequate evidence of benefit and therefore should not generally be considered appropriate uses for pacemakers in the absence of indications cited in the above two groups.

1. Syncope of undetermined cause.
2. Sinus bradycardia without significant symptoms.
3. Sinoatrial block or sinus arrest without significant symptoms.
4. Prolonged R-R intervals with atrial fibrillation (without third degree AV block) or with other causes of transient ventricular pause.
5. Bradycardia during sleep.
6. Right bundle branch block with left axis deviation (and other forms of fascicular or bundle branch block) without syncope or other symptoms of intermittent AV block.
7. Asymptomatic second degree AV block of Mobitz Type I.

*Note:* This table is based upon recommendations in references 5 and 12.

Confused patients or those with a high level of anxiety during the preoperative evaluation should be sedated just prior to pacemaker implantation. Triazolam, diazepam, lorazepam, haloperidol, or thioridazine work well in most patients.

If there is a history of angina pectoris or heart failure, the status of each patient should be carefully reviewed. Additional nitrate or diuretic therapy might be required to enhance comfort and to reduce risk during the operation. If there is unstable angina and an unreliable intrinsic mechanism to support adequate heart rate, a temporary pacemaker is preferable to isoproterenol or atropine for rate control during placement of a permanent pacer. The history of allergy should specify local anesthetics, sedatives, analgesics, adhesive tape, antibiotics, x-ray contrast medium, and iodine. Each of these agents might be used in the course of a pacemaker implantation.

The cardiovascular examination should emphasize issues relevant to pacer placement. Physical findings of tricuspid regurgitation prepare the operator to use a fixation ventricular electrode. The preliminary assessment should include an estimate of the need for physiologic pacing. If the patient's condition permits, the physical examination should include a determination of blood pressure in the supine, sitting, and standing positions. Knowledge of orthostatic hypotension could be crucial to selecting a physiologic pacing system, especially if sole ventricular excitation also causes relative hypotension. Significant mitral stenosis or aortic stenosis prepares the operator to use a physiologic pacing system. If there is a systolic murmur and carotid pulse contour, both characteristic of IHSS, an echocardiogram should be obtained to confirm the diagnosis and the probable need for a physiologic pacing system. The finding of varicose veins suggests the possibility of orthostatic hypotension.

The areas of venous access should be examined carefully. The presence or absence of external jugular, internal jugular, and cephalic veins should be noted. A large distended vein might result from partial venous obstruction, as might a prominent plexus of veins over the shoulder area. The thickness and integrity of the skin overlying potential sites for placing the pacemaker bear close examination. Abrasions and excoriations are potential sources of infection and should be avoided. The clavicles and overlying skin should be carefully inspected; if the clavicle is prominent and the skin thin, the catheter should be placed in the cephalic vein or subclavian vein. A neck placement might eventually result in necrosis of the skin overlying the clavicular portion of the pacing catheter. In addition, the breasts of female patients are examined carefully for pathologic conditions. If there is a suspicious lump, the pacemaker should be placed from the contralateral approach.

Laboratory data are checked for potential problems: there should be correction of abnormal levels of glucose, hematocrit, potassium gas exchange, clotting parameters, and toxic levels of drugs such as digitalis. The chest roentgenogram is carefully reviewed for evidence of pneumonia or other pathologic conditions. Is there evidence of infection such as fever or unexplained high white blood count?

The preoperative orders might include the considerations in Table 32-5. Operative consent includes a description of the patient's rhythm disturbance, the best pacemaker modality for correction, and the technical requirements for pacemaker placement. The benefits and risks of the operation are detailed, as well as other therapeutic options and the risks of not having the operation. Operative risks include the possibility of death, infection, arrhythmias, including bradyarrhythmias and catheter-induced tachyarrhythmias; the possible need for cardioversion in the event of a tachyarrhythmia; perforation of the heart and its consequences; displacement of the electrode with pacemaker failure; the possible need for a reoperation; and a discussion of secondary approaches for venous access in the event of failure of the initial approach.

***Permanent Pacemaker Procedure.***
The pacemaker implantation is usually performed in an operating room or cardiac catheterization laboratory. The patient is made as comfortable as possible on the x-ray table, with his/her head and shoulders elevated slightly. If left heart failure is present, the shoulders are elevated higher and nasal oxygen is administered. The patient's hands are restrained loosely at the sides of the table to prevent inadvertent movement and possible contamination of the operative field. If there is restlessness, confusion, or a general inability to cooperate, the legs are restrained by a binder across the knees.

There are highly visible cardiac monitors to display and record the electrocardiographic events during the pacemaker implantation. An audio "beep" capability to signal each heart beat is helpful. A control 12-lead ECG recording is taken at the start of the operation as a reference in the event of change during the course of the procedure. Our laboratory monitors ECG leads II and $V_1$. A defibrillator is in a state of readiness within the room, and an emergency drug cart is in the vicinity. An external transcutaneous pacemaker capability is recommended in the event of unexpected asystole prior to permanent placement of the pacing catheter. A sterile drape covers the fluoroscopic tube.

The operative field is shaved; the neck veins are marked; the entire field, including the axilla, chest, and neck, is cleansed with surgical skin scrubs. An elevated bar is positioned at the level of the neck and parallel to the shoulders so that when sterile drapes are properly positioned across the bar, the patient's face is screened from the sterile field.

The skin is infiltrated with a local anesthetic in preparation for the incision. Only enough lidocaine to achieve a state of satisfactory anesthesia is administered, for lidocaine is absorbed systemically to levels that can suppress subsidiary intrinsic pacemaker activity. If the cephalic vein is sought, its course is constant in the deltopectoral groove. A small artery frequently crosses the vein; it must be anticipated and may require division. The diameter of the cephalic vein is often small. As it courses in a superior and medial direction towards the subclavian vein, the cephalic vein becomes larger. At times, some pectoralis muscle must be dissected from the clavicle to expose a large segment of the vein. A length of vein is isolated and cleansed of fat and adventitia. The

---

**TABLE 32-5.**  *Pre- and Postoperative Orders for Permanent Pacemaker Placement*

| Preoperative | Postoperative |
|---|---|
| • Coagulation blood screen | • Bed rest for 24 hours with graded increase in subsequent activity |
| • Chest roentgenogram | • Portable chest roentgenogram—same day |
| • Surgical skin scrubs to the chest and neck 24 hours before procedure | • EKG—same day |
| • Functioning intravenous or heparin lock | • Cardiac monitor until ambulating |
| • Consent for operation | • Analgesia |
| • Transportation by stretcher with portable cardiac monitor | • Chest roentgenograms P-A and lateral prior to discharge |

distal end of the vein segment can be ligated, and a loose silk should be placed on the proximal end to control bleeding. Suction should be available in the event of brisk arterial or venous bleeding.

A subcutaneous "pocket" must be prepared for the pacemaker generator before or after the pacing catheter is placed in the vein. The subcutaneous space is created by sharp or blunt dissection in the fascial plane just above the pectoralis muscle. Adequate local anesthesia is required, for this is usually the most uncomfortable part of the operation. An antibiotic-soaked radioopaque sponge is placed within the pocket, and the size of the created space should correspond to the size of the pacemaker generator.

The vein should be incised near its ligated end with a blade or a fine sharp-tipped scissors. A vein introducer will facilitate the entrance of the pacing catheter. Bathing the vein and the electrode tip in lidocaine may prevent venospasm. If the cephalic vein is thick-walled but too small to accept the pacing catheter, a vein dilator or small snap may be introduced to stretch the vein to a larger diameter. When the tip of the pacing catheter cannot completely enter the vein, a curved snap can gently tease the edges over the catheter tip's largest diameter.

A variety of pacing catheters are suitable for the uncomplicated or the problem patient. There are thin leads for small veins, screw-in active fixation electrodes that minimize the risks of dislodgement, and tined-tip leads that acquire excellent fixation, so good, in fact, that in time removal by traction may be impossible—a vexing problem if there is an infected pacer system.

The permanent pacing catheter is very flexible and very "floppy." The catheter is guided through the venous system and right heart chambers by a stiffening wire stylet that is placed in a central channel extending throughout the catheter and stopping at the tip electrode of the catheter. The stylet can be shaped into any desired curve or combination of curves by the operator. A single gentle curve of the distal 2 inches is usually all that is required.

The pacing catheter enters the cephalic vein with a straight or curved stylet in place, and the catheter is advanced several inches into the vein without rotation. The stylet is then withdrawn 1 to 2 inches to give the catheter a more flexible tip, and the catheter is now advanced further to negotiate curves en route to the subclavian vein. Further advance should be with fluoroscopic assistance. Difficulty may be encountered in entering the subclavian vein. The pacing catheter may turn back toward the axilla or enter the subclavian vein pointing laterally toward the arm rather than medially toward the heart. The stylet should be withdrawn and a single curve or variety of curves fashioned until the catheter takes the correct route. Experience and skill are necessary in manipulating the stylet and catheter. One hand slowly advances or withdraws the pacing catheter at the point of entry to the vein. The thumb and index finger of the other hand turn the stylet while the body of the catheter is held firmly between the palm and the remaining fingers (Fig. 32-3).

The pacing catheter is guided into the subclavian vein and superior vena cava. If the catheter cannot be advanced along the proper route, it must be withdrawn and a venogram must be performed from the cephalic vein to demonstrate the true route or the stenosis-thrombosis that is preventing passage. If the cephalic approach fails, there are two options. The skin incision can be extended medially to prepare for the placement of a subclavian introducer, or the sterile drapes can be readjusted to expose the neck where external and internal jugular veins are accessible.

The gentle curve of the stylet permits smooth passage of the catheter from the subclavian vein to the superior vena cava and helps direct passage from the right atrium to the ventricle. When the tricuspid valve is difficult to traverse, success may be achieved by looping the tip of the catheter against the lateral atrial wall and then rotating the loop medially against the atrial septum with the catheter tip just above the tricuspid valve. Gentle withdrawal of the catheter will straighten the loop and direct the tip inferiorly past the tricuspid valve.

Difficulty crossing the tricuspid valve can be expected when there is a large right atrium or when there is tricuspid regurgitation. In the latter condition, the regurgitant jet may reject the catheter from the ventricle back to the atrium. Entry of the catheter into the ventricle will often result in ventricular ectopy, ventricular couplets, and occasional nonsustained or sustained ventricular tachycardia. The pacing catheter should be perma-

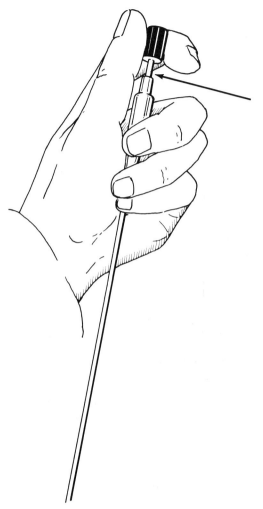

**Fig. 32-3.** Stylet and pacing catheter. See text for explanation. For illustrative purposes, the diameter of the stylet guide wire (arrow) is exaggerated and the hand is not gloved.

routinely pass the catheter to the pulmonary artery to be certain of a right ventricular position. The ideal catheter placement is on the diaphragmatic surface or "floor" of the right ventricle between its midpoint and its apex. The "floor" of the proximal ventricle is a second choice. The least desirable option is in the midventricle or apex with the catheter tip pointing toward the outflow tract (Fig. 32-4).

When the pacing catheter has been advanced to the right ventricle, the stylet is rotated to direct the tip inferiorly. The stylet is then withdrawn about 2 inches, and the catheter is advanced toward the cardiac apex. When the catheter tip is advanced to the endocardial wall of the ventricle or to a trabeculated muscle bridge, the operator feels some resistance, and a buckling is seen in the unstiffened distal part of the catheter. A slight forward movement of the catheter tip could indicate a "wedging" of the tip under a trabeculum. If the pacing catheter tip fails to follow the desired intraventricular route, or will not "wedge," the curved stylet is exchanged for a straight stylet while the pacing catheter remains in the right ventricle. The straight stylet will usually direct the catheter tip to the diaphragmatic surface of the ventricle.

Once the pacing catheter has a satisfactory intracardiac position by fluoroscopic appearance, other studies and maneuvers are undertaken to test adequate position and fixation. A catheter with fixation or "wedging" of the tip can be slowly withdrawn until the atrial curve straightens and a slight "tug" is felt during diastole similar to that of a fish nibble on a hand-held fishing line. This maneuver is helpful only when the catheter moves very freely within the vein. If there is venous spasm or if there is an excessively tortuous route from the cephalic vein to the ventricle, the "tug" test should not be used. If the catheter tip is not "wedged," the mere reduction of the atrial arc of the pacing catheter will usually displace the tip electrode from its position. Conversely, if the atrial curve is straightened without movement of the tip, the electrode is most likely in a "wedged" position.

Respiratory maneuvers are also helpful in determining proper placement, stability, and arc of a pacing catheter. During deep inspiration, the diaphragm moves downward, the mediastinum elongates, and the heart moves

nently positioned at a distance from any arrhythmogenic areas. The operator observes the fluoroscopic image during catheter manipulations; thus laboratory personnel must observe the heart rhythm on the cardiac monitor. If ectopy is excessive, intravenous lidocaine can be safely administered if there is no danger of suppressing a subsidiary pacemaker or if there is a temporary pacer in place.

Because entry into an inferior branch of the coronary vein can occasionally mimic a right ventricular position, some operators

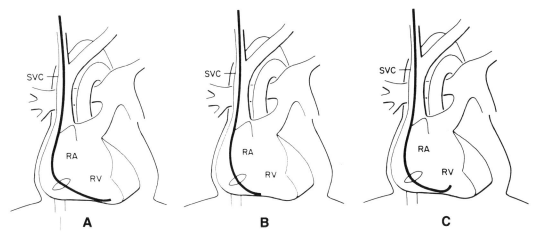

**Fig. 32-4.** Common catheter positions for right ventricular pacing (see text). A. Most desirable position. B. Acceptable position. C. Acceptable but least desirable position SVC = superior vena cava; RA = right atrium; RV = right ventricle.

inferiorly. When the tip and atrial curve of the pacing catheter are fluoroscopically observed during deep inspiration, the tip should not move but the arc of the atrial curve should reduce and move away from the lateral wall (Fig. 32-5). As this maneuver is being performed to determine stability of the catheter, a judgment can be made regarding the proper amount of atrial curve, or catheter slack, required in the system (Fig. 32-6). During ventricular systole there is often a desirable gentle upward bowing in the catheter segment between the tricuspid valve and the tip electrode. If there is excess catheter in the right atrium, the catheter often hugs the lateral wall and projects more inferiorly into the atrium than is usually the case. In this circumstance, the catheter segment from the tricuspid valve to electrode tip will have an exaggerated upward bowing during systole (Fig. 32-6). Some patients have an exaggerated mediastinal excursion during inspiration, which requires that an excessive amount of right atrial catheter curvature be retained to prevent tip dislodgement during cough, stretch, or exercise.

Perforation is the major risk of an excessive arc in the right atrial portion of the catheter, since a pacemaker catheter that hugs the right atrial wall can direct excessive force toward the tip electrode and perforate the ventricle (Fig. 32-7).

Another determinant of a satisfactory placement of a ventricular pacing catheter is the intracardiac electrogram. The electro-

gram is helpful in documenting constant contact between the electrode and the endocardial wall. An electrogram is displayed by attaching the central V lead terminal of the patient's ECG cable to the distal electrode terminal pin of the pacemaker catheter with a sterile connecting cable. A variety of intraventricular patterns may be displayed, the most typical of which is a negative complex

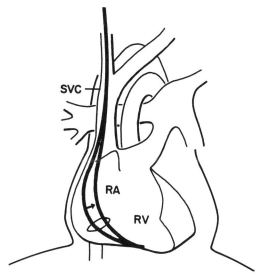

**Fig. 32-5.** Catheter motion during respiration. The catheter's arc decreases during inspiration (arrow) as the heart descends during diaphragmatic excursion; however, the pacing tip does not move.

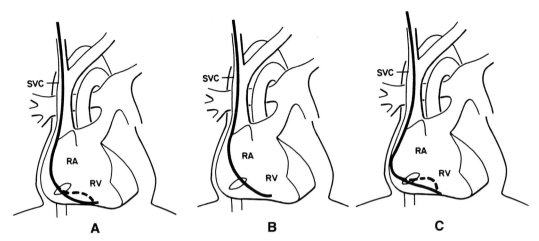

**Fig. 32-6.** Adjusting the arc of the catheter. A. The catheter has a gentle arc through the atrium to the ventricle. There is a slight upward bow during ventricular systole (dotted line). B. The catheter is too straight. Displacement of the tip is likely. Adjustment is required. C. The catheter has too much slack (arc). It is hugging the wall of the atrium and has an exaggerated upward bow (dotted line) during systole. Adjustment is required.

with a current of injury (Fig. 32-8). ST segment elevation should persist when the catheter's loop is reduced to relieve pressure at the interface between the tip electrode and the endocardial wall. The current of injury should also remain unchanged during respiratory maneuvers. Loss of ST elevation could indicate withdrawal of the electrode from good contact with the endocardial surface, and an atypical electrogram pattern could suggest ventricular perforation, especially if the electrode tip had advanced to the lateral

border of the heart on the fluoroscopic image as in Figure 32-7.

The electrical properties of the pacemaker system represent the most crucial test of an acceptable pacing catheter position. A pacemaker system analyzer is used to test the electrical properties of the catheter and the generator. The electrical properties are measured in terms of voltage, current, and resistance. The electrical threshold for stimulating the heart is an important measurement. Historically, the early pacemakers had

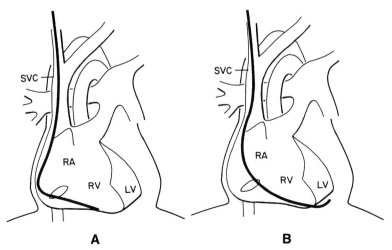

**Fig. 32-7.** Cardiac perforation by pacing catheter. A. Catheter positioned near apex of the right ventricle with abundant slack and an excessive arc to the catheter segment in right atrium. B. The catheter tip has perforated the myocardial wall and is overlying the left ventricle between the epicardium and pericardium.

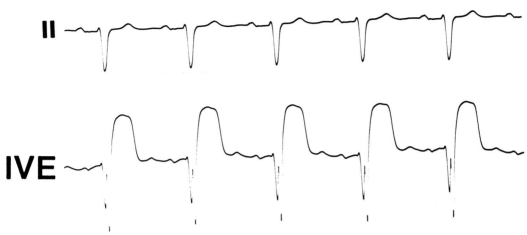

**Fig. 32-8.** Intraventricular electrogram (IVE) recorded from the tip of a permanent pacemaker catheter being positioned in the right ventricle. Two-channel simultaneous recording of ECG lead II (top) and IVE (bottom) reveals R:S ratio of less than one with current of injury.

a stimulus duration of 2.0 msec. Most modern pacemakers have multiprogrammable stimulus durations with a nominal factory setting of 0.5 msec. Our laboratory continues to threshold test at 2.0 msec as well as the nominal stimulus duration at 0.5 msec. At a 2.0 msec duration of stimulus, we accept a threshold measurement for ventricular pacing of 1.0 mA current, 500 to 600 ohms resistance, and 0.5 volts. During electrical testing of the pacing threshold, a subcutaneous needle placed in the lower margin of the skin incision is used for the grounding (anode) electrode of a monopolar system. Other workers use a metal disk placed within the subcutaneous pocket. If a threshold determination is unacceptable, the connecting cable, grounding needle, analyzer system, and all electrical connections must be checked. If each is in good order and the threshold remains poor, the pacing catheter must be repositioned. The pacing threshold can be rigorously stressed by setting the energy level slightly above threshold while the patient takes several deep breaths. Failure to maintain continuous pacing during respiratory maneuvers suggests poor contact between the tip electrode and the endocardium.

A low pacing threshold at the time of pacemaker implantation is essential because it usually increases sharply during the first few weeks before returning to a lower level. As fibrosis develops about the electrode's tip, the threshold again gradually rises to two or three times the original value before stabiliz-

ing. Since a slowing of pacemaker rate is one indicator of the approaching end of battery life, there should be a large margin of safety between the energy level that indicates the impending end of battery life and the energy level required to continuously pace the heart. Most generators have a 5.0 volt discharge or 10 mA current (assuming a 500-ohm resistance). The rate-slowing warning that signals the near end of battery life usually occurs when the voltage drops to approximately 3.5 volts, or a current of 7.0 mA. If the threshold for cardiac stimulation is greater than 7.0 mA, there will be no warning prior to failure of effective pacing. Therefore, only optimal thresholds should be accepted at the time of permanent pacer implantation.

Several helpful physical and electrophysiolgic observations may be made during ventricular pacing. Standard cuff blood pressure determinations are recorded during sinus or intrinsic rhythm and during ventricular pacing. If there is a marked reduction in blood pressure during the transition from sinus rhythm to ventricular paced rhythm, a physiologic pacing system may be required.[18-19]

During ventricular pacing, the dual channel oscilloscope recorder is scrutinized for evidence of atrial activity. P waves may follow each pacemaker-induced complex indicating retrograde V-A conduction, during which time the heart is at a hemodynamic disadvantage, or the P waves may be independent and totally dissociated from the paced ventricular beats. The dual channel ECG oscilloscope/recorder is also scrutinized for the pattern of the paced beats. If the pacing catheter is situated on the "floor" of the right ventricle, simultaneous leads II and $V_1$ will display a pattern of left bundle branch block with left axis deviation. An anteroposterior fluoroscopic field could show a pacing catheter in apparently acceptable position even though such was not the case. Examples include the catheter in an inferior branch of the coronary sinus, perforating the free right ventricular wall or septum, and overlying or being within the left ventricle. Pacing in each circumstance initiates left ventricular excitation and late excitation of the right ventricle, which will yield an ECG pattern of right bundle branch block.

After the pacing catheter is well positioned and has satisfactory electrical properties for stimulating the ventricle, the fluoroscopic image is directed to the left diaphragm, and 5.0 volts of energy, or an equivalent of the maximum energy of the selected permanent pacemaker, are used to stimulate the right ventricle. The fluoroscopic image and patient are observed for evidence of extracardiac stimulation, such as contraction of the diaphragm or chest wall, in synchrony with pacemaker-induced cardiac stimulation. If such occurs, the catheter must be repositioned.

Competition between pacemaker stimuli and intrinsic spontaneous cardiac excitation is prevented by the pacemaker's ability to sense the latter. The pacemaker generator can easily sense an endocardial electrogram with at least a 3.0 millivolt (mv) maximum signal and a 1 mv per msec rate of rise (slew rate).[20] A marginal sensing threshold is sufficient cause to reposition the pacing catheter unless the pacer generator can be reprogrammed to low threshold sensing capability. Some pacer systems have late sensing failure because the elevated ST segment current of injury is being sensed rather than an R or S wave. Sensing fails when the injury current diminishes. Sensing failure may also occur because of delay in either the maximal signal or slew rate as the tip electrode is enveloped in fibrous tissue.

After the electrical properties are fully tested and found to be adequate, a gentle tie secures the catheter within the vein. The pacing catheter is also fixed to the pectoralis muscle or its overlying fascia with a butterfly

or similar plastic anchoring apparatus. A tie should not be placed directly on the body of the polyurethane pacing catheter because of the risk of material fracture.

The pacemaker is then reprogrammed to the patient's needs while still within its sterile packaging. Prior to implantation, the pacemaker unit is tested with the system analyzer to assure against a rare component failure between the last factory review and placement. The pacing generator is then attached to the pacing catheter. After removal of the antibiotic-soaked irrigating sponges, both the catheter and pacemaker generators are arranged in the subcutaneous pocket with the catheter on the underside of the pacemaker generator. If the pacing system is unipolar and the generator has a noninsulated and an insulated surface, the noninsulated side of the generator (anode) should be positioned against the undersurface of the skin to minimize the likelihood of pectoralis muscle stimulation from the pacemaker's electrical field. Once the pacemaker generator is positioned, the implantation site should be carefully scrutinized. Local muscle stimulation, if present, might be eliminated by placing an insulating cover about the pacemaker-generator.

The system should be reviewed fluoroscopically before skin closure. The catheter should not have changed orientation or position. Radiopaque sponges should not be in the pacemaker pocket, and there should be no sharp angulations in the extravascular catheter segment. The wound is then closed in layers and dressed. A strip chart recording should be made to document proper permanent pacemaker function. The patient is then discharged from the procedure room with a portable monitor.

The post-pacemaker orders depend on hospital custom and personal preference. Because pacemaker failure is highest in the first few days, there should be close surveillance during this period. Typical postoperative orders are listed in Table 32-5.

***Postoperative Evaluation.*** A daily postoperative evaluation of the patient and the pacemaker is performed at the bedside. The cardiac monitor is observed for failure of pacing or sensing. If the pacemaker is inhibited by a fast intrinsic rate, a magnet placed over the pacemaker generator will activate its asynchronous fixed rate mode and demonstrate the pacemaker's ability to stimulate the ventricle. During paced rhythm, the chest wall and costal margin are observed for extracardiac stimulation of the pectoralis or the diaphragm. The wound is examined for evidence of infection and bleeding.

The examiner should be attentive to the presence of a new pericardial friction rub or a pacemaker click during cardiac auscultation. These findings could result from cardiac perforation. Signs of cardiac tamponade, such as distended neck veins and pulsus paradoxus, should be sought. The examiner should also palpate the pulse while observing the cardiac monitor. If the pulse amplitude becomes weak during paced beats that are not preceded by P waves, the heart may be demonstrating a strong dependence on the atrial contribution to ventricular filling, which was not present or was not appreciated at the time of pacemaker implantation.

Chart and laboratory data are scrutinized carefully. The temperature chart is reviewed for fever, the hematocrit should be stable, and the position of the pacing catheter on a chest roentgenogram should resemble that seen on fluoroscopy during implantation. The postoperative electrocardiogram should maintain a left bundle branch block pattern during ventricular pacing.

### Physiologic Permanent Pacing.
Preservation of the normal A-V sequence to maintain optimal cardiac performance is required in a variety of conditions, most of which are associated with a noncompliant "stiff" left ventricle or V-A conduction. Recent or old myocardial infarction and significant mitral or aortic stenosis are classic examples of conditions in which there is left ventricular dependence on atrial transport. Other conditions associated with such a dependence include hypertrophic, obstructive, hypertensive, and ischemic cardiomyopathies. Sick sinus syndrome without A-V conduction abnormality is also a relatively common indication for A-V sequential pacemaker placement. Such patients might fare better with physiologic pacing. Patients with rare conditions such as recurrent carotid sinus, vasovagal, and glossopharyngeal (swallowing) syncope might also receive consideration for a physiologic pacing system because of its ability to counter the vasodepressor effects of the vagal reflex.

Technical advances in atrial lead design have made permanent atrial and dual cham-bered pacing practical. If the cephalic vein is used for the ventricular lead, the atrial lead is most often introduced into a jugular vein. The other options for the atrial lead include the cephalic vein if it is large or the subclavian vein. The use of a percutaneous subclavian vein introducer is currently very popular because it is rapid and relatively safe and permits introduction of a single or dual catheter.[21-22]

Although the right atrium does not have many trabeculations in its free wall, the atrial appendage is richly endowed with trabeculae. Atrial leads with a distal end curved in the shape of the letter J permit the tip electrode to be positioned in the atrial appendage, where fixation can be accomplished with a tine or screw-in tip. The screw-in lead can also be secured to the atrial free wall.

A pacing catheter properly positioned in the right atrial appendage has a distinctive fluoroscopic appearance. During atrial systole, the loop moves medially and the tip moves laterally (Fig. 32-9). When placing the atrial pacing catheter in the appendage, the tip must be anterior and the J loop posterior. It is difficult to determine on the standard A-P fluoroscopic projection if the tip electrode is properly oriented anteriorly or improperly oriented posteriorly. Clockwise rotation of a properly oriented electrode will force the loop medially toward the septum and will direct the tip laterally as in the systolic frame of Figure 32-9. The amount of free catheter in the right atrium is crucial, since an excessive length of atrial catheter can result in its loop projecting through the tricuspid valve and causing ventricular ectopy. In contrast, insufficient catheter slack in the right atrium can result in displacement during deep inspiratory effort or stretching of the upper body.

The atrial catheter is tested for electrical properties of stimulation, resistance, and sensing. The atrial electrogram has a low amplitude, which explains why failure to sense is the most common problem of atrial pacing systems. The phrenic nerve overlies the right atrium and is susceptible to stimulation through the thin atrial wall. Therefore, the catheter must be tested with a 5.0 volt stimulus prior to accepting a final position.

Potential problems with dual chamber pacing include a greater chance of malfunction because of the system's complexity. Retrograde P waves may trigger ventricular ex-

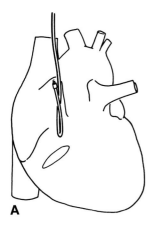 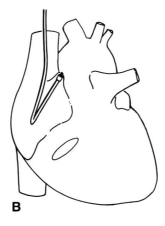

**A**   **B**

**Fig. 32-9.** Motion of pacing catheter in the right atrial appendage. A. During atrial systole the catheter tip appears to move in a lateral direction and the loop moves in a medial direction. B. During atrial diastole the catheter tip moves medially and the loop laterally.

citation in the DDD mode. Dual pacemaker catheters double the risk of catheter failure and increase the chance of venous thrombosis in the upper body. All modern dual chamber pacemakers are programmable to sole ventricular pacing; thus, a malfunctioning atrial component can be eliminated.

Programming a pacemaker between a physiologic mode (VAT) and sole ventricular pacing (VVI) has permitted hemodynamic and subjective comparisons in the same patient. In general, there is a significant improvement in hemodynamic state, exercise tolerance, and subjective state of well-being during physiologic pacing.[23] Physiologic pacing can be achieved either by atrial pacing in the presence of an intact A-V node or by DDD pacing in the presence of a pathologic A-V node. If there is fixed atrial fibrillation or if there is no perceived advantage to physiologic pacing, a conventional ventricular pacemaker should be placed.

### Acknowledgment

For many years, I have observed Dr. Howard A. Frank's skilled surgical approach to pacemaker implantation. Many of his techniques are described in this chapter.

## REFERENCES

1. Zoll PM: Resuscitation of the heart in ventricular standstill by external electrical stimulation. N Engl J Med 247:768, 1952.
2. Furman S, Schweidel JB: An intracardiac pacemaker for Stokes-Adams seizures. N Engl J Med 261:943, 1959.
3. Elmquist R, Senning A: An implantable pacemaker for the heart. Proceedings of the Second International Conference on Medical Electronics. Paris, June 24, 1979.
4. Parsonett V: The proliferation of cardiac pacing; medical technology and socioeconomic dilemmas. Circulation 65:841, 1982.
5, Parsonnet V, Furman S, Smyth N, Bilitch M: Inter-Society Commission for Heart Disease Resources (ICHD): Optimal resources for implantable cardiac pacemakers. Pacemaker Study Group. Circulation 68:227A, 1983.
6. Ludmer PL, Goldschlager N: Cardiac pacing in the 1980s. N Engl J Med 311:1671, 1984.
7. Zoll PM, et al: External non-invasive temporary cardiac pacing: clinical trials. Circulation 71:937, 1985.
8. Boal BH, Keller BD, Ascheim RS, Kaltman AJ: Complications of intracardiac electrical pacing—knotting together of temporary and permanent electrodes. N Engl J Med 280:650, 1969.
9. Bing OHL, McDowell JW, Hantman J, Messer JV: Pacemaker placement by electrocardiographic monitoring. N Engl J Med 287:651, 1972.
10. Kramer DH, Moss AJ: Permanent atrial pacing from the coronary vein. Circulation 42:427, 1970.
11. Berens SC, Kolin A, MacAlpin RN, Lenz MW: New stable temporary atrial pacing loop. Am J Cardiol 34:325, 1974.
12. Guidelines for permanent cardiac pacemaker

implantation May 1984, Joint American College of Cardiology/American Heart Association Task Force on Assessment of Cardiovascular Procedures (Subcommittee on Pacemaker Implantation) J Am Coll Cardiol 4:434, 1984. and Circulation 70:331A, 1984.

13. Parsonnet V: Technique for implantation and replacement of permanent pacemakers. In Modern Techniques in Cardiac/Thoracic Surgery. New York; Futura, 1979, Chapter 12.

14. Meere C, Lesperance J: Surgical techniques in cardiac pacing. In Thalen HJ, Meere C. editors: Fundamentals of Cardiac Pacing. Hague/Boston/London, Martinus Nijhoff, 1979, pp. 127–169.

15. Smyth NPD: Techniques of pacemaker implantation: atrial and ventricular, thoractomy and transvenous. Prog Cardiovasc Dis 23:435, 1981.

16. Martinis AJ: Pacemaker insertion. In Dillard DH, Miller DW: Atlas of Cardiac Surgery. New York, Macmillan 1983, pp. 156–163.

17. Mond HG: The Cardiac Pacemaker: Function and Malfunction. New York, Grune and Stratton, 1983, pp. 191–232.

18. Cohen SI, Frank H: Preservation of active atrial transport. An important clinical consideration in cardiac pacing. Chest 81:51, 1982.

19. Ogawa S, et al: Hemodynamic consequences of atrioventricular and ventriculoatrial pacing. Pace 1:8, 1978.

20. Furman S. Hurzler P, Decaprio V: The ventricular endocardial electrogram and pacemaker sensing. J Thorac Cardiovasc Surg 73:258, 1977.

21. Friesen A, et al: Percutaneous insertion of a permanent transvenous pacemaker electrode throughout the subclavian vein. Can J Surg 20:131, 1977.

22. Janss B: Two leads in one introducer technique for A-V sequential implantations. Pace 5:217, 1982.

23. Kruse I, Arman K, Conradson TB, Ryden L: A comparison of the acute and long-term hemodynamic effects of ventricular inhibited and atrial synchronous ventricular inhibited pacing. Circulation 65:846, 1982.

*chapter thirty three*

# Potential Role of Lasers in the Cardiac Catheterization Laboratory

J. RICHARD SPEARS

ᴬᵀᵀᴱᴹᴾᵀˢ to apply laser technology to the management of cardiovascular disorders have been made only recently, long after the successful application of lasers in a variety of other medical-surgical disciplines.[1] Along with the advent of percutaneous transluminal coronary angioplasty (PTCA) and intracoronary thrombolytic therapy has come the realization that instrumentation can be safely used in a coronary artery, even in clinically unstable patients. In this setting, investigators have been encouraged to pursue potentially useful therapeutic catheterization techniques utilizing the rapidly evolving technology of the laser-fiberoptic industry.

At the present time, it is premature to surmise the precise role of lasers in the cardiac catheterization laboratory of the future, but at least four different laser approaches to the treatment of obstructive coronary atherosclerosis are currently being investigated (Table 33-1): (1) direct laser vaporization; (2) photodynamic therapy with light-sensitive dyes; (3) hyperthermia without vaporization; and (4) laser welding of plaque-arterial wall separations following PTCA.

## DIRECT LASER VAPORIZATION

The spatially and temporally coherent nature of monochromatic laser light makes it

**TABLE 33-1.** *Potential Cardiovascular Applications of Lasers*

I. Vaporization of tissues: ablation of atheromatous plaques, thrombi, stenotic valves, A-V conduction and accessory pathways, hypertrophied septum of IHSS; myocardial revascularization with transmural channels.

II. Photodynamic therapy: selective ablation of atheromatous plaques, vegetations of infectious endocarditis with light-sensitive dye.

III. Hyperthermia: enhancement of alternative techniques for ablation of atheromatous plaque.

IV. Fusion of disrupted arterial tissues (laser balloon angioplasty): prevention of abrupt reclosure and restenosis from balloon angioplasty, treatment of spontaneous dissections (e.g., aortic).

possible to concentrate great quantities of light onto a small region of interest, such as the core of a flexible optical fiber. The latter, of course, can then be used to transmit the energy to tissues, such as atheromatous plaques, located remotely from the laser

536

source. Sufficiently great absorption of laser energy at a variety of different wavelengths will result in vaporization of atheromatous plaque tissue.[2-6] The primary mechanism of tissue vaporization by lasers operating in the visible or infrared spectrum is conversion of laser energy to thermal energy. A photodecomposition process involving disruption of molecular bonds also has been proposed as a possible mechanism for tissue ablation by excimer lasers, emitting pulsed ultraviolet radiation.[7] Although laser-arterial wall interactions require considerably more study, reported studies in experimental models to date indicate that nonperforating laser-induced thermal injury may be well tolerated acutely and chronically by the normal arterial wall.[8]

The optimal wavelength for vaporizing atheromatous obstructions is unclear. Ideally, absorption of laser radiation should dominate scattering in order to minimize thermal damage adjacent to a well-defined, shallow region of vaporization; the radiation should be transmissible through a clinically usable waveguide; and some degree of greater selective absorption by the plaque, compared to adjacent normal arterial tissue, would be useful to reduce thermal injury to normal tissues. Strong absorption of infrared and ultraviolet radiation by soft tissues, such as atheromatous plaques, which are not heavily calcified, would theoretically favor the use of lasers that produce energy at these wavelengths such as the $CO_2$ laser (10.6 $\mu$) and excimer lasers (<0.4 $\mu$). However, flexible, inexpensive waveguides for transmitting wavelengths <3 $\mu$ coaxially through standard-sized coronary catheters are not, at present, commercially available despite the recent fabrication of waveguides from novel materials,[9] and excimer lasers may need further development before they can be used safely in the clinical setting. An alternative technique for reducing the amount of thermal injury to tissues adjacent to vaporized regions with visible wavelengths would be to pulse the laser energy rather than apply continuous wave (cw) energy.

In practice, a variety of different lasers can be used to effectively vaporize all but heavily calcified atheromatous plaques. Recanalization of peripheral arteries with atheromatous obstructions in patients has been achieved with an argon-ion laser (principal lines = 488

and 515 nm) by Ginsburg et al[10] and with a Nd:YAG laser (1.06 $\mu$) by Geschwind et al,[11] although the long-term patency rate has been inadequate for the former and unknown at present for the latter. Choy et al[12] likewise have attempted to open atheromatous coronary obstructions located just proximal to the arteriotomy site with an argon-ion laser during otherwise conventional coronary bypass surgical procedures in 9 patients, but only 1 patient demonstrated patency of the treated vessel at angiographic follow-up approximately 1 month after the procedure. The limiting factor in vaporizing atheromatous plaques with lasers is, very likely, not the inability to deliver the optimal wavelength of radiation. Despite the fact that plaques absorb light poorly at the argon-ion and Nd:YAG laser wavelengths, these lasers and many others can be used to effectively vaporize plaque tissue when a thin layer of blood, preferably diluted with a crystalloid solution, covers the plaque surface.[11] Whole blood is an efficient chromophore at all wavelengths, although this fact may be overlooked when only the relative absorption spectrum of hemoglobin is examined.[13]

The inability to discriminate between atheromatous plaque and the plaque-free arterial wall is the major technical problem that currently limits the practical application of laser vaporization of coronary artery obstructions during cardiac catheterization. As a result, vessel perforation could occur either by vaporizing a thin rim of normal arterial wall constituting a portion of the lumen cross section compromised by an eccentrically located plaque or by vaporizing medial and adventitial layers of tissue external to a targeted plaque.[14] Perforation of the coronary artery on the epicardial surface could, of course, quickly result in lethal cardiac tamponade.[15]

Multiple techniques, which could be used to discriminate between atheromatous plaque and the normal arterial wall, are being developed. For example, hollow optical fibers with a concentric core-cladding arrangement may soon allow transmission of laser energy around a guide wire located coaxially within a fiber. The guide wire would facilitate alignment of the optical fiber tip with the long axis of the vessel and, hence, the orientation between the optical fiber tip and the plaque. Unfortunately, it is unlikely that the development of any fiber-guiding system, whether passive (e.g., the hollow fiber) or active, such as a steerable optical fiber tip, will be sufficient to eliminate the possibility of vessel perforation. Even if a stereofluoroscopic system can be made practical, delineation of blood-arterial wall boundaries by angiography cannot be used to reliably differentiate atheromatous plaque from the plaque-free arterial wall, especially in highly tortuous coronary arteries.

Angioscopy has been proposed as an alternative imaging modality for discrimination between atheromatous plaques and the normal arterial wall.[16] Ultrathin imaging bundles consisting of >3000 optical fibers, coherently arranged at two ends, can be made less than 1 mm in diameter. The feasibility of performing coronary angioscopy during both open heart surgery and cardiac catheterization has been demonstrated.[17,18] Translucent crystalloid solutions were used to transiently displace blood during the procedures, and the findings could be continuously recorded on a videoendoscopic system (Fig. 33-1). However, a number of technical improvements would have to be made in order to render angioscopy a useful imaging modality for laser vaporization of atheromatous plaques, including smaller dimensions, greater flexibility, and incorporation of an angulation system for directional control of the distal tip. Additional problems include:

(1) the similar spectral reflectance of light from the surface of most plaques and the normal arterial wall, i.e., inability to reliably identify the plaque-normal wall boundary within the lumen; and (2) the fact that lumen cross-sectional size varies in a nonlinear manner with the distance between the lens mounted at the distal end of the angioscope and a cross section of interest, i.e., angioscopy provides qualitative information alone unless the exact distance between the lens and cross section is known. Fluoroscopy could provide the latter information, but the integration of information from two different imaging techniques would, very likely, be cumbersome. Regarding the problem of plaque identification, one or more of a potential variety of plaque-seeking vital dyes might be used. Should all such problems be solved, it might still be difficult in tortuous vessels to simultaneously visualize a cross section quantitatively and vaporize a lesion within the cross section from a position sufficiently upstream from the lesion to avoid damage to the distal end of the angioscope.

Plaque-seeking vital dyes might be used to enhance preferential absorption of laser energy in plaques compared to that of the normal arterial wall, since the absorption spectrum of plaques otherwise often differs little from that of the normal arterial wall. A wavelength for lasing then could be matched to the absorption maxima of the chromophore.

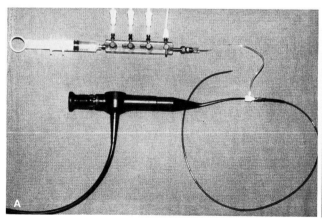
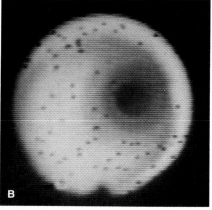

**Fig. 33-1.** (A) Catheterization system for angioscopy. Displacement of blood by injection of normal saline between an Olympus ultrathin fiberscope (1.8 mm outer diameter) and a modified 8.3 French USCI woven Dacron angioplasty guiding catheter is performed manually during videoendoscopic recording. (B) Videoangioscopic frame showing proximal segment of stump of occluded right coronary artery. The thin crescent shape is the end of the guiding catheter. Whitish plaque is seen to encroach upon the residual lumen. Black dots represent broken optical fibers. (From Spears JR, et al: Coronary angioscopy during cardiac catheterization. J Am Coll Cardiol 6:93, 1985. Reproduced with permission of J Amer Coll Cardiol.)

Examples of potential chromophores include hematoporphyrin derivative, Evan's blue dye, and tetracycline.[19]

## PHOTODYNAMIC THERAPY (PDT)

The viability of mammalian cells is generally unaffected by direct exposure to ambient light. However, in the presence of an appropriate photosensitizer, irreversible cell damage can occur upon exposure to light. This principle has been used in the treatment of malignant neoplasms with hematoporphyrin derivative (HPD),[20–23] a photosensitive material, which produces cytotoxic singlet oxygen upon light exposure.[22] HPD is given intravenously 1 to 3 days before light exposure and appears to be retained in neoplasms selectively compared to normal adjacent tissue.[23] Red light generated by an argon-ion pumped dye laser tuned to 631 nm is commonly used to photoactivate HPD because of the relatively deep (1 to 2 cm) penetration into tissues compared to that of other shorter wavelengths in the absorption spectrum of HPD. Tumor necrosis ensues 2 to 3 days after light exposure. The possibility exists that HPD-PDT might also be applied to atheromatous plaques, since all plaques appear to selectively concentrate intravenously administered HPD compared to the normal arterial wall[24] (Fig. 33-2). HPD-laden atheromatous plaques could be exposed to light with an intraarterial optical fiber that terminates in a diffusing tip for directing light radially and homogeneously along the length of the diffusing tip. The interaction of light and HPD would specifically target plaques for a photodynamic effect. Several important problems that may limit the applicability of HPD-PDT to atheromatous plaques currently are being addressed. The absorption of light at 631 nm by whole blood is far greater than by other tissues, including hemoglobin solutions,[13] so that either displacement of blood with a translucent balloon or hemodilution with translucent liquids is necessary, when a >2 mm thickness of blood at a normal hematocrit must be penetrated sufficiently by 631 nm light at a conventional dose of 100 to 600 mW of CW laser output to produce a photodynamic response.[25] Since intermittent light exposure appears to work as well as or better than a continuous one for eliciting a photodynamic response in tissues, blood dis-

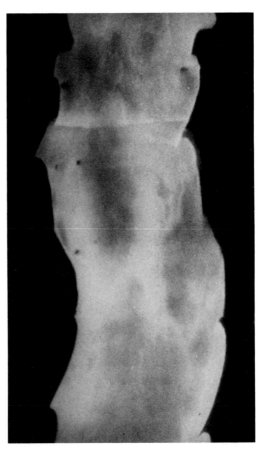

**Fig. 33-2.** Fluorescence of hypercholesterolemia-induced atheromatous plaques of rabbit aorta, the luminal surface of which was exposed to ultraviolet light and photographed through a Corning 3-68 orange filter.

placement or hemodilution could be performed intermittently for ≦1 minute periods in a coronary artery[26] in order to achieve the total of 5 to 15 minutes of cumulative duration of light exposure routinely used for treatment of other tissues.

A more difficult problem in applying HPD-PDT technology to ablation of atheromatous plaques relates to the fact that a vascular reaction (either hemorrhage or, more commonly, blanching) of HPD-containing tissues occurs shortly after light exposure and that this reaction may be the primary mechanism for tissue necrosis.[27] It is likely that the capillary endothelial cell is injured by PDT and that pericapillary edema, resulting from leakage of plasma, produces capillary closure. In the normal and atheromatous rabbit aorta, it is likely that destruction of the vasa vasorum may contribute to the observed necrosis of portions of the media of the former and neo-intima of the latter 2 to 30 days after HPD-PDT.[28] Since human atheromatous plaques are richly invested with a network of vasa vasorum,[29,30] a HPD-PDT vascular reaction is expected to occur. Whether this reaction will result in plaque ablation and a larger lumen in patients is unknown and cannot be tested easily in experimental models of atherosclerosis, where plaque vascularity is usually minimal. Direct cytolysis of cultured arterial smooth muscle cells, which are phenotypically analogous to the proliferating smooth muscle cells of experimental atheromatous plaques,[31] can be achieved with HPD-PDT,[32] and subtle direct effects of HPD-PDT on experimental plaques in vivo have been observed, but widespread necrosis of plaques from this therapy, in the absence of a vascular reaction, may be unlikely. Except for the endothelial cells of the vasa vasorum, much of the viable plaque tissue may be quite hypoxic,[33,34] and oxygen availability may be the rate-limiting factor in eliciting HPD-mediated photodynamic reactions in tissues. Further studies are needed in this regard.

## HYPERTHERMIA

Rather than vaporizing atheromatous plaques with lasers, it may be possible to produce cytolysis of viable plaque tissue with milder degrees of laser-induced hyperthermia. The fact that atheromatous plaques contain much viable tissue is not widely appreciated, but studies of both experimental and human plaques show that plaques have a higher rate of anaerobic glycolysis than the normal arterial wall per gram of tissue.[35,36] The vascularity of human plaques, as noted above, also attests to an important viable component.

Mild degrees of hyperthermia (41°C to 45°C) have been used with some success in the treatment of malignant neoplasms and may be useful for potentiating the effect of radiation therapy and chemotherapy.[37] Although ultrasound and microwaves each can be used to induce local hyperthermia in specific sites, these techniques do not lend themselves to a catheterization application. However, the 1.06 $\mu$ radiation of the Nd:YAG laser can be used efficaciously for volume heating because of relatively deep penetra-

tion into tissues, and this radiation can be transmitted through conventional fiberoptics. In addition to the use of the Nd:YAG laser to treat diseased tissues with hyperthermia per se, the 1.06 $\mu$ radiation has been used to produce hyperthermia in conjunction with HPD-PDT in order to enhance the effect of the latter.[38]

A potential major advantage in the use of lasers, compared to alternative energy sources, for heating atheromatous plaques may be the use of a plaque-seeking chromophore that strongly absorbs the specific wavelength(s) of the laser, such as hematoporphyrin derivative. Differential heating of plaques, compared to that of the normal, dye-free arterial wall, may then be possible. Practical application of hyperthermia to treat atheromatous plaques during a catheterization procedure would require a far shorter treatment period than that used for neoplasms. By increasing tissue temperature to much greater temperatures (60 to 90°C) than is currently used for the treatment of neoplasms, it may be possible to shorten the exposure period to the duration of balloon occlusion tolerated during PTCA procedures. In regard to the latter, it may be possible to occlude a coronary artery for longer periods than currently used ($\leq$ 1 minute) by perfusion of either arterial blood or oxygenated perfluorochemicals through the central channel of the balloon catheter. Moreover, intermittent thermal exposure might also be used to circumvent the problem of myocardial ischemia during thermal exposure from a laser-emitting optical fiber terminating within an occluding balloon.

It is important to recognize that any injury of the arterial wall, even if successful in producing necrosis of viable tissue within atheromatous plaques, may potentially accelerate plaque growth in the region of injury.[39] Thus, although the arterial wall appears to tolerate laser-induced thermal injury remarkably well experimentally,[8] any laser-induced injury to the plaque, including hyperthermia, may potentially accelerate plaque growth.

## LASER ENHANCEMENT OF PTCA (LASER BALLOON ANGIOPLASTY)

The application of PTCA to the treatment of obstructive coronary atherosclerosis is currently limited by the 5% incidence of abrupt reclosure and the >30 percent incidence of restenosis 3 to 6 months after the procedure.[40-42] Plaque fracture and arterial wall dissections resulting from balloon inflation may be important mechanisms for lumen enlargement, but propagation of a dissection and collapse of an intimal fragment, with or without an associated thrombus, may result in abrupt reclosure, representing an adverse extension of these mechanisms. In addition, disruption of the arterial wall and lumen architecture by balloon inflation may predispose to local deposition of platelets and to unfavorable hydrodynamic flow patterns that may both contribute to accelerated plaque growth and restenosis.

A variety of lasers have been recently used to fuse adjacent tissues together in order to create sutureless anastomoses of arteries and veins.[43] We have recently shown that the 1.06 $\mu$ radiation of the Nd:YAG laser is effective in fusing plaque-arterial wall separations of human atherosclerotic arteries in vitro.[44] Since the laser radiation could be delivered to the arterial wall from a diffusing tip within a prototype balloon during balloon inflation, laser-induced thermal fusion of plaque-media separations resulted in obliteration of false channels and produced a smooth lumen, which resembled the shape and size of the balloon upon subsequent balloon deflation (Fig. 33-3). Theoretically, this

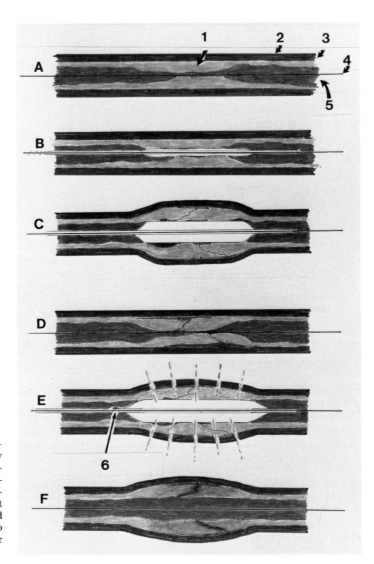

**Fig. 33-3.** Laser balloon angioplasty. Nd:YAG laser energy may be useful for fusing disrupted elements of the arterial wall following conventional PTCA. An acoustic sensor could be used to detect high frequency sounds generated by tissue vaporization in order to automatically terminate the laser exposure.

technique—laser balloon angioplasty—may be useful in the catheterization laboratory for the treatment of abrupt reclosure. In addition, if the thermal injury is found to be well tolerated by the arterial wall, the technique might produce a lumen geometry which could favorably affect the incidence of restenosis associated with conventional PTCA. Additional applications of this technique might include the treatment of spontaneous aortic dissections and arterial perforations.

## OTHER POTENTIAL LASER APPLICATIONS

In addition to laser treatment of obstructive coronary artery disease, tissue ablation with a laser catheter might be useful for the treatment of a variety of other cardiovascular disorders. Thus, the use of laser energy has been proposed for performing valvulotomy of stenosed pulmonic valves,[45] treatment of arrhythmias,[46,47] and photodynamic therapy of infectious endocarditis.[48] The photocoagulation properties of the Nd:YAG laser may be useful for treatment of spontaneous aortic dissection with a balloon catheter in addition to its proposed use for enhancing PTCA.[44] For each such application, whether the laser-based technique will be as safe, effective, and easy to implement as alternative techniques will determine its potential clinical utility. Many preclinical studies will be required before any of these techniques can be applied in the clinical setting.

## BIBLIOGRAPHY

1. Goldman L (ed): The Biomedical Laser: Technology and Clinical Application. New York, Springer-Verlag, 1981.
2. Lee G, Ikeda RM, Kozina J, Mason DT: Laser-dissolution of coronary atherosclerotic obstruction. Am Heart J 102:1074, 1981.
3. Abela GS, et al: Effects of carbon dioxide, Nd-YAG and argon laser radiation coronary atheromatous plaques. Am J Cardiol 50:1199, 1982.
4. Choy DSJ, Stertzer SH, Rotterdam HZ, Bruno MS: Laser coronary angioplasty: Experience with 9 cadaver hearts. Am J Cardiol 50:1209, 1982.
5. Grundfest W, et al: Pulsed ultraviolet lasers provide precise control of atheroma ablation. Circulation 70 (Suppl II):II-35, 1984 (abstr).
6. Isner JM, et al: The excimer laser: gross, light microscopic, and ultrastructural analysis of potential advantages for use in laser therapy of cardiovascular disease. Circulation 70 (Suppl II):II-35, 1984 (abstr).
7. Lane RJ, Wynne JJ: Medical applications of excimer lasers. Lasers Applic 3:59, 1984.
8. Abela GS, et al: No evidence for accelerated atherosclerosis following laser ablation. Circulation 70 (Suppl II):II-323, 1984.
9. Tebo AR: Infrared optical fibers: the promise of the future. Electro-Optics, June 1983, pp 41–36.
10. Ginsburg R, et al: Salvage of an ischemic limb by laser angioplasty. Clinical Cardiol 7:54, 1983.
11. Geschwind H, Boussignac G, Teisseire B: Transluminal laser angioplasty in man. Circulation 70 (Supply II):II-298, 1984.
12. Choy DSJ, et al: Human coronary laser recanalization. Clin Cardiol 7:377, 1984.
13. Spokojny AM, et al: Intravascular application of hematoporphyrin derivative photodynamic therapy. Proc SPIE 494:61, 1984.
14. Isner JM, et al: Simulated intra-operative laser coronary angioplasty using intact postmortem specimens: high incidence of perforation related to calcific deposits, branch points, and coronary tortuosities. Circulation 70 (Suppl II):II-104, 1984.
15. Crea F, et al: Transluminal laser irradiation of coronary arteries in live dogs. Circulation 70 (Suppl II):II-36, 1984.
16. Lee G, et al: Intraoperative use of dual fiberoptic catheter for simultaneous in vivo visualization and laser vaporization of peripheral atherosclerotic obstructive disease. Cathet Cardiovasc Diagn 10:II-16, 1984.
17. Spears JR, et al: In vivo coronary angioscopy. J Am Coll Cardiol 1:1311, 1983.
18. Spears JR, Spokojny A, Marais HJ: Coronary angioscopy during cardiac catheterization. J Am Coll Cardiol 6:93, 1985.
19. Murphy-Chutorian D, et al: Selective absorption of ultraviolet laser energy by human atherosclerotic plaque treated with tetracycline. Am J Cardiol 55:1293, 1985.
20. Dougherty TJ, et al: Photoradiation therapy for

the treatment of malignant rumors. Cancer Res 38:2628, 1978.

21. Dougherty TJ, et al: Photoradiation in the treatment of recurrent breast carcinoma. J Natl Cancer Inst 62:231, 1979.

22. Weishaupt KR, Gomer CJ, Dougherty TJ: Identification of singlet oxygen as the cytotoxic agent in photoinactivation of a murine tumor. Cancer Res 36:2326, 1976.

23. Lipson RI, Balders EJ, Olsen AM: The use of a derivative of hematoporphyrin in tumor detection. J Natl Cancer Inst 26:1, 1961.

24. Spears JR, Serur J, Shropshire D, Paulin S: Fluorescence of experimental atheromatous plaques with hematoporphyrin derivative. J Clin Invest 71:395, 1983.

25. Spears JR, et al: Intraarterial hematoporphyrin photodynamic therapy in the Fluosol-DA exchanged rabbit. Circulation 70 (Suppl II):II-245, 1984.

26. Spears JR, Gruntzig AR, Simpson J, Principal Investigators: Fluosol-DA 20% in percutaneous transluminal coronary angioplasty. Norma McIntosh, Clinical Project Manager. Alpha Therapeutic Corporation clinic protocol ATC 83-03, FDA interim summary, May 28, 1984.

27. Castellani A, Pace GP, Concioli M: Photodynamic effect of hematoporphyrin on blood microcirculation. J Pathol Bacteriol 86:99, 1963.

28. Spears Jr, et al: Effect of hematoporphyrin derivative photodynamic therapy on the normal and atheromatous rabbit aorta. J Clin Invest 71:395, 1983.

29. Winternitz MC, Thomas RM, LeCompte PM: The relation of vascularity to disease of the vessel wall. *In* The Biology of Arteriosclerosis. Springfield, IL, Charles C Thomas, pp 68–79, 1938.

30. Barger AC, Beeuwkes III R, Lainey LL, Silverman KJ: Hypothesis: vasa vasorum and neovascularization of human coronary arteries. A possible role in the pathophysiology of atherosclerosis. N Engl J Med 310:175, 1984.

31. Ross R, Glomset JE: Atherosclerosis and the arterial smooth muscle cell. Science 180:1332, 1973.

32. Hundley RP, Spears JR, Weinstein R: Photodynamic cytolysis of arterial smooth muscle cells in vitro. J Am Coll Cardiol 5:408, 1985.

33. Zemplenyi T: Arterial hypoxia and lactate dehydrogenase enzymes as related to atherosclerosis. *In* Enzyme Biochemistry of the Arterial Wall as Related to Atherosclerosis. London, Lloyd-Luke Ltd, pp 161–167, 1968.

34. Heughen C, Niinikoski J, Hunt TK: Oxygen tensions in lesions of experimental atherosclerosis in rabbits. Atherosclerosis 17:361, 1973.

35. Kirk JR: Intermediary metabolism of human arterial tissue and its changes with age and atherosclerosis. *In* Sandler M, Baurne GH (eds): Atherosclerosis and Its Origin. New York, Academic Press, pp 67–117, 1963.

36. Morrison ES, Scott RF, Kroms M, Freck J: Glucose degradation in normal and atherosclerotic aortic intima-media atherosclerosis 16:175, 1972.

37. Hahn GM. Effects of hyperthermia against spontaneous cancers. *In* Hyperthermia and Cancer. New York, Plenum Press, pp 227–256, 1982.

38. Dougherty TJ: Personal communication.

39. Moore J: Endothelial injury and atherosclerosis Exp Mol Pathol 31:182, 1979.

40. Kent KM, et al: Percutaneous transluminal coronary angioplasty: report from the Registry of the National Heart, Lung, and Blood Institute. Am J Cardiol 49:2011, 1982.

41. Gruntzig AR, Meier B: Percutaneous transluminal coronary angioplasty. The first five years and the future. Int J Cardiol 2:319, 1983.

42. Meier B, et al: Repeat coronary angioplasty. J Am Coll Card 4:463, 1984.

43. Gomes OM, et al: Vascular anastomosis by argon laser beam. Tex Heart Inst J 10:145, 1983.

44. Hiehle JF, Shapshay S, Schoen FJ, Spears JR: Nd:YAG laser fusion of human atheromatous plaque-arterial wall separations in vitro. J Am Coll Cardiol in press, 1985.

45. Macruz R, et al: The use of laser beam as a surgical tool for correction of experimental pulmonary stenosis during catheterization procedure. Circulation 64 (Suppl IV):IV-235, 1981.

46. Narula DS, Boreja BK, Cohen DM, Tarjan PP: Laser catheter induced A-V nodal delays and block: Acute and chronic studies. Circulation 70 (Suppl II):II-99, 1984.

47. Lee BI, Gottdiemer JS, Notargiacano A, Fletcher RD: Effects of laser vs. electrical transcatheter endocardial ablation on regional and global LV function: assessment by 2D echocardiography. Circulation 70 (Suppl II):V-413, 1984.

48. Spokojny AM, Mattson DL, Paulin S, Spears JR: Selective uptake of hematoporphyrin derivative by valvular vegetations in rabbits. Circulation 70 (Suppl II):II-144, 1984.

# Appendix
# Normal Values*

A. Pressures (mm Hg)
  1. Systemic arterial:
      peak systolic/end diastolic           100–140/60–90
      mean           70–105
      systolic mean           80–130
  2. Left ventricle:
      peak systolic/end diastolic           100–140/3–12
      systolic mean/diastolic mean           80–130/1–10
  3. Left atrium (or pulmonary
    capillary wedge):
      mean           2–10
      "a" wave           3–15
      "v" wave           3–15
      diastolic mean           1–10
  4. Pulmonary artery:
      peak systolic/end diastolic           15–30/4–12
      mean           9–18
      systolic mean           10–20
  5. Right ventricle:
      peak systolic/end diastolic           15–30/2–8
      systolic mean/diastolic mean           10–20/0–4
  6. Right atrium:
      mean           2–8
      "a" wave           2–10
      "v" wave           2–10
B. Resistances (dynes-sec-cm$^{-5}$)
  1. systemic vascular resistance           700–1600
  2. total pulmonary resistance           100–300
  3. pulmonary vascular resistance           20–130
C. Flows
  1. cardiac output           Varies with patient's size
  2. cardiac index (L/min/M$^2$)           2.6–4.2
  3. stroke index (ml/beat/M$^2$)           30–65
D. Oxygen consumption (L/min/M$^2$)           110–150
E. Arteriovenous oxygen difference (ml/L)           30–50
F. Time intervals (sec)
  1. Left ventricle:
      systolic ejection period/beat           0.22–0.32
      systolic ejection period/min           13.2–32
      diastolic filling period/beat           0.38–0.50
      diastolic filling period/min           22.8–50

*Normal values should be determined in each individual laboratory. The values listed here represent the normal range in the author's laboratory.

G.  Left ventricular volumes, mass, wall thickness,                    See Table 19-2,
    and ejection fraction                                              p. 292
H.  Left ventricular myocardial mechanics
    1.  isovolumic indices
    2.  ejection phase indices                                         See Table 20-2,
I.  Left ventricular work                                              p. 308
    1.  stroke work index† (gram-meters/$M^2$)                         30–90
    2.  left ventricular minute work‡ index (Kg-meters/$M^2$/min)      1.8–6.6

†Computed as (LVSM − LVEDP) (SI) (.0136), where LVSM = left ventricular systolic mean, LVEDP = left ventricular end diastolic pressure, SI = left ventricular stroke index, and .0136 is the factor for converting mm Hg × ml/$M^2$ into gram-meters/$M^2$. In the presence of mitral or aortic regurgitation, SI must be the *total* LV stroke index, determined by angiography or other method, not the forward (Fick) stroke volume.

‡Computed as LVSWI × HR/1000, where LVSWI = left ventricular stroke work index, HR = heart rate, and 1000 is factor for converting grams to kilograms.

# Index

![Index decorative rule]

Page numbers in *italics* indicate illustrations; page numbers followed by "t" indicate tables.